Michael J. Edel (Ed.)

iPS Cells for Modelling and Treatment of Human Diseases

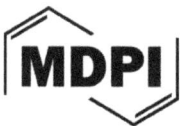

MDPI

This book is a reprint of the special issue that appeared in the online open access journal *Journal of Clinical Medicine* (ISSN 2077-0383) in 2014 and 2015 (available at: http://www.mdpi.com/journal/jcm/special_issues/iPS).

Guest Editor
Michael J. Edel
Departament de Ciències Fisiològiques I
Facultat de Medicina
Universitat de Barcelona
Spain
The University of Western Australia
Centre for Cell Therapy and Regenerative Medicine (CCTRM)

Editorial Office
MDPI AG
Klybeckstrasse 64
Basel, Switzerland

Publisher
Shu-Kun Lin

Managing Editor
Maple Lv

1. Edition 2015

MDPI • Basel • Beijing • Wuhan

ISBN 978-3-03842-121-4 (PDF)
ISBN 978-3-03842-122-1 (Hbk)

Table of Contents

Chapter 1: Neuronal

Chapter 2: Cardiac

Chapter 3: Eye

Chapter 4: Spinal Cord Injury

Chapter 5: Liver

Chapter 6: Muscle

Chapter 7: Bone

Chapter 8: Germ Cells

Chapter 9: Genetic Disorders

Chapter 10: Immune Response

List of Contributors

Ana Belén Alvarez-Palomo: Control of Pluripotency Laboratory, Department of Physiological Sciences I, Faculty of Medicine, University of Barcelona, Hospital Clinic, Casanova 143, 08036, Barcelona, Spain

Gillian Blue: Heart Centre for Children, The Children's Hospital at Westmead, Westmead NSW 2145, Australia; Sydney Medical School, University of Sydney, Sydney NSW 2006, Australia

Alexis Bosman: Victor Chang Cardiac Research Institute, Lowy Packer Building, 405 Liverpool St., Darlinghurst NSW 2010, Australia; St. Vincent's Clinical School and School of Biotechnology and Biomolecular Sciences, University of New South Wales, Kensington NSW 2052, Australia

Ricardo P. Casaroli-Marano: Department of Surgery, School of Medicine and Hospital Clínic de Barcelona (IDIBAPS), University of Barcelona, Calle Sabino de Arana 1 (2nd floor), E-08028 Barcelona, Spain; CellTec-UB and the Clinic Foundation for Biomedical Research (FCRB), University of Barcelona, Avda. Diagonal 643, E-08028 Barcelona, Spain; Tissue Bank of BST (GenCat), Calle Dr Antoni Pujadas 42, SSMM Sant Joan de Déu, Edifici Pujadas, E-08830 Sant Boi de Llobregat, Spain

Fred Kuanfu Chen: Centre for Ophthalmology and Visual Science (Incorporating Lions Eye Institute), The University of Western Australia, Perth WA 6009, Australia; Ophthalmology Department, Royal Perth Hospital, Perth WA 6009, Australia

I-Ping Chen: Department of Oral Health and Diagnostic Sciences, University of Connecticut Health Center, 263 Farmington Avenue, Farmington, CT 06030, USA

Peter Coffey: Division of Cellular Therapy, Institute of Ophthalmology, University College of London, London EC1V 9EL, UK

Antonella Consiglio: Institute for Biomedicine of the University of Barcelona (IBUB), Barcelona Science Park, Barcelona 08028, Spain; Department of Molecular and Translational Medicine, Fibroblast Reprogramming Unit, University of Brescia, Brescia 25123, Italy

Stefania Corti: Dino Ferrari Centre, Neuroscience Section, Department of Pathophysiology and Transplantation (DEPT), University of Milan, Neurology Unit, IRCCS Foundation Ca'Granda Ospedale Maggiore Policlinico, via Francesco Sforza 35, 20122 Milan, Italy

Lyndon Da Cruz: Department of Vitreoretinal Surgery, Moorfields Eye Hospital, London EC1V 2PD, UK; Division of Cellular Therapy, Institute of Ophthalmology, University College of London, London EC1V 9EL, UK

Francesca de Angelis Rigotti: Institute for Biomedicine of the University of Barcelona (IBUB), Barcelona Science Park, Barcelona 08028, Spain

Patrizia Dell'Era: Department of Molecular and Translational Medicine, Fibroblast Reprogramming Unit, University of Brescia, Brescia 25123, Italy

Rodney J. Dilley: Ear Science Institute Australia, Centre for Cell Therapy and Regenerative Medicine and School of Surgery, University of Western Australia, Nedlands WA 6009, Australia

Michael J. Edel: Control of Pluripotency Laboratory, Department of Physiological Sciences I, Faculty of Medicine, University of Barcelona, Hospital Clinic, Casanova 143, Barcelona 08036, Spain; Developmental and Stem Cell Biology, Victor Chang Cardiac Research Institute, Sydney NSW 2145, Australia; Faculty of Medicine, Westmead Children's Hospital, Division of Paediatrics and Child Health, University of Sydney Medical School, Sydney NSW 2145, Australia; School of Anatomy, Physiology and Human Biology, and the Harry Perkins Institute for Medical Research (CCTRM), The University of Western Australia, Western Australia 6009

Irene Faravelli: Dino Ferrari Centre, Neuroscience Section, Department of Pathophysiology and Transplantation (DEPT), University of Milan, Neurology Unit, IRCCS Foundation Ca'Granda Ospedale Maggiore Policlinico, via Francesco Sforza 35, 20122 Milan, Italy

Michael G. Fehlings: Department of Genetics and Development, Toronto Western Research Institute, University Health Network, Toronto, M5T 2S8, ON, Canada; Department of Surgery, University of Toronto, Toronto, M5T 1P5, ON, Canada; Institute of Medical Sciences, University of Toronto, Toronto, M5S 1A8, ON, Canada

Anis Feki: Department of Obstetrics and Gynecology, Cantonal Hospital of Fribourg, Chemin des Pensionnats 2-6, 1708 Fribourg, Switzerland

Emanuele Frattini: Dino Ferrari Centre, Neuroscience Section, Department of Pathophysiology and Transplantation (DEPT), University of Milan, Neurology Unit, IRCCS Foundation Ca'Granda Ospedale Maggiore Policlinico, via Francesco Sforza 35, 20122 Milan, Italy

Kristine Freude: Department of Veterinary Clinical and Animal Sciences, Faculty of Health and Medical Sciences, University of Copenhagen, Gronnegaardsvej 7, Frederiksberg C DK-1870, Denmark

Stephanie Friedrichs: Institute of Physiology I, Life and Brain Center, University of Bonn, Bonn 53127, Germany

Masahiro J. Go: Research and Development Center for Cell Therapy, Foundation for Biomedical Research and Innovation, TRI#308 1-5-4, Minatojima-Minamimachi, Chuo-ku, Kobe 650-0047, Japan

Tomer Halevy: Stem Cell Unit, Department of Genetics, Institute of Life Sciences, The Hebrew University of Jerusalem, Jerusalem 91904, Israel

Vanessa Jane Hall: Department of Veterinary Clinical and Animal Sciences, Faculty of Health and Medical Sciences, University of Copenhagen, Gronnegaardsvej 7, Frederiksberg C DK-1870, Denmark

Alan R. Harvey: School of Anatomy, Physiology and Human Biology, The University of Western Australia, Crawley, Western Australia 6009, Australia

Richard P. Harvey: Victor Chang Cardiac Research Institute, Lowy Packer Building, 405 Liverpool St., Darlinghurst NSW 2010, Australia; St. Vincent's Clinical School and School of Biotechnology and Biomolecular Sciences, University of New South Wales, Kensington NSW 2052, Australia

Meilyn Hew: Department of Clinical Immunology, Pathwest Laboratory Medicine, Queen Elizabeth II Medical Centre, Perth 6009, Western Australia, Australia

Youssef Hibaoui: Department of Genetic Medicine and Development, University of Geneva Medical School and Geneva University Hospitals, 1 Rue Michel-Servet, CH-1211 Geneva, Switzerland

Stuart I. Hodgetts: School of Anatomy, Physiology and Human Biology, The University of Western Australia, Crawley, Western Australia 6009, Australia

Poul Hyttel: Department of Veterinary Clinical and Animal Sciences, Faculty of Health and Medical Sciences, University of Copenhagen, Gronnegaardsvej 7, Frederiksberg C DK-1870, Denmark

Tetsuya Ishii: Office of Health and Safety, Hokkaido University, Sapporo 060-0808, Japan

Hoshimi Kanemura: Research and Development Center for Cell Therapy, Foundation for Biomedical Research and Innovation, TRI#308 1-5-4, Minatojima-Minamimachi, Chuo-ku, Kobe 650-0047, Japan; Laboratory for Retinal Regeneration, RIKEN Center for Developmental Biology, 2-2-3, Minatojima-Minamimachi, Chuo-ku, Kobe 650-0047, Japan

Shin Kawamata: Research and Development Center for Cell Therapy, Foundation for Biomedical Research and Innovation, TRI#308 1-5-4, Minatojima-Minamimachi, Chuo-ku, Kobe 650-0047, Japan

Mohamad Khazaei: Department of Genetics and Development, Toronto Western Research Institute, University Health Network, Toronto, M5T 2S8, ON, Canada

Cheuk-Yiu Law: Cardiology Division, Department of Medicine, Rm. 1928, Block K, Queen Mary Hospital, the University of Hong Kong, Hong Kong SAR, China; Research Center of Heart, Brain, Hormone and Healthy Aging, Li Ka Shing Faculty of Medicine, the University of Hong Kong, Hong Kong SAR, China

Yao Li: Department of Ophthalmology, Columbia University, 635 W 165th St, New York, NY 10032, USA

Michaela Lucas: Department of Clinical Immunology, Pathwest Laboratory Medicine, Queen Elizabeth II Medical Centre, Perth 6009, Western Australia, Australia; School of Medicine and Pharmacology and School of Pathology and Laboratory Medicine, The University of Western Australia, Harry Perkins Institute of Medical Research, Perth, 6009, Western Australia, Australia; Institute for Immunology and Infectious Diseases, Murdoch University, Perth, 6150, Western Australia

David A. Mackey: Centre for Ophthalmology and Visual Science (Incorporating Lions Eye Institute), The University of Western Australia, Perth WA 6009, Australia

Daniela Malan: Institute of Physiology I, Life and Brain Center, University of Bonn, Bonn 53127, Germany

Eva M. Martínez-Conesa: Tissue Bank of BST (GenCat), Calle Dr Antoni Pujadas 42, SSMM Sant Joan de Déu, Edifici Pujadas, E-08830 Sant Boi de Llobregat, Spain

Samuel McLenachan: Centre for Ophthalmology and Visual Science (Incorporating Lions Eye Institute), The University of Western Australia, Perth WA 6009, Australia

Maurizio Memo: Department of Molecular and Translational Medicine, Fibroblast Reprogramming Unit, University of Brescia, Brescia 25123, Italy

Kwong-Man Ng: Cardiology Division, Department of Medicine, Rm. 1928, Block K, Queen Mary Hospital, the University of Hong Kong, Hong Kong SAR, China; Research Center of Heart, Brain, Hormone and Healthy Aging, Li Ka Shing Faculty of Medicine, the University of Hong Kong, Hong Kong SAR, China

Huy V. Nguyen: College of Physicians and Surgeons, Columbia University, 100 Haven Ave, Apt 14B, New York, NY 10032, USA

Núria Nieto-Nicolau: CellTec-UB and the Clinic Foundation for Biomedical Research (FCRB), University of Barcelona, Avda. Diagonal 643, E-08028 Barcelona, Spain

Monica Nizzardo: Dino Ferrari Centre, Neuroscience Section, Department of Pathophysiology and Transplantation (DEPT), University of Milan, Neurology Unit, IRCCS Foundation Ca'Granda Ospedale Maggiore Policlinico, via Francesco Sforza 35, 20122 Milan, Italy

Scott Nyberg: Division of Experimental Surgery, Mayo Clinic College of Medicine, Rochester, MN 55905, USA

Kevin O'Connor: Department of Clinical Immunology, Royal Perth Hospital, Perth 6000, Western Australia, Australia

Dmitry A. Ovchinnikov: Stem Cell Engineering Group, Australian Institute for Bioengineering and Nanotechnology, The University of Queensland, St. Lucia 4072, Australia

Carlota Pires: Department of Veterinary Clinical and Animal Sciences, Faculty of Health and Medical Sciences, University of Copenhagen, Gronnegaardsvej 7, Frederiksberg C DK-1870, Denmark

Agnese Ramirez: Dino Ferrari Centre, Neuroscience Section, Department of Pathophysiology and Transplantation (DEPT), University of Milan, Neurology Unit, IRCCS Foundation Ca'Granda Ospedale Maggiore Policlinico, via Francesco Sforza 35, 20122 Milan, Italy

Angel Raya: Control of Stem Cell Potency Group, Institute for Bioengineering of Catalonia (IBEC), Barcelona 08028, Spain; Institució Catalana de Recerca i Estudis Avançats (ICREA), Barcelona 08010, Spain; Center for Networked Biomedical Research on Bioengineering, Biomaterials and Nanomedicine (CIBER-BBN), Madrid 28029, Spain; Center of Regenerative Medicine in Barcelona, Dr. Aiguader 88, Barcelona 08003, Spain

Jordi Requena: Control of Pluripotency Laboratory, Department of Physiological Sciences I, Faculty of Medicine, University of Barcelona, Hospital Clinic, Casanova 143, 08036, Barcelona, Spain

Isart Roca: Control of Pluripotency Laboratory, Department of Physiological Sciences I, Faculty of Medicine, University of Barcelona, Hospital Clinic, Casanova 143, 08036, Barcelona, Spain

Noriko Sakai: Laboratory for Retinal Regeneration, RIKEN Center for Developmental Biology, 2-2-3, Minatojima-Minamimachi, Chuo-ku, Kobe 650-0047, Japan

Philipp Sasse: Institute of Physiology I, Life and Brain Center, University of Bonn, Bonn 53127, Germany

Ahad M. Siddiqui: Department of Genetics and Development, Toronto Western Research Institute, University Health Network, Toronto, M5T 2S8, ON, Canada

Giulia Stuppia: Dino Ferrari Centre, Neuroscience Section, Department of Pathophysiology and Transplantation (DEPT), University of Milan, Neurology Unit, IRCCS Foundation Ca'Granda Ospedale Maggiore Policlinico, via Francesco Sforza 35, 20122 Milan, Italy

Masayo Takahashi: Laboratory for Retinal Regeneration, RIKEN Center for Developmental Biology, 2-2-3, Minatojima-Minamimachi, Chuo-ku, Kobe 650-0047, Japan

Roger Torrent: Institute for Biomedicine of the University of Barcelona (IBUB), Barcelona Science Park, Barcelona 08028, Spain

Stephen H. Tsang: Department of Ophthalmology, Columbia University, 635 W 165th St, New York, NY 10032, USA

Hung-Fat Tse: Cardiology Division, Department of Medicine, Rm. 1928, Block K, Queen Mary Hospital, the University of Hong Kong, Hong Kong SAR, China; Research Center of Heart, Brain, Hormone and Healthy Aging, Li Ka Shing Faculty of Medicine, the University of Hong Kong, Hong Kong SAR, China; Hong Kong-Guangdong Joint Laboratory on Stem Cell and Regenerative Medicine, the University of Hong Kong and Guangzhou Institutes of Biomedicine and Health, Hong Kong SAR, China; Shenzhen Institutes of Research and Innovation, the University of Hong Kong, Hong Kong SAR, China

Achia Urbach: Mina and Everard Goodman Faculty of Life Sciences, Bar-Ilan University, Ramat Gan 5290002, Israel

Yvonne Voss: Institute of Physiology I, Life and Brain Center, University of Bonn, Bonn 53127, Germany; Physical Chemistry I, University of Siegen, Siegen 57076, Germany

Xuehao Wang: Key Laboratory of Living Donor Liver Transplantation, Ministry of Public Health, Nanjing, Jiangsu Province 210029, China; Liver Transplantation Center, The First Affiliated Hospital of Nanjing Medical University, Nanjing, Jiangsu Province 210029, China

David S. Winlaw: Heart Centre for Children, The Children's Hospital at Westmead, Westmead NSW 2145, Australia; Sydney Medical School, University of Sydney, Sydney NSW 2006, Australia

Ernst J. Wolvetang: Stem Cell Engineering Group, Australian Institute for Bioengineering and Nanotechnology, The University of Queensland, St. Lucia 4072, Australia

Yue Yu: Key Laboratory of Living Donor Liver Transplantation, Ministry of Public Health, Nanjing, Jiangsu Province 210029, China; Liver Transplantation Center, The First Affiliated Hospital of Nanjing Medical University, Nanjing, Jiangsu Province 210029, China

About the Guest Editor

Dr. **Michael Edel** has specialised his university studies in the basic and fundamental principles of Anatomy, Embryology and Human Physiology, completing his PhD in Pathology in 2000 at the University of Western Australia, Perth, Australia. He moved to Barcelona in 2004, and works with his wife, Dr. Ana Belen Alvarez Palomo, to develop new clinical grade cell reprogramming technology to make stem cells to study and treat human disease.

He is currently a Group Leader/Ramon y Cajal Investigator and accredited Associate Professor, based at the University of Barcelona, Faculty of Medicine. He is a senior researcher in the field of IPSCs, hESC, gene regulation, epigenetics, cell cycle, direct cell reprogramming to neurons, lung or cardiac muscle cells for the use of such cells as a cell replacement therapy. He has 46 publications to date, a book on the state of the art of iPSC technology (Journal of Clinical Medicine, 2015), he is an Editorial Board Member for the *Journal of Clinical Medicine*, ten years post-doctoral experience and five years as a group leader. He is affiliated as a Senior Research Fellow at the University of Western Australia, Centre for Cell Therapy and Regenerative Medicine (CCTRM), School of Medicine and Pharmacology, as well as at the University of Sydney, Faculty of Medicine, and Visiting International Research Fellow at the Victor Chang Cardiac Research Institute, Sydney, Australia.

Dr. Edel has a number of current research project grants as chief investigator to develop new clinical grade stem cell technology, including a University of Western Australia near miss grant to develop a project on bioengineering cardiac muscle from iPSC to treat heart disease. He has been invited as a guest speaker as part of the distinguished faculty or co-chair for over 20 congresses the past ten years. For more information see his Lab Web Page: http://pluripotencylaboratory.wordpress.com/

Preface

Dear Colleagues,

The field of reprogramming somatic cells into induced pluripotent stem cells (iPSC) has moved very quickly, from bench to bedside in just eight years since its first discovery in humans. The best example of this is the RIKEN clinical trial this year in Japan, which will use iPSC-derived retinal pigmented epithelial (RPE) cells to treat macular degeneration (MD). This is the first human disease to be tested for regeneration and repair by iPSC-derived cells and others will follow in the near future.

Currently, there is an intense worldwide research effort to bring stem cell technology to the clinic for application to treat human diseases and pathologies. Human tissue diseases, including those of the lung, heart, brain, spinal cord, and muscle, drive organ bioengineering to the forefront of technology concerning cell replacement therapy. Given the critical mass of research and translational work being performed, iPSCs may very well be the cell type of choice for regenerative medicine in the future.

Basic science questions, such as efficient differentiation protocols to the correct cell type for regenerating human tissues, the immune response of iPSC replacement therapy, gene editing for disease modeling and genetic stability of iPSC-derived cells, are currently being investigated for future clinical applications. New methodologies to change cell fate are being developed. The field of direct cell reprogramming is also gaining momentum with over five different cell types generated to date including central nervous system cells, spinal motor neurons, RPE cells, pericytes, monocytes and hepatocytes. As this field develops, new applications not previously thought possible before will open up to take advantage to treat human diseases and conditions.

Please join us in presenting this Special Issue on the state of the art research currently being performed worldwide to bring iPSC to the clinic so as to help understand and treat various human diseases. It is my pleasure to thank the authors and reviewers for contributing to this special issue and am sure it will become an excellent reference text for iPSC research covering ten different human disease/conditions.

Dr. Michael J. Edel

Guest Editor

Editorial Board Member

University of Barcelona: michaeledel@ub.edu

University of Western Australia: Michael.edel@uwa.edu.au

Centre for Cell Therapy and Regenerative Medicine (CCTRM)

Chapter 1:
Neuronal

Using iPS Cells toward the Understanding of Parkinson's Disease

Roger Torrent, Francesca De Angelis Rigotti, Patrizia Dell'Era, Maurizio Memo, Angel Raya and Antonella Consiglio

Abstract: Cellular reprogramming of somatic cells to human pluripotent stem cells (iPSC) represents an efficient tool for *in vitro* modeling of human brain diseases and provides an innovative opportunity in the identification of new therapeutic drugs. Patient-specific iPSC can be differentiated into disease-relevant cell types, including neurons, carrying the genetic background of the donor and enabling *de novo* generation of human models of genetically complex disorders. Parkinson's disease (PD) is the second most common age-related progressive neurodegenerative disease, which is mainly characterized by nigrostriatal dopaminergic (DA) neuron degeneration and synaptic dysfunction. Recently, the generation of disease-specific iPSC from patients suffering from PD has unveiled a recapitulation of disease-related cell phenotypes, such as abnormal α-synuclein accumulation and alterations in autophagy machinery. The use of patient-specific iPSC has a remarkable potential to uncover novel insights of the disease pathogenesis, which in turn will open new avenues for clinical intervention. This review explores the current Parkinson's disease iPSC-based models highlighting their role in the discovery of new drugs, as well as discussing the most challenging limitations iPSC-models face today.

Reprinted from *J. Clin. Med.* Cite as: Torrent, R.; De Angelis Rigotti, F.; Dell'Era, P.; Memo, M.; Raya, A.; Consiglio, A. Using iPS Cells toward the Understanding of Parkinson's Disease. *J. Clin. Med.* **2015**, *4*, 548–566.

1. Parkinson's Disease

Parkinson's disease (PD) is the second most common neurodegenerative disease in the world after Alzheimer's disease (AD), affecting 2% of the population over the age of 60. The mean duration of the disease from the time of diagnosis to death is approximately 15 years, with a mortality ratio of 2 to 1 in the affected subjects [1].

PD is characterized by debilitating motor deficits, such as tremor, limb rigidity and slowness of movements (bradykinesia) although non-motor features, such as hyposmia, cognitive decline, depression, and disturbed sleep are also present in later stages of the disease [1–3]. Neuropathologically, these motor deficits are caused by the progressive preferential loss of striatal-projecting neurons of the substantia nigra pars compacta; more specifically a subtype of dopaminergic neurons (DAn) patterned for the ventral midbrain (vmDAn). Neuronal loss is typically accompanied by the presence of intra-cytoplasmic ubiquitin-positive inclusions in surviving neurons. These structures are known as Lewy bodies and Lewy neurites and they are mainly composed of the neuronal protein α-synuclein (α-syn). These protein inclusions are not only found throughout the brain but also outside of the CNS. Moreover, microglial activation and an increase in astroglia and lymphocyte infiltration also occur in PD [4].

Approximately 90%–95% of all PD cases are sporadic with no family history. Although disease onset and age are highly correlated, PD occurs when complex mechanisms such as mitochondrial activity, autophagy or degradation via proteasome are dysregulated by environmental influence or PD-specific mutation susceptibility [5].

Studies of rare large families showing classical Mendelian inherited PD have allowed for the identification of 11 genes out of 16 identified disease *loci*. They include dominant mutations in Leucine-rich repeat kinase 2 (*LRRK2*), recessive mutations in Parkin (coded by *PARK2*) and PTEN-induced putative kinase (*PINK1*) [6], as well as both rare dominant mutations and multiplications in the gene encoding α-synuclein (*SNCA*).

Current treatment for PD is limited to targeting only the symptoms of the disease and does not cure or delay disease progression. Therefore, the identification of new and more effective drugs to slow down, stop and even reverse PD is critical. This limited symptomatic treatment is due to the lack of clear understanding of the underlying mechanisms affected during PD. Using patient-specific iPSC-based models to recapitulate the disease from start to finish delivers a more detailed picture of the mechanisms involved in the progression of Parkinson's disease and will aid in the discovery of disease-targeted therapies in the future.

2. Models of Parkinson's Disease

Despite advances in the identification of genes and proteins involved in PD, there are still gaps in our understanding of the underlying mechanisms involved [7,8]. The lack of PD models fully representing the complex mechanisms involved in disease progression, as well as the near impossible task of extracting live neurons from patients has proven the investigation of PD difficult [8]. In general, genetic mouse models do not represent the pathophysiological neurodegeneration and protein aggregation pattern observed in PD patients [9,10], and are thus limited [11,12]. On the other hand, PD animal models of administration of neurotoxins systemically or locally have successfully replicated DAn neurodegeneration, however they fail to recapitulate the degeneration in a slow and progressive manner, nor the formation of Lewy body-like inclusions which occur in PD human pathology [13].

Although the cellular models of PD, mostly based on human neuronal tumor cell lines, have provided helpful insights into alterations in specific subcellular components (such as proteasome, lysosome and mitochondrion), the relevance of these findings for PD pathogenesis is not always immediate. These models do not, however, investigate the defective mechanisms within the predominantly affected cell in PD, the DAn [14]. In addition, all studies involving human tissue have been performed with post-mortem samples, which can only allow for a limited analysis.

The recent discovery of cellular reprogramming to generate induced pluripotent stem cells (iPSC) from patient somatic cells offers a remarkable opportunity to generate disease-specific iPSC [15], and to reproduce at a cellular and molecular level the mechanisms involved in disease progression. The use of iPSC offers not only the possibility of addressing important questions such as the functional relevance of the molecular findings, the contribution of individual genetic variations, patient-specific response to specific interventions, but also helps to recapitulate the prolonged time-course of the disease (Figure 1).

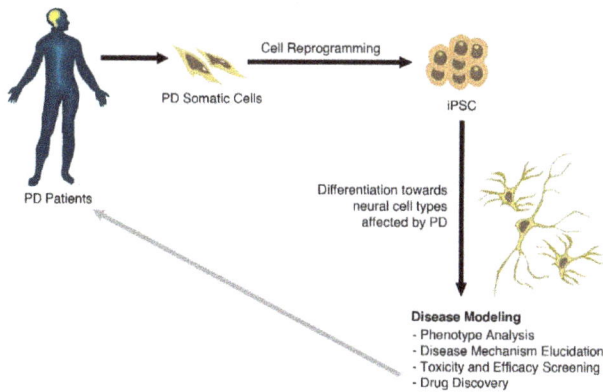

Figure 1. Generation and use of iPSC modelling in PD. Somatic cells from a diseased patient are isolated and then reprogrammed to a pluripotent state (iPSCs). iPSCs can be maintained in culture or induced to differentiate along tissue- and cell-type specific pathways. Differentiated cells can be used to elucidate disease mechanism pathways, as well as for the development of novel therapies.

3. Generation of PD-Specific iPSCs

In recent years, neurodegenerative disease research has quickly advanced with the help of stem cell technology reprogramming somatic cells, such as fibroblasts, into induced pluripotent stem cells (iPSC) [15]. Human iPSC share many characteristics with human embryonic stem cells (hESC), including similarities in their morphologies, gene expression profiles, self-renewal ability, and capacity to differentiate into cell types of the three embryonic germ layers *in vitro* and *in vivo* [16]. An important advantage of induced cell reprogramming is represented by the possibility of generating iPSC from patients showing sporadic or familial forms of the disease. These *in vitro* models are composed of cells that carry the patients' genetic variants, some known and others not, that are key to the contribution of disease onset and progression. Moreover, given that iPSC can be further differentiated into neurons, this technology potentially provides, for the first time, an unlimited source of native phenotypes of cells specifically involved in the process related to neuronal death in neurodegeneration *in vitro.*

One issue found in modeling PD with the use of iPSC is to correctly reproduce its late-onset characteristics, since aging is a crucial risk factor. Indeed, at first it was unclear whether disease-specific features of neurodegenerative disorders that usually progressively appear over several years were reproducible *in vitro* over a period of only a few days to a few months. As a consequence, iPSC were initially used to model neurodevelopmental phenotypes and a variety of monogenic early-onset diseases [17–24]. However, studies using iPSC derived from patients with monogenic and sporadic forms of PD have illustrated these key features of PD pathophysiology, as a late-onset neurodegenerative disorder, after differentiating these iPSC into dopaminergic neurons. Moreover, several inducible factors that cause cell stress, such as mitochondrial toxins [25], growth factor deficiency, or even modulated aging with induced expression of progerin (a protein causing premature aging) [26], have also been used to accelerate and reproduce the phenotypes found during disease progression.

In this review, the recent work on iPSC-based PD modeling for both sporadic and familial cases will be discussed, as well as how iPSC-based studies are helping in the advancement of novel drug discoveries. These studies give insight for the fundsamental understanding of PD pathogenesis, which is critical for the development of new treatments.

4. Modeling Sporadic and Familial PD Using iPSC

Over the last few years, several studies have reported the generation of iPSC from patients suffering from sporadic and genetic forms of PD (Table 1). The first group generated PD-specific iPSC from a sporadic PD patient in 2008 [27]. Over the following year, the Jaenisch's group was able to demonstrate that iPSC derived from PD patients were able to differentiate towards DAn, however, no characteristic signs of progressive neurodegeneration or disease-related phenotypes were observed in those cells [28]. The Jaenisch group generated gene-free iPSC lines from skin fibroblasts of five idiopathic PD patients. Using *in vivo* experiments, they showed that PD-specific iPSC-derived DAn were able to survive and engraft in the rodent striatum for at least 12 weeks. A small number of these cells co-expressed tyrosine hydroxylase (TH) and G-protein-gated inwardly rectifying K+ channel subunit (GIRK2), which are the hallmark characteristics of vmDAn. Remarkably, injection of these iPSC-derived DAn into the brains of 6-OHDA-lesioned rats resulted in motor symptoms improvement [29].

Many laboratories have now successfully recapitulated *in vitro* some of the characteristics of PD, using iPSC as a model compared to the aforementioned studies in which no signs of Parkinson's disease were observed. However, given that PD is a progressive aging disease that affects several cellular mechanisms involving different cell types, each iPSC model highlights only some PD-associated characteristics. Nevertheless, each one of these models has helped to understand some of the fundamental underlying mechanisms as a proof-of-concept. In the last few years, iPSC-model reliability has rapidly improved and has paved the way for the discovery of new complex biomolecular interactions in the pathogenesis of PD. Thus, iPSC modeling has shown to be promising as a tool for drug-screening platforms in the future.

Table 1. Summary of the described PD iPSC modeling publications in this review.

Gene	Publication	Mutation	Number of patients	Isogenic Controls	Cell Type Differentiation	Findings
	Devine *et al.*, 2011 [30]	Triplication	1	NO	Floor-plate DAn differentiation (21–30 days): 28%–37% TH⁺/TUJ1⁻	mRNA doubled expression of SNCA
	Byers *et al.*, 2011 [31]	Triplication	1	NO	DAn differentiation (50 days): 6%–11% TH⁺	Double expression of SNCA, increased susceptibility to OS
SNCA	Chung *et al.*, 2013 [32]	A53T	2	YES	Neuronal differentiation (56–84 days): DAn yield not specified	Increased nitrosative stress, and ER stress, reversed by adding NAB2.
	Ryan *et al.*, 2013 [25]	A53T	1	YES	Kriks's Floor-plate DAn differentiation: ~80% A9 DAn of total neurons.	Diminished spare respiration mitochondrial capacity; increased ROS/RNS and attenuation of MEF2/PGC1α neuroprotective pathway
GBA1	Mazzulli *et al.*, 2011 [33]	N370S/84GG insertion	1	NO	DAn diff. (30 days): 80% TUJ1⁺, 10% TH⁺/TUJ1⁺	Formation of soluble α-syn oligomers, correlated with a decline of lysosomal proteolysis.
	Schöndorf *et al.*, 2014 [34]	GBA1 (RecNcil/wt) GD (N370S; L444P)	4 GBA1 4 GD	YES	Kriks's Floor-plate DAn differentiation: 15%–20% TH⁺/GIRK2⁺/FOXA2⁺/VMAT2⁺ There is also further purification of DAn by FACS	Causal relation of GBA1 mutations with increased a-syn and LB inclusions, correlated with autophagic/lysosomal system impairment
PARK2	Jiang *et al.*, 2012 [35]	Exon 3/5 deletion	2	NO	DAn differentiation (70 days): yield not specified	Loss of Parkin function; decreased DA uptake and incorrectly folded DAT protein, with increased OS susceptibility Transduction of WT PARK2 reversed OS sensitiveness.
	Imaizumi *et al.*, 2012 [36]	Exons 2–4 and 6,7 homozygous deletion	2	NO	DAn differentiation (10 days): yield not specified	Abnormal mitochondrial morphology and impaired mitochondrial homeostasis.
PARK2 PINK1	Miller *et al.*, 2013 [26]	PINK1 (Q456X) Parkin (V324a)	1 1	NO	Kriks's Floor-plate DAn differentiation yield not specified	Loss of dendrite lenght and decreased neuronal survival, as seen by decreased p-ATK values, when exposing mDA neurons to progerin.

Table 1. *Cont.*

Gene	Publication	Mutation	Number of patients	Isogenic Controls	Cell Type Differentiation	Findings
PINK1	Seibler *et al.*, 2013 [37]	C1366T, C509G	3	NO	Floor-plate DAn differentiation: 11%–16% TH⁺/TUJ1⁺	Endogenous mutant PINK1 diminished Parkin recruitment to the mitochondrial membrane under the presence of valynomycin. WT PINK1 rescued Parkin recruitment.
(PINK1)	Cooper *et al.*, 2012 [38]	Q456X	2	NO	DAn differentiation (22 days): 35% TUJ1⁺; 10% TH⁺	Increased vulnerability of neural cells to chemical stressors, with common defects to protect against OS.
	Nguyen *et al.*, 2011 [39]	G2019S, R1441C	2	NO	Floor-plate DAn differentiation (30–35 days): 3.6%–5% TH⁺	α-syn accumulation, increased OS genes, and increased susceptibility to hydrogen peroxide.
LRRK2	Sánchez-Danes *et al.*, 2012 [40]	G2019S	7 Sporadic 4 LRRK2 (G2019S)	NO	DAn diff (Lentiviral-mediated forced expression LMX1A in neural precursors) (75 days): 55% TH⁺/TUJ1⁺ (Majority TH⁺GIRK2⁺)	Reduced neurite lenght and number. Accumulation of α-syn in LRRK2 DAn. Reduction of autophagic flux and accumulation of early autophagosomes.
	Orenstein *et al.*, 2013 [41]	G2019S	4 LRRK2 (G2019S)	NO	As described in [40]	Blockage of the CMA degradation pathway due to accumulated α-syn with correlated increased expression of LAMP-2A.
	Reinhardt *et al.*, 2013 [42]	G2019S	2	YES	Floor-plate DAn differentiation (30–35 days): 20% TH/TUJ1/DAPI	Decreased neurite lenght levels. Increased ERK activation levels, and discover of novel genes dysregulated in LRRK2 DAn.

Recently, iPSC-derived DA neurons carrying a triplication of *SNCA*, the coding gene for α-syn protein, have been generated [30,31]. These cells showed enhanced α-syn mRNA and protein levels [30] and increased cell death vulnerability when exposed to oxidative-stress inducers [31]. Using an iPSC model based on the rare missense A53T *SNCA* mutation, Chung *et al.* observed early pathogenic phenotype in patient-derived neurons, compared to isogenic gene-corrected controls. In particular, they observed a connection between nitrosative and ER stress in the context of α-syn toxicity. Interestingly, the levels of CHOP (CCAAT enhancer binding protein homologous protein), a component of ER stress-induced apoptosis, did not change, indicating that in this model cellular pathology was still at an early stage [32]. iPSC-derived DAn, carrying the A53T *SNCA* mutation, also showed α-syn aggregation, altered mitochondrial machinery, thus enhancing basal ROS/RNS production [25]. The increase of RNS production leads to *S*-nitrosylation of the *pro*-survival transcription factor MEF2 and its consequent inhibition, reducing the expression of the mitochondrial master regulator PGC1α and genes that are important for the development and survival of A9 DAn [43]. Interestingly, Ryan *et al.*, postulated that the MEF2-PGC1α pathway contributes to the appearance of late-onset phenotypes in PD due to the complex interaction between environmental factors and gene expression. Indeed, when PD-associated pesticides were added below EPA-accepted levels, this was enough to exacerbate oxidative/nitrosative stress, inhibiting MEF2-PGC1α and inducing apoptosis, a late-onset phenotype [25].

Interestingly, α-syn is one of the main pathological readouts for many of the sporadic and familial PD cases that are not related with mutations in *SNCA* [44]. For example, the clinical link between the lysosomal storage disorder Gaucher disease (GD) and PD appears to be based on the fact that mutations in acid *GBA1* gene, which causes GD, contributes to the pathogenesis of synucleinopathies [33,34]. *GBA1* encodes the lysosomal enzyme β-Glucocerebrocidase (GCase), which cleaves the β-glucosyl linkage of GlcCer. Functional loss of GCase activity in iPSC-derived neurons has been associated with compromised lysosomal protein degradation, which in turn induces α-syn accumulation, resulting in neurotoxicity through aggregation-dependent mechanisms [33]. In addition, iPSC-derived neurons carrying the heterozygous mutation in *GBA1* also have shown increased levels of GlcCer, changes in the autophagic/lysosomal system and calcium homeostasis, which may cause a selective threat to DA neurons in PD [34].

Similarly to mutations in *GBA1*, mutations in *PINK1* and *PARK2* are also associated with early onset recessive forms of familial PD [45]. Both proteins, PINK1 and Parkin, are involved in the clearance of mitochondrial damage. Therefore their mutations cause a PD characterized by mitochondrial stress as main feature [46–48]. Under physiological conditions, Parkin, which is localized in the cytoplasm, is translocated to damaged mitochondria in a PINK-dependent manner triggering mitophagy [49]. This has been confirmed in iPSC-derived DA neurons carrying a mutation in *PINK1*. In these cells, Parkin recruitment to mitochondria was impaired and only over-expression of WT *PINK1* was able to rescue the function [37]. On the other hand, iPSC models for mutation in *PARK2* revealed an increase of oxidative stress. Jiang and colleagues showed that iPSC from patients carrying mutations in *PARK2* enhanced the transcription of monoamine oxidase, the spontaneous release of dopamine and significantly decreased dopamine uptake, increasing susceptibility to reactive oxygen species [35]. Although the incremented oxidative stress has been confirmed in a parallel study, in this study no difference in monoamine oxidase was observed [36]. On the contrary, the oxidative stress was accompanied by a compensation mechanism that involved the activation of the reducing Nrf2A pathway [36].

Mutations in *LRRK2* have been one of the most studied mutations in PD, not only because they are the most common cause of familial PD, but also because clinical symptoms of *LRRK2*-PD are similar to those of idiopathic PD [50]. The most common mutation is the G2019S, which results in hyper-activity of the LRRK2 kinase domain. Although penetrance of this gene has shown to be variable between individuals' age, iPSC model of a G2019S *LRRK2*-PD has recapitulated characteristic features of PD, such as accumulation of α-syn, increase in genes responsible for oxidative stress and enhanced susceptibility to hydrogen peroxide, which is displayed through caspase-3 activation [39]. Furthermore, the expression of key oxidative stress-response genes and α-syn were found to be increased in neurons from *LRRK2*-iPSC, when compared to those differentiated from control iPSC or hESC.

Our group has generated iPSC lines from seven patients with idiopathic PD and four patients carrying G2019S mutation in the *LRRK2* gene [40]. We observed morphological alterations in PD-derived iPSC vmDAn (fewer and shorter neurites) as well as an increase in the number of apoptotic neurons over a long-time culture (2.5 months). Moreover, we found an accumulation of α-syn in *LRRK2*-iPSC derived DAn after a 30 days culture.

Sporadic forms of PD are not as well defined, given that they may be caused by several genetic variants, as well as a strong environmental effect. However, our study revealed that DAn, which were derived from idiopathic PD patients, also showed an increased susceptibility to degeneration *in vitro* after long-term culture [40].

Importantly, the appearance of the neurodegenerative phenotypes in differentiated DAn from either idiopathic or *LRRK2*-associated PD was shown to be the consequence, at least in part, of impaired autophagy. Blockade of autophagy by lysosomal inhibition showed a specific reduction in autophagic flux by LC3-II immunoblotting, suggesting that the clearance of autophagosomes was compromised [40]. Proteins may also enter the autophagic process directly at the lysosome level, via chaperone-mediated autophagy (CMA). Increased co-localization of α-syn with LAMP2A puncta in iPSC-derived *LRRK2* DAn, revealed a compromised degradation of α-syn by CMA [41]. Although both wild-type and mutant LRRK2 inhibit CMA, G2019S LRRK2 protein was more resistant to the CMA-mediated degradation, resulting in α-syn accumulation [41]. Furthermore, the same phenotype was induced by over-expression of wild-type or G2019S *LRRK2* in control iPSC-derived cultures [40] and rescued by LRRK2 inhibition [42]. Indeed, iPSC-derived DAn cultures from isogenic G2019S *LRRK2* lines (mutation being the sole experimental variable) exhibited an increased mutant-specific apoptosis and decreased neurite outgrowth, as well as alterations in the expression of several pERK (phosphorylated ERK) controlled genes, all of which could be rescued by the inhibition of LRRK2 [42]. Moreover, the genetic correction of LRRK2 mutation resulted in the phenotypic rescue of differentiated neurons with improved neurite length to levels comparable to those of controls.

5. Patient-Derived Stem Cells Could Improve Drug Research for PD

An important goal of humanized stem cell-based PD model systems is the screening of potential new drugs that could affect the neurodegenerative process at several levels during its development in specifically affected human cells. Moreover, the availability of such patient-specific stem cell-based model systems could help identifying new pharmacological strategies for the design of personalized therapies. Recently, iPSC-derived forebrain neurons have been used as a platform to screen disease-modifying drugs, highlighting the possibilities of iPSC technology as an *in vitro* cell-based assay system for AD research [51]. A recent study has also taken a significant leap towards personalized medicine for PD patients, by investigating signs of the disease in patient-specific iPSC-derived neurons and testing how the cells respond to drug treatments [38]. The study showed that neurons derived from PD patients carrying mutations in the *PINK1* or *LRRK2* genes display common signs of distress and vulnerability such as abnormalities in mitochondria and increased vulnerability to oxidative stress. However, they found that oxygen consumption rates were lower in cells with mutations in *LRRK2* and higher in cells with the mutations in *PINK1*. Notably, they were able to rescue the phenotype caused by toxins to which the cells were exposed to with various drug treatments, including the antioxidant coenzyme Q10 and rapamycin. Most importantly, the response of iPSC-derived neurons was different depending on the type of familial PD, since drugs that prevented damage to neurons with mutations in *LRRK2*, did not protect neurons with mutations in *PINK1* [38].

In addition, Ryan and colleagues performed a high-throughput screening (HTS) to identify molecules that are capable of protecting DAn from the toxic effect of PD-associated pesticides. They observed that the MEF2-PGC1α pathway contributes to the late-onset PD phenotypes due to the interaction between environmental factors and gene expression [25]. They performed HTS for small molecules capable of targeting the MEF2-PGC1α pathway and they identify isoxazole as new potential therapeutic drug. Isoxazole, not only drove the expression of both MEF2 and PGC1α, but also protected A53T DAn from pesticide-induced apoptosis [25].

Chung and colleagues investigated yeast and iPSC PD models in parallel to discover and reverse phenotypic responses to α-syn. In conjunction to what was previously reported, they showed a connection between α-syn toxicity, accumulation of NO and ER stress [32]. With these results, they took a step further by screening for possible α-syn toxicity suppressors in their iPSC model, to compare with their previous yeast screenings [52–54]. In particular they showed that the ubiquitin ligase Nedd4 and its chemical activator NAB2 [53] are able to rescue the α-syn toxicity in patient-derived neurons [32], opening a door to a new potential drug treatment.

These results encourage the use of iPSC technology as a tool to discover potential therapeutic drugs. However, concluding for what recent studies have unveiled up until now focusing only on genetic forms of PD, it remains to be determined whether this advanced technology can be used also in sporadic patients with uncertain genetic cause of the disease.

6. Limitations of Using iPSC in Disease Modeling: From Overall Neurodegeneration to the Detailed Mechanisms Involved

6.1. Reprogramming and Epigenetic Signatures

Reprogramming increases cell variability due to the introduction of mutations in the genomic DNA [55] and the insertion of exogenous reprogramming genes. Moreover reprogrammed cells maintain a residual DNA methylation signature characteristic of the somatic tissue of origin [56–59] affecting also gene expression [60]. These issues can affect the predisposition of a given line to differentiate into particular cell type independently of the patient's genotype, and will abrogate the possibility of using these lines for cell therapy treatment in the future. To decrease the impact of these technical limitations, more than one clone for each iPSC line is usually analyzed. However, the use of integrating methods, such as lenti- and retro-virus infection for gene transduction, not only increases cell variability, but also maintains residual expression of exogenous reprogramming genes that is only partially lost through cell passaging. The residual expression of reprogramming genes can, not only create problems during cell differentiation, but overall iPSC do not need a constant over expression of reprogramming genes. Indeed, the reprogramming process by which a somatic cell acquires pluripotent potential is not a genetic transformation, but an epigenomic one [61], therefore only a transient expression of reprogramming genes needs to be activated. Alternative methods to the retro- or lenti-viral infection, have been recently adopted. These include the use of non-integrating viral vectors such as Sendai virus [62], episomal vectors [63], protein transduction [64], or transfection of modified mRNA transcripts [65]. These methods of reprogramming are relevant in the context of any future clinical applications of iPSCs in the field of transplantable replacement cell therapies.

As aforementioned, one of the major concerns in iPSC modeling through the reprogramming of somatic cells into iPSCs has been that of resetting the identity of these cells back to an embryonic stage, therefore having to consider the generated iPSC-derived neurons as fetal neurons. Given the slow progression of neurodegenerative diseases, the idea of modeling this type of disease in a dish has been highly doubted. However, despite the typical late-onset of PD, the key cellular and molecular pathological mechanisms may have started before the onset of the disease. Therefore, α-syn accumulation, autophagic clearance and mitochondrial dysfunctions, among other pathological mechanisms afforested, could have been active in the early stages of the disease. The cumulative effect of these abnormalities along with the effect of environmental influence, have been shown to progressively encourage neurodegeneration [25]. In addition the use of cell stressors and inducible aging [26] also have shown the possibility of accelerating the appearance of diseased phenotypes in a dish.

6.2. Reliable Control Lines and Gene-Editing

Comparative studies require an appropriate control that accounts for differences between lines due only to the genotypic background that exists between individuals. This is especially crucial in diseases whose causative mutations do not have a high penetrance. For example, when complex diseases, such as PD, are modeled with patient- and healthy donor-derived iPSC, the patient iPSC tend to show subtle phenotypes that can be masked by genetic background effects [66]. For this reason, it is imperative to remove the excess genetic variation between iPSC clones and controls, to ensure a more reliable comparative analysis. Given that to obtain iPSC from unaffected siblings or parental controls is not often possible, a solution is to generate isogenic controls directly from the patient iPSCs. In the last years, several research groups have used this approach to correct known mutations [25,26,32,34,42,67], or even utilizing the introduction of the same mutation in control iPSC lines to see the effect of just the mutation itself [42,67]. For this reason, isogenic controls have claimed to be crucial when it comes to assess the impact of any mutation on specific cellular processes. Therefore, editing technologies based on Zinc Fingers Nucleases, TALENs or CRISPR [68], have become indispensable tools in developing comparative studies in iPSC models, allowing for the reduction of iPSC cohorts.

6.3. Cell Differentiation and Sorting

The efficacy of Parkinson's disease iPSC models depends highly on their ability to correctly differentiate neurons into the specific cell type that is affected by the disease (in this case A9 dopaminergic neuronal subtype). Indeed this is critical in order to recapitulate disease features *in vitro* and observe comparative differences between diseased and healthy control lines. Neuronal differentiation of iPSC into DA neurons is not only subjected to high variability of efficiency, depending on the techniques used in a laboratory, but also on the specific ability of each iPSC line. For example, by comparing the studies reported in this review, the percentage of DA neurons compared to the total number of cells varies depending on each cell line, differentiation method and even laboratory group (Table 1). Throughout the field, groups encountered problems in yielding a high percentage of DA neurons within the differentiated population. Therefore, although a number of results are based on the disease phenotype through the identification of TH positive cells by immunocytochemistry, protein immunoblots in which all cell populations are considered skews the data. More specifically, the levels of affected protein in the few TH positive cells may be diluted and missed when mixed with the whole population of differentiate cells when analyzed. Interpretation of these results have been, thus, controversial, especially in the cases in which PD iPSC-derived models have low yield in DA differentiation, which probably cannot go beyond the gross neurodegeneration mechanisms that they have observed. Thus, delving deep inside the biomolecular pathways affected in PD will require a more fine-tuned differentiation protocol that allows the enrichment of the cell type of interest. To achieve this, a novel floor-plate-based strategy described by Kriks and colleagues has become the gold standard in the generation of human A9 vmDA neurons for both transplantation and research purposes [69]. The protocol is based on the concurrent inhibition of two parallel SMAD/TGF-β (transforming growth factor-β) superfamily-signaling pathways, which during CNS development induce no neuronal fates such as endoderm or mesoderm. This inhibition directs the cell culture to a predetermined neural progenitor fate with an efficiency of at least 80% of PAX6$^+$ neural cells among total cells [70]. Differentiation of these neuronal stem cells into mature vmDAn is then instructed through the molecular guidance of Sonic Hedgehog (SHH), FGF8 and more importantly Wnt signaling pathway induction, which enhances expression of the transcription factors FOXA2 and LMX1A [71,72]. The final step of neuronal maturation is achieved through the use of a cocktail of neurotrophic factors, including BDNF, GDNF, TGFβ3, dbcAMP, and ascorbic acid (Figure 2). Interestingly, the most recent papers reviewed here have started to implement the A9 vmDAn enrichment protocol [25,26,34] with the addition of isogenic-corrected controls [25,34]. Moreover, Schöndorf and colleagues improved the Kriks differentiation protocol thanks to the use of a cell sorting method (Fluorescence-activated cell sorting), which allowed for a 6.1-fold enrichment of the neuronal population. This step of sorting was necessary to assess reliable biomolecular changes that could not have been assessed with an unsorted heterogenic population [34].

On the other hand, to unveil the mechanisms behind pathophysiological processes such as neuroinflammation, the investigation of all cells responsible for the maintenance of CNS homeostasis, such as astrocytes and microglia, is crucial. Nevertheless, the study of a more isolated system may allow investigators to detect early events of a disease that would otherwise be missed.

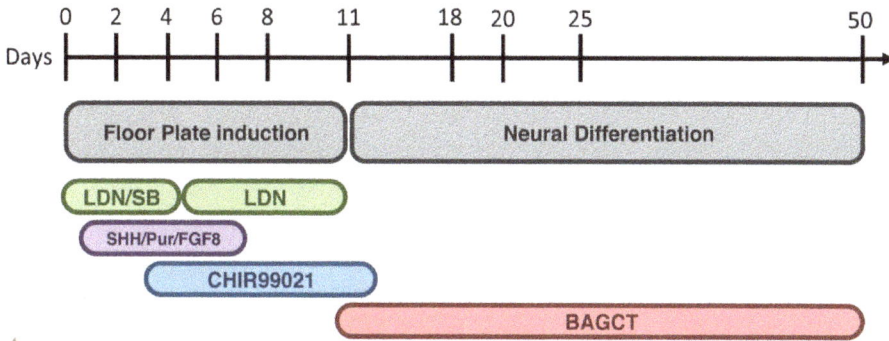

Figure 2. Schematic summary of the novel floor-plate A9 vmDAn differentiation protocol by Kriks [69]. The first stage illustrates floor-plate induction [70], with the appropriate modification in order to reach a more specialized A9 midbrain DA neuronal identity. Exposure to LDN (LDN193189) and SB (SB431542) triggers the Dual-SMAD inhibition. Purmorphamine (Pur), which activates Sonic Hedgehog (SHH) signaling, together with SHH and FGF8 is not sufficient to trigger a selective enrichment of midbrain DA precursors. However, SHH/Pur/FGF8 in combination with exposure to CHIR99021 (a potent GSK3β inhibitor known to strongly activate WNT signaling) allows for a complete enrichment of DA precursors with A9 midbrain identity, by inducing the expression of FOXA2 and LMX1A. Neural differentiation and maturation is achieved through the use of a cocktail of neurotrophic factors BAGCT (BDNF + ascorbic acid + GDNF + dbcAMP + TGFβ3).

7. Conclusions and Challenges

PD is a progressive neurodegenerative disease resulting in the gradual loss of vmDA neurons, as well as cytoplasmic inclusions called Lewy Bodies. The exact mechanisms leading to vmDA neuronal death in PD are still unclear, although pathogenic protein aggregation of α-synuclein, mitochondrial dysfunction, oxidative and nitrosative stress, or altered autophagy have been proposed as mechanisms that contribute to this devastating neurodegenerative process. The generation of reliable iPSC-based models for late-onset neurodegenerative disorders, in which the etiology is yet to be uncovered, has proven to be difficult to overcome. However, recent advances in the field have demonstrated the feasibility of developing experimental models of PD based on iPSC from patients of both genetic and idiopathic forms of PD that recapitulate the key features of the disease. The successful generation of these genetic and idiopathic PD models has opened the door bringing to light some of the crucial pathogenic mechanisms responsible for the initiation and progression of PD, as well as aid in the development of novel drugs that may prevent or rescue neurodegeneration in PD. Recent findings in the field have moved far beyond the proof-of-principle stage, and have started to optimize and standardize these models for the discovery of new aspects of disease biology and new targets for therapeutic intervention. The use of isogenic-corrected controls, more reliable differentiation protocols [25,26,34] and efficient cell-sorting methods [34], have strongly validated the reliability of iPSC models in the context of complex diseases such as PD. Within the field of neuroscience, the opportunity and challenge to combine patient-derived disease-specific stem cells with drug screening technologies with the aim of finding new therapies is now a possibility. In addition, the combination of establishing optimal neuronal differentiation protocols of iPSC using genetic reporters, together with software analysis algorithms, allows for the possibility of automatically tracking each cell over time and to assess any feature of interest, thus providing this system with a powerful tool in drug discovery in the near future.

Moreover, by studying symptomatic and asymptomatic mutation carriers, iPSC technology could also provide a unique opportunity for identifying putative gene-linked PD biomarkers in pre-symptomatic individuals, opening a new novel window for the early diagnosis and individualized treatment in the preclinical phase of the disease.

Acknowledgments

The authors would like to thank all the laboratory members for their helpful discussion and in particular Angelique Di Domenico for editorial comments. Roger Torrent was partially supported by a pre-doctoral fellowship from MINECO. Work in the authors' laboratories is funded by grants from MINECO (RyC-2008-02772, BFU2010-21823), and the ERC-2013-StG grant of the European Research Council (ERC) to Antonella Consiglio, SAF2012-33526, PLE2009-0144, and ACI2010-1117 to Ángel Raya, and a CIBERNED Cooperative Project (to Ángel Raya).

Author Contributions

All the authors contributed to conception and design, data collection and manuscript writing. All the authors approved submission.

Conflicts of Interest

The authors declare no conflict of interest.

References

1. Lees, A.J.; Hardy, J.; Revesz, T. Parkinson's disease. *Lancet* **2009**, *373*, 2055–2066.
2. Obeso, J.A.; Rodriguez-Oroz, M.C.; Goetz, C.G.; Marin, C.; Kordower, J.H.; Rodriguez, M.; Hirsch, E.C.; Farrer, M.; Schapira, A.H.; Halliday, G. Missing pieces in the Parkinson's disease puzzle. *Nat. Med.* **2010**, *16*, 653–661.
3. Schapira, A.H.; Tolosa, E. Molecular and clinical prodrome of Parkinson disease: Implications for treatment. *Nat. Rev. Neurol.* **2010**, *6*, 309–317.
4. Glass, C.K.; Saijo, K.; Winner, B.; Marchetto, M.C.; Gage, F.H. Mechanisms underlying inflammation in neurodegeneration. *Cell* **2010**, *140*, 918–923.
5. Dauer, W.; Przedborski, S. Parkinson's disease: Mechanisms and models. *Neuron.* **2003**, *39*, 889–909.

6. Kim, J.; Byun, J.W.; Choi, I.; Kim, B.; Jeong, H.K.; Jou, I.; Joe, E. PINK1 Deficiency Enhances Inflammatory Cytokine Release from Acutely Prepared Brain Slices. *Exp. Neurobiol.* **2013**, *22*, 38–44.

7. Melrose, H.; Lincoln, S.; Tyndall, G.; Dickson, D.; Farrer, M. Anatomical localization of leucine-rich repeat kinase 2 in mouse brain. *Neuroscience* **2006**, *139*, 791–794.

8. Dawson, T.M.; Ko, H.S.; Dawson, V.L. Genetic animal models of Parkinson's disease. *Neuron* **2010**, *66*, 646–661.

9. Gispert, S.; del Turco, D.; Garrett, L.; Chen, A.; Bernard, D.J.; Hamm-Clement, J.; Korf, H.W.; Deller, T.; Braak, H.; Auburger, G.; *et al.* Transgenic mice expressing mutant A53T human alpha-synuclein show neuronal dysfunction in the absence of aggregate formation. *Mol. Cell Neurosci.* **2003**, *24*, 419–429.

10. Gispert, S.; Ricciardi, F.; Kurz, A.; Azizov, M.; Hoepken, H.H.; Becker, D.; Voos, W.; Leuner, K.; Müller, W.E.; Kudin, A.P.; *et al.* Parkinson phenotype in aged PINK1-deficient mice is accompanied by progressive mitochondrial dysfunction in absence of neurodegeneration. *PLoS ONE* **2009**, *4*, e5777.

11. Chesselet, M.F.; Richter, F. Modelling of Parkinson's disease in mice. *Lancet Neurol.* **2011**, *10*, 1108–1118.

12. Magen, I.; Chesselet, M.F. Genetic mouse models of Parkinson's disease. The state of the art. Prog. *Brain Res.* **2010**, *184*, 53–87

13. Tieu, K. A guide to neurotoxic animal models of Parkinson's disease. *Cold Spring Harb. Perspect. Med.* **2011**, doi:10.1101/cshperspect.a009316.

14. Kume, T.; Kawato, Y.; Osakada, F.; Izumi, Y.; Katsuki, H.; Nakagawa, T.; Kaneko, S.; Niidome, T.; Takada-Takatori, Y.; Akaike, A. Dibutyryl cyclic AMP induces differentiation of human neuroblastoma SH-SY5Y cells into a noradrenergic phenotype. *Neurosci. Lett.* **2008**, *443*, 199–203.

15. Takahashi, K.; Tanabe, K.; Ohnuki, M.; Narita, M.; Ichisaka, T.; Tomoda, K.; Yamanaka, S. Induction of pluripotent stem cells from adult human fibroblasts by defined factors. *Cell* **2007**, *131*, 861–872.

16. Rodríguez-Pizà, I.; Richaud-Patin, Y.; Vassena, R.; González, F.; Barrero, M.J.; Veiga, A.; Raya, A.; Izpisúa Belmonte, J.C. Reprogramming of human fibroblasts to induced pluripotent stem cells under xeno-free conditions. *Stem Cells* **2010**, *28*, 36–44.

17. Ebert, A.D.; Yu, J.; Rose, F.F., Jr.; Mattis, V.B.; Lorson, C.L.; Thomson, J.A.; Svendsen, C.N. Induced pluripotent stem cells from a spinal muscular atrophy patient. *Nature* **2009**, *457*, 277–280.

18. Lee, G.; Papapetrou, E.P.; Kim, H.; Chambers, S.M.; Tomishima, M.J.; Fasano, C.A.; Ganat, Y.M.; Menon, J.; Shimizu, F.; Viale, A.; *et al.* Modelling pathogenesis and treatment of familial dysautonomia using patient-specific iPSCs. *Nature* **2009**, *461*, 402–406.

19. Raya, A.; Rodriguez-Piza, I.; Guenechea, G.; Vassena, R.; Navarro, S.; Barrero, M.J.; Consiglio, A.; Castella, M.; Rio, P.; Sleep, E.; *et al.* Disease-corrected haematopoietic progenitors from Fanconi anaemia induced pluripotent stem cells. *Nature* **2009**, *460*, 53–55.

20. Carvajal-Vergara, X.; Sevilla, A.; D'Souza, S.L.; Ang, Y.S.; Schaniel, C.; Lee, D.F.; Yang, L.; Kaplan, A.D.; Adler, E.D.; Rozov, R.; *et al.* Patient-specific induced pluripotent stem-cell-derived models of LEOPARD syndrome. *Nature* **2010**, *465*, 808–812.

21. Ku, S.; Soragni, E.; Campau, E.; Thomas, E.A.; Altun, G.; Laurent, L.C.; Loring, J.F.; Napierala, M.; Gottesfeld, J.M. Friedreich's ataxia induced pluripotent stem cells model intergenerational GAATTC triplet repeat instability. *Cell Stem Cell* **2010**, *7*, 631–637.

22. Moretti, A.; Bellin, M.; Welling, A.; Jung, C.B.; Lam, J.T.; Bott-Flugel, L.; Dorn, T.; Goedel, A.; Hohnke, C.; Hofmann, F.; *et al.* Patient-specific induced pluripotent stem-cell models for long-QT syndrome. *N. Engl. J. Med.* **2010**, *363*, 1397–1409.

23. Rashid, S.T.; Corbineau, S.; Hannan, N.; Marciniak, S.J.; Miranda, E.; Alexander, G.; Huang-Doran, I.; Griffin, J.; Ahrlund-Richter, L.; Skepper, J.; *et al.* Modeling inherited metabolic disorders of the liver using human induced pluripotent stem cells. *J. Clin. Invest.* **2010**, *120*, 3127–3136.

24. Zhang, J.; Lian, Q.; Zhu, G.; Zhou, F.; Sui, L.; Tan, C.; Mutalif, R.A.; Navasankari, R.; Zhang, Y.; Tse, H.F.; *et al.* A human iPSC model of Hutchinson Gilford Progeria reveals vascular smooth muscle and mesenchymal stem cell defects. *Cell Stem Cell* **2011**, *8*, 31–45.

25. Ryan, S.D.; Dolatabadi, N.; Chan, S.F.; Zhang, X.; Akhtar, M.W.; Parker, J.; Soldner, F.; Sunico, C.R.; Nagar, S.; Talantova, M.; *et al.* Isogenic human iPSC Parkinson's model shows nitrosative stress-induced dysfunction in mef2-pgc1alpha transcription. *Cell* **2013**, *155*, 1351–1364.

26. Miller, J.D.; Ganat, Y.M.; Kishinevsky, S.; Bowman, R.L.; Liu, B.; Tu, E.Y.; Mandal, P.K.; Vera, E.; Shim, J.W.; Kriks, S.; *et al.* Human iPSC-based modeling of late-onset disease via progerin-induced aging. *Cell Stem Cell* **2013**, *13*, 691–705.

27. Park, I.H.; Arora, N.; Huo, H.; Maherali, N.; Ahfeldt, T.; Shimamura, A.; Lensch, M.W.; Cowan, C.; Hochedlinger, K.; Daley, G.Q. Disease-specific induced pluripotent stem cells. *Cell* **2008**, *134*, 877–886.

28. Soldner, F.; Hockemeyer, D.; Beard, C.; Gao, Q.; Bell, G.W.; Cook, E.G.; Hargus, G.; Blak, A.; Cooper, O.; Mitalipova, M.; *et al.* Parkinson's disease patient-derived induced pluripotent stem cells free of viral reprogramming factors. *Cell* **2009**, *136*, 964–977.

29. Hargus, G.; Cooper, O.; Deleidi, M.; Levy, A.; Lee, K.; Marlow, E.; Yow, A.; Soldner, F.; Hockemeyer, D.; Hallett, P.J.; *et al.* Differentiated Parkinson patient-derived induced pluripotent stem cells grow in the adult rodent brain and reduce motor asymmetry in Parkinsonian rats. *Proc. Natl. Acad. Sci. USA* **2010**, *107*, 15921–15926.

30. Devine, M.J.; Ryten, M.; Vodicka, P.; Thomson, A.J.; Burdon, T.; Houlden, H.; Cavaleri, F.; Nagano, M.; Drummond, N.J.; Taanman, J.W.; *et al.* Parkinson's disease induced pluripotent stem cells with triplication of the alpha-synuclein locus. *Nat. Commun.* **2011**, *2*, doi:10.1038/ncomms1453.

31. Byers, B.; Cord, B.; Nguyen, H.N.; Schüle, B.; Fenno, L.; Lee, P.C.; Deisseroth, K.; Langston, J.W.; Pera, R.R.; Palmer, T.D. SNCA triplication Parkinson's patient's iPSC-derived DA neurons accumulate α-synuclein and are susceptible to oxidative stress. *PLoS ONE* **2011**, *6*, e26159.

32. Chung, C.Y.; Khurana, V.; Auluck, P.K.; Tardiff, D.F.; Mazzulli, J.R.; Soldner, F.; Baru, V.; Lou, Y.; Freyzon, Y.; Cho, S.; *et al.* Identification and rescue of α-synuclein toxicity in Parkinson patient-derived neurons. *Science* **2013**, *342*, 983–987.

33. Mazzulli, J.R.; Xu, Y.H.; Sun, Y.; Knight, A.L.; McLean, P.J.; Caldwell, G.A.; Sidransky, E.; Grabowski, G.A.; Krainc, D. Gaucher disease glucocerebrosidase and α-synuclein form a bidirectional pathogenic loop in synucleinopathies. *Cell* **2011**, *146*, 37–52.

34. Schöndorf, D.C.; Aureli, M.; McAllister, F.E.; Hindley, C.J.; Mayer, F.; Schmid, B.; Sardi, S.P.; Valsecchi, M.; Hoffmann, S.; Schwarz, L.K.; *et al.* iPSC-derived neurons from GBA1-associated Parkinson's disease patients show autophagic defects and impaired calcium homeostasis. *Nat. Commun.* **2014**, *5*, doi:10.1038/ncomms5028.

35. Jiang, H.; Ren, Y.; Yuen, E.Y.; Zhong, P.; Ghaedi, M.; Hu, Z.; Azabdaftari, G.; Nakaso, K.; Yan, Z.; Feng, J. Parkin controls dopamine utilization in human midbrain dopaminergic neurons derived from induced pluripotent stem cells. *Nat. Commun.* **2012**, *3*, doi:10.1038/ncomms1669.

36. Imaizumi, Y.; Okada, Y.; Akamatsu, W.; Koike, M.; Kuzumaki, N.; Hayakawa, H.; Nihira, T.; Kobayashi, T.; Ohyama, M.; Sato, S.; *et al.* Mitochondrial dysfunction associated with increased oxidative stress and α-synuclein accumulation in PARK2 iPSC-derived neurons and postmortem brain tissue. *Mol. Brain.* **2012**, *5*, doi:10.1186/1756-6606-5-35.

37. Seibler, P.; Graziotto, J.; Jeong, H.; Simunovic, F.; Klein, C.; Krainc, D. Mitochondrial Parkin recruitment is impaired in neurons derived from mutant PINK1 induced pluripotent stem cells. *J. Neurosci.* **2011**, *31*, 5970–5976.

38. Cooper, O.; Seo, H.; Andrabi, S.; Guardia-Laguarta, C.; Graziotto, J.; Sundberg, M.; McLean, J.R.; Carrillo-Reid, L.; Xie, Z.; Osborn, T.; *et al.* Pharmacological rescue of mitochondrial deficits in iPSC-derived neural cells from patients with familial Parkinson's disease. *Sci. Transl. Med.* **2012**, *4*, doi:10.1126/scitranslmed.3003985.

39. Nguyen, H.N.; Byers, B.; Cord, B.; Shcheglovitov, A.; Byrne, J.; Gujar, P.; Kee, K.; Schule, B.; Dolmetsch, R.E.; Langston, W.; *et al.* LRRK2 Mutant iPSC-Derived DA Neurons Demonstrate Increased Susceptibility to Oxidative Stress. *Cell Stem Cell* **2011**, *8*, 267–280.

40. Sanchez-Danes, A.; Richaud-Patin, Y.; Carballo-Carbajal, I.; Jimenez-Delgado, S.; Caig, C.; Mora, S.; Di Guglielmo, C.; Ezquerra, M.; Patel, B.; Giralt, A.; *et al.* Disease-specific phenotypes in dopamine neurons from human iPS-based models of genetic and sporadic Parkinson's disease. *EMBO Mol. Med.* **2012**, *4*, 380–395.

41. Orenstein, S.J.; Kuo, S.-H.; Tasset, I.; Arias, E.; Koga, H.; Fernandez Carasa, I.; Cortes, E.; Honig, L.S.; Dauer, W.; Consiglio, A.; *et al.* Interplay of LRRK2 with chaperone-mediated autophagy. *Nat. Neurosci.* **2013**, *16*, 394–406.

42. Reinhardt, P.; Schmid, B.; Burbulla, L.F.; Schöndorf, D.C.; Wagner, L.; Glatza, M.; Höing, S.; Hargus, G.; Heck, S.A.; Dhingra, A.; *et al.* Genetic correction of a LRRK2 mutation in human iPSCs links parkinsonian neurodegeneration to ERK-dependent changes in gene expression. *Cell Stem Cell* **2013**, *12*, 354–367.

43. Clark, J.; Simon, D.K. Transcribe to survive: Transcriptional control of antioxidant defense programs for neuroprotection in Parkinson's disease. *Antiox. Redox Signal.* **2009**, *11*, 509–528.

44. Chan, P.; Jiang, X.; Forno, L.S.; Di Monte, D.A.; Tanner, C.M.; Langston, J.W. Absence of mutations in the coding region of the alpha-synuclein gene in pathologically proven Parkinson's disease. *Neurology* **1998**, *50*, 1136–1137.

45. Klein, C.; Djarmati, A.; Hedrich, K.; Schäfer, N.; Scaglione, C.; Marchese, R.; Kock, N.; Schüle, B.; Hiller, A.; Lohnau, T.; *et al.* PINK1, Parkin, and DJ-1 mutations in Italian patients with early-onset parkinsonism. *Eur. J. Hum. Genet.* **2005**, *13*, 1086–1093.

46. Singleton, A.B.; Farrer, M.J.; Bonifati, V. The genetics of Parkinson's disease: Progress and therapeutic implications. *Mov. Disord.* **2013**, *28*, 14–23.

47. Tan, J.M.M.; Dawson, T.M. Parkin blushed by PINK1. *Neuron* **2006**, *50*, 527–529.

48. Okatsu, K.; Oka, T.; Iguchi, M.; Imamura, K.; Kosako, H.; Tani, N.; Kimura, M.; Go, E.; Koyano, F.; Funayama, M.; *et al.* PINK1 autophosphorylation upon membrane potential dissipation is essential for Parkin recruitment to damaged mitochondria. *Nat. Commun.* **2012**, *3*, doi:10.1038/ncomms2016.

49. Narendra, D.P.; Jin, S.M.; Tanaka, A.; Suen, D.F.; Gautier, C.A.; Shen, J.; Cookson, M.R.; Youle, R.J. PINK1 is selectively stabilized on impaired mitochondria to activate Parkin. *PLoS Biol.* **2010**, *8*, e1000298.

50. Haugarvoll, K.; Rademakers, R.; Kachergus, J.M.; Nuytemans, K.; Ross, O.A.; Gibson, J.M.; Tan, E.K.; Gaig, C.; Tolosa, E.; Goldwurm, S.; *et al.* LRRK2 R1441C parkinsonism is clinically similar to sporadic Parkinson disease. *Neurology* **2008**, *70*, 1456–1460.

51. Yahata, N.; Asai, M.; Kitaoka, S.; Takahashi, K.; Asaka, I.; Hioki, H.; Kaneko, T.; Maruyama, K.; Saido, T.C.; Nakahata, T.; *et al.* Anti-Aβ drug screening platform using human iPS cell-derived neurons for the treatment of Alzheimer's disease. *PLoS ONE* **2011**, *6*, e25788.

52. Gitler, A.D.; Chesi, A.; Geddie, M.L.; Strathearn, K.E.; Hamamichi, S.; Hill, K.J.; Caldwell, K.A.; Caldwell, G.A.; Cooper, A.A.; Rochet, J.S.; *et al.* α-Synuclein is part of a diverse and highly conserved interaction network that includes PARK9 and manganese toxicity. *Nat. Genet.* **2009**, *41*, 308–315.

53. Tardiff, D.F.; Jui, N.T.; Khurana, V.; Tambe, M.A.; Thompson, M.L.; Chung, C.Y.; Kamadurai, H.B.; Kim, H.T.; Lancaster, A.K.; Caldwell, K.A.; *et al.* Yeast Reveal a "Druggable" Rsp5/Nedd4 Network that Ameliorates α-synuclein Toxicity in Neurons. *Science* **2013**, *343*, 979–983.

54. Cooper, A.A.; Gitler, A.D.; Cashikar, A.; Haynes, C.M.; Hill, K.J.; Bhullar, B.; Liu, K.; Xu, K.; Strathearn, K.E.; Liu, F.; *et al.* α-synuclein blocks ER-Golgi traffic and Rab1 rescues neuron loss in Parkinson's models. *Science* **2006**, *313*, 324–328.

55. Gore, A.; Li, Z.; Fung, H.L.; Young, J.E.; Agarwal, S.; Antosiewicz-Bourget, J.; Canto, I.; Giorgetti, A.; Israel, M.A.; Kiskinis, E.; *et al.* Somatic coding mutations in human induced pluripotent stem cells. *Nature* **2011**, *471*, 63–67.

56. Kim, K.; Doi, A.; Wen, B.; Ng, K.; Zhao, R.; Cahan, P.; Kim, J.; Aryee, M.J.; Ji, H.; Ehrlich, L.I.; *et al.* Epigenetic memory in induced pluripotent stem cells. *Nature* **2010**, *467*, 285–290.

57. Marchetto, M.C.; Yeo, G.W.; Kainohana, O.; Marsala, M.; Gage, F.H.; Muotri, A.R. Transcriptional signature and memory retention of human-induced pluripotent stem cells. *PLoS ONE* **2009**, *4*, e7076.

58. Hussein, S.M.; Batada, N.N.; Vuoristo, S.; Ching, R.W.; Autio, R.; Närvä, E.; Ng, S.; Sourour, M.; Hämäläinen, R.; Olsson, C.; *et al.* Copy number variation and selection during reprogramming to pluripotency. *Nature* **2011**, *471*, 58–62.

59. Lister, R.; Pelizzola, M.; Kida, Y.S.; Hawkins, R.D.; Nery, J.R.; Hon, G.; Antosiewicz-Bourget, J.; O'Malley, R.; Castanon, R.; Klugman, S.; *et al.* Hotspots of aberrant epigenomic reprogramming in human induced pluripotent stem cells. *Nature* **2011**, *471*, 68–73.

60. Laurent, L.C.; Ulitsky, I.; Slavin, I.; Tran, H.; Schork, A.; Morey, R.; Lynch, C.; Harness, J.V.; Lee, S.; Barrero, M.J.; *et al.* Dynamic changes in the copy number of pluripotency and cell proliferation genes in human escs and ipscs during reprogramming and time in culture. *Cell Stem Cell* **2011**, *8*, 106–118.

61. Ma, H.; Morey, R.; O'Neil, R.C.; He, Y.; Daughtry, B.; Schultz, M.D.; Hariharan, M.; Nery, J.R.; Castanon, R.; Sabatini, K.; *et al.* Abnormalities in human pluripotent cells due to reprogramming mechanisms. *Nature* **2014**, *511*, 177–183.

62. Ban, H.; Nishishita, N.; Fusaki, N.; Tabata, T.; Saeki, K.; Shikamura, M.; Takada, N.; Inoue, M.; Hasegawa, M.; Kawamata, S.; *et al.* Efficient generation of transgene-free human induced plutipotent stem cells (iPSCs) by temperature-sensitive Sendai virus vectors. *Proc. Natl. Acad. Sci. USA* **2011**, *108*, 13234–14239.

63. Okita, K.; Matsumura, Y.; Sato, Y.; Okada, A.; Morizane, A.; Okamoto, S.; Hong, H.; Nakagawa, M.; Tanabe, K.; Tezuka, K.; *et al.* A more efficient method to generate integration-free human iPS cells. *Nat. Methods* **2011**, *8*, 409–412.

64. Kim, D.; Kim, C.H.; Moon, J.I.; Chung, Y.G.; Chang, M.Y.; Han, B.S.; Ko, S.; Yang, E.; Cha, K.Y.; Lanza, R.; *et al.* Generation of human induced pluripotent stem cells by direct delivery of reprogramming proteins. *Cell Stem Cell* **2009**, *4*, 472–476.

65. Warren, L.; Manos, P.D.; Ahfeldt, T.; Loh, Y.H.; Li, H.; Lau, F.; Ebina, W.; MAndal, P.K.; Smith, Z.D.; Meissner, A.; *et al.* Highly efficient reprogramming to pluripotency and directed differentiation of human cells with synthetic modified mRNA. *Cell Stem Cell* **2010**, *7*, 618–630.

66. International Parkinson Disease Genomics Consortium; Nalls, M.A.; Plagnol, V.; Hernandez, D.G.; Sharma, M.; Sheerin, U.M.; Saad, M.; Simón-Sánchez, J.; Schulte, C.; Lesage, S.; *et al.* Imputation of sequence variants for identification of genetic risks for Parkinson's disease: A meta-analysis of genome-wide association studies. *Lancet* **2011**, *377*, 641–649.

67. Liu, G.H.; Qu, J.; Suzuki, K.; Nivet, E.; Li, M.; Montserrat, N.; Yi, F.; Xu, X.; Ruiz, S.; Zhang, W.; *et al.* Progressive degeneration of human neural stem cells caused by pathogenic LRRK2. *Nature* **2012**, *491*, 603–607.

68. Kim, H.S.; Bernitz, J.; Lee, D.F.; Lemischka, I.R. Genomic editing tools to model human diseases with isogenic pluripotent stem cells. *Stem Cells Dev.* **2014**, *23*, 2673–2686.

69. Kriks, S.; Shim, J.W.; Piao, J.; Ganat, Y.M.; Wakeman, D.R.; Xie, Z.; Carrillo-Reid, L.; Auyeung, G.; Antonacci, C.; Buch, A.; *et al.* Dopamine neurons derived from human ES cells efficiently engraft in animal models of Parkinson's disease. *Nature* **2011**, *480*, 547–551.

70. Chambers, S.M.; Fasano, C.A.; Papapetrou, E.P.; Tomishima, M.; Sadelain, M.; Studer, L. Highly efficient neural conversion of human ES and iPS cells by dual inhibition of SMAD signaling. *Nat. Biotechnol.* **2001**, *27*, 275–280.

71. Muroyama, Y.; Fujihara, M.; Ikeya, M.; Kondoh, H.; Takada, S. Wnt signaling plays an essential role in neuronal specification of the dorsal spinal cord. *Genes Dev.* **2002**, *16*, 548–553.

72. Joksimovic, M.; Yun, B.A.; Kittappa, R.; Anderegg, A.M.; Chang, W.W.; Taketo, M.M.; McKay, R.D.; Awatrami, R.B. Wnt antagonism of Shh facilitates midbrain floor plate neurogenesis. *Nat. Neurosci.* **2009**, *12*, 125–131.

Opportunities and Limitations of Modelling Alzheimer's Disease with Induced Pluripotent Stem Cells

Dmitry A. Ovchinnikov and Ernst J. Wolvetang

Abstract: Reprogramming of somatic cells into induced pluripotent stem cells (iPSCs) has opened the way for patient-specific disease modelling. Following their differentiation into neuronal cell types, iPSC have enabled the investigation of human neurodegenerative diseases, such as Alzheimer's disease (AD). While human iPSCs certainly provide great opportunities to repeatedly interrogate specific human brain cell types of individuals with familial and sporadic forms of the disease, the complex aetiology and timescale over which AD develops in humans poses particular challenges to iPSC-based AD models. Here, we discuss the current state-of-play in the context of these and other iPSC model-related challenges and elaborate on likely future developments in this field of research.

Reprinted from *J. Clin. Med.*. Cite as: Ovchinnikov, D.A.; Wolvetang, E.J. Opportunities and Limitations of Modelling Alzheimer's Disease with Induced Pluripotent Stem Cells. *J. Clin. Med.* **2014**, *3*, 1357–1372.

1. Opportunities and Limitations of Modelling Alzheimer's Disease with Induced Pluripotent Stem Cells

The ability to generate patient-specific induced pluripotent stem cells (iPSCs) through reprogramming of somatic cells and, following their differentiation into neuronal cell types, investigate the aetiology of human neurodegenerative diseases, such as Alzheimer's disease (AD), has created much excitement about this new *in vitro* disease modelling paradigm. While human iPSCs certainly provide great opportunities to repeatedly interrogate specific human brain cell types of individuals with familial and sporadic forms of the disease, the complex aetiology and timescale over which AD develops in humans poses particular challenges to iPSC-based AD models. Here, we discuss the current state-of-play in the context of these and other iPSC model-related challenges and elaborate on likely future developments in this field of research.

2. iPSCs as a Model System

Following the ground-breaking work by Takahashi, Yamanaka and others [1], the concept of personalized disease modelling with induced pluripotent stem cells, generated from a patient's own somatic tissues, is now firmly established (e.g., see [2–6]). While larger cohorts of iPSCs from various diseases are being generated worldwide through various consortia, industry or iPSC banks, a survey of the literature indicates that the vast majority of studies are limited to the comparison of a few disease and control samples (Table 1). While this in no way invalidates the data obtained thus far, there is evidence that iPSCs, even from the same individual, can vary in terms of both DNA mutation load [7], gene expression [8] and epigenetic signatures [9–15], often resulting in differences that may affect their propensity to differentiate into particular cell types [16]. Others, however, report no or only a few differences in gene expression between different hESC and iPSC lines [17–19]. Some of the variability appears to be driven by the method chosen to reprogram the somatic cells, with non-integrating methods showing the least variability [20–22], allelic variation [23,24], the age and type of cells used for reprogramming [25] and the culture time and method used to expand iPSC following establishment [26]. Rarely, researchers have shown, however, that three independent clonal iPSC lines from multiple patients with the same disease statistically differ from controls and that this does not change with increased passage number. Given what we now know about the erosion of imprinting at affected loci, as well as the variability (and erosion) of X-chromosome inactivation [27,28], parameters that can profoundly affect neurally-differentiated cell types, these are important factors to consider when embarking on or interpreting iPSC disease modelling studies. Similarly, the issue of choosing the appropriate controls for comparative studies of human samples is not a trivial one. While unaffected sibling or parental control samples are preferable, these are not always available or come from family members of different age or gender and different genetic make-up. We predict that with time, there is likely to be an increasing demand for the isogenic gene-corrected controls (if the mutation is known [4]) or verification of the causality of single or compounded disease-associated alleles through the introduction of such mutations into control ("disease-unaffected") iPSC lines through genome editing technologies (e.g., using CRISPRs (Clustered Regularly Interspaced Short Palindromic Repeats) or TALENs (Transcription Activator-Like Nucleases) [29,30]), thereby reducing the need for very large (and costly) disease and patient-specific iPSC cohorts.

Table 1. iPSc models of Alzheimer's disease.

Genetic Defect	Affected Process(es)	Disease Type, iPS/hES N and n *	Transgene-Free?	Investigated Cell Type(s)	Ref.
APP	Aβ production and aggregation, MAPT	Familial early-onset ($N = 2$, father + daughter; $n = 2$ pre-selected)	N	Neurons	[31]
APP	Aβ production, ER stress	Familial early-onset ($N = 2$, $n = 2$ and 3) and sporadic ($N = 2$; $n = 2$)	Y	Cortical neurons, astrocytes	[32]
PSEN1	β-amyloid processing	Early-onset AD, OE model in $N = 1$ hES and $N = 1$ iPS	Y/N	Neurons	[33]
PSEN1, PSEN2	β-amyloid processing	Early-onset AD, $N = 2$ PSEN1&2; $n = 2$	N	Neurons	[34]
ApoE(4)	Aβ levels	Early and late-onset DA, familial ($N = 2$) and sporadic ($N = 3$)	N	Basal forebrain cholinergic neuron	[35]
PSEN1	Aβ production and aggregation, MAPT	Familial AD, $N = 4$	N	Neural stem cells, neurons	[36]
APP and PSEN1 OE	Aβ production and processing	OE models of familial AD mutations	N	Neural precursor cells, neurons	[37]

OE, Overexpression; * N, Number of analysed individuals (unrelated, unless stated otherwise), *i.e.*, population size; n, Number of independently-generated iPS clones, *i.e.*, sample size, N = No; Y = Yes; Y/N = Undetermined.

3. Making the Right Cell Type

AD is characterized by progressive dementia accompanied by the occurrence of neuritic plaques (NP), mainly comprised of extracellular deposits of amyloid beta (Aβ) protein and neurofibrillary tangles (NFT), consisting of intracellularly-aggregated hyperphosphorylated tau protein [38]. With the exception of familial forms of the disease, constituting approximately 2%–5% of disease burden, the vast majority of clinically seen AD is the sporadic form of the disease, and despite many decades of research, its aetiology remains largely enigmatic. Sporadic AD can vary in its time of onset, severity and clinical read-outs and may in fact encompass multiple AD-like diseases with distinct aetiologies. Glutamatergic and basal forebrain cholinergic neurons in the cerebral cortex and the hippocampus are thought to be cells that are affected at early stages and lost during AD pathogenesis, with further loss of GABAergic and other neuronal cell types during the advanced stages of the disease [39]. These AD tell-tale signs further appear to be invariably associated with, and perhaps driven by, astrocyte and microglial activation, as well as changes in local vasculature [40]. Given that AD development is clearly a gradual process involving the interaction of multiple cell types in a complex three-dimensional milieu and typically first observed in specific regions of the ageing brain, what is the correct iPSC-derived cell type that will most faithfully model AD *in vitro* (Figure 1)? Thus far, most iPSC-AD modelling studies have employed either embryoid body/ neurosphere or small molecule-based neuronal differentiation protocols that are known to generate mainly glutamatergic cortical forebrain neurons [32–34,41–43]. In terms of gene and neuronal marker expression, these largely cortical neuronal cultures at 4–9 weeks still consist of a mixture of different cell types of variable maturity levels, most closely resembling early human foetal neurons (a conclusion largely based on gene expression and functional analyses of their action potentials and calcium-handling ability). Despite these facts, and perhaps as a testament to the robustness and expressivity of certain AD phenotypes, increased Aβ42 amyloid production and tau-phosphorylation changes have been observed in such cultures. There is a clear need, however, to develop protocols that will allow the generation of specific and relevant cell types (e.g., basal forebrain cholinergic neurons) and purify such neurons away from differently patterned neuronal cell types if we are to decipher the gene-regulatory networks involved in disease initiation. There is a similar need for the development of protocols that will mimic or accelerate the maturation and "ageing" processes of such neurons *in vitro*. Researchers have started to explore this concept through subjecting neural cells to prolonged culture [44], the transient delivery of progerin [45], telomere shortening [46], chronic exposure to oxidative stress [47], DNA damaging agents [48] or proteasome inhibitors [49,50]. Similarly, the field has started to embrace the concept that AD is not a solely neuron-driven disease, but involves an interaction between neurons and astrocytes [51] (and likely microglia [52] and the local microvasculature [40]) that, while initially beneficial, upon reaching a certain threshold, becomes deleterious to neuronal function and survival [53]. Even though it is difficult to envisage that we will be able to artificially recreate such a complex, three-dimensional tissue as the human brain at this stage, iPSC technology is well suited to study paracrine interactions in the dish [54,55], particularly since astrocytes can be readily isolated from control or AD neuronal cultures using flow cytometry or magnetic bead technology and co-cultured with neurons from control or AD patients.

Experiments of this type recently identified astrocytes as an important contributor to neuro-degeneration in Down syndrome iPSC-derived neuronal cultures, a condition that displays AD with a 100% penetrance [56]. Adding microglia, the third cell type of the AD pathogenesis "triad", to such an *in vitro* model is now achievable. While differentiation of microglia from mouse pluripotent stem cells is achievable [57–59], the generation of this yolk sack haematopoiesis-derived macrophage cell type [60] from human pluripotent stem cells has thus far not been reported. The biggest advantage of any iPSC-based AD modelling exercise will remain the ability to gene-edit the cells by the introduction of the specific mutations or transgenes and corroborate the causality of newly-discovered cell-cell or gene-gene interactions. Combining such an approach with single-cell sequencing technology may be the key to uncovering whether increasing cellular heterogeneity, occurring over time, and possibly induced by normal neuronal activity, is a contributing factor in AD pathogenesis.

Figure 1. Modelling Alzheimer disease with iPSC-derived cell types has the potential to reveal cell-cell and paracrine signalling events underlying disease aetiology.

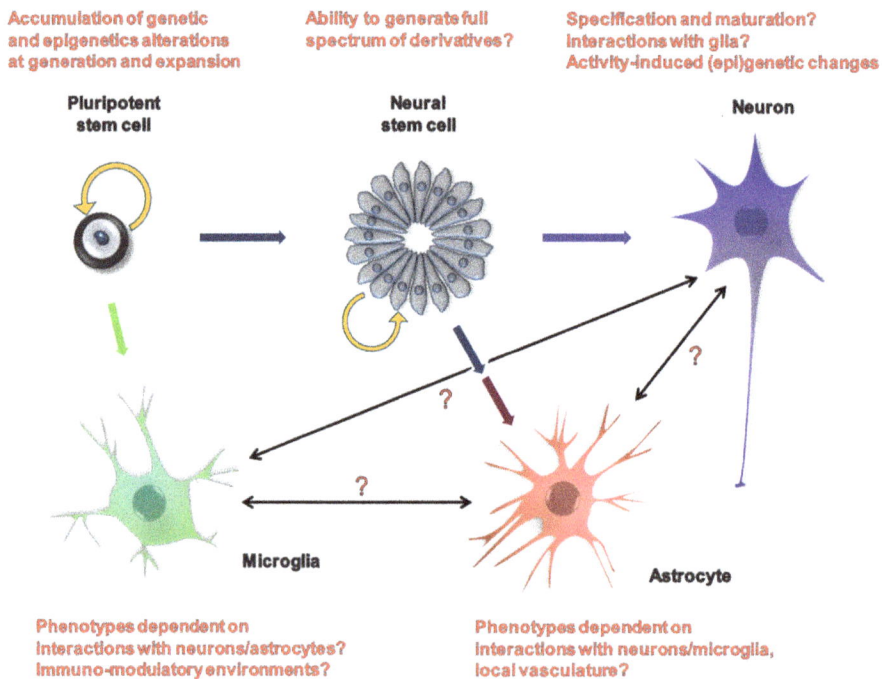

4. AD Phenotypes Which Can be Reliably Modelled *in Vitro*

There appears to be forming an increasing consensus that AD-like pathological changes involve early alterations in phosphorylation of the neuronal protein, tau, and its aggregation into neurofibrillary tangles (NFTs), followed and exacerbated by beta-amyloid toxicity and plaque formation [61–63]. In AD patients, cognitive decline correlates closely with the decreased thickness of cortical layers in various regions of the brain and predicts progression to AD [64,65]. At a superficial level, subjecting

AD iPSC-derived neurons to cell survival assays before and after noxious stimuli, such as oxidative stress, appears sensible and is, thus, commonly used [66]. A correlate that closely matches the cognitive decline in AD is the occurrence of NFTs, rather than beta-amyloid plaques [67]. Determining the level of the microtubule-associated protein, tau, the main constituent of NFT, and the prevalence and subcellular localisation of its different phosphorylated forms would therefore seem essential, since tau appears to act as a key mediator or enabler of both Aβ- and apoE4-dependent AD pathogenesis. In one study [34], the expression of tau or phospho-tau isoforms was not observed, whereas others [41] did observe this in familial and one sporadic AD-iPSC-derived neurons [31]. Measuring the activity and phosphorylation status of GSK3β, one of the key kinases involved in tau-phosphorylation [68], is also commonly a part of the analysis [69]. Although it has become clear that the role of β-amyloid in AD pathogenesis is much more complex than was initially appreciated, with perhaps early neuro-protective roles for APP and clear neuro-degenerative effects of aggregated processed forms, such as Aβ42 during later stages, measurements of the expression of APP and its processed forms remains a highly relevant parameter to examine. Indeed, elevated levels of extracellular Aβ42, as well as the presence of intracellular aggregates have been reported in iPSC-based models of AD [32]. There is further increasing evidence that APP and β-amyloid are linked to enlargement and altered localisation of early endosomal compartments marked by RAB5, and this has indeed been reported in AD iPSC-derived neurons [41]. Both tau and β-amyloid have been linked to a loss of dendritic spines and synapses in mice and humans, and this is another parameter that closely matches the cognitive decline in AD [70]. While these can be readily measured in neurons generated *in vitro* from AD-iPSCs, this approach has so far been under-used, perhaps owing to the fact that identification and binning of different neuronal subtypes is still difficult to achieve. Notably, there is evidence in mouse models of AD that synapto-dendritic degeneration is often preceded by an aberrant neuronal network activity [71,72], suggesting that inappropriate synaptic wiring or network stimulation may be an early contributor to AD pathogenesis. While rabies virus-based synaptic connectivity assays have been used to good effect in iPSC models of schizophrenia [73] and neuronal connectivity in the dish can be readily assessed through dye injection (Figure 2, [74]), these have thus far not been used to any extent in iPSC-based AD research. Given emerging evidence that neuronal activity may stimulate retrotransposon mobility [75], induce double-stranded DNA breaks [76], elicit epigenetic changes in neurons [77–82] and trigger the expression of activity-dependent long non-coding RNAs (lncRNAs) [83–85], this may provide a fertile "hunting ground" for finding novel AD-linked pathogenic mechanisms.

Figure 2. A Day 70 neuronal culture from control iPSCs, imaged 30 min after one cell was micro-injected with NeuroBiotin™ and detected using Streptavidin-Cy3, reveals the highly interconnected nature of neurons and astrocytes generated *in vitro*. Image courtesy of Patrick Fortuna and Refik Kanjhan (University of Queensland, Brisbane, Australia).

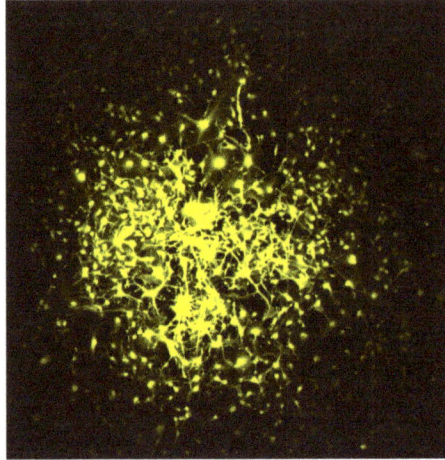

5. Down Syndrome iPSC as a Model for AD

All individuals with Down syndrome develop an early-onset AD. An obvious candidate gene for this phenomenon is APP (amyloid precursor protein), which resides on chromosome 21. Although increased *APP* gene dosage can certainly be a major driver of AD, as indicated by the fact that families with *APP* gene duplications develop early onset AD [86–88] and the lack of discernible AD pathology in partial trisomy 21 patients lacking the gene [89], this does not mean that other *HSA21* genes do not contribute to AD in DS. Indeed, mouse models and clinical data clearly indicate important AD enhancing roles for the DYRK1A kinase (because of its ability to directly phosphorylate tau, APP and RCAN1) [90–92], RCAN1 (a calcium regulated phosphatase able to increase tau-phosphorylation through inhibition of the phosphatase calcineurin and to regulate vesicle fusion kinetics) [93,94], ETS2 (a transcription factor upregulated by oxidative stress that transactivates APP) [95–97] and BACE2 (a non-amyloidogenic θ-secretase) [98–100].

Since the genetic defect in Down syndrome is known (trisomy 21), iPSCs from DS individuals present an attractive model to test hypotheses of AD pathogenesis. Indeed, we and others have shown that neuronally-differentiated DS iPSCs exhibit a number of phenotypes akin to AD, including: Increased neuronal cell death that can be rescued by anti-oxidants, reduced neurite extension numbers [66], reduced synapse formation, increased Aβ42 production and hyperphosphorylated tau [42]. DS iPSCs subjected to neural differentiation also show enhanced gliogenesis, generating astrocytes that exhibit an activated phenotype and increased ROS production levels, upregulation of iNOS, yet reduced expression of NFE2L2, TSP-1 and TSP-2, consistent with the reduced neuroprotective and neurotrophic ability of such astrocytes [56]. It is therefore evident that DS iPSC-derived neural cell types recapitulate key features of AD. Importantly, we and others were able to isolate isogenic euploid iPSC from reprogrammed DS fibroblast cultures, providing the ideal isogenic controls needed for gene regulatory network analysis. Advanced genome interrogation tools, such as CRISPR, can now be used to delete specific genes or gene cohorts on chromosome 21, and delivery of XIST to HSA21 has already been used to epigenetically silence the supernumerary trisomy 21 genes [101]. We anticipate that such genome modifying technologies in iPSC will rapidly provide novel insights into the cell-autonomous and non-cell autonomous processes underlying AD pathogenesis in DS. This will be of great relevance to understanding the bases of the sporadic AD in the general population. The time is now ripe for testing the effect of susceptibility loci identified through GWAS studies, such as ApoE ε4 allele PICALM, BIN1, SORL1, clusterin/ApoJ and CR1 [102] using, for example, CRISPR technology in iPSC models of AD disease and testing their contribution to *in vitro*-assessable phenotypes.

6. Drug Screening Utilizing AD iPSC-Derived Cell Types

AD iPSC-derived neurons are currently being used to screen for drugs that could be of potential benefit to patients. Encouragingly, compounds that inhibit gamma-secretase activity were effective at reducing beta-amyloid production in AD iPSC-derived neuronal cultures. Non-steroidal anti-inflammatory drugs, such as sulindac sulphide, show effectiveness in presenilin 1-overexpressing cells, albeit not for the L166P mutant [43]. Similarly, minocycline was able to normalize the pathological phenotypes of DS astroglia [56], emerging as a promising drug candidate for DS-associated AD and possibly familial AD, as well. In order to enable the high-throughput capability required for screening large chemical libraries, the field will need to address the issue of identifying, generating and culturing the correct cell types (discussed above), make informed choices about what cellular readout will be most informative in terms of preventing early AD changes in the brain and consider the fact that a combination of drugs will affect multiple cell types that are functionally inter-linked to the disease process, providing challenges to image analysis and culture platforms alike. A recent study by Choi *et al.* [37] demonstrated that the generation of three-dimensional cultures of familial AD-recapitulating human neurons was essential and sufficient to reproduce some aspects of the AD phenotype, such as extracellular amyloid-β plaque and neurofibrillary tangle formation. While the study did not utilize the iPS cells per se, the multipotent neural progenitor cell line used closely resembles neural progenitor cells generated during standard neural iPS differentiation [66].

7. Conclusions

Although it is still a relatively young field of research, the iPSC-based disease modelling of AD has made great progress in a short time, and it is anticipated that, as more AD researchers come to appreciate both the value and limitations of this platform, exciting new discoveries that will ultimately benefit dementia patients are likely to be forthcoming. Recent advances in footprint-free iPSC generation, single cell and epigenome analysis technology and the ability to introduce or correct combinations of sequence variants in iPSC are set to accelerate this process.

Acknowledgments

Patrick Fortuna and Refik Kanjhan are greatly acknowledged for providing the figure illustrating neuronal connectivity *in vitro*. The ARC Centre of Excellence "Stem Cells Australia" is gratefully acknowledged for financial support.

Author Contributions

Dmitry A. Ovchinnikov: Manuscript writing and editing; Ernst J. Wolvetang: Manuscript writing, editing and final approval.

Conflicts of Interest

The authors declare no conflict of interest.

References

1. Takahashi, K.; Tanabe, K.; Ohnuki, M.; Narita, M.; Ichisaka, T.; Tomoda, K.; Yamanaka, S. Induction of pluripotent stem cells from adult human fibroblasts by defined factors. *Cell* **2007**, *131*, 861–872.

2. Yu, J.; Hu, K.; Smuga-Otto, K.; Tian, S.; Stewart, R.; Slukvin, I.I.; Thomson, J.A. Human induced pluripotent stem cells free of vector and transgene sequences. *Science* **2009**, *324*, 797–801.

3. Hwang, D.Y.; Kim, D.S.; Kim, D.W. Human ES and iPS cells as cell sources for the treatment of parkinson's disease: Current state and problems. *J. Cell. Biochem.* **2010**, *109*, 292–301.

4. Ryan, S.D.; Dolatabadi, N.; Chan, S.F.; Zhang, X.; Akhtar, M.W.; Parker, J.; Soldner, F.; Sunico, C.R.; Nagar, S.; Talantova, M.; *et al.* Isogenic human iPSC parkinson's model shows nitrosative stress-induced dysfunction in MEF2-PGC1α transcription. *Cell* **2013**, *155*, 1351–1364.

5. Reinhardt, P.; Schmid, B.; Burbulla, L.F.; Schondorf, D.C.; Wagner, L.; Glatza, M.; Hoing, S.; Hargus, G.; Heck, S.A.; Dhingra, A.; *et al.* Genetic correction of a LRRK2 mutation in human iPSCs links parkinsonian neurodegeneration to ERK-dependent changes in gene expression. *Cell Stem Cell* **2013**, *12*, 354–367.

6. Schondorf, D.C.; Aureli, M.; McAllister, F.E.; Hindley, C.J.; Mayer, F.; Schmid, B.; Sardi, S.P.; Valsecchi, M.; Hoffmann, S.; Schwarz, L.K.; *et al.* IPSC-derived neurons from GBA1-associated Parkinson's disease patients show autophagic defects and impaired calcium homeostasis. *Nat. Commun.* **2014**, *5*, 4028.

7. Gore, A.; Li, Z.; Fung, H.L.; Young, J.E.; Agarwal, S.; Antosiewicz-Bourget, J.; Canto, I.; Giorgetti, A.; Israel, M.A.; Kiskinis, E.; *et al.* Somatic coding mutations in human induced pluripotent stem cells. *Nature* **2011**, *471*, 63–67.

8. Laurent, L.C.; Ulitsky, I.; Slavin, I.; Tran, H.; Schork, A.; Morey, R.; Lynch, C.; Harness, J.V.; Lee, S.; Barrero, M.J.; *et al.* Dynamic changes in the copy number of pluripotency and cell proliferation genes in human ESCs and iPSCs during reprogramming and time in culture. *Cell Stem Cell* **2011**, *8*, 106–118.

9. Kim, K.; Doi, A.; Wen, B.; Ng, K.; Zhao, R.; Cahan, P.; Kim, J.; Aryee, M.J.; Ji, H.; Ehrlich, L.I.; *et al.* Epigenetic memory in induced pluripotent stem cells. *Nature* **2010**, *467*, 285–290.

10. Marchetto, M.C.; Yeo, G.W.; Kainohana, O.; Marsala, M.; Gage, F.H.; Muotri, A.R. Transcriptional signature and memory retention of human-induced pluripotent stem cells. *PLoS ONE* **2009**, *4*, e7076.

11. Hussein, S.M.; Batada, N.N.; Vuoristo, S.; Ching, R.W.; Autio, R.; Narva, E.; Ng, S.; Sourour, M.; Hamalainen, R.; Olsson, C.; *et al.* Copy number variation and selection during reprogramming to pluripotency. *Nature* **2011**, *471*, 58–62.

12. Lister, R.; Pelizzola, M.; Kida, Y.S.; Hawkins, R.D.; Nery, J.R.; Hon, G.; Antosiewicz-Bourget, J.; O'Malley, R.; Castanon, R.; Klugman, S.; *et al.* Hotspots of aberrant epigenomic reprogramming in human induced pluripotent stem cells. *Nature* **2011**, *471*, 68–73.

13. Deng, J.; Shoemaker, R.; Xie, B.; Gore, A.; LeProust, E.M.; Antosiewicz-Bourget, J.; Egli, D.; Maherali, N.; Park, I.H.; Yu, J.; *et al.* Targeted bisulfite sequencing reveals changes in DNA methylation associated with nuclear reprogramming. *Nat. Biotechnol.* **2009**, *27*, 353–360.

14. Doi, A.; Park, I.H.; Wen, B.; Murakami, P.; Aryee, M.J.; Irizarry, R.; Herb, B.; Ladd-Acosta, C.; Rho, J.; Loewer, S.; *et al.* Differential methylation of tissue- and cancer-specific CPG island shores distinguishes human induced pluripotent stem cells, embryonic stem cells and fibroblasts. *Nat. Genet.* **2009**, *41*, 1350–1353.

15. Bock, C.; Kiskinis, E.; Verstappen, G.; Gu, H.; Boulting, G.; Smith, Z.D.; Ziller, M.; Croft, G.F.; Amoroso, M.W.; Oakley, D.H.; *et al.* Reference maps of human ES and iPS cell variation enable high-throughput characterization of pluripotent cell lines. *Cell* **2011**, *144*, 439–452.

16. Nazor, K.L.; Altun, G.; Lynch, C.; Tran, H.; Harness, J.V.; Slavin, I.; Garitaonandia, I.; Muller, F.J.; Wang, Y.C.; Boscolo, F.S.; *et al.* Recurrent variations in DNA methylation in human pluripotent stem cells and their differentiated derivatives. *Cell Stem Cell* **2012**, *10*, 620–634.

17. Kim, H.; Lee, G.; Ganat, Y.; Papapetrou, E.P.; Lipchina, I.; Socci, N.D.; Sadelain, M.; Studer, L. Mir-371-3 expression predicts neural differentiation propensity in human pluripotent stem cells. *Cell Stem Cell* **2011**, *8*, 695–706.

18. Guenther, M.G.; Frampton, G.M.; Soldner, F.; Hockemeyer, D.; Mitalipova, M.; Jaenisch, R.; Young, R.A. Chromatin structure and gene expression programs of human embryonic and induced pluripotent stem cells. *Cell Stem Cell* **2010**, *7*, 249–257.

19. Mallon, B.S.; Chenoweth, J.G.; Johnson, K.R.; Hamilton, R.S.; Tesar, P.J.; Yavatkar, A.S.; Tyson, L.J.; Park, K.; Chen, K.G.; Fann, Y.C.; *et al.* Stemcelldb: The human pluripotent stem cell database at the national institutes of health. *Stem Cell Res.* **2013**, *10*, 57–66.

20. Hartjes, K.A.; Li, X.; Martinez-Fernandez, A.; Roemmich, A.J.; Larsen, B.T.; Terzic, A.; Nelson, T.J. Selection via pluripotency-related transcriptional screen minimizes the influence of somatic origin on iPSC differentiation propensity. *Stem Cells* **2014**, *32*, 2350–2359.

21. Sommer, C.A.; Christodoulou, C.; Gianotti-Sommer, A.; Shen, S.S.; Sailaja, B.S.; Hezroni, H.; Spira, A.; Meshorer, E.; Kotton, D.N.; Mostoslavsky, G. Residual expression of reprogramming factors affects the transcriptional program and epigenetic signatures of induced pluripotent stem cells. *PLoS One* **2012**, *7*, e51711.

22. Ma, H.; Morey, R.; O'Neil, R.C.; He, Y.; Daughtry, B.; Schultz, M.D.; Hariharan, M.; Nery, J.R.; Castanon, R.; Sabatini, K.; *et al.* Abnormalities in human pluripotent cells due to reprogramming mechanisms. *Nature* **2014**, *511*, 177–183.

23. Lo, H.S.; Wang, Z.; Hu, Y.; Yang, H.H.; Gere, S.; Buetow, K.H.; Lee, M.P. Allelic variation in gene expression is common in the human genome. *Genome Res.* **2003**, *13*, 1855–1862.

24. Yan, H.; Yuan, W.; Velculescu, V.E.; Vogelstein, B.; Kinzler, K.W. Allelic variation in human gene expression. *Science* **2002**, *297*, 1143.

25. Polo, J.M.; Liu, S.; Figueroa, M.E.; Kulalert, W.; Eminli, S.; Tan, K.Y.; Apostolou, E.; Stadtfeld, M.; Li, Y.; Shioda, T.; *et al.* Cell type of origin influences the molecular and functional properties of mouse induced pluripotent stem cells. *Nat. Biotechnol.* **2010**, *28*, 848–855.

26. Wutz, A. Epigenetic alterations in human pluripotent stem cells: A tale of two cultures. *Cell Stem Cell* **2012**, *11*, 9–15.

27. Mekhoubad, S.; Bock, C.; de Boer, A.S.; Kiskinis, E.; Meissner, A.; Eggan, K. Erosion of dosage compensation impacts human iPSC disease modeling. *Cell Stem Cell* **2012**, *10*, 595–609.

28. Shen, Y.; Matsuno, Y.; Fouse, S.D.; Rao, N.; Root, S.; Xu, R.; Pellegrini, M.; Riggs, A.D.; Fan, G. X-inactivation in female human embryonic stem cells is in a nonrandom pattern and prone to epigenetic alterations. *Proc. Natl. Acad. Sci. USA* **2008**, *105*, 4709–4714.

29. Kim, H.S.; Bernitz, J.M.; Lee, D.F.; Lemischka, I.R. Genomic editing tools to model human diseases with isogenic pluripotent stem cells. *Stem Cells Dev.* **2014**, *23*, 2673–2686.

30. Li, M.; Suzuki, K.; Kim, N.Y.; Liu, G.H.; Izpisua Belmonte, J.C. A cut above the rest: Targeted genome editing technologies in human pluripotent stem cells. *J. Biol. Chem.* **2014**, *289*, 4594–4599.

31. Muratore, C.R.; Rice, H.C.; Srikanth, P.; Callahan, D.G.; Shin, T.; Benjamin, L.N.; Walsh, D.M.; Selkoe, D.J.; Young-Pearse, T.L. The familial Alzheimer's disease APPV717I mutation alters APP processing and tau expression in iPSC-derived neurons. *Hum. Mol. Genet.* **2014**, *23*, 3523–3536.

32. Kondo, T.; Asai, M.; Tsukita, K.; Kutoku, Y.; Ohsawa, Y.; Sunada, Y.; Imamura, K.; Egawa, N.; Yahata, N.; Okita, K.; *et al.* Modeling Alzheimer's disease with iPSCs reveals stress phenotypes associated with intracellular abeta and differential drug responsiveness. *Cell Stem Cell* **2013**, *12*, 487–496.

33. Koch, P.; Tamboli, I.Y.; Mertens, J.; Wunderlich, P.; Ladewig, J.; Stuber, K.; Esselmann, H.; Wiltfang, J.; Brustle, O.; Walter, J. Presenilin-L l166P mutant human pluripotent stem cell-derived neurons exhibit partial loss of γ-secretase activity in endogenous amyloid-β generation. *Am. J. Pathol.* **2012**, *180*, 2404–2416.

34. Yagi, T.; Ito, D.; Okada, Y.; Akamatsu, W.; Nihei, Y.; Yoshizaki, T.; Yamanaka, S.; Okano, H.; Suzuki, N. Modeling familial Alzheimer's disease with induced pluripotent stem cells. *Hum. Mol. Genet.* **2011**, *20*, 4530–4539.

35. Duan, L.; Bhattacharyya, B.J.; Belmadani, A.; Pan, L.; Miller, R.J.; Kessler, J.A. Stem cell derived basal forebrain cholinergic neurons from Alzheimer's disease patients are more susceptible to cell death. *Mol. Neurodegener.* **2014**, *9*, doi:10.1186/1750-1326-9-3.

36. Liu, Q.; Waltz, S.; Woodruff, G.; Ouyang, J.; Israel, M.A.; Herrera, C.; Sarsoza, F.; Tanzi, R.E.; Koo, E.H.; Ringman, J.M.; *et al.* Effect of potent γ-secretase modulator in human neurons derived from multiple presenilin 1-induced pluripotent stem cell mutant carriers. *JAMA Neurol.* **2014**, doi:10.1001/jamaneurol.2014.2482.

37. Choi, S.H.; Kim, Y.H.; Hebisch, M.; Sliwinski, C.; Lee, S.; D'Avanzo, C.; Chen, H.; Hooli, B.; Asselin, C.; Muffat, J.; *et al.* A three-dimensional human neural cell culture model of Alzheimer's disease. *Nature* **2014**, *515*, 274–278.

38. Musiek, E.S.; Holtzman, D.M. Origins of Alzheimer's disease: Reconciling cerebrospinal fluid biomarker and neuropathology data regarding the temporal sequence of amyloid-β and tau involvement. *Curr. Opin. Neurol.* **2012**, *25*, 715–720.

39. Braak, H.; Braak, E. Morphological criteria for the recognition of Alzheimer's disease and the distribution pattern of cortical changes related to this disorder. *Neurobiol. Aging* **1994**, *15*, 355–356.

40. Zlokovic, B.V. Neurovascular pathways to neurodegeneration in Alzheimer's disease and other disorders. *Nat. Rev. Neurosci.* **2011**, *12*, 723–738.

41. Israel, M.A.; Yuan, S.H.; Bardy, C.; Reyna, S.M.; Mu, Y.L.; Herrera, C.; Hefferan, M.P.; van Gorp, S.; Nazor, K.L.; Boscolo, F.S.; *et al.* Probing sporadic and familial Alzheimer's disease using induced pluripotent stem cells. *Nature* **2012**, *482*, 216–220.

42. Shi, Y.; Kirwan, P.; Smith, J.; MacLean, G.; Orkin, S.H.; Livesey, F.J. A human stem cell model of early Alzheimer's disease pathology in down syndrome. *Sci. Transl. Med.* **2012**, *4*, doi:10.1126/scitranslmed.3003771.

43. Yahata, N.; Asai, M.; Kitaoka, S.; Takahashi, K.; Asaka, I.; Hioki, H.; Kaneko, T.; Maruyama, K.; Saido, T.C.; Nakahata, T.; *et al.* Anti-abeta drug screening platform using human iPS cell-derived neurons for the treatment of Alzheimer's disease. *PLoS ONE* **2011**, *6*, e25788.

44. Sanchez-Danes, A.; Richaud-Patin, Y.; Carballo-Carbajal, I.; Jimenez-Delgado, S.; Caig, C.; Mora, S.; di Guglielmo, C.; Ezquerra, M.; Patel, B.; Giralt, A.; *et al.* Disease-specific phenotypes in dopamine neurons from human iPS-based models of genetic and sporadic Parkinson's disease. *EMBO Mol. Med.* **2012**, *4*, 380–395.

45. Miller, J.D.; Ganat, Y.M.; Kishinevsky, S.; Bowman, R.L.; Liu, B.; Tu, E.Y.; Mandal, P.K.; Vera, E.; Shim, J.W.; Kriks, S.; *et al.* Human iPSC-based modeling of late-onset disease via progerin-induced aging. *Cell Stem Cell* **2013**, *13*, 691–705.

46. Batista, L.F.; Pech, M.F.; Zhong, F.L.; Nguyen, H.N.; Xie, K.T.; Zaug, A.J.; Crary, S.M.; Choi, J.; Sebastiano, V.; Cherry, A.; *et al.* Telomere shortening and loss of self-renewal in dyskeratosis congenita induced pluripotent stem cells. *Nature* **2011**, *474*, 399–402.

47. Finkel, T.; Holbrook, N.J. Oxidants, oxidative stress and the biology of ageing. *Nature* **2000**, *408*, 239–247.

48. Moskalev, A.A.; Shaposhnikov, M.V.; Plyusnina, E.N.; Zhavoronkov, A.; Budovsky, A.; Yanai, H.; Fraifeld, V.E. The role of DNA damage and repair in aging through the prism of koch-like criteria. *Ageing Res. Rev.* **2013**, *12*, 661–684.

49. Keller, J.N.; Gee, J.; Ding, Q. The proteasome in brain aging. *Ageing Res. Rev.* **2002**, *1*, 279–293.

50. Mao, L.; Romer, I.; Nebrich, G.; Klein, O.; Koppelstatter, A.; Hin, S.C.; Hartl, D.; Zabel, C. Aging in mouse brain is a cell/tissue-level phenomenon exacerbated by proteasome loss. *J. Proteome Res.* **2010**, *9*, 3551–3560.

51. Wyss-Coray, T.; Rogers, J. Inflammation in Alzheimer disease—A brief review of the basic science and clinical literature. *Cold Spring Harb. Perspect. Med.* **2012**, *2*, doi:10.1101/cshperspect.a006346.

52. Norden, D.M.; Godbout, J.P. Review: Microglia of the aged brain: Primed to be activated and resistant to regulation. *Neuropathol. Appl. Neurobiol.* **2013**, *39*, 19–34.

53. Steele, M.L.; Robinson, S.R. Reactive astrocytes give neurons less support: Implications for Alzheimer's disease. *Neurobiol. Aging* **2012**, *33*, doi:10.1016/j.neurobiolaging.2010.09.018.

54. Di Giorgio, F.P.; Carrasco, M.A.; Siao, M.C.; Maniatis, T.; Eggan, K. Non-cell autonomous effect of glia on motor neurons in an embryonic stem cell-based als model. *Nat. Neurosci.* **2007**, *10*, 608–614.

55. Marchetto, M.C.; Muotri, A.R.; Mu, Y.; Smith, A.M.; Cezar, G.G.; Gage, F.H. Non-cell-autonomous effect of human SOD1 G37R astrocytes on motor neurons derived from human embryonic stem cells. *Cell Stem Cell* **2008**, *3*, 649–657.

56. Chen, C.; Jiang, P.; Xue, H.; Peterson, S.E.; Tran, H.T.; McCann, A.E.; Parast, M.M.; Li, S.; Pleasure, D.E.; Laurent, L.C.; *et al.* Role of astroglia in down's syndrome revealed by patient-derived human-induced pluripotent stem cells. *Nat. Commun.* **2014**, *5*, doi:10.1038/ncomms5430.

57. Beutner, C.; Roy, K.; Linnartz, B.; Napoli, I.; Neumann, H. Generation of microglial cells from mouse embryonic stem cells. *Nat. Protoc.* **2010**, *5*, 1481–1494.

58. Napoli, I.; Kierdorf, K.; Neumann, H. Microglial precursors derived from mouse embryonic stem cells. *Glia* **2009**, *57*, 1660–1671.

59. Tsuchiya, T.; Park, K.C.; Toyonaga, S.; Yamada, S.M.; Nakabayashi, H.; Nakai, E. Characterization of microglia induced from mouse embryonic stem cells and their migration into the brain parenchyma. *J. Neuroimmunol.* **2005**, *160*, 210–218.

60. Ginhoux, F.; Greter, M.; Leboeuf, M.; Nandi, S.; See, P.; Gokhan, S.; Mehler, M.F.; Conway, S.J.; Ng, L.G.; Stanley, E.R.; *et al.* Fate mapping analysis reveals that adult microglia derive from primitive macrophages. *Science* **2010**, *330*, 841–845.

61. Giacobini, E.; Gold, G. Alzheimer disease therapy—Moving from amyloid-β to tau. *Nat. Rev. Neurol.* **2013**, *9*, 677–686.

62. Ittner, L.M.; Gotz, J. Amyloid-β and tau—A toxic pas de deux in Alzheimer's disease. *Nat. Rev. Neurosci.* **2011**, *12*, 65–72.

63. Spires-Jones, T.L.; Hyman, B.T. The intersection of amyloid beta and tau at synapses in Alzheimer's disease. *Neuron* **2014**, *82*, 756–771.

64. Frisoni, G.B.; Fox, N.C.; Jack, C.R., Jr.; Scheltens, P.; Thompson, P.M. The clinical use of structural MRI in Alzheimer disease. *Nat. Rev. Neurol.* **2010**, *6*, 67–77.

65. Putcha, D.; Brickhouse, M.; O'Keefe, K.; Sullivan, C.; Rentz, D.; Marshall, G.; Dickerson, B.; Sperling, R. Hippocampal hyperactivation associated with cortical thinning in Alzheimer's disease signature regions in non-demented elderly adults. *J. Neurosci.: Off. J. Soc. Neurosci.* **2011**, *31*, 17680–17688.

66. Briggs, J.A.; Sun, J.; Shepherd, J.; Ovchinnikov, D.A.; Chung, T.L.; Nayler, S.P.; Kao, L.P.; Morrow, C.A.; Thakar, N.Y.; Soo, S.Y.; *et al.* Integration-free induced pluripotent stem cells model genetic and neural developmental features of down syndrome etiology. *Stem Cells* **2013**, *31*, 467–478.

67. Giannakopoulos, P.; Herrmann, F.R.; Bussiere, T.; Bouras, C.; Kovari, E.; Perl, D.P.; Morrison, J.H.; Gold, G.; Hof, P.R. Tangle and neuron numbers, but not amyloid load, predict cognitive status in Alzheimer's disease. *Neurology* **2003**, *60*, 1495–1500.

68. Cho, J.H.; Johnson, G.V. Primed phosphorylation of tau at Thr231 by glycogen synthase kinase 3β (GSK3β) plays a critical role in regulating tau's ability to bind and stabilize microtubules. *J. Neurochem.* **2004**, *88*, 349–358.

69. Israel, M.A.; Goldstein, L.S. Capturing Alzheimer's disease genomes with induced pluripotent stem cells: Prospects and challenges. *Genome Med.* **2011**, *3*, doi:10.1186/gm265.

70. Palop, J.J.; Chin, J.; Mucke, L. A network dysfunction perspective on neurodegenerative diseases. *Nature* **2006**, *443*, 768–773.

71. Marchetti, C.; Marie, H. Hippocampal synaptic plasticity in Alzheimer's disease: What have we learned so far from transgenic models? *Rev. Neurosci.* **2011**, *22*, 373–402.

72. Palop, J.J.; Mucke, L. Amyloid-beta-induced neuronal dysfunction in Alzheimer's disease: From synapses toward neural networks. *Nat. Neurosci.* **2010**, *13*, 812–818.

73. Brennand, K.J.; Simone, A.; Jou, J.; Gelboin-Burkhart, C.; Tran, N.; Sangar, S.; Li, Y.; Mu, Y.; Chen, G.; Yu, D.; *et al.* Modelling schizophrenia using human induced pluripotent stem cells. *Nature* **2011**, *473*, 221–225.

74. Huang, Q.; Zhou, D.; DiFiglia, M. Neurobiotin, a useful neuroanatomical tracer for *in vivo* anterograde, retrograde and transneuronal tract-tracing and for *in vitro* labeling of neurons. *J. Neurosci. Methods* **1992**, *41*, 31–43.

75. Muotri, A.R.; Marchetto, M.C.; Coufal, N.G.; Oefner, R.; Yeo, G.; Nakashima, K.; Gage, F.H. L1 retrotransposition in neurons is modulated by MECP2. *Nature* **2010**, *468*, 443–446.

76. Suberbielle, E.; Sanchez, P.E.; Kravitz, A.V.; Wang, X.; Ho, K.; Eilertson, K.; Devidze, N.; Kreitzer, A.C.; Mucke, L. Physiologic brain activity causes DNA double-strand breaks in neurons, with exacerbation by amyloid-β. *Nat. Neurosci.* **2013**, *16*, 613–621.

77. Guo, J.U.; Ma, D.K.; Mo, H.; Ball, M.P.; Jang, M.H.; Bonaguidi, M.A.; Balazer, J.A.; Eaves, H.L.; Xie, B.; Ford, E.; *et al.* Neuronal activity modifies the DNA methylation landscape in the adult brain. *Nat. Neurosci.* **2011**, *14*, 1345–1351.

78. Miller, C.A.; Sweatt, J.D. Covalent modification of DNA regulates memory formation. *Neuron* **2007**, *53*, 857–869.

79. Schor, I.E.; Rascovan, N.; Pelisch, F.; Allo, M.; Kornblihtt, A.R. Neuronal cell depolarization induces intragenic chromatin modifications affecting ncam alternative splicing. *Proc. Natl. Acad. Sci. USA* **2009**, *106*, 4325–4330.

80. Sharma, R.P.; Tun, N.; Grayson, D.R. Depolarization induces downregulation of DNMT1 and DNMT3a in primary cortical cultures. *Epigenetics* **2008**, *3*, 74–80.

81. Feng, J.; Zhou, Y.; Campbell, S.L.; Le, T.; Li, E.; Sweatt, J.D.; Silva, A.J.; Fan, G. DNMT1 and DNMT3a maintain DNA methylation and regulate synaptic function in adult forebrain neurons. *Nat. Neurosci.* **2010**, *13*, 423–430.

82. Graff, J.; Woldemichael, B.T.; Berchtold, D.; Dewarrat, G.; Mansuy, I.M. Dynamic histone marks in the hippocampus and cortex facilitate memory consolidation. *Nat. Commun.* **2012**, *3*, doi:10.1038/ncomms1997.

83. Barry, G.; Briggs, J.A.; Vanichkina, D.P.; Poth, E.M.; Beveridge, N.J.; Ratnu, V.S.; Nayler, S.P.; Nones, K.; Hu, J.; Bredy, T.W.; *et al.* The long non-coding RNA gomafu is acutely regulated in response to neuronal activation and involved in schizophrenia-associated alternative splicing. *Mol. Psychiatry* **2014**, *19*, 486–494.

84. Kim, T.K.; Hemberg, M.; Gray, J.M.; Costa, A.M.; Bear, D.M.; Wu, J.; Harmin, D.A.; Laptewicz, M.; Barbara-Haley, K.; Kuersten, S.; *et al.* Widespread transcription at neuronal activity-regulated enhancers. *Nature* **2010**, *465*, 182–187.

85. Lipovich, L.; Dachet, F.; Cai, J.; Bagla, S.; Balan, K.; Jia, H.; Loeb, J.A. Activity-dependent human brain coding/noncoding gene regulatory networks. *Genetics* **2012**, *192*, 1133–1148.

86. Sleegers, K.; Brouwers, N.; Gijselinck, I.; Theuns, J.; Goossens, D.; Wauters, J.; del-Favero, J.; Cruts, M.; van Duijn, C.M.; van Broeckhoven, C. APP duplication is sufficient to cause early onset Alzheimer's dementia with cerebral amyloid angiopathy. *Brain: A J. Neurol.* **2006**, *129*, 2977–2983.

87. Rovelet-Lecrux, A.; Frebourg, T.; Tuominen, H.; Majamaa, K.; Campion, D.; Remes, A.M. APP locus duplication in a finnish family with dementia and intracerebral haemorrhage. *J. Neurol. Neurosurg. Psychiatry* **2007**, *78*, 1158–1159.

88. Kasuga, K.; Shimohata, T.; Nishimura, A.; Shiga, A.; Mizuguchi, T.; Tokunaga, J.; Ohno, T.; Miyashita, A.; Kuwano, R.; Matsumoto, N.; *et al.* Identification of independent APP locus duplication in Japanese patients with early-onset Alzheimer disease. *J. Neurol. Neurosurg. Psychiatry* **2009**, *80*, 1050–1052.

89. Korbel, J.O.; Tirosh-Wagner, T.; Urban, A.E.; Chen, X.N.; Kasowski, M.; Dai, L.; Grubert, F.; Erdman, C.; Gao, M.C.; Lange, K.; *et al.* The genetic architecture of down syndrome phenotypes revealed by high-resolution analysis of human segmental trisomies. *Proc. Natl. Acad. Sci. USA* **2009**, *106*, 12031–12036.

90. Ryoo, S.R.; Cho, H.J.; Lee, H.W.; Jeong, H.K.; Radnaabazar, C.; Kim, Y.S.; Kim, M.J.; Son, M.Y.; Seo, H.; Chung, S.H.; *et al.* Dual-specificity tyrosine(Y)-phosphorylation regulated kinase 1A-mediated phosphorylation of amyloid precursor protein: Evidence for a functional link between down syndrome and Alzheimer's disease. *J. Neurochem.* **2008**, *104*, 1333–1344.

91. Liu, F.; Liang, Z.; Wegiel, J.; Hwang, Y.W.; Iqbal, K.; Grundke-Iqbal, I.; Ramakrishna, N.; Gong, C.X. Overexpression of DYRK1A contributes to neurofibrillary degeneration in down syndrome. *FASEB J.* **2008**, *22*, 3224–3233.

92. Jung, M.S.; Park, J.H.; Ryu, Y.S.; Choi, S.H.; Yoon, S.H.; Kwen, M.Y.; Oh, J.Y.; Song, W.J.; Chung, S.H. Regulation of rcan1 protein activity by DYRK1A protein-mediated phosphorylation. *J. Biol. Chem.* **2011**, *286*, 40401–40412.

93. Martin, K.R.; Corlett, A.; Dubach, D.; Mustafa, T.; Coleman, H.A.; Parkington, H.C.; Merson, T.D.; Bourne, J.A.; Porta, S.; Arbones, M.L.; *et al.* Over-expression of RCAN1 causes down syndrome-like hippocampal deficits that alter learning and memory. *Hum. Mol. Genet.* **2012**, *21*, 3025–3041.

94. Lloret, A.; Badia, M.C.; Giraldo, E.; Ermak, G.; Alonso, M.D.; Pallardo, F.V.; Davies, K.J.; Vina, J. Amyloid-β toxicity and tau hyperphosphorylation are linked via RCAN1 in Alzheimer's disease. *JAD* **2011**, *27*, 701–709.

95. Wolvetang, E.J.; Bradfield, O.M.; Hatzistavrou, T.; Crack, P.J.; Busciglio, J.; Kola, I.; Hertzog, P.J. Overexpression of the chromosome 21 transcription factor ETS2 induces neuronal apoptosis. *Neurobiol. Dis.* **2003**, *14*, 349–356.

96. Wolvetang, E.W.; Bradfield, O.M.; Tymms, M.; Zavarsek, S.; Hatzistavrou, T.; Kola, I.; Hertzog, P.J. The chromosome 21 transcription factor ETS2 transactivates the beta-APP promoter: Implications for down syndrome. *BBA* **2003**, *1628*, 105–110.

97. Helguera, P.; Pelsman, A.; Pigino, G.; Wolvetang, E.; Head, E.; Busciglio, J. ETS-2 promotes the activation of a mitochondrial death pathway in down's syndrome neurons. *J. Neurosci.* **2005**, *25*, 2295–2303.

98. Ahmed, R.R.; Holler, C.J.; Webb, R.L.; Li, F.; Beckett, T.L.; Murphy, M.P. BACE1 and BACE2 enzymatic activities in Alzheimer's disease. *J. Neurochem.* **2010**, *112*, 1045–1053.

99. Holler, C.J.; Webb, R.L.; Laux, A.L.; Beckett, T.L.; Niedowicz, D.M.; Ahmed, R.R.; Liu, Y.; Simmons, C.R.; Dowling, A.L.; Spinelli, A.; *et al.* BACE2 expression increases in human neurodegenerative disease. *Am. J. Pathol.* **2012**, *180*, 337–350.

100. Sun, X.; He, G.; Song, W. BACE2, as a novel APP theta-secretase, is not responsible for the pathogenesis of Alzheimer's disease in down syndrome. *FASEB J.* **2006**, *20*, 1369–1376.

101. Jiang, J.; Jing, Y.; Cost, G.J.; Chiang, J.C.; Kolpa, H.J.; Cotton, A.M.; Carone, D.M.; Carone, B.R.; Shivak, D.A.; Guschin, D.Y.; *et al.* Translating dosage compensation to trisomy 21. *Nature* **2013**, *500*, 296–300.

102. Medway, C.; Morgan, K. Review: The genetics of Alzheimer's disease; putting flesh on the bones. *Neuropathol. Appl. Neurobiol.* **2014**, *40*, 97–105.

Induced Plursipotent Stem Cells Derived from Alzheimer's Disease Patients: The Promise, the Hope and the Path Ahead

Kristine Freude, Carlota Pires, Poul Hyttel and Vanessa Jane Hall

Abstract: The future hope of generated induced pluripotent stem cells (iPS cells) from Alzheimer's disease patients is multifold. Firstly, they may help to uncover novel mechanisms of the disease, which could lead to the development of new and unprecedented drugs for patients and secondly, they could also be directly used for screening and testing of potential new compounds for drug discovery. In addition, in the case of familial known mutations, these cells could be targeted by use of advanced gene-editing techniques to correct the mutation and be used for future cell transplantation therapies. This review summarizes the work so far in regards to production and characterization of iPS cell lines from both sporadic and familial Alzheimer's patients and from other iPS cell lines that may help to model the disease. It provides a detailed comparison between published reports and states the present hurdles we face with this new technology. The promise of new gene-editing techniques and accelerated aging models also aim to move this field further by providing better control cell lines for comparisons and potentially better phenotypes, respectively.

Reprinted from *J. Clin. Med.* Cite as: Freude, K.; Pires, C.; Hyttel, P.; Hall, V.J. Induced Pluripotent Stem Cells Derived from Alzheimer's Disease Patients: The Promise, the Hope and the Path Ahead. *J. Clin. Med.* **2014**, *3*, 1402–1436.

1. Introduction

Alzheimer's disease (AD) is an incurable age-associated disorder characterized by progressive neurodegeneration and is the most common type of dementia, currently affecting 35.6 million people worldwide, which is a figure that is expected to triple by 2050 [1]. The majority of cases have a development of late-onset symptoms (after the age of ~65), which include personality/behaviour changes and memory deficits, hindering general, everyday activities [2]. This late-onset form is most often the sporadic form of AD (SAD), whereby increasing age is the greatest risk factor, but may also be associated with unknown environmental exposures, or a family history of AD. Mutations in the polymorphic apolipoprotein E (*APOE*) gene are known to increase the risk in developing late-onset AD and it is further believed that this complex disease involves other susceptibility genes and/or spontaneous mutations in unknown genes [3–5]. Genetic factors account for approximately 80% of the risk for AD, and genome-wide association studies (GWAS) have identified several candidate genes besides *APOE* that may be associated with late-onset disease, including *ABCA7, BIN1, CD33, CLU, CR1, CD2AP, EPHA1, MS4A6A-MS4A4E, PICALM, HLA-DRB5-DRB1, SORL1, FERMT2, CASS4, PTK2B*, amongst others [6–10]. However, these susceptibility loci explain only around half of the total genetic variance and extensive further analyses are still necessary to characterize these candidate genes and elucidate their association with AD risk. Less than 5% of AD patients manifest symptoms at an earlier stage (before the age of 65), *i.e.*, familial AD (FAD), which is linked to genetic mutations in one of three genes, including, amyloid precursor protein (APP), presenilin1

(PSEN1) and presenilin 2 (PSEN2) [11]. PSEN1 accounts for the majority of FAD cases, whereas, PSEN2 and APP mutations are rarer and some FAD cases are not caused by mutations on any of these genes [12]. In this review, we provide an overview of the current status in the development of patient-specific induced pluripotent stem (iPS) cells derived from AD patients and how these cells may help sufferers of the disease, with respect to basic research findings, drug discovery and other treatments that may prospectively benefit the patients.

2. AD Pathology and Progression

The pathophysiology of the disease is not well understood and considering the prevalence and poor prognosis of AD, there has been a research priority in developing disease models for studying pathogenicity and to aid in development of therapeutic approaches. The difficulty in accessing brain samples from patients, along with the fact that only post-mortem brain analysis allows a definite AD diagnosis, makes iPS cells technology highly relevant in this context. That is, these cells, which are produced from directly reprogrammed AD patient somatic cells (e.g., dermal fibroblasts) into neuronal cells [13], will help us gain access to the disease in a dish, which would be much easier to study.

Two pathological hallmarks are known to occur in the patient's brain, however, it remains unclear which of these appear first and/or is mainly responsible for the disease's progress [11,14]. One hallmark is the development of senile neuritic plaques, composed of extracellular accumulation of Amyloid-β (Aβ). These are formed from the extracellular deposition of Aβ monomers, which aggregate as amyloid fibrils outside of the neurons. There is much evidence to support the Amyloid hypothesis, which suggests these plaques are largely responsible for extensive synaptic loss and neuronal death in the disease [15,16]. Tauopathy, the second hallmark, refers to intracellular neurofibrillary tangles (NFTs) of hyperphosphorylated cytoskeletal protein tau, which are known to destabilize axonal microtubules and lead to cell loss [17]. These tangles are also considered by many to be the leading cause of the disease and which is described as the tau hypothesis. Both the Amyloid hypothesis and the tau hypothesis remain leading contenders for the underlying cause of the disease.

Staging of AD progression based on cortical neurofibrillary changes and increased expression of abnormal tau on postmortem brains reveal that Stage I (asymptomatic) initiates first in the periallococortical transentorhinal region of the temporal mesocortex located on the medial surface of the rhinal or collateral sulcus [18]. Stage II (asymptomatic) is evident to have spread to the layer pre-α or layer II of the entorhinal region and even deeper into the transentorhinal region. In stage III, lesions have progressed into the hippocampus, the layers pre-α and pri-α of the deep entorhinal layers, the temporal mesocortex and the high order sensory association areas of the temporal neocortex. In stage IV, the Ammon's horn, the insular cortex and the medial temporal gyrus become affected [18]. Stage V is characterized by progression of lesions into the superior temporal gyrus and slightly affecting the premotor and first order sensory association areas of the neocortex [18]. The peristriate region and parastriate area of the occipital lobe are also affected. The final stage VI ultimately resulting in death, is characterized by progression to the parastriate area and Brodman area of the first order sensory association areas and primary areas of the neocortex [18].

As a consequence, varying neural cells are affected, including, glia and neurons, such as pyramidal neurons, interneurons and specific neurons such as basal forebrain cholinergic neurons (BFCNs) [18–24]. In addition, extensive inflammation, glycation defects, deficiencies in the cell cycle in primary neurons, oxidative stress and endoplasmic reticulum stress-induced apoptosis have also been implicated in the disease [25–33].

3. Requirement for Further Basic Research into the Disease

With the difficulties in obtaining patient brain samples and a lack of adequate animal models of the disease, AD research is considerably hampered. Since discovering genetic mutations within FAD, several transgenic animal models (mostly rodent) containing single mutations (in PSEN, APP and tau) have been made [34–37]. These models have explained, to some extent, the pathogenicity of soluble Aβ oligomers and the connection between amyloidopathy and tauopathy, but failed to recapitulate the complete pathology observed in humans. For example, the transgenic AD mouse model (the PDAPP mouse), which overexpresses human APP containing the Indiana mutation (V717F) [34], has senile plaques, age-related Aβ accumulation and synaptic loss, however fails to show the presence of NFTs. Hsiao and colleagues developed the most studied AD transgenic model (Tg2576 mice), which overexpresses the human APP transgene containing the Swedish mutation (K670N/M671L) [35]. These mice also show age-related Aβ deposition, an increased Aβ1-42/ Aβ1-40 soluble ratio, plus senile plaques, however, fail to show any neuronal loss [38]. Several other transgenic models have since been generated [39–42] and Aβ deposits and cognitive decline were widely reported in these models, but not NFTs or neuronal loss. The crossing of lines or production of double, triple or multiple mutations appear to mimic AD pathology even better, including in some cases, NFT-like lesions and neuronal death [43–47]. Unfortunately, the use of this multiple gene-strategy to induce widespread pathological features in the rodent differs considerably to familial human AD patients, which carry only single mutations. Furthermore, the use of these rodent models for pharmacological testing and evaluation of candidate drug targets has not led to the development of many successful drugs to date [48,49]. Staggeringly, it has been reported that hundreds of candidate drugs have failed during drug development [50] and it may simply be that our animal models are currently not optimal for either drug discovery or drug testing [49]. Emerging research indicates that *in vitro* human cell models of the disease may serve as more suitable models for recapitulating both the amyloid and tau hallmarks of the disease. One recent paper has reported that human neural progenitors cultured *in vitro* in 3D overexpressing either or both human *APP* and *PSEN1* genes containing *FAD* mutations could display both increased Aβ40 and Aβ42 expression, increased extracellular Aβ deposits, increased insoluble Aβ and increased phosphorylated tau (*p*-tau) in a proportion of differentiated neurons. Such evidence definitely helps to pave the way for future research into disease modeling using human-based cell culture systems.

Currently, there is no cure for AD or available drugs for the disease that can prevent progression long-term. Healthcare systems are over-loaded with dementia patients, which costs the society globally, around $604 billion (US dollars, 2010), making the disease a heavy economic burden on society [1]. With the ever-increasing age of the population and lack of highly successful clinical trials, it has become an urgent necessity to find enhanced treatments for AD. The prospect of even a slight improvement and delay in clinical onset of the disease within patients would have a great economic and social impact [51]. Reliable biomarkers are also very much needed since they allow for the *in vivo* detection of AD pathology in "normal" asymptomatic individuals [51]. Imaging technologies (*i.e.*, PET scans) and cerebrospinal fluid biomarkers have been developed and can detect certain indications of AD pathology in humans, but their predictive capacity at an individual level is still not reliable [11]. Moreover, these tests have been mainly used in a research environment and the question of whether they should be applied widely in clinics is still debatable, due to the lack of adequate testing in preclinical and clinical trials [11].

4. Hope in Modeling Alzheimer's Disease Using Patient-Specific Induced Pluripotent Stem Cells

The development of iPS cells emerged in 2006, when mouse fibroblasts were successfully reprogrammed into pluripotent stem cells by retroviral-delivery of four transcription factors (Oct3/4, Sox2, c-Myc and Klf4), which activated an endogenous pluripotent state in somatic cells [52]. These iPS cells resembled embryonic stem cells (ESCs) [53], both in their expression profile, their ability to grow indefinitely and their ability to differentiate into all cell lineages of the body, including ectoderm, mesoderm and endoderm [52]. These cells have the potential to contribute to chimeras and to be transmitted through these chimeras into the germline, further proving their pluripotency [54]. The same and similar sets of factors were then applied to adult human fibroblasts [55–57]. It is reported these cells truthfully mimic human ESCs, however the reprogramming process is thought to induce some disparity at both the genetic and epigenetic levels [58–61]. Viral-delivery methods have shown good efficiency but also result in random integration of the transgenes into the genome, potentially leading to insertional mutagenesis and tumorigenicity, therefore restricting its use for future potential clinical trials [62]. More recently, integration-free reprogramming systems, including episomal plasmids containing the reprogramming factors, Sendai virus, direct mRNA, protein and small molecules, have all been successfully used for generation of potentially transgene-free human iPS cells [56,63–65]. Moreover, xeno- and feeder-free culture methods have also helped to decrease variability between lines generated [66,67]. In addition, other cell types from patients have been successfully and safely used for reprogramming. As an alternate to dermal skin fibroblasts (acquired from surgical skin biopsies), peripheral blood mononuclear cells (PBMCs) (which are easy to harvest from routine peripheral blood samples) have been used to isolate T cells and generate human iPS cells [68,69]. One advantage is that the reprogramming of these cells can also be done quickly, with no need for prior expansion. These protocols therefore facilitate the production of human iPS cells from human somatic cells with minimal invasiveness. Together, these mentioned advances in production of human iPS cells might allow research to fulfill the restricted guidelines of Good Manufacturing Practices (GMPs) for the development of clinically-approved iPS cells required in the regenerative medicine field [70].

5. Therapeutic Benefits

The discovery of iPS cells is groundbreaking, as it means that patient-specific cell lines can be established easily. Contrary to human iPS cells, human ESCs have been surrounded by ethical controversy due to the use of human embryos, which is a serious problem in terms of sample availability and public acceptance [71]. Human iPS cells are also clinically advantageous since the use of autologous tissue ideally surpasses the patient's immune rejection, contrary to the allogeneic barriers of human ESCs [72]. Therapeutic cloning also allows the generation of pluripotent stem cells that are genetically similar to patients, however this requires the destruction of donor eggs or embryos and still has several technical issues [73,74]. Moreover, considering the unavailability of *in vitro* human disease models, human iPS cells could help to provide large numbers of patient-specific neuronal cells for research and clinical objectives. Pairing of both human iPS cell technology and advances in genome-editing technologies may also provide more robust findings since isogenic cell lines could lead to the replacement of age- and sex-matched controls [75–78]. Experimentally, this would allow for more phenotypic findings attributed to the genetic difference causing the disease, which would not be influenced by individual epigenetic differences [79]. Moreover, disease and population heterogeneity can also be diminished due to singular-patient origin of human iPS cells.

Regenerative medicine, including testing of transplantation of cells into live tissues and organs is ongoing for AD models of rodents, such as neural progenitor cells (NPCs) [80–86] and mesenchymal stem cells [87–89], but remains restricted in relation to transplantation of ESC or iPS-derived neural cells [80,90]. Some research, however, does suggest that implanted cells do not survive and that the beneficial effect may likely come from their secretion of BDNF (brain-derived neurotrophic factor) and GDNF (glial cell-derived neurotrophic factor) [82]. Due to improved immunocompatibility in the use of autologous iPS cells, there is considerable hope that differentiated progeny of patient-specific iPS cells may be favorable for transplantation.

In addition, human iPS cells are already being used for drug development and screening in various diseases [91] to identify new and superior targets relevant for production of new drugs. In the future, it may even be possible to provide patient-customized cell screens from the iPS-derived cells to screen a panel of drugs in order to identify the most beneficial treatment plan for each individual patient [92]. This could have significant impact in treating this disease where patient variability is wide in response to certain drugs [93]. The development of patient-specific iPS cells may also help researchers to identify new mechanisms/biomarkers which may help lead to earlier diagnoses of the disease [94] as it is possible to culture early neurons or NPCs which may have underlying deficits related to the disease. It is also believed that earlier intervention is a key factor for a successful therapeutic strategy and an earlier diagnosis would be of extreme benefit to patients, as the initial stages of the disease could be treated whilst the patients are still early symptomatic [51]. It is crucial for clinical trials to target these early symptomatic patients, therefore facilitating therapeutic procedures to succeed in delaying, stopping or even preventing the cognitive decline [51]. We summarize the implications patient-specific iPS cells have on basic research as well as therapeutic benefits for AD in Figure 1.

Figure 1. Schematic illustration of the use of induced pluripotent stem (iPS) cells in relation to Alzheimer's disease (AD). (**A**) iPS cells are derived from a skin biopsy from an AD patient and differentiated into neural progenitor cells and neurons; (**B**) In familial cases, the disease-causing mutation can be corrected by gene-editing of the iPS cells, and neural progenitor cells and neurons can be used for research and drug screening; (**C**) The patients can in the long run benefit from these activities by cell therapy, better diagnostic procedures, customized treatments and novel medical approaches.

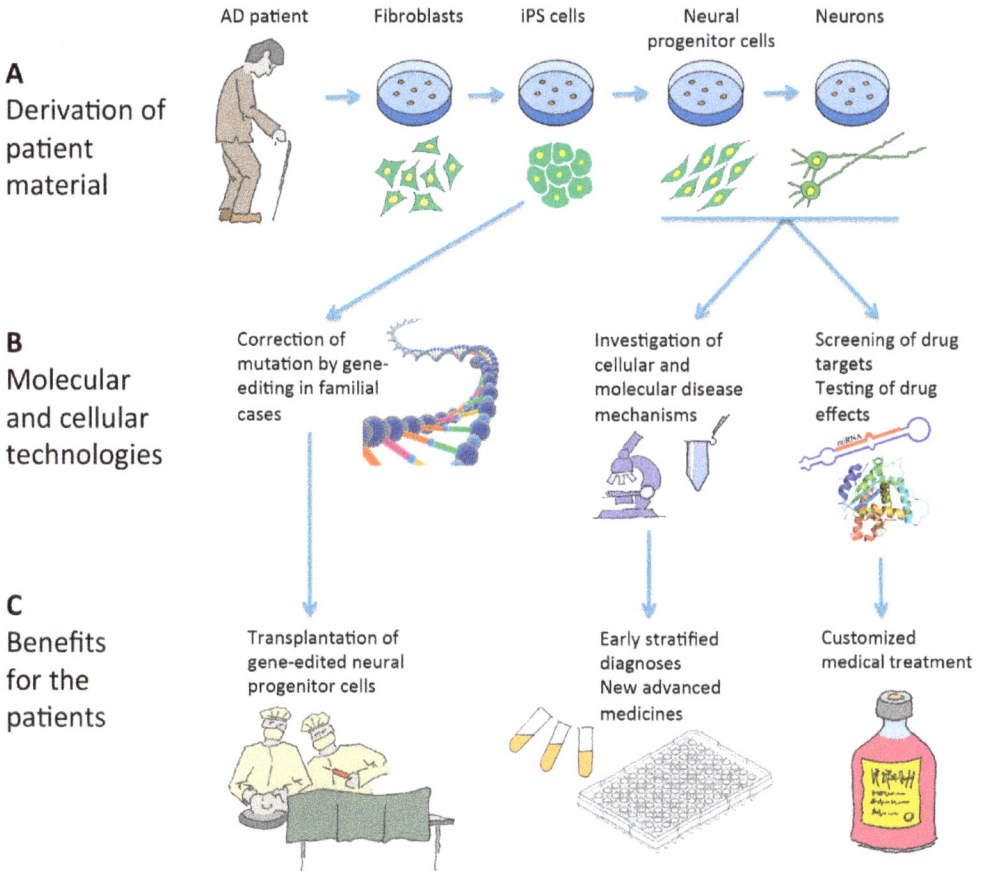

6. Induced Pluripotent Stem Cells and Neural Cell Derivatives Have Been Produced from Several AD Patients

The discovery of iPS cells paved the way to model diseases by using patient-specific cells which can then be differentiated into disease relevant cell types. However, despite this breakthrough, there have been surprisingly only a handful of studies published on Alzheimer's disease [95–102,103]. Induced pluripotent stem cells have now been derived from both familial and sporadic patients and these iPS cells have been differentiated into varying neurons and glia, which have been studied in respect to specific AD pathology. Here, we summarize the types of cells analyzed and the extent of their characterization (Table 1). The genetic backgrounds of patients that have been used to date, include, duplication or mutations of *APP*, mutations of *PSEN1* and *PSEN2*, in the case of familial AD [96–99,101,102] and mutations in APOE3/E4 resulting in both early sporadic and late sporadic forms of the disease [95]. It should be stated that in the case of one study [98], the *APP* (E693Δ) mutation background (which is responsible for Alzheimer-type dementia [104]) showed no evident tau pathology and lack of fibrilization of Aβ peptides. Therefore not all hallmark pathologies would be anticipated in the iPSC-derived neurons. We also include a study where a Down-syndrome iPS cell line was used to model features of AD [100], since it could clearly model varying pathological features of the disease.

In each article, different types of neural cells have been analyzed, which have been derived using various differentiation protocols (see overview of protocols in Table 2). Cortical neurons have been studied by both Shi and colleagues and Kondo and colleagues [98,100]. Forebrain neurons have been studied by Muratore and colleagues [103]. Astrocytes (GFAP+) have also been studied by Kondo and colleagues [98] and basal forebrain cholinergic neurons (BFCNs) have been studied by Duan and colleagues [95]. GABAergic neurons have been studied by Koch and colleagues [97], whereas, more less-defined neurons (βIIITubulin+/MAP2+) have been studied by Israel and colleagues, Yagi and colleagues, Liu and colleagues and Sproul and colleagues [96,99,101,102]. Whilst some protocols used FACS to sort and purify the neural cell populations (e.g., sorting of CD24+CD184−CD44− neurons [96,101] and Lhx8+/Gbx1+ neurons [95]), it is without doubt that all the final cell populations analyzed had some degree of cell heterogeneity, as often observed by the percentages of positive cells stated. Three particular articles performed extensive characterization of the types of neurons generated. In the case of the generation of BFCNs, immunocytochemistry confirmed their mature features, since a large proportion expressed ChAT and VaChT, and all were found to be HB9 negative (a selective marker of motor neurons in the vertebrates) (Table 2).

Table 1. Phenotypes of neural cells analyzed from differentiated patient-specific induced pluripotent stem cells for studying Alzheimer's disease.

Mutation	Cell Type Analyzed	Analyses Performed	Phenotype	Reference
Familial PSEN1 (A246E) 2 clones	Neurons (βIIITubulin+ MAP2+)	Extracellular Aβ Tau accumulation (HT7 antibody) Tangle formation Treatment with γ-secretase inhibitor and modulator of γ-secretase-mediated APP cleavage	Increased Aβ42:Aβ40 No Tau accumulation No tangle formation Decreased Aβ40+Aβ42 with γ-secretase inhibitor and modulator of APP cleavage	[99]
Familial PSEN2 (N141I) 2 clones				
Familial APP dup'n APP^{Dp}1 3 clones	Neurons (βIII-Tubulin+ MAP2+) >90%	Genome-wide mRNA seq. Extracellular Aβ p-tau (Thr231) GSK-3β activity Treatment with γ-secretase and β-secretase inhibitors Endosome markers Synaptic markers	Increased Aβ40, Increased p-tau (Thr231), Increased aGSK-3β γ-/β-secretase inhibitors reduced Aβ40	[96]
Familial APP dup'n APP^{Dp}2 3 clones			Increased Aβ40 Increased p-tau (Thr231), Increased aGSK-3β γ-/β-secretase inhibitors reduced Aβ40 β-secretase inhibitor reduced aGSK-3β+p-tau had large/very large Rab5 + early endosomes No change in synapsin I + puncta on dendrites	
Sporadic sAD1 3 clones			No change in Aβ40, No increase of p-tau (Thr231), No increase aGSK-3β γ-/β-secretase inhibitors reduced Ab40	
Sporadic sAD2 3 clones			No change in Aβ40 Increased p-tau (Thr^{231}) and aGSK-3β γ-/β-secretase inhibitors reduced Aβ40 β-secretase inhibitor reduced aGSK-3β+p-tau had large/very large Rab5 + early endosomes No change in synapsin I + puncta on dendrites	

Table 1. *Cont.*

Mutation	Cell Type Analyzed	Analyses Performed	Phenotype	Reference
Familial PSEN1 (D385N)	It-NES progenitor cells (NESTIN+SOX2+)	Expression APP+ γ-secretase components Extracellular Aβ Aβ length qPCR	Dominant-negative effect on S3 cleavage of Notch in progenitors, decreased HES5	[97]
	Neurons (βIII-Tubulin+MAP2ab+ GABA+) + <10% Astrocyte (GFAP+)		Increased full-length APP Decreased Aβ40	
Familial PSEN1 (L166P)	It-NES cells (NESTIN+SOX2+)		Dominant-negative effect on S3 cleavage of Notch in progenitors, decreased HES5	
	Neurons (βIII-Tubulin+MAP2ab+ GABA+) <10% Astrocyte (GFAP+)		Decreased Aβ40	
Trisomy 21 DS1-iPS4	Cortical neurons; Early born, (TBR1+ βIII-Tubulin+ /CTIP2+ βIII-Tubulin+) 30% Late born, (BM2+ βIII-Tubulin+/SATB2+ βIII-Tubulin+) 20%–25% Functional synapses Glutamatergic (PSD95+)	Extracellular Aβ Aggregation of Aβ Treatment with γ-secretase inhibitor p-tau expression Cell death	Increased Aβ40 Increased Aβ42 (>70 days cultures) Increased Aβ42:Aβ40 Intracellular and extracellular Aβ42 aggregates Decreased Aβ40+Aβ42 with γ-secretase inhibitor p-tau localized in cell bodies and dendrites Increased secretion of total tau and p-tau Increased cell death (2 fold)	[100]

Table 1. *Cont.*

Mutation	Cell Type Analyzed	Analyses Performed	Phenotype	Reference
Familial APP(E693Δ) 3 clones	Cortical neurons (SATB2+TBR1+)	Extracellular Aβ Intracellular Aβ Aβ Oligomers Gene expression profiling ROS expression Aβ Oligomers ROS expression	Decreased Aβ40 and Aβ42 Elevated Aβ oligomers in neural cells Elevated levels of oxidative stress-related genes Elevated ROS	[98]
	Astrocytes		Elevated Aβ oligomers Elevated ROS	
Familial APP(V717L) 2 clones	Cortical neurons (SATB2+TBR1+)		Increased Aβ42, increased Aβ42:Aβ40 Elevated levels of oxidative stress-related genes	
Sporadic AD3E211 1 clone	Cortical neurons (SATB2+TBR1+)		No change in Aβ40 or Aβ42 Elevated levels of oxidative stress-related genes	
Sporadic AD8K213 1 clone	Cortical neurons (SATB2+TBR1+)		No change in Aβ40 or Aβ42 Elevated Aβ oligomers in neural cells Elevated levels of oxidative stress-related genes and ROS	
	Astrocytes		Elevated Aβ oligomers, Elevated ROS	
Sporadic Early ApoE3/E4 AG04402 (2 clones)	Basal forebrain cholinergic neurons (MAP2+ChAT+ VaChT+P75R+NKX2.1+HB9−) Expressed tetrodotoxin-sensitive voltage-activated currents and voltage-gated calcium channels	Extracellular Aβ Treatment with γ-secretase inhibitors Treatment with ionomycin + glutamate Fura-2 calcium imaging	Elevated Aβ42, Increased Aβ40 with γ-secretase inhibitor Increased susceptibility to glutamate-induced excitotoxic death Increased calcium transient	[95]
Sporadic Early, APOE3/E4 AG11414			Elevated Aβ42 Increased Aβ40 with γ-secretase inhibitor Susceptibility to cell death following calcium influx	
Sporadic Late APOE3/E4 AG05810			No elevated Aβ42 Increased susceptibility to glutamate-induced excitotoxic death Increased calcium transient	
Familial AG07872			Elevated Aβ42 Reduced Ab40 with γ-secretase inhibitor	
Familial PSEN1 (A246E) AG066848			No elevated Aβ42 Reduced Aβ40 with γ-secretase inhibitor	

Table 1. *Cont.*

Mutation	Cell Type Analyzed	Analyses Performed	Phenotype	Reference
Familial APP (V717I) (fAD1) (2 clones)	Forebrain neurons (MAP2−Tau+ βIII-Tubulin+Cux1+ TBR1+PSD95+ VGLUT1+)	Extracellular Aβ APP cleavage product expression Treatment with γ-secretase inhibitor Expression of tau Treatment with Aβ antibodies	APP holoprotein 1.4× increased Increased Aβ42:Aβ40 Increased Aβ42 Increased Aβ38 Decreased APPsα:APPsβ (Increased APPsβ) γ-secretase inhibitor blocked APPsβ cleavage Increased total tau Increased p-tau (Ser^{262}) d100 Aβ antibodies blocked increased total tau (early differentiated neurons only)	[103]
(fAD2) asymptomatic (2 clones)				
Familial PSEN1 (A246E) (2 patients)	Neurons (βIII-Tubulin+MAP2+)	Extracellular Aβ Treatment with γ-secretase inhibitors	Increased Aβ42:Aβ40 Increased Aβ42 γ-secretase inhibitor lowered total Aβ, Aβ40, Aβ42, Aβ38	[101]
PSEN1 (H163R) asymptomatic			Increased Aβ42:Aβ40 Increased Aβ42 γ-secretase inhibitor lowered Aβ42	
PSEN1 (M146L)			Increased Aβ42:Aβ40 Increased Aβ42 γ-secretase inhibitor lowered Aβ42	
Familial; PSEN1 (A246E) (2 clones) 7671C/7768C	D14 immature neurons (79% NESTIN+ small pop'n TUJ1+)	Extracellular Aβ Total Aβ	Increased Aβ42:Aβ40 Increased NLRP2, ASB9, NDP	[102]
	Neurons Electrical signaling properties		Increased Aβ42:Aβ40	
PSEN1 (M146L) (2 clones) 8446B/8446D	D14 immature neurons (79% NESTIN+ small pop'n TUJ1+)		Increased Aβ42:Aβ40 Increased NLRP2, ASB9, NDP	
	Neurons Electrical signaling properties		Increased Aβ42:Aβ40	

Table 2. Reprogramming and differentiation strategies for induction of induced pluripotent stem cells and their neural progeny.

Reprogramming Strategy	Differentiation Protocol	Cell Type Formed	Reference
Retrovirus *OCT4, SOX2, KLF4, LIN28, NANOG* Human dermal fibroblasts	EB induction w/o bFGF 8 days EBs plated gelatin w/o bFGF 8 days Neuron induction w/o growth factors 2 weeks Added compound E or compound W 48 h	Neurons βIII-Tubulin+MAP2+	[99]
Retrovirus *OCT4, SOX2, KLF4, cMYC* Human dermal fibroblasts	Neuronal rosette induction on PA6 stromal cells 11 days NPCs isolated by FACS CD184+CD15−CD44−CD271− NPC cultured 4 weeks Neuron induction-BDNF/GDNF/cAMP 3 weeks CD24+CD184−CD44− neurons selected by FACS Cultured in BDNF/GDNF/cAMP 5 days	Neurons βIII-Tubulin+MAP2+ >90% VGluT1+ 15% GABA+ 8% Expressed tetrodotoxin-sensitive voltage-activated currents GABA+AMPA receptors Spontaneous inhibitory/excitatory synaptic currents	[96]
hESC (I3) transduced with lentivirus containing mutations in PS1 iPSC—Retrovirus Human dermal fibroblasts (PKa)	lt-NES induction with bFGF+EGF+B27 Neuron induction—Matrigel w/o factors, +N2+B27+cAMP 4 weeks	Neurons βIII-Tubulin+ 80% Astrocytes 6%	[97]
Trisomy 21 Retrovirus *OCT4, SOX2, KLF4, cMYC* Human dermal fibroblasts	Matrigel+N2+B27+Noggin+SB431542 Dissociated and cultured with 3N+bFGF 100 days	Cortical neurons; Early born, TBR1+βIII-Tubulin+ CTIP2+βIII-Tubulin+ 30% Late born, BM2+βIII-Tubulin+ SATB2+βIII-Tubulin+ 20%–25% Functional synapses Glutamatergic+ PSD95+	[100]

Table 2. *Cont.*

Reprogramming Strategy	Differentiation Protocol	Cell Type Formed	Reference
Episomal vectors SOX2, KLF4, OCT4, L-MYC, LIN28, shRNA p53 Human dermal fibroblasts	EB induction DMEM/HamsF12+ 5% KSR+SB431542 8 days Neural induction—plated on Matrigel+N2+SB431542 16 days Cortical neuron induction—dissociated and cultured in NB media+B27+BDNF+GDNF+NT3 48 days As above, but on day 58 cortical neuron induction, cells passaged Repeated passages on day 96, 126, 156, 176	Cortical neurons SATB2+TBR1+ Astrocytes	[98]
Retroviral vector Klf4, Oct4, Sox2, cMyc Human fibroblasts	RA+bFGF 7 days Neurosphere formation w/o bFGF 7 days Neurospheres cultured with bFGF+EGF 4 days Neurospheres cultured with SHH+FGF8 3 days Dissociated and transfected with Lhx8/Gbx1-IRES-EGFP 2 days Lhx8+/Gbx1+ cells selected by FACS and cultured in NB media+ bFGF+NGF 2 weeks (+arabinoside from day 5–10 of NB culture step)	Basal forebrain cholinergic neurons 95% MAP2 66% ChAT VaChT+P75R+, NKX2.1+HB9– Expessed tetrodotoxin-sensitive voltage-activated currents, voltage-gated calcium channels	[95]
Lentivirus OCT4, SOX2, cMYC, KLF4 Human dermal fibroblasts	Aggregates with iPS cell media 4 days + neural media+N2 2 days Aggregates plated on matrigel, Neural media + N2 10 days Suspension culture, neural media+B27+N2+cAMP+IGF1 7 days Neural rosettes selected manually or Neural Rosette selection agent Dissociated+plated on Matrigel+NBmedia+N2+B27+ cAMP+BDNF+GDNF+IGF1 35 days–76 days	Neurons 90% MAP2 Tau+, βIII-Tubulin+Cux1+Tbr1+PSD95+VGLUT1+ Spontaneous activity from microelectrode array	[103]

Table 2. *Cont.*

Reprogramming Strategy	Differentiation Protocol	Cell Type Formed	Reference
MMLV retrovirus Oct4, Sox2, Klf4, cMyc Human dermal fibroblasts	Neuronal rosette induction on PA6 stromal cells +Noggin and SB431542 6 days –Noggin and SB431542 8 days CD24+/CD184+/CD271–/CD44– cells selected by FACS Cultured in neural media (DMEM:F12+N2+B27+BDNF+GDNF+dcAMP) for 3 weeks w/o bFGF CD24+/CD184–/CD44– neurons selected by FACS	Neurons βIII-Tubulin+MAP2+	[101]
Retrovirus OCT4, KLF4, SOX2, cMYC Human dermal fibroblasts	Neuronal progenitor induction using dual-SMAD inhibition 9 days NB media 26 days–46 days	Neural progenitors 79% NESTIN+, small pop'n βIII-Tubulin+ Neurons Active Na+ channels K+ channels Produce action potentials 40% neurons Ca²+ spikes	[102]

Electrophysiological recordings also confirmed these cells to express tetrodotoxin sensitive voltage-activated currents and have active voltage-gated calcium channels. Together, this gave very convincing evidence for functional BFCNs with a relatively high purity. Israel and colleagues also performed extensive characterization of their neurons, including electrophysiological recordings. However, although 90% of the neurons were βIIITubulin+/MAP2+, the specific types of neurons produced remain unclear, with only 15% of neurons expressing VGluT1 and 8% expressing GABA. In the case of the cortical neurons generated by Shi and colleagues, these were found to include populations of both early and late born cortical neurons. These also formed functional synapses and expressed the glutamatergic marker PSD95 [100].

7. Modeling Impaired APP Processing from Patient-Specific Induced Pluripotent Stem Cells Reveals Considerable Variability

Varying AD pathologies were analyzed in these articles and all articles had in common an analysis of extracellular Aβ. Although some studies were unable to detect Aβ42 (as levels were below the detectable limits of the ELISA), it was striking to see how variable levels of Aβ40 were in the patient lines in comparison to the control/healthy cells. The familial lines carrying the APP duplication (APP[Dp]1/2) had increased Aβ40, although some sporadic lines (sAD1/2) reported no change in Aβ40 levels [96], and decreased Aβ40 was reported in at least three other familial lines carrying either a mutation in APP or PSEN1 [97,98]. Furthermore, increased Aβ42 was only reported in approximately one third of the patients [95,98,101,103]. Increased Aβ42:40 was noted in several familial PSEN1 and two familial APP(V717I) patient-derived neurons and it was apparent in at least two studies, that this elevation was due to increased Aβ42 [101–103]. The variation in observed secreted Aβ products may be dependent on the neuronal subtype analyzed, as elevated Aβ42 was observed in three of the five patients, where BFCNs were analyzed [95] and in both APP (V717I) patients, where forebrain neurons were produced [103]. In addition, increased Aβ42 was also observed in one AD patient, where cortical neurons were analyzed [98]. It was only the Down-syndrome-derived cortical neurons that displayed both increased secreted Aβ40 and Aβ42 levels [100]. In addition, in the same study, the increased Aβ42 was only detectable in neuron cultures that were older than 70 days and in APP (V717I)-derived neurons differentiated for 40–50 days, an increase in Aβ42 was also detectable [103]. Interestingly, in the case of PSEN1 (E280A) a screening of young pre-symptomatic carriers showed increased levels of Aβ42 in both plasma and CSF [105]. These studies therefore report a wide range of results for both Aβ40 and Aβ42 and may suggest that it could be necessary to have long-term culture protocols in order to see potentially relevant phenotypes. In the case of AD patients, we also know that a variation in expression levels of short Aβ peptides exists. For example, Aβ42 levels have been reported to be reduced in cerebral spinal fluid of patients compared to controls [106,107], whereas another study reported both increased and decreased Aβ42 in AD patients carrying PSEN mutations and decreased Aβ40 in the AD patient's cerebral spinal fluids [108]. It was also interesting to see that the APP (V717I) iPS cell-derived neurons had an increase in Aβ38 [103]. Thus, it may be important for future studies on AD-derived iPS cells to perform long-term neuronal cultures and compare these directly to the Aβ levels in the original patient.

The evaluation for the presence of Aβ oligomers has been performed in only one study to date. Kondo and colleagues could detect the positive expression of the Aβ oligomer marker, NU1 and expression of the low weight oligomer marker, 11A1, in their cortical neurons, specifically localized as puncta throughout the neurons from both a familial APP and sporadic AD patient [98]. This was also the case for astrocytes generated from the same backgrounds. However, Aβ oligomers were not observed in another line, which had increased extracellular Aβ42:Aβ40. Postulation for this difference was made by the authors to support a hypothesis that AD may be classified as displaying either an extracellular or an intracellular phenotype.

APP processing was also studied in the AD iPS cell-derived cells by evaluating the effects that γ-secretase or β-secretase inhibitors had on the cultured cells. In general, most studies reported a decrease of Aβ40 or Aβ42 following treatment of the cells with a γ-secretase or β-secretase inhibitor [95–97,99–101]. One study also reported that a γ-secretase inhibitor decreased the production of APPsβ [103]. As an exception, two sporadic background iPS cell lines were reported to have increased Aβ40 levels following treatment with γ-secretase inhibitors [95]. The authors claimed that this may reflect the potential differences in APP processing in early onset disease *vs.* late onset disease as these two lines were derived from patients exhibiting early onset AD, or alternately, it may reflect patient-specific differences.

8. Tau Processing, Cell Death and Oxidative Stress in iPS Cell Lines Modeling AD

Levels of total and *p*-tau have been studied in only four of the reports to date. In one study, increased *p*-tau (Thr^{231}) was reported in βIIITubulin$^+$/MAP2$^+$ neurons in two familial AD-iPS carrying APP duplications and one sporadic AD-iPS cell line, however, this was not observed in a second sporadic AD-iPSC line when compared to control cells [96]. A second study has shown that Down-syndrome iPS cell-derived cortical neurons re-localized *p*-tau (Ser^{202} and Thr^{205}) to the dendrites and cell bodies, which was not observed in the control cortical neurons, where diffuse staining was only observed in the axons [100]. Furthermore, this study showed that these neurons also secreted higher levels of total tau and *p*-tau (pSer^{396} and pThr^{231}) over a 48 h period compared to the control neurons. Another study has reported both increased total tau and *p*-tau (Ser^{262}), however the increase in pSer^{262} was only detectable in iPS cell-derived neurons differentiated for 100 days [103]. The final study revealed that no abnormal tau protein accumulation could be detected, or led to the production of tangles in two PSEN1-iPS cell neurons [99]. Interestingly, the tau pathology was noted in cells obtained from patients carrying mutations in the APP gene and not in the patient cells carrying PSEN1 mutations. However, given the limited numbers of studies analyzing *p*-tau, it may be difficult to conclude anything from this outcome. Again, it may be important that longer-term cultured cells are studied for such pathology as the latter study of *p*-tau on PSEN1-iPS was performed on neurons that were only 2 weeks old.

Cell death has only been reported in one study, namely in the Down-syndrome iPS cell-derived cortical neurons [100]. Cell death in the neurons was reportedly two-fold higher compared to the control neurons and was considered to be due to the secretion of tau into the medium. It was interesting to observe that despite some studies reporting increased levels of the toxic Aβ peptide Aβ42, this did not lead to increased cell death. In one study, a test on increased susceptibility to cell death by use of glutamate-induced excitation was performed on early sporadic AD iPS cell-derived BFCNs which had increased Aβ42 revealing that increased susceptibility could be seen, however this was also observed in a late sporadic AD iPS cell line which did not have elevated Aβ42 [95], meaning that the levels of increased Aβ42 alone could not be the primary reason for this susceptibility to cell death.

AD-iPS cell models may also be useful for studying oxidative stress. Whilst reports remain limited to date, one report showed that both familial and sporadic AD-iPS lines had increased levels of oxidative stress genes [98]. Elevated reactive oxygen species (ROS) was also detected both in the analyzed cortical neurons and astrocytes that were generated. Further research is clearly needed to further investigate the role of oxidative stress in these cell types compared to other AD *in vitro* cell models.

9. Hunting for New Genes of Interest in AD

It is apparent, that with current global gene/protein/lipid expression profiling technologies, human cells models of disease could be used to identify potentially new mechanisms. One recent study performed gene expression profiling (GEP) on immature neurons carrying PSEN1 FAD mutations and discovered several dysregulated genes [102]. Ten upregulated genes and four downregulated genes were validated and three upregulated genes, namely *NLRP2*, *ASB9* and *NDP* were investigated further by analyzing publically available GEPs performed on AD hippocampus and cDNA from the temporal pole of AD patients. *NLRP2*, a gene involved in inflammation was actually found to be downregulated in human AD temporal pole and no significant difference determined in the AD hippocampus. The gene *ASB9*, an ubiquitin ligase, was found to be upregulated in some AD patient temporal lobes, but not in the hippocampi. Finally, *NDP*, a gene thought to play an important role in CNS development was actually found to be significantly decreased in the AD patient hippocampi. Together, this study highlights that new genes can be discovered that could be used to pursue new mechanisms related to the disease, however, validation in the human brain is still an important and necessary measure to confirm the *in vitro* cell model findings.

10. Current Use of AD-Modeling Stem Cells for Compound Screening and Drug Testing

Only a rare cohort of studies has applied the use of stem cells derived from AD models to screen for novel compounds of interest or for testing recently identified drugs. These, to date, remain mostly restricted to mouse studies and primarily involve ESCs [109] although one study has used a non-AD human iPS cell model that is sensitive to Aβ aggregation for such purposes [110]. In one promising mouse study, ESCs were differentiated from a mouse model of AD (Tg2576) into an enriched population of pyramidal neurons and were subjected to a small molecule library to detect for inhibitors of Aβ40 [109]. Four candidate inhibitors were detected to induce over a 40% reduction in Aβ40 levels compared to controls, which included amiridine, icariin, phenelzine and progesterone. In the human study, healthy iPS cells were differentiated into forebrain neurons and subjected to an Aβ1-42 toxicity assay. These cells were then used to screen a GSK proprietary compound library for improvement in cell viability, which resulted in 19 hits, including a Cdk2 inhibitor. This field no doubt will grow in the coming years and will encompass AD-derived iPS cell lines which will help not only to discover new compounds of interest, but could also pave the way for patient-specific therapies.

11. Production of AD Isogenic Controls for Potential Gene/Cell Therapy

With the new revolution in gene editing, research has approached a new frontier for the generation of patient-specific cell therapies by correcting the patient's diseased cells. This of course remains relevant for familial cases of AD and cases of known and diagnosed mutations. New techniques in genome-editing have been developed, which can be used to repair the particular disease causing mutation in a relatively simple manner by using transcription activator-like factor nucleases (TALENs), which are artificially produced restriction enzymes that specifically detect and bind to a desired nucleotide sequence in the genome and which initiate a double stranded break in the DNA. Homologous DNA fragments with the correct sequence need to be provided, so the cells can use these as a template to generate the correct sequence and thereby replacing the mutation. This method facilitates the generation of isogenic controls and control cell lines, which are absolutely identical to the patient iPS cells except for the repaired disease-causing mutation. Another such method is facilitated by clustered regularly interspaced short palindromic repeats (CRISPRs). This method is potentially faster and easier than the TALEN method. Correction of varying disease-related mutations in specific cell types has recently been performed and has even resulted in the correction of the disease in new progeny (in mice) when targeted in oocytes [111–117]. Some of these involve correction of frame-shifts [116], but it may also be possible to correct for single base pair mutations. One of the considered benefits of TALENs and CRISPRs is that there may be no residual ectopic sequences at the site of correction, although this depends on the strategy used for selecting for targeted clones, which may involve insertion of a selectable cassette. One potential drawback with this strategy is the potential to induce off-targeting genetic changes to other genomic sites that have either a similar or the same genetic sequence as that of the targeted sequence. The potential of targeting these other sites of course may lead to potential alteration in other genes throughout the genome. Such off-targeting has been observed in a handful of these studies [112,115,117], and therefore improvements in the design of the TALENs and CRISPRs for only the desired recognition target site may be needed before the next step to clinical transplantation is taken. To date, there is no literature on successful correction of an AD phenotype using either of these technologies; however, this area will no doubt be the focus of the next generation of research. Not only will it be important for the generation of healthy patient-specific cells that could be potentially transplanted, but corrected cell lines will form the ideal control cells needed for a more accurate interpretation of the AD phenotype in the diseased cells, due to the variation observed both between patients, but also between healthy age-matched controls.

12. Current General Limitations of Use of iPS Cells for Disease Modeling

There are several general limitations regarding the generation of iPS cells and differentiation into specific cellular subtypes, which are challenging and not very well understood. General limitations are caused by the limited understanding of the nature of iPS cells themselves and by their differentiation potential. In particular, the differentiation into a defined neural cell population is currently quite challenging. This is mainly because the developmentally relevant proteins and transcription factors, which are needed to mimic differentiation into a specific neural cell type, are not yet fully understood.

One general problem of using patient-specific iPS cells is the different epigenetic make-up and exposure to diverse environmental conditions every individual is facing. These differences have implications on comparative studies involving different patient-specific iPS cells, even between patients carrying the same pathological mutation. Despite these inter-patient differences, it has also been described that the reprogramming event itself can result in significant clone-to-clone variations, resulting in non-desired experimental background noise and even generation of non-disease related artifacts [118]. Currently, most studies involving the generation of patient-specific iPS cells involve the use of age- and gender-matched controls, which results in comparing epigenetically mismatched iPS cells. Isogenic controls generated via TALEN or CRISPR gene editing will be much more ideal for the study of disease-related cellular phenotypes and for pharmacological screens, which would help overcome this limitation.

Another general challenge is that only some of the aspects of a differentiated, aged cell can be restored to the state of pluripotency following reprogramming. Some of these may include an elongation of telomeres and restoration of functional mitochondria [119,120]. Other features pertaining to the original cell persist following reprogramming, such as acquired mutations, DNA damage, epigenetic changes and protein aggregation [121–123]. To date, it is still unclear what effect this has on the overall reprogramming efficiency and subsequent differentiation of iPS cells into the desired mature cell types. Moreover, iPS cells seem to retain an epigenetic memory, which makes them preferentially differentiate into their tissue of origin [124].

13. Hurdles Needed to be Overcome in Order to Recapitulate AD Faithfully in a Dish

One hurdle that needs to be overcome in order to accurately mimic the disease *in vitro* is the ability to produce the most relevant neurons for study. In order to develop *in vitro* models that can be used to screen for novel compounds for possible future treatments, it may be important to focus on areas of the brain that are affected earliest, and attempt to model the disease even before the symptoms first arise. One hope may be that iPS cells may be able to recapitulate earlier stages of the disease. Since Alzheimer's disease pathology can first be detected in the entorhinal cortex, it might therefore be of interest to focus on differentiation of iPS cells into cell types affected in this area of the brain, namely pyramidal neurons with glutamate excitation and the varying GABAergic interneurons. It appears that it is the long projection neurons that are most vulnerable to developing pathology [18]. Short-axon projection cells such as spiny stellate cells apparently resist the pathology [18]. Short-axon local circuit cells also avoid pathology with the exception of the axo-axonic cells. It is particularly interesting that the vulnerable neurons are either un-myelinated or have only a thin sheath of myelin, as for e.g. heavily myelinated Betz cells and Meynert pyramidal cells also resist the pathology [18]. It may even be possible in the future to treat pre-symptomatic patients by large-scale screenings of the population. This would of course require earlier diagnostic tools for the disease for patients, which are still in general lacking, but of which several efforts are being undertaken [125–128]. In the case of the hippocampus, it is the CA1 neurons from the temporal medial lobe that are heavily affected by the disease, and ideally cross-comparisons with *in vitro* produced CA3 neurons, which are not affected as severely as the CA1 neurons would be ideal, however recapitulating these neurons *in vitro* is no easy task. In the CA1 region, which includes pyramidal neurons of at least three subtypes, there is also the supportive GABAergic interneuron population of which at least 20 different types are known [129]. Calretinin positive interneurons and somatostatin/parvalbumin positive interneurons (bistratified interneurons) in the CA1 are both affected in earlier stages of the disease [20]. In order to develop such protocols, a better understanding of the development of these neurons *in vivo* is required in order to mimic this process *ex vivo*. In the case of cortical pyramidal neurons, these are produced from progenitors located in the neocortical germinal zone in the dorsolateral wall of the telencephalon [130]. One recent report has shown the successful generation of cortical pyramidal neurons from both human ESC and iPS cells, which could successfully innervate the mouse brain [131], indicating there may be a strong future for developing efficient protocols for these cell types. In the case of the interneurons, these are generated in the ventral telencephalon and migrate to the neocortex [130]. Furthermore, although some markers can be used to distinguish pyramidal neurons from interneurons [129], additional markers of these neurons, in particularly, surface-specific markers are needed in order to improve selection and purification of these by use of FACS. Even though the brain regions affected by AD are composed of several neuronal subtypes as mentioned above, most differentiation protocols focus on the derivation of specific neural subtypes, which are mostly affected by the disease. These current protocols achieve in some cases good enrichment of a certain neural subpopulation (see Table 2). Despite the varying outcomes of different protocols there is also the problem of different results from the different iPS cell clones from the same patient cell line. Furthermore, neural differentiation is a complex scenario, which is dependent on internal and external morphogenic cues, gene expression and transcription factor activity in a spatio-temporal manner [132].

Another significant hurdle is overcoming the lack of knowledge of the types of cells that are currently being used for analyses. Heterogeneity itself may not be a problem, if we can re-create the same heterogeneity observed in the specific regions of the brain affected. However, several different approaches and protocols currently exist for differentiation of ESC and iPS cells into cortical neurons [100], BFCNs [95], other neurons like dopaminergic neurons mostly affected in Parkinson's disease [133] and astrocytes [134,135]. Some of these differentiation protocols may show variation in differentiation efficiency between cell lines, but even from experiment to experiment using the same clone but at different time points [136].

Many of the differentiation protocols in the AD iPS cell papers to date have produced neurons which are βIIITubulin$^+$ and MAP2$^+$ [95–97,99,101] using neuronal induction factors, such as, BDNF, GDNF, N2 and B27 (see Table 2). Although it is promising to see phenotypic hallmarks of AD recapitulated at a cellular level using these differentiation protocols, there remain variations in the phenotypes created. This may be due to the differences in timing of differentiation, some degree of cell heterogeneity and the lack of clear understanding of the types of neurons generated. It therefore remains difficult to make a direct comparison of the conducted approaches and analyses of AD iPS cells. For example, it might well be possible that the observed elevated expression of stress-related genes and ROS as well as the formation of Aβ oligomers found in the SATB2$^+$ and TBR1$^+$ neurons is only observable in this specific sub-population and not detectable in other βIIITubulin$^+$ and MAP2$^+$ neurons.

In conclusion, there are many differences amongst the final neural cell population generated by the differentiation protocols, as well as in the final composition of neural subtypes generated. The reproducible detection of an AD related phenotype is very much dependent on the generation of predictable and fully matured brain region-specific neurons. Therefore, it would be relevant to combine the phenotypic observations so far gathered and routinely check all AD iPS cell models for the presence or absence of all of these disease hallmarks.

Even though tremendous advances have been made in the generation of AD iPS cells and subsequent differentiation into cortical neurons, other neurons and glia, the analysis of the cellular disease phenotype is still the most challenging aspect of this cellular model of AD. One of the most profound problems is the lack of reliable reproducibility of the differentiation protocols and the clonal variation even amongst iPS cell clones from the same patient, which could be responsible for the varying outcomes in the results. One explanation could be the incomplete reset of the cellular epigenetic landscape to the pluripotent state and current limitations of differentiation protocols, which fail to produce functional and specific neuronal subtypes. This could possibly be contributing to the observed lack of a disease phenotype and also the diversity in the observed disease phenotypes.

One of the sporadic AD iPS cell lines showed no phenotype whatsoever, which could mean that there are either unknown phenotypic hallmarks related to AD, or simply, in this case, the neurons were not matured enough to display a disease phenotype. The lack of mature neuronal differentiation is supported by the findings that another APP related mutation (APPV717I) showed a marked increase in Aβ42 levels, which increased during the course of the differentiation protocol. A comparative analysis of APP and APP cleavage products starting from day 9 until day 100 clearly showed that a significant increase of Aβ42 was not detectable before day 40 during the terminal differentiation protocol [103]. These two approaches underline the necessity of optimized differentiation protocols in terms of duration and timepoint of analyses of the disease phenotype. Another plausible explanation for the absence of a cellular SAD phenotype could be due to altered Aβ clearance in the patients. It has been shown by several groups that astrocytes may contribute to the Aβ clearance by restricting the inflammatory response in the brain [137,138]. Interestingly, APOE4, which is a risk factor for SAD, is expressed in astrocytes implying an important functional role of these cells in the neurodegenerative progression in the patients [139]. Microglia certainly also play an important role in Aβ clearance [140]. These cell types and their impact in AD *in vitro* systems remain largely unexplored. Nevertheless, it was also possible to observe an increase in phosphorylation of tau (Thr^{231}) and an increase in GSK3 beta activity, in the two APP duplication iPS cell models and in one of the sporadic AD iPS cell models [96]. The use of more defined neural subtypes could be more beneficial in dissecting the underlying causes of AD progression. These are also encouraging findings for validation in using these cellular models to identify cellular changes in AD. Different groups have reported the production of AD iPS cells and used different approaches to perform neural differentiation and analyses of these cells. This makes it difficult to establish a common cellular phenotype to set as a baseline for AD iPS cell models. However, this is very necessary in order to ensure that a lack of phenotype or a novel phenotype is not caused by insufficient neural subtype differentiation.

Overcoming the variation in the AD pathologies of analyzed AD-iPS-derived neural cells is important. Whether this variation is reflective of patient variability or cell line variability remains unclear. However, one way to overcome this problem would be to make sure at least three clones of each patient are produced, and that these produced identical phenotypes. It may also be important to have patient medical history that can verify pathology observed when first analyzing results. It is evident that not all iPS cell clones recapitulate results, and those that do not should be discarded or eliminated from analyses and interpretation. It is also clear that our lack of understanding of the cell types that are being analyzed could impede dramatically on our results and interpretations of them. This is a difficult task to overcome, as the complexity of the brain is colossal. It requires significant years of basic research into identifying the development cues of the neurons and neural cells of interest for the disease. Although, a recent promising study has revealed that 3D brain structures can be recreated *in vitro* from differentiated human embryonic stem cells [141], revealing that it may be possible to even recreate specific sub-regions of the brain within a dish in the future.

14. Future Induction of an AD Phenotype Using Components that Introduce Cellular Stress

Issues in resetting the biological clock during reprogramming could quite possibly explain the difficulties observed in obtaining ideal phenotypes in some AD iPS cell models. This does not come as a surprise since AD is a disease in which not only the malfunction of AD related genes, but also the aging of cells, as well as the whole organism is involved. This potentially makes the fundamental use of *in vitro* AD iPS cell systems questionable. However, some research groups have started to use cellular stresses to provoke accelerated aging in *in vitro* produced neural cells and have even introduced systems, which overexpress genes related to premature aging. This could lead to the development of shorter differentiation protocols, which would be of extreme benefit both for researchers and for the eventual benefits for patients.

In one study, it was possible to alleviate Aβ oligomer-induced cellular stress using docosahexaenoic acid (DHA) in neurons derived from iPS cells [98]. Since it is known that oxidative stress is a key hallmark of Alzheimer's disease and accelerates the diseases progression [142], ROS could be useful in triggering a disease phenotype in SAD iPS cell-derived neurons where no disease phenotype is observable or to accelerate the cellular disease and aging process itself. Mitochondria generate energy via oxidative phosphorylation and ROS is the byproduct for this energy generation. This observation led to the free radical hypothesis of ageing, which makes ROS species responsible for accumulative cellular damage over lifetime [143]. Currently, aerobic metabolism and the corresponding generation of ROS is still the most widely accepted cause of ageing, but little is known about the intracellular targets of ROS and how oxygen manipulation of these influences lifespan [144]. Another widely used ROS species is hydrogen peroxide (H_2O_2), which belongs to the exogenous ROS species, causing mostly DNA damage and which induced an apoptotic cellular response at high doses. The usage of this kind of stressor has therefore a lasting effect due to the DNA damage; however, it is not clear if these mutations directly cause a phenotype. On the other hand, a recent study showed that exposure of rat NPCs to H_2O_2 may actually be beneficial and induce neurogenesis [145], which is in contrast to the proposed damaging effect H_2O_2. This report also showed that low dosages of H_2O_2 induced proliferation of rat NPC cells, and even modified their differentiation potential towards an oligodendrocyte fate. This is a particularly interesting aspect since inflammation processes in the brain caused by H_2O_2 have been reported [146]. Unfortunately, the preferred differentiated neural subtype by low dosage exposure to H_2O_2 are oligodendrocytes, which would not be useful in replacing the degenerated pyramidal, cortical or cholinergic neurons, which are mostly affected by neurodegeneration in AD. Another technique, which is widely used to stress cells, includes serum starvation (which in the case of neural cells involves withdrawal of B27). This has been shown to robustly induce autophagy and neural death [147] and therefore a reduction of B27 in the neural media could be used to mimic stress and induce autophagy. Currently, none of the AD iPS cell published studies have used ROS species or serum starvation to provoke a more profound disease phenotype.

15. Induction of an AD Phenotype by Manipulating the Gene Expression of Age Inducing Genes

Another possible approach to mimic ageing in a dish could be to activate or repress key regulatory genes involved in the ageing process. A recent report revealed that overexpression of progerin (which when occurs in humans, causes Hutchinson-Gilford progeria) in an iPS cell model of Parkinson's disease resulted in an accelerated aged phenotype [148]. This cell model revealed pronounced dendritic degeneration, progressive loss of tyrosine hydroxylase expression, enlarged mitochondria and Lewy-body-precursor inclusions, which are indicative to the fact that the induced ageing was successful.

Other strategies to induce accelerated aging could involve RNAi-mediated knockdown of relevant targets such as sirtuin 1 (SIRT1), repressor element 1-silencing transcription factor (REST) or vacuolar protein sorting 41 (VPS41). Further genes of interest have been identified in *C. elegans*, which are also involved in autophagy lysosomal trafficking and shown to convey neuroprotective features. Amongst these are autophagy related 7 (ATG7) and PDZ domain containing family, member 1 (GIPC) [149]. SIRT1 has been shown to be involved in healthy ageing and longevity [150,151] and appears to be neuroprotective in AD [152]. Moreover, REST induces the expression of stress response genes and is neuroprotective [153]. VPS41 is involved in lysosomal trafficking and overexpression of this protein has been shown to enhance clearance of misfolded alpha synuclein [154]. A knockdown of VPS41 appears to hinder the lysosomal complex function and formation and accelerate accumulation of toxic misfolded proteins including Aβ. In particular, genes involved in autophagy could be of interest since the clearing of misfolded Aβ is believed to occur via autophagy and a downregulation or ablation of genes in this pathway could induce ageing as well as enhance the AD phenotype related to autophagy. Other studies have implied an important role for Beclin1 in autophagy and even APP processing [155], which makes this gene an interesting target as well. Clearly a systematic knockdown approach via RNAi targeting components of the autophagy and lysosomal pathways would be an amenable approach for identifying suitable targets that could induce ageing and accelerate the cellular pathology of AD iPS cell-derived neurons.

16. Conclusions and Future Perspectives

There are obviously still some hurdles that need to be overcome before science can faithfully recapitulate AD in a dish using iPS cells that might provide benefit to AD patients. It also remains to be seen if cell therapy by transplantation of AD-corrected iPS-derived neural cells could be of benefit to patients, by assessing integration of grafts into the brain and/or other related effects such as inflammation, or if AD-iPS derived disease models could help to deliver new and more advanced therapies to the patients. It is clear from the studies performed so far that more research is required. In keeping perspective, this research is aimed for the development of new and better medicines that can treat the disease long-term, rather than medicines that apply temporary brakes on it, and ultimately we are searching for a cure, which may totally alleviate the disease. The benefits to the community both at a societal level, but also at an economical level, are tremendous and would positively benefit millions of people around the globe.

What is evident, however, is that there is a clear step towards translational medicine for pluripotent stem cells, and in particular for treatment of disease. This is most striking in the case of other neurodegenerative disease such as Parkinson's disease [156,157]. Ultimately, human iPS cells will help to contribute detailed knowledge on AD mechanisms and might even lead to breakthroughs that could allow clinicians to develop earlier diagnoses, or be used for patient individualized medication and potentially for future cell transplantations. In considering how far we have come with the advancement of iPS technologies, and in the few years since the implementation of the technology, it is likely that the path ahead will unveil potentially significant advances in the treatment of the disease.

Acknowledgments

We would like to thank the financial support of the Danish Research Council for Independent Research, Technology and Production for their financial support on research pertaining to Alzheimer's disease. We also thank the financial support from the People Programme (Marie Curie Actions) of the European Union's Seventh Framework Programme FP7/2007-2013/ under REA grant agreement No. PIAPP-GA-2012-324451 (STEMMAD) and the Copenhagen University 2016 award on Precise Genetic Engineering.

Author Contributions

Kristine Freude, Carlota Pires and Vanessa Hall contributed towards writing of the manuscript. Poul Hyttel contributed to production of the figure in the manuscript.

Abbreviations

B27 (B27 supplement); BDNF (brain-derived neurotrophic factor); bFGF (basic fibroblast growth factor); cAMP (cyclic AMP); dcAMP (dibutryl cyclic AMP); EB (embryoid body); EGF (epidermal growth factor); EGFP (enhanced green fluorescent protein); FACS (fluorescence activated cell sorting); GDNF (glial cell-derived neurotrophic factor); IGF (insulin growth factor); IPS cell (induced pluripotent stem cells); It-NES (neuroepithelial stem cells); KSR (knockout serum replacement); N2 (N2 supplement); NB (neural basal media); NGF (nerve growth factor); NPC (neural progenitor cell); RA (retinoic acid); seq. (sequencing); SHH (sonic hedgehog); wks (weeks); w/o (without); 3N (modified bold 3N medium).

Conflicts of Interest

The authors declare no conflict of interest.

References

1. World Health Organization and Alzheimer's Disease International. *Dementia: A Public Health Priority*; WHO Press: Geneva, Switzerland, 2012; p. 103.

2. Aalten, P.; Verhey, F.R.; Boziki, M.; Brugnolo, A.; Bullock, R.; Byrne, E.J.; Camus, V.; Caputo, M.; Collins, D.; de Deyn, P.P.; *et al.* Consistency of neuropsychiatric syndromes across dementias: Results from the European Alzheimer Disease Consortium. Part II. *Dement. Geriatr. Cogn. Disord.* **2008**, *25*, 1–8.

3. Kamboh, M.I. Molecular genetics of late-onset Alzheimer's disease. *Ann. Hum. Genet.* **2004**, *68*, 381–404.

4. Roses, A.D.; Saunders, A.M. Perspective on a pathogenesis and treatment of Alzheimer's disease. *Alzheimer's Dement.* **2006**, *2*, 59–70.

5. Bertram, L.; McQueen, M.B.; Mullin, K.; Blacker, D.; Tanzi, R.E. Systematic meta-analyses of Alzheimer disease genetic association studies: The AlzGene database. *Nat. Genet.* **2007**, *39*, 17–23.

6. Harold, D.; Abraham, R.; Hollingworth, P.; Sims, R.; Gerrish, A.; Hamshere, M.L.; Pahwa, J.S.; Moskvina, V.; Dowzell, K.; Williams, A.; *et al.* Genome-wide association study identifies variants at CLU and PICALM associated with Alzheimer's disease. *Nat. Genet.* **2009**, *41*, 1088–1093.

7. Seshadri, S.; Fitzpatrick, A.L.; Ikram, M.A.; DeStefano, A.L.; Gudnason, V.; Boada, M.; Bis, J.C.; Smith, A.V.; Carassquillo, M.M.; Lambert, J.C.; *et al.* Genome-wide analysis of genetic loci associated with Alzheimer disease. *JAMA* **2010**, *303*, 1832–1840.

8. Hollingworth, P.; Harold, D.; Sims, R.; Gerrish, A.; Lambert, J.C.; Carrasquillo, M.M.; Abraham, R.; Hamshere, M.L.; Pahwa, J.S.; Moskvina, V.; *et al.* Common variants at ABCA7, MS4A6A/MS4A4E, EPHA1, CD33 and CD2AP are associated with Alzheimer's disease. *Nat. Genet.* **2011**, *43*, 429–435.

9. Cruchaga, C.; Kauwe, J.S.; Harari, O.; Jin, S.C.; Cai, Y.; Karch, C.M.; Benitez, B.A.; Jeng, A.T.; Skorupa, T.; Carrell, D.; *et al.* GWAS of cerebrospinal fluid tau levels identifies risk variants for Alzheimer's disease. *Neuron* **2013**, *78*, 256–268.

10. Lambert, J.C.; Ibrahim-Verbaas, C.A.; Harold, D.; Naj, A.C.; Sims, R.; Bellenguez, C.; DeStafano, A.L.; Bis, J.C.; Beecham, G.W.; Grenier-Boley, B.; *et al.* Meta-analysis of 74,046 individuals identifies 11 new susceptibility loci for Alzheimer's disease. *Nat. Genet.* **2013**, *45*, 1452–1458.

11. Holtzman, D.M.; Morris, J.C.; Goate, A.M. Alzheimer's disease: The challenge of the second century. *Sci. Transl. Med.* **2011**, *3*, doi:10.1126/scitranslmed.3002369.

12. Rao, A.T.; Degnan, A.J.; Levy, L.M. Genetics of Alzheimer disease. *Am. J. Neuroradiol.* **2014**, *35*, 457–458.

13. Takahashi, K.; Yamanaka, S. Induced pluripotent stem cells in medicine and biology. *Development* **2013**, *140*, 2457–2461.

14. Bird, T.D. Genetic aspects of Alzheimer disease. *Genet. Med.* **2008**, *10*, 231–239.

15. Iwatsubo, T.; Odaka, A.; Suzuki, N.; Mizusawa, H.; Nukina, N.; Ihara, Y. Visualization of A beta 42(43) and A beta 40 in senile plaques with end-specific A beta monoclonals: Evidence that an initially deposited species is A beta 42(43). *Neuron* **1994**, *13*, 45–53.

16. Selkoe, D.J. Alzheimer's disease is a synaptic failure. *Science* **2002**, *298*, 789–791.

17. Alonso, A.C.; Li, B.; Grundke-Iqbal, I.; Iqbal, K. Mechanism of tau-induced neurodegeneration in Alzheimer disease and related tauopathies. *Curr. Alzheimer Res.* **2008**, *5*, 375–384.

18. Braak, H.; Rub, U.; Schultz, C.; del Tredici, K. Vulnerability of cortical neurons to Alzheimer's and Parkinson's diseases. *J. Alzheimer's Dis.* **2006**, *9*, 35–44.

19. Mann, D.M. Pyramidal nerve cell loss in Alzheimer's disease. *Neurodegeneration* **1996**, *5*, 423–427.

20. Baglietto-Vargas, D.; Moreno-Gonzalez, I.; Sanchez-Varo, R.; Jimenez, S.; Trujillo-Estrada, L.; Sanchez-Mejias, E.; Torres, M.; Romero-Acebal, M.; Ruano, D.; Vizuete, M.; *et al.* Calretinin interneurons are early targets of extracellular amyloid-beta pathology in PS1/AbetaPP Alzheimer mice hippocampus. *J. Alzheimer's Dis.* **2010**, *21*, 119–132.

21. Verret, L.; Mann, E.O.; Hang, G.B.; Barth, A.M.; Cobos, I.; Ho, K.; Devidze, N.; Masliah, E.; Kreitzer, A.C.; Mody, I.; *et al.* Inhibitory interneuron deficit links altered network activity and cognitive dysfunction in Alzheimer model. *Cell* **2012**, *149*, 708–721.

22. Whitehouse, P.J.; Price, D.L.; Struble, R.G.; Clark, A.W.; Coyle, J.T.; Delon, M.R. Alzheimer's disease and senile dementia: Loss of neurons in the basal forebrain. *Science* **1982**, *215*, 1237–1239.

23. West, M.J.; Coleman, P.D.; Flood, D.G.; Troncoso, J.C. Differences in the pattern of hippocampal neuronal loss in normal ageing and Alzheimer's disease. *Lancet* **1994**, *344*, 769–772.

24. Schliebs, R.; Arendt, T. The cholinergic system in aging and neuronal degeneration. *Behav. Brain Res.* **2011**, *221*, 555–563.

25. Dickson, D.W.; Lee, S.C.; Mattiace, L.A.; Yen, S.H.; Brosnan, C. Microglia and cytokines in neurological disease, with special reference to AIDS and Alzheimer's disease. *Glia* **1993**, *7*, 75–83.

26. Griffin, W.S.; Sheng, J.G.; Roberts, G.W.; Mrak, R.E. Interleukin-1 expression in different plaque types in Alzheimer's disease: Significance in plaque evolution. *J. Neuropathol. Exp. Neurol.* **1995**, *54*, 276–281.

27. White, J.A.; Manelli, A.M.; Holmberg, K.H.; van Eldik, L.J.; Ladu, M.J. Differential effects of oligomeric and fibrillar amyloid-beta 1–42 on astrocyte-mediated inflammation. *Neurobiol. Dis.* **2005**, *18*, 459–465.

28. Munch, G.; Thome, J.; Foley, P.; Schinzel, R.; Riederer, P. Advanced glycation endproducts in ageing and Alzheimer's disease. *Brain Res. Rev.* **1997**, *23*, 134–143.

29. McShea, A.; Harris, P.L.; Webster, K.R.; Wahl, A.F.; Smith, M.A. Abnormal expression of the cell cycle regulators P16 and CDK4 in Alzheimer's disease. *Am. J. Pathol.* **1997**, *150*, 1933–1939.

30. McShea, A.; Lee, H.G.; Petersen, R.B.; Casadesus, G.; Vincent, I.; Linford, N.J.; Funk, J.O.; Shapiro, R.A.; Smith, M.A. Neuronal cell cycle re-entry mediates Alzheimer disease-type changes. *Biochim. Biophys. Acta* **2007**, *1772*, 467–472.

31. Markesbery, W.R. Oxidative stress hypothesis in Alzheimer's disease. *Free Radic. Biol. Med.* **1997**, *23*, 134–147.

32. Perry, G.; Castellani, R.J.; Hirai, K.; Smith, M.A. Reactive Oxygen Species Mediate Cellular Damage in Alzheimer Disease. *J. Alzheimer's Dis.* **1998**, *1*, 45–55.

33. Unterberger, U.; Hoftberger, R.; Gelpi, E.; Flicker, H.; Budka, H.; Voigtlander, T. Endoplasmic reticulum stress features are prominent in Alzheimer disease but not in prion diseases *in vivo*. *J. Neuropathol. Exp. Neurol.* **2006**, *65*, 348–357.

34. Games, D.; Adams, D.; Alessandrini, R.; Barbour, R.; Berthelette, P.; Blackwell, C.; Carr, T.; Clemens, J.; Donaldson, T.; Gillespie, F.; *et al*. Alzheimer-type neuropathology in transgenic mice overexpressing V717F beta-amyloid precursor protein. *Nature* **1995**, *373*, 523–527.

35. Hsiao, K.; Chapman, P.; Nilsen, S.; Eckman, C.; Harigaya, Y.; Younkin, S.; Yang, F.; Cole, G. Correlative memory deficits, Abeta elevation, and amyloid plaques in transgenic mice. *Science* **1996**, *274*, 99–102.

36. Sturchler-Pierrat, C.; Abramowski, D.; Duke, M.; Wiederhold, K.H.; Mistl, C.; Rothacher, S.; Ledermann, B.; Burki, K.; Frey, P.; Paganetti, P.A.; *et al*. Two amyloid precursor protein transgenic mouse models with Alzheimer disease-like pathology. *Proc. Natl. Acad. Sci. USA* **1997**, *94*, 13287–13292.

37. Duff, K.; Eckman, C.; Zehr, C.; Yu, X.; Prada, C.M.; Perez-tur, J.; Hutton, M.; Buee, L.; Harigaya, Y.; Yager, D.; *et al*. Increased amyloid-beta42(43) in brains of mice expressing mutant presenilin 1. *Nature* **1996**, *383*, 710–713.

38. Irizarry, M.C.; McNamara, M.; Fedorchak, K.; Hsiao, K.; Hyman, B.T. APPSw transgenic mice develop age-related A beta deposits and neuropil abnormalities, but no neuronal loss in CA1. *J. Neuropathol. Exp. Neurol.* **1997**, *56*, 965–973.

39. Holcomb, L.; Gordon, M.N.; McGowan, E.; Yu, X.; Benkovic, S.; Jantzen, P.; Wright, K.; Saad, I.; Mueller, R.; Morgan, D.; *et al*. Accelerated Alzheimer-type phenotype in transgenic mice carrying both mutant amyloid precursor protein and presenilin 1 transgenes. *Nat. Med.* **1998**, *4*, 97–100.

40. Chishti, M.A.; Yang, D.S.; Janus, C.; Phinney, A.L.; Horne, P.; Pearson, J.; Strome, R.; Zuker, N.; Loukides, J.; French, J.; *et al*. Early-onset amyloid deposition and cognitive deficits in transgenic mice expressing a double mutant form of amyloid precursor protein 695. *J. Biol. Chem.* **2001**, *276*, 21562–21570.

41. Davis, J.; Xu, F.; Deane, R.; Romanov, G.; Previti, M.L.; Zeigler, K.; Zlokovic, B.V.; van Nostrand, W.E. Early-onset and robust cerebral microvascular accumulation of amyloid beta-protein in transgenic mice expressing low levels of a vasculotropic Dutch/Iowa mutant form of amyloid beta-protein precursor. *J. Biol. Chem.* **2004**, *279*, 20296–20306.

42. Knobloch, M.; Konietzko, U.; Krebs, D.C.; Nitsch, R.M. Intracellular Abeta and cognitive deficits precede beta-amyloid deposition in transgenic arcAbeta mice. *Neurobiol. Aging* **2007**, *28*, 1297–1306.

43. Oddo, S.; Caccamo, A.; Shepherd, J.D.; Murphy, M.P.; Golde, T.E.; Kayed, R.; Metherate, R.; Mattson, M.P.; Akbari, Y.; LaFerla, F.M. Triple-transgenic model of Alzheimer's disease with plaques and tangles: Intracellular Abeta and synaptic dysfunction. *Neuron* **2003**, *39*, 409–421.

44. Casas, C.; Sergeant, N.; Itier, J.M.; Blanchard, V.; Wirths, O.; van der Kolk, N.; Vingtdeux, V.; van de Steeg, E.; Ret, G.; Canton, T.; *et al.* Massive CA1/2 neuronal loss with intraneuronal and *N*-terminal truncated Abeta42 accumulation in a novel Alzheimer transgenic model. *Am. J. Pathol.* **2004**, *165*, 1289–1300.

45. Lim, F.; Hernandez, F.; Lucas, J.J.; Gomez-Ramos, P.; Moran, M.A.; Avila, J. FTDP-17 mutations in tau transgenic mice provoke lysosomal abnormalities and Tau filaments in forebrain. *Mol. Cell. Neurosci.* **2001**, *18*, 702–714.

46. Oakley, H.; Cole, S.L.; Logan, S.; Maus, E.; Shao, P.; Craft, J.; Guillozet-Bongaarts, A.; Ohno, M.; Disterhoft, J.; van Eldik, L.; *et al.* Intraneuronal beta-amyloid aggregates, neurodegeneration, and neuron loss in transgenic mice with five familial Alzheimer's disease mutations: Potential factors in amyloid plaque formation. *J. Neurosci.* **2006**, *26*, 10129–10140.

47. Lewis, J.; Dickson, D.W.; Lin, W.L.; Chisholm, L.; Corral, A.; Jones, G.; Yen, S.H.; Sahara, N.; Skipper, L.; Yager, D.; *et al.* Enhanced neurofibrillary degeneration in transgenic mice expressing mutant tau and APP. *Science* **2001**, *293*, 1487–1491.

48. Shineman, D.W.; Basi, G.S.; Bizon, J.L.; Colton, C.A.; Greenberg, B.D.; Hollister, B.A.; Lincecum, J.; Leblanc, G.G.; Lee, L.B.; Luo, F.; *et al.* Accelerating drug discovery for Alzheimer's disease: Best practices for preclinical animal studies. *Alzheimer's Res. Ther.* **2011**, *3*, doi:10.1186/alzrt90.

49. Franco, R.; Cedazo-Minguez, A. Successful therapies for Alzheimer's disease: Why so many in animal models and none in humans? *Front. Pharmacol.* **2014**, *5*, doi:10.3389/fphar.2014.00146.

50. Becker, R.E.; Greig, N.H. Increasing the success rate for Alzheimer's disease drug discovery and development. *Exp. Opin. Drug Discov.* **2012**, *7*, 367–370.

51. Sperling, R.A.; Karlawish, J.; Johnson, K.A. Preclinical Alzheimer disease-the challenges ahead. *Nat. Rev. Neurol.* **2013**, *9*, 54–58.

52. Takahashi, K.; Yamanaka, S. Induction of pluripotent stem cells from mouse embryonic and adult fibroblast cultures by defined factors. *Cell* **2006**, *126*, 663–676.

53. Thomson, J.A.; Itskovitz-Eldor, J.; Shapiro, S.S.; Waknitz, M.A.; Swiergiel, J.J.; Marshall, V.S.; Jones, J.M. Embryonic stem cell lines derived from human blastocysts. *Science* **1998**, *282*, 1145–1147.

54. Okita, K.; Ichisaka, T.; Yamanaka, S. Generation of germline-competent induced pluripotent stem cells. *Nature* **2007**, *448*, 313–317.

55. Takahashi, K.; Tanabe, K.; Ohnuki, M.; Narita, M.; Ichisaka, T.; Tomoda, K.; Yamanaka, S. Induction of pluripotent stem cells from adult human fibroblasts by defined factors. *Cell* **2007**, *131*, 861–872.

56. Yu, J.; Vodyanik, M.A.; Smuga-Otto, K.; Antosiewicz-Bourget, J.; Frane, J.L.; Tian, S.; Nie, J.; Jonsdottir, G.A.; Ruotti, V.; Stewart, R.; *et al.* Induced pluripotent stem cell lines derived from human somatic cells. *Science* **2007**, *318*, 1917–1920.

57. Park, I.H.; Lerou, P.H.; Zhao, R.; Huo, H.; Daley, G.Q. Generation of human-induced pluripotent stem cells. *Nat. Protoc.* **2008**, *3*, 1180–1186.

58. Malchenko, S.; Galat, V.; Seftor, E.A.; Vanin, E.F.; Costa, F.F.; Seftor, R.E.; Soares, M.B.; Hendrix, M.J. Cancer hallmarks in induced pluripotent cells: New insights. *J. Cell. Physiol.* **2010**, *225*, 390–393.

59. Bock, C.; Kiskinis, E.; Verstappen, G.; Gu, H.; Boulting, G.; Smith, Z.D.; Ziller, M.; Croft, G.F.; Amoroso, M.W.; Oakley, D.H.; *et al.* Reference Maps of human ES and iPS cell variation enable high-throughput characterization of pluripotent cell lines. *Cell* **2011**, *144*, 439–452.

60. Nishino, K.; Toyoda, M.; Yamazaki-Inoue, M.; Fukawatase, Y.; Chikazawa, E.; Sakaguchi, H.; Akutsu, H.; Umezawa, A. DNA methylation dynamics in human induced pluripotent stem cells over time. *PLoS Genet.* **2011**, *7*, e1002085.

61. Wang, A.; Huang, K.; Shen, Y.; Xue, Z.; Cai, C.; Horvath, S.; Fan, G. Functional modules distinguish human induced pluripotent stem cells from embryonic stem cells. *Stem Cells Dev.* **2011**, *20*, 1937–1950.

62. Bellin, M.; Marchetto, M.C.; Gage, F.H.; Mummery, C.L. Induced pluripotent stem cells: The new patient? *Nat. Rev. Mol. Cell Biol.* **2012**, *13*, 713–726.

63. Stadtfeld, M.; Nagaya, M.; Utikal, J.; Weir, G.; Hochedlinger, K. Induced pluripotent stem cells generated without viral integration. *Science* **2008**, *322*, 945–949.

64. Kim, D.; Kim, C.H.; Moon, J.I.; Chung, Y.G.; Chang, M.Y.; Han, B.S.; Ko, S.; Yang, E.; Cha, K.Y.; Lanza, R.; *et al.* Generation of human induced pluripotent stem cells by direct delivery of reprogramming proteins. *Cell Stem Cell* **2009**, *4*, 472–476.

65. Okita, K.; Matsumura, Y.; Sato, Y.; Okada, A.; Morizane, A.; Okamoto, S.; Hong, H.; Nakagawa, M.; Tanabe, K.; Tezuka, K.; *et al.* A more efficient method to generate integration-free human iPS cells. *Nat. Methods* **2011**, *8*, 409–412.

66. Amit, M.; Itskovitz-Eldor, J. Feeder-free culture of human embryonic stem cells. *Methods Enzymol.* **2006**, *420*, 37–49.

67. Chen, G.; Gulbranson, D.R.; Hou, Z.; Bolin, J.M.; Ruotti, V.; Probasco, M.D.; Smuga-Otto, K.; Howden, S.E.; Diol, N.R.; Propson, N.E.; *et al.* Chemically defined conditions for human iPSC derivation and culture. *Nat. Methods* **2011**, *8*, 424–429.

68. Loh, Y.H.; Hartung, O.; Li, H.; Guo, C.; Sahalie, J.M.; Manos, P.D.; Urbach, A.; Heffner, G.C.; Grskovic, M.; Vigneault, F.; *et al.* Reprogramming of T cells from human peripheral blood. *Cell Stem Cell* **2010**, *7*, 15–19.

69. Seki, T.; Yuasa, S.; Oda, M.; Egashira, T.; Yae, K.; Kusumoto, D.; Nakata, H.; Tohyama, S.; Hashimoto, H.; Kodaira, M.; *et al.* Generation of induced pluripotent stem cells from human terminally differentiated circulating T cells. *Cell Stem Cell* **2010**, *7*, 11–14.

70. Nakagawa, M.; Taniguchi, Y.; Senda, S.; Takizawa, N.; Ichisaka, T.; Asano, K.; Morizane, A.; Doi, D.; Takahashi, J.; Nishizawa, M.; *et al.* A novel efficient feeder-free culture system for the derivation of human induced pluripotent stem cells. *Sci. Rep.* **2014**, *4*, doi:10.1038/srep03594.

71. Hyun, I. The bioethics of stem cell research and therapy. *J. Clin. Investig.* **2010**, *120*, 71–75.

72. Charron, D.; Suberbielle-Boissel, C.; Al-Daccak, R. Immunogenicity and allogenicity: A challenge of stem cell therapy. *J. Cardiovasc. Transl. Res.* **2009**, *2*, 130–138.

73. Noggle, S.; Fung, H.L.; Gore, A.; Martinez, H.; Satriani, K.C.; Prosser, R.; Oum, K.; Paull, D.; Druckenmiller, S.; Freeby, M.; *et al.* Human oocytes reprogram somatic cells to a pluripotent state. *Nature* **2011**, *478*, 70–75.

74. Jaenisch, R. Human cloning—The science and ethics of nuclear transplantation. *N. Engl. J. Med.* **2004**, *351*, 2787–2791.

75. Costa, M.; Dottori, M.; Sourris, K.; Jamshidi, P.; Hatzistavrou, T.; Davis, R.; Azzola, L.; Jackson, S.; Lim, S.M.; Pera, M.; *et al.* A method for genetic modification of human embryonic stem cells using electroporation. *Nat. Protoc.* **2007**, *2*, 792–796.

76. Zou, J.; Maeder, M.L.; Mali, P.; Pruett-Miller, S.M.; Thibodeau-Beganny, S.; Chou, B.K.; Chen, G.; Ye, Z.; Park, I.H.; Daley, G.Q.; *et al.* Gene targeting of a disease-related gene in human induced pluripotent stem and embryonic stem cells. *Cell Stem Cell* **2009**, *5*, 97–110.

77. Miller, J.C.; Tan, S.; Qiao, G.; Barlow, K.A.; Wang, J.; Xia, D.F.; Meng, X.; Paschon, D.E.; Leung, E.; Hinkley, S.J.; *et al.* A TALE nuclease architecture for efficient genome editing. *Nat. Biotechnol.* **2011**, *29*, 143–148.

78. Yang, L.; Yang, J.L.; Bryne, S.; Pan, J.; Church, G.M. CRISPR/Cas9-directed genome editing of cultured cells. In *Current Protocols in Molecular Biology*; John Wiley & Sons Inc.: Hoboken, NJ, USA, 2014; Volume 107, pp. 1–17.

79. Cherry, A.B.; Daley, G.Q. Reprogrammed cells for disease modeling and regenerative medicine. *Ann. Rev. Med.* **2013**, *64*, 277–290.

80. Wang, Q.; Matsumoto, Y.; Shindo, T.; Miyake, K.; Shindo, A.; Kawanishi, M.; Kawai, N.; Tamiya, T.; Nagao, S. Neural stem cells transplantation in cortex in a mouse model of Alzheimer's disease. *J. Med. Investig.* **2006**, *53*, 61–69.

81. Yamasaki, T.R.; Blurton-Jones, M.; Morrissette, D.A.; Kitazawa, M.; Oddo, S.; LaFerla, F.M. Neural stem cells improve memory in an inducible mouse model of neuronal loss. *J. Neurosci.* **2007**, *27*, 11925–11933.

82. Blurton-Jones, M.; Kitazawa, M.; Martinez-Coria, H.; Castello, N.A.; Muller, F.J.; Loring, J.F.; Yamasaki, T.R.; Poon, W.W.; Green, K.N.; LaFerla, F.M. Neural stem cells improve cognition via BDNF in a transgenic model of Alzheimer disease. *Proc. Natl. Acad. Sci. USA* **2009**, *106*, 13594–13599.

83. Park, D.; Lee, H.J.; Joo, S.S.; Bae, D.K.; Yang, G.; Yang, Y.H.; Lim, I.; Matsuo, A.; Tooyama, I.; Kim, Y.B.; *et al.* Human neural stem cells over-expressing choline acetyltransferase restore cognition in rat model of cognitive dysfunction. *Exp. Neurol.* **2012**, *234*, 521–526.

84. Tong, L.M.; Djukic, B.; Arnold, C.; Gillespie, A.K.; Yoon, S.Y.; Wang, M.M.; Zhang, O.; Knoferle, J.; Rubenstein, J.L.; Alvarez-Buylla, A.; *et al.* Inhibitory Interneuron Progenitor Transplantation Restores Normal Learning and Memory in ApoE4 Knock-In Mice without or with Abeta Accumulation. *J. Neurosci.* **2014**, *34*, 9506–9515.

85. Xuan, A.G.; Luo, M.; Ji, W.D.; Long, D.H. Effects of engrafted neural stem cells in Alzheimer's disease rats. *Neurosci. Lett.* **2009**, *450*, 167–171.

86. Kern, D.S.; Maclean, K.N.; Jiang, H.; Synder, E.Y.; Sladek, J.R., Jr.; Bjugstad, K.B. Neural stem cells reduce hippocampal tau and reelin accumulation in aged Ts65Dn Down syndrome mice. *Cell Transplant.* **2011**, *20*, 371–379.

87. Babaei, P.; Soltani Tehrani, B.; Alizadeh, A. Transplanted bone marrow mesenchymal stem cells improve memory in rat models of Alzheimer's disease. *Stem Cells Int.* **2012**, *2012*, doi.:10.1155/2012/369417.

88. Kim, S.; Chang, K.A.; Kim, J.; Park, H.G.; Ra, J.C.; Kim, H.S.; Suh, Y.H. The preventive and therapeutic effects of intravenous human adipose-derived stem cells in Alzheimer's disease mice. *PLoS ONE* **2012**, *7*, e45757.

89. Lee, H.J.; Lee, J.K.; Lee, H.; Carter, J.E.; Chang, J.W.; Oh, W.; Yang, Y.S.; Suh, J.G.; Lee, B.H.; Jin, H.K.; *et al.* Human umbilical cord blood-derived mesenchymal stem cells improve neuropathology and cognitive impairment in an Alzheimer's disease mouse model through modulation of neuroinflammation. *Neurobiol. Aging* **2012**, *33*, 588–602.

90. Moghadam, F.H.; Alaie, H.; Karbalaie, K.; Tanhaei, S.; Nasr Esfahani, M.H.; Baharvand, H. Transplantation of primed or unprimed mouse embryonic stem cell-derived neural precursor cells improves cognitive function in Alzheimerian rats. *Differ. Res. Biol. Divers.* **2009**, *78*, 59–68.

91. Yahata, N.; Asai, M.; Kitaoka, S.; Takahashi, K.; Asaka, I.; Hioki, H.; Kaneko, T.; Maruyama, K.; Saido, T.C.; Nakahata, T.; *et al.* Anti-Abeta drug screening platform using human iPS cell-derived neurons for the treatment of Alzheimer's disease. *PLoS One* **2011**, *6*, e25788.

92. Ebert, A.D.; Liang, P.; Wu, J.C. Induced pluripotent stem cells as a disease modeling and drug screening platform. *J. Cardiovasc. Pharmacol.* **2012**, *60*, 408–416.

93. Noetzli, M.; Eap, C.B. Pharmacodynamic, pharmacokinetic and pharmacogenetic aspects of drugs used in the treatment of Alzheimer's disease. *Clin. Pharmacokinet.* **2013**, *52*, 225–241.

94. Tan, C.C.; Yu, J.T.; Tan, L. Biomarkers for preclinical Alzheimer's disease. *J. Alzheimer's Dis.* **2014**, *42*, 1051–1069.

95. Duan, L.; Bhattacharyya, B.J.; Belmadani, A.; Pan, L.; Miller, R.J.; Kessler, J.A. Stem cell derived basal forebrain cholinergic neurons from Alzheimer's disease patients are more susceptible to cell death. *Mol. Neurodegener.* **2014**, *9*, doi:10.1186/1750-1326-9-3.

96. Israel, M.A.; Yuan, S.H.; Bardy, C.; Reyna, S.M.; Mu, Y.; Herrera, C.; Hefferan, M.P.; van Gorp, S.; Nazor, K.L.; Boscolo, F.S.; *et al.* Probing sporadic and familial Alzheimer's disease using induced pluripotent stem cells. *Nature* **2012**, *482*, 216–220.

97. Koch, P.; Tamboli, I.Y.; Mertens, J.; Wunderlich, P.; Ladewig, J.; Stuber, K.; Esselmann, H.; Wiltfang, J.; Brustle, O.; Walter, J. Presenilin-1 L166P mutant human pluripotent stem cell-derived neurons exhibit partial loss of gamma-secretase activity in endogenous amyloid-beta generation. *Am. J. Pathol.* **2012**, *180*, 2404–2416.

98. Kondo, T.; Asai, M.; Tsukita, K.; Kutoku, Y.; Ohsawa, Y.; Sunada, Y.; Imamura, K.; Egawa, N.; Yahata, N.; Okita, K.; *et al.* Modeling Alzheimer's disease with iPSCs reveals stress phenotypes associated with intracellular Abeta and differential drug responsiveness. *Cell Stem Cell* **2013**, *12*, 487–496.

99. Yagi, T.; Ito, D.; Okada, Y.; Akamatsu, W.; Nihei, Y.; Yoshizaki, T.; Yamanaka, S.; Okano, H.; Suzuki, N. Modeling familial Alzheimer's disease with induced pluripotent stem cells. *Hum. Mol. Genet.* **2011**, *20*, 4530–4539.

100. Shi, Y.; Kirwan, P.; Smith, J.; MacLean, G.; Orkin, S.H.; Livesey, F.J. A human stem cell model of early Alzheimer's disease pathology in Down syndrome. *Sci. Transl. Med.* **2012**, *4*, doi:10.1126/scitranslmed.3003771.

101. Liu, Q.; Waltz, S.; Woodruff, G.; Ouyang, J.; Israel, M.A.; Herrera, C.; Sarsoza, F.; Tanzi, R.E.; Koo, E.H.; Ringman, J.M.; *et al.* Effect of Potent gamma-Secretase Modulator in Human Neurons Derived From Multiple Presenilin 1-Induced Pluripotent Stem Cell Mutant Carriers. *JAMA Neurol.* **2014**, doi:10.1001/jamaneurol.2014.2482.

102. Sproul, A.A.; Jacob, S.; Pre, D.; Kim, S.H.; Nestor, M.W.; Navarro-Sobrino, M.; Santa-Maria, I.; Zimmer, M.; Aubry, S.; Steele, J.W.; *et al.* Characterization and molecular profiling of PSEN1 familial Alzheimer's disease iPSC-derived neural progenitors. *PLoS ONE* **2014**, *9*, e84547.

103. Muratore, C.R.; Rice, H.C.; Srikanth, P.; Callahan, D.G.; Shin, T.; Benjamin, L.N.; Walsh, D.M.; Selkoe, D.J.; Young-Pearse, T.L. The familial Alzheimer's disease APPV717I mutation alters APP processing and Tau expression in iPSC-derived neurons. *Hum. Mol. Genet.* **2014**, *23*, 3523–3536.

104. Tomiyama, T.; Nagata, T.; Shimada, H.; Teraoka, R.; Fukushima, A.; Kanemitsu, H.; Takuma, H.; Kuwano, R.; Imagawa, M.; Ataka, S.; *et al.* A new amyloid beta variant favoring oligomerization in Alzheimer's-type dementia. *Ann. Neurol.* **2008**, *63*, 377–387.

105. Reiman, E.M.; Quiroz, Y.T.; Fleisher, A.S.; Chen, K.; Velez-Pardo, C.; Jimenez-Del-Rio, M.; Fagan, A.M.; Shah, A.R.; Alvarez, S.; Arbelaez, A.; *et al.* Brain imaging and fluid biomarker analysis in young adults at genetic risk for autosomal dominant Alzheimer's disease in the presenilin 1 E280A kindred: A case-control study. *Lancet. Neurol.* **2012**, *11*, 1048–1056.

106. Boss, M.A. Diagnostic approaches to Alzheimer's disease. *Biochim. Biophys. Acta* **2000**, *1502*, 188–200.

107. Palumbo, B.; Siepi, D.; Sabalich, I.; Tranfaglia, C.; Parnetti, L. Cerebrospinal fluid neuron-specific enolase: A further marker of Alzheimer's disease? *Funct. Neurol.* **2008**, *23*, 93–96.

108. Kumar-Singh, S.; Theuns, J.; van Broeck, B.; Pirici, D.; Vennekens, K.; Corsmit, E.; Cruts, M.; Dermaut, B.; Wang, R.; van Broeckhoven, C. Mean age-of-onset of familial alzheimer disease caused by presenilin mutations correlates with both increased Abeta42 and decreased Abeta40. *Hum. Mutat.* **2006**, *27*, 686–695.

109. McIntire, L.B.; Landman, N.; Kang, M.S.; Finan, G.M.; Hwang, J.C.; Moore, A.Z.; Park, L.S.; Lin, C.S.; Kim, T.W. Phenotypic assays for beta-amyloid in mouse embryonic stem cell-derived neurons. *Chem. Biol.* **2013**, *20*, 956–967.

110. Xu, X.; Lei, Y.; Luo, J.; Wang, J.; Zhang, S.; Yang, X.J.; Sun, M.; Nuwaysir, E.; Fan, G.; Zhao, J.; *et al.* Prevention of beta-amyloid induced toxicity in human iPS cell-derived neurons by inhibition of Cyclin-dependent kinases and associated cell cycle events. *Stem Cell Res.* **2013**, *10*, 213–227.

64

111. Yin, H.; Xue, W.; Chen, S.; Bogorad, R.L.; Benedetti, E.; Grompe, M.; Koteliansky, V.; Sharp, P.A.; Jacks, T.; Anderson, D.G. Genome editing with Cas9 in adult mice corrects a disease mutation and phenotype. *Nat. Biotechnol.* **2014**, *32*, 551–553.

112. Wu, Y.; Liang, D.; Wang, Y.; Bai, M.; Tang, W.; Bao, S.; Yan, Z.; Li, D.; Li, J. Correction of a genetic disease in mouse via use of CRISPR-Cas9. *Cell Stem Cell* **2013**, *13*, 659–662.

113. Low, B.E.; Krebs, M.P.; Joung, J.K.; Tsai, S.Q.; Nishina, P.M.; Wiles, M.V. Correction of the Crb1rd8 allele and retinal phenotype in C57BL/6N mice via TALEN-mediated homology-directed repair. *Investig. Ophthalmol. Visual Sci.* **2014**, *55*, 387–395.

114. Ma, N.; Liao, B.; Zhang, H.; Wang, L.; Shan, Y.; Xue, Y.; Huang, K.; Chen, S.; Zhou, X.; Chen, Y.; *et al.* Transcription activator-like effector nuclease (TALEN)-mediated gene correction in integration-free beta-thalassemia induced pluripotent stem cells. *J. Biol. Chem.* **2013**, *288*, 34671–34679.

115. Sun, N.; Zhao, H. Seamless correction of the sickle cell disease mutation of the *HBB* gene in human induced pluripotent stem cells using TALENs. *Biotechnol. Bioeng.* **2014**, *111*, 1048–1053.

116. Ousterout, D.G.; Perez-Pinera, P.; Thakore, P.I.; Kabadi, A.M.; Brown, M.T.; Qin, X.; Fedrigo, O.; Mouly, V.; Tremblay, J.P.; Gersbach, C.A. Reading frame correction by targeted genome editing restores dystrophin expression in cells from Duchenne muscular dystrophy patients. *Mol. Ther.* **2013**, *21*, 1718–1726.

117. Osborn, M.J.; Starker, C.G.; McElroy, A.N.; Webber, B.R.; Riddle, M.J.; Xia, L.; DeFeo, A.P.; Gabriel, R.; Schmidt, M.; von Kalle, C.; *et al.* TALEN-based gene correction for epidermolysis bullosa. *Mol. Ther.* **2013**, *21*, 1151–1159.

118. Liang, G.; Zhang, Y. Embryonic stem cell and induced pluripotent stem cell: An epigenetic perspective. *Cell Res.* **2013**, *23*, 49–69.

119. Agarwal, S.; Loh, Y.H.; McLoughlin, E.M.; Huang, J.; Park, I.H.; Miller, J.D.; Huo, H.; Okuka, M.; dos Reis, R.M.; Loewer, S.; *et al.* Telomere elongation in induced pluripotent stem cells from dyskeratosis congenita patients. *Nature* **2010**, *464*, 292–296.

120. Prigione, A.; Hossini, A.M.; Lichtner, B.; Serin, A.; Fauler, B.; Megges, M.; Lurz, R.; Lehrach, H.; Makrantonaki, E.; Zouboulis, C.C.; *et al.* Mitochondrial-associated cell death mechanisms are reset to an embryonic-like state in aged donor-derived iPS cells harboring chromosomal aberrations. *PLoS One* **2011**, *6*, e27352.

121. Lapasset, L.; Milhavet, O.; Prieur, A.; Besnard, E.; Babled, A.; Ait-Hamou, N.; Leschik, J.; Pellestor, F.; Ramirez, J.M.; de Vos, J.; *et al.* Rejuvenating senescent and centenarian human cells by reprogramming through the pluripotent state. *Genes Dev.* **2011**, *25*, 2248–2253.

122. Suhr, S.T.; Chang, E.A.; Rodriguez, R.M.; Wang, K.; Ross, P.J.; Beyhan, Z.; Murthy, S.; Cibelli, J.B. Telomere dynamics in human cells reprogrammed to pluripotency. *PLoS ONE* **2009**, *4*, e8124.

123. Yagi, T.; Kosakai, A.; Ito, D.; Okada, Y.; Akamatsu, W.; Nihei, Y.; Nabetani, A.; Ishikawa, F.; Arai, Y.; Hirose, N.; *et al.* Establishment of induced pluripotent stem cells from centenarians for neurodegenerative disease research. *PLoS ONE* **2012**, *7*, e41572.

124. Kim, K.; Doi, A.; Wen, B.; Ng, K.; Zhao, R.; Cahan, P.; Kim, J.; Aryee, M.J.; Ji, H.; Ehrlich, L.I.; *et al.* Epigenetic memory in induced pluripotent stem cells. *Nature* **2010**, *467*, 285–290.

125. Cohen, A.D.; Klunk, W.E. Early detection of Alzheimer's disease using PiB and FDG PET. *Neurobiol. Dis.* **2014**.

126. Lista, S.; Garaci, F.G.; Ewers, M.; Teipel, S.; Zetterberg, H.; Blennow, K.; Hampel, H. CSF Abeta 1–42 combined with neuroimaging biomarkers in the early detection, diagnosis and prediction of Alzheimer's disease. *Alzheimer's Dement.* **2014**, *10*, 381–392.

127. Caselli, R.J.; Reiman, E.M. Characterizing the preclinical stages of Alzheimer's disease and the prospect of presymptomatic intervention. *J. Alzheimer's Dis.* **2013**, *33* (Suppl. 1), 405–416.

128. Koronyo, Y.; Salumbides, B.C.; Black, K.L.; Koronyo-Hamaoui, M. Alzheimer's disease in the retina: Imaging retinal abeta plaques for early diagnosis and therapy assessment. *Neurodegener. Dis.* **2012**, *10*, 285–293.

129. Szilagyi, T.; Orban-Kis, K.; Horvath, E.; Metz, J.; Pap, Z.; Pavai, Z. Morphological identification of neuron types in the rat hippocampus. *Rom. J. Morphol. Embryol.* **2011**, *52*, 15–20.

130. Molyneaux, B.J.; Arlotta, P.; Menezes, J.R.; Macklis, J.D. Neuronal subtype specification in the cerebral cortex. *Nat. Rev. Neurosci.* **2007**, *8*, 427–437.

131. Espuny-Camacho, I.; Michelsen, K.A.; Gall, D.; Linaro, D.; Hasche, A.; Bonnefont, J.; Bali, C.; Orduz, D.; Bilheu, A.; Herpoel, A.; *et al.* Pyramidal neurons derived from human pluripotent stem cells integrate efficiently into mouse brain circuits *in vivo*. *Neuron* **2013**, *77*, 440–456.

132. De la Torre-Ubieta, L.; Bonni, A. Transcriptional regulation of neuronal polarity and morphogenesis in the mammalian brain. *Neuron* **2011**, *72*, 22–40.

133. Badger, J.L.; Cordero-Llana, O.; Hartfield, E.M.; Wade-Martins, R. Parkinson's disease in a dish—Using stem cells as a molecular tool. *Neuropharmacology* **2014**, *76*, 88–96.

134. Roybon, L.; Lamas, N.J.; Garcia-Diaz, A.; Yang, E.J.; Sattler, R.; Jackson-Lewis, V.; Kim, Y.A.; Kachel, C.A.; Rothstein, J.D.; Przedborski, S.; *et al.* Human stem cell-derived spinal cord astrocytes with defined mature or reactive phenotypes. *Cell Rep.* **2013**, *4*, 1035–1048.

135. Juopperi, T.A.; Kim, W.R.; Chiang, C.H.; Yu, H.; Margolis, R.L.; Ross, C.A.; Ming, G.L.; Song, H. Astrocytes generated from patient induced pluripotent stem cells recapitulate features of Huntington's disease patient cells. *Mol. Brain* **2012**, *5*, doi:10.1186/1756-6606-5-17.

136. Hu, B.Y.; Weick, J.P.; Yu, J.; Ma, L.X.; Zhang, X.Q.; Thomson, J.A.; Zhang, S.C. Neural differentiation of human induced pluripotent stem cells follows developmental principles but with variable potency. *Proc. Natl. Acad. Sci. USA* **2010**, *107*, 4335–4340.

137. Xiao, Q.; Yan, P.; Ma, X.; Liu, H.; Perez, R.; Zhu, A.; Gonzales, E.; Burchett, J.M.; Schuler, D.R.; Cirrito, J.R.; *et al.* Enhancing astrocytic lysosome biogenesis facilitates Abeta clearance and attenuates amyloid plaque pathogenesis. *J. Neurosci.* **2014**, *34*, 9607–9620.

138. Kraft, A.W.; Hu, X.; Yoon, H.; Yan, P.; Xiao, Q.; Wang, Y.; Gil, S.C.; Brown, J.; Wilhelmsson, U.; Restivo, J.L.; *et al.* Attenuating astrocyte activation accelerates plaque pathogenesis in APP/PS1 mice. *FASEB J.* **2013**, *27*, 187–198.

139. Sun, Y.; Wu, S.; Bu, G.; Onifade, M.K.; Patel, S.N.; LaDu, M.J.; Fagan, A.M.; Holtzman, D.M. Glial fibrillary acidic protein-apolipoprotein E (apoE) transgenic mice: Astrocyte-specific expression and differing biological effects of astrocyte-secreted apoE3 and apoE4 lipoproteins. *J. Neurosci.* **1998**, *18*, 3261–3272.

140. Doens, D.; Fernandez, P.L. Microglia receptors and their implications in the response to amyloid beta for Alzheimer's disease pathogenesis. *J. Neuroinflamm.* **2014**, *11*, doi:10.1186/1742-2094-11-48.

141. Lancaster, M.A.; Renner, M.; Martin, C.A.; Wenzel, D.; Bicknell, L.S.; Hurles, M.E.; Homfray, T.; Penninger, J.M.; Jackson, A.P.; Knoblich, J.A. Cerebral organoids model human brain development and microcephaly. *Nature* **2013**, *501*, 373–379.

142. Dumont, M.; Beal, M.F. Neuroprotective strategies involving ROS in Alzheimer disease. *Free Radic. Biol. Med.* **2011**, *51*, 1014–1026.

143. Harman, D. Aging: A theory based on free radical and radiation chemistry. *J. Gerontol.* **1956**, *11*, 298–300.

144. Balaban, R.S.; Nemoto, S.; Finkel, T. Mitochondria, oxidants, and aging. *Cell* **2005**, *120*, 483–495.

145. Perez Estrada, C.; Covacu, R.; Sankavaram, S.R.; Svensson, M.; Brundin, L. Oxidative Stress Increases Neurogenesis and Oligodendrogenesis in Adult Neural Progenitor Cells. *Stem Cells Dev.* **2014**, *23*, 2311–2327.

146. Su, B.; Wang, X.; Nunomura, A.; Moreira, P.I.; Lee, H.G.; Perry, G.; Smith, M.A.; Zhu, X. Oxidative stress signaling in Alzheimer's disease. *Curr. Alzheimer Res.* **2008**, *5*, 525–532.

147. Young, J.E.; Martinez, R.A.; la Spada, A.R. Nutrient deprivation induces neuronal autophagy and implicates reduced insulin signaling in neuroprotective autophagy activation. *J. Biol. Chem.* **2009**, *284*, 2363–2373.

148. Miller, J.D.; Ganat, Y.M.; Kishinevsky, S.; Bowman, R.L.; Liu, B.; Tu, E.Y.; Mandal, P.K.; Vera, E.; Shim, J.W.; Kriks, S.; *et al.* Human iPSC-based modeling of late-onset disease via progerin-induced aging. *Cell Stem Cell* **2013**, *13*, 691–705.

149. Hamamichi, S.; Rivas, R.N.; Knight, A.L.; Cao, S.; Caldwell, K.A.; Caldwell, G.A. Hypothesis-based RNAi screening identifies neuroprotective genes in a Parkinson's disease model. *Proc. Natl. Acad. Sci. USA* **2008**, *105*, 728–733.

150. Herranz, D.; Munoz-Martin, M.; Canamero, M.; Mulero, F.; Martinez-Pastor, B.; Fernandez-Capetillo, O.; Serrano, M. Sirt1 improves healthy ageing and protects from metabolic syndrome-associated cancer. *Nat. Commun.* **2010**, *1*, doi:10.1038/ncomms1001.

151. Giblin, W.; Skinner, M.E.; Lombard, D.B. Sirtuins: Guardians of mammalian healthspan. *Trends Genet.* **2014**, *30*, 271–286.

152. Braidy, N.; Jayasena, T.; Poljak, A.; Sachdev, P.S. Sirtuins in cognitive ageing and Alzheimer's disease. *Curr. Opin. Psychiatry* **2012**, *25*, 226–230.

153. Lu, T.; Aron, L.; Zullo, J.; Pan, Y.; Kim, H.; Chen, Y.; Yang, T.H.; Kim, H.M.; Drake, D.; Liu, X.S.; *et al.* REST and stress resistance in ageing and Alzheimer's disease. *Nature* **2014**, *507*, 448–454.

154. Harrington, A.J.; Yacoubian, T.A.; Slone, S.R.; Caldwell, K.A.; Caldwell, G.A. Functional analysis of VPS41-mediated neuroprotection in Caenorhabditis elegans and mammalian models of Parkinson's disease. *J. Neurosci.* **2012**, *32*, 2142–2153.

155. Salminen, A.; Kaarniranta, K.; Kauppinen, A.; Ojala, J.; Haapasalo, A.; Soininen, H.; Hiltunen, M. Impaired autophagy and APP processing in Alzheimer's disease: The potential role of Beclin 1 interactome. *Prog. Neurobiol.* **2013**, *106–107*, 33–54.

156. Morizane, A.; Doi, D.; Kikuchi, T.; Okita, K.; Hotta, A.; Kawasaki, T.; Hayashi, T.; Onoe, H.; Shiina, T.; Yamanaka, S.; *et al.* Direct Comparison of Autologous and Allogeneic Transplantation of iPSC-Derived Neural Cells in the Brain of a Nonhuman Primate. *Stem Cell Rep.* **2013**, *1*, 283–292.

157. Doi, D.; Samata, B.; Katsukawa, M.; Kikuchi, T.; Morizane, A.; Ono, Y.; Sekiguchi, K.; Nakagawa, M.; Parmar, M.; Takahashi, J. Isolation of human induced pluripotent stem cell-derived dopaminergic progenitors by cell sorting for successful transplantation. *Stem Cell Rep.* **2014**, *2*, 337–350.

iPSC-Based Models to Unravel Key Pathogenetic Processes Underlying Motor Neuron Disease Development

Irene Faravelli, Emanuele Frattini, Agnese Ramirez, Giulia Stuppia, Monica Nizzardo and Stefania Corti

Abstract: Motor neuron diseases (MNDs) are neuromuscular disorders affecting rather exclusively upper motor neurons (UMNs) and/or lower motor neurons (LMNs). The clinical phenotype is characterized by muscular weakness and atrophy leading to paralysis and almost invariably death due to respiratory failure. Adult MNDs include sporadic and familial amyotrophic lateral sclerosis (sALS-fALS), while the most common infantile MND is represented by spinal muscular atrophy (SMA). No effective treatment is ccurrently available for MNDs, as for the vast majority of neurodegenerative disorders, and cures are limited to supportive care and symptom relief. The lack of a deep understanding of MND pathogenesis accounts for the difficulties in finding a cure, together with the scarcity of reliable *in vitro* models. Recent progresses in stem cell field, in particular in the generation of induced Pluripotent Stem Cells (iPSCs) has made possible for the first time obtaining substantial amounts of human cells to recapitulate *in vitro* some of the key pathogenetic processes underlying MNDs. In the present review, recently published studies involving the use of iPSCs to unravel aspects of ALS and SMA pathogenesis are discussed with an overview of their implications in the process of finding a cure for these still orphan disorders.

Reprinted from *J. Clin. Med.* Cite as: Faravelli, I.; Frattini, E.; Ramirez, A.; Stuppia, G.; Nizzardo, M.; Corti, S. iPSC-Based Models to Unravel Key Pathogenetic Processes Underlying Motor Neuron Disease Development. *J. Clin. Med.* **2014**, *3*, 1124–1145.

1. Introduction

Motor Neuron Diseases (MNDs) are incurable neurological disorders characterized by the progressive loss of pyramidal cells in the primary motor cortex (upper motor neurons, UMNs) and/or cells in the anterior horns of the spinal cord and their homologues in the motor nuclei of the brainstem (lower motor neurons, LMNs). Concerning their epidemiology, the prevalence of MNDs accounts for about 5–7 cases in every 100,000 people, with an annual incidence of approximately two new cases per 100,000 people [1]. MNDs are not equally distributed between genders, being more common in males, with a male to female ratio of 2:1 [1]. There is a great variability in life expectancy of patients affected by MNDs, for reasons that remain unknown for the most part: death usually occurs within 3–5 years after the onset of symptoms (such as for amyotrophic lateral sclerosis—ALS), but cases with either a slower (*i.e.*, spinobulbar muscular atrophy—SBMA) or a more rapid course have been described (*i.e.*, spinal muscular atrophy—SMA type 1) [2].

The biological substrate of MNDs is responsible for the extremely disabling clinical phenotype, characterized by progressive weakness with muscle wasting, eventually leading to paralysis and death, mostly secondary to respiratory insufficiency [3]. No effective therapy is currently available and the only possible treatments are limited to palliative care. Besides affecting life expectancy,

MNDs highly impact on patients' quality of life: they are usually dependent on the use of respiratory aids and wheelchairs, requiring 24-h assistance [4].

MNDs are usually differentiated relating to the subset of motor neurons that are mainly involved in the disease course. Upper motor neurons are especially affected in primary lateral sclerosis (PLS) and hereditary spastic paraplegias (HSP). On the other hand, SMA, progressive muscular atrophy (PMA), SBMA and hereditary motor neuropathies (HMNs) involve mainly lower motor neurons.

ALS is the most common adult form of MND, characterized by the simultaneous degeneration of UMNs and LMNs. ALS can be divided into a sporadic form (sALS), representing 90%–95% of all cases, and a familial form (fALS), accounting for the remaining 5%–10% of cases [5]. It is well accepted that genetic factors play a determinant role also in the sporadic ALS cases [6]. The sporadic form presents a rather uniform distribution in Western countries: in Europe and North America, the incidence is 1.5–2.7 cases per 100,000 persons every year [5], with a prevalence of 2.7–7.4 cases per 100,000 persons [7]. The incidence increases considerably every decade of life, reaching a peak at 74 years of age, and then progressively decreases [8]. The lifetime risk to develop ALS is 1:350 for males and 1:400 for females [9]. The age of onset is around 50–60 years, and the mean survival of ALS patients is 2–3 years after the diagnosis. 5%–10% of patients affected by ALS have a familial history of MNDs (fALS), in most cases presenting a mendelian autosomal dominant pattern of inheritance [6]. The clinical phenotype of fALS is usually considered indistinguishable from sALS. Nevertheless, fALS is characterized by an equal male to female ratio, a more precocious age of onset and, oftentimes, a longer life expectancy. At present, more than 16 loci have been associated with ALS or other atypical forms of MNDs, and two loci have been associated to ALS with frontotemporal dementia (ALS-FTD) [6]. In about 60% of fALS patients, a causative gene can be identified. Mutations of *C9ORF72* are found in 40% of cases, followed by mutations of superoxide dismutase-1 (*SOD1*) (20% of cases), *TARDBP* (4% of cases), *FUS* (4% of cases) and other genes [10].

The group of SMAs comprises a series of LMN disorders characterized by extreme heterogeneity in both clinical presentation and genetic condition.

The most prevalent forms of SMAs go under the name of "Proximal Spinal Muscular Atrophy", often referred to simply as "SMA", and are caused by genetic mutations on chromosome 5q (hence the term "5q-SMA"). SMA is the most common MND during childhood: with an incidence of 1:6000–1:10,000 live births and a carrier frequency of 1:40–1:60, it is the leading genetic cause of infantile mortality [11,12]. SMA selectively affects LMNs, being characterized by the degeneration of alpha MNs in the ventral horns of the spinal cord and MNs in the motor nuclei of cranial nerves in the brainstem. SMA patients exhibit a progressive and symmetric involvement of various muscle groups, which present hypotonic, hyposthenic and atrophic, with a preferential distribution in the proximal compartments of the lower limb. Based on the degree of severity of the disease, different forms of SMA can be identified (types I–IV). Children with type I SMA, the most severe and common form, are affected at birth or, at the latest, by the age of 6 months, thus never becoming able to sit [13]. The other types of SMA present a progressively milder phenotype. Life expectancy is extremely variable in the spectrum of the different forms of the disease, ranging from less than 2 years of age in type I, to an unaffected lifespan in type IV. The genetic condition accounting for the disease displays homozygous deletions or mutations of the survival motor neuron (*SMN*) gene mapped in 5q11.2–q13.3 [14]. In the human genome, two almost identical copies of *SMN* are localized on chromosome 5q13: the telomeric *SMN1* gene and its inverted centromeric homologue *SMN2*. *SMN2* only differs from *SMN1* for five base pair changes, of which a C to T substitution at +6 of exon 7 (c.840C > T) is the only nucleotide change in the coding region [15]. This is localized in an exonic splicing enhancer, thus causing an alternative splicing of *pre*-mRNA of *SMN2* that excludes exon 7 from the majority of *SMN2* transcripts. The result is the production of 10%–50% of the full-length functional protein and 50%–90% of a truncated, non-functional and unstable transcript (SMNΔ7) [16]. All individuals affected by SMA retain a variable number of copies of *SMN2*, which correlates to the severity of the disease. The exact functions of the SMN protein, as much as the reasons accounting for the disruption of MNs in SMA, are yet to be fully disclosed.

Further, less common forms of SMAs recognize defects in genes other than *SMN1* and present with early denervation weakness, but different clinical symptoms than those stated above, including joint contractures (infantile SMA with arthrogryposis—XL-SMA), distal rather than proximal weakness (distal SMA or HMNs), diaphragmatic paralysis (SMA with respiratory distress 1—SMARD1), and pontocerebellar degeneration (SMA with pontocerebellar hypoplasia—SMA-PCH) [17,18].

The inaccessibility to the cell type of interest majorly involved in MNDs and the lack of established models for the elucidation of pathogenetic mechanisms underlying such disorders represent a fundamental obstacle for progresses to be made in the field of therapies development. In order to resolve these issues and make durable discoveries, new strategies should be taken into account. In this respect, stem cell technology may represent a valuable solution.

Induced pluripotent stem cells (iPSCs) are originated from patients' differentiated cells (oftentimes fibroblasts) through the use of reprogramming factors, first identified by Yamanaka in 2006 [19]. IPSCs are able to differentiate towards cell types of the three germ layers *in vitro* and give rise to teratomas *in vivo*. They can be identified with stem cell markers and resemble embryonic stem cells (ESCs) both in morphology and behaviour, but they are not burdened by ethical concerns [20]. IPSCs are patients' specific cells, thus avoiding more likely immunoreactions if transplantation strategies were taken into account. Moreover, iPSCs can be produced in substantial amounts, providing an optimal cell source for regenerative therapeutic approaches. The possibility of differentiating iPSCs towards any cell type of interest represents a great advantage in the context of MNDs, which affect MNs rather selectively [21]. Indeed, in recent years, protocols for the differentiation of iPSCs towards MNs have been developed and optimized, since obtaining human relevant cells appears pivotal for the development of *in vitro* models that recapitulate mechanisms responsible for the establishment of pathologies [21]. Obtained results could be crucial in guiding the process of finding an effective treatment for ALS, SMA and other MNDs. Fibroblasts can be easily obtained from skin biopsies and grown in culture, thus making the premises for a simple disease model [22]. Furthermore, MNDs with a genetic background may benefit from *in vitro* models obtained from iPSC-derived differentiated cells, like iPSC-MNs, exhibiting the affected genotype peculiar to the disease. So far, the great potential of iPSCs led to the generation of patient-specific cells for several neurodegenerative disorders, including Alzheimer's Disease [23], Huntington's Disease [24], Parkinson's Disease [25] and Amyotrophic Lateral Sclerosis [26]. These considerations suggest that iPSCs could be the key to unravel pathogenetic processes behind human diseases which are challenging to study in the animal models for their specific features (Figure 1). Obtained results may pave the way to the development of effective treatments targeting specific disease mechanisms. Here, we review the recent advances in the field of iPSCs as regards their use in modeling and studying MNDs, with a focus on ALS and SMA pathogenesis.

Figure 1. iPSC-based platforms for motor neuron disease modeling. Patients-derived somatic cells can be reprogrammed into iPSCs. Obtained cells can be differentiated towards the subtype of interest and studied in their development. Further analyses include the investigation of the transcriptional profile and the elucidation of molecular pathogenetic pathways. Human iPSCs are also a valuable tool for the identification of molecular targets and the screening of potential therapeutic compounds.

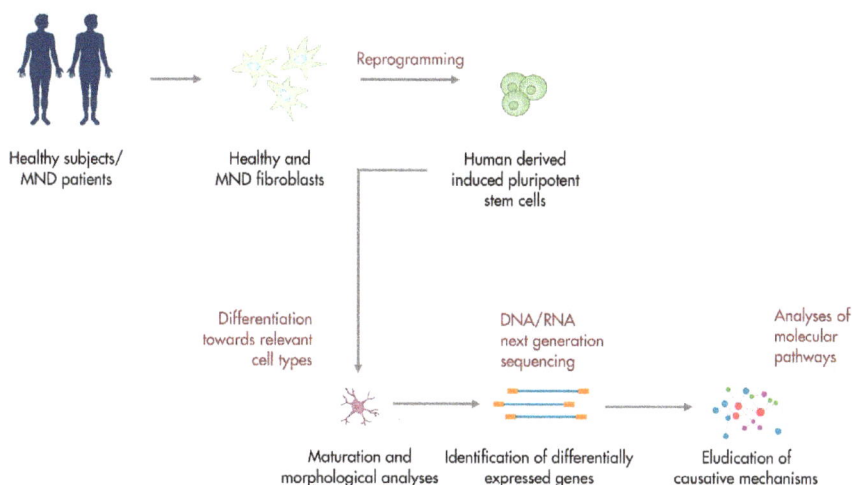

2. Modeling and Studying Amyotrophic Lateral Sclerosis Using IPSCs

Amyotrophic lateral sclerosis (ALS) is a fatal neurodegenerative disease with adult onset. Symptoms reflect the dysfunction and death of motor neurons (MNs) and are characterized by muscular weakness and atrophy progressively leading to paralysis [27]. Upper and lower MNs appear to be particularly vulnerable to the disease process since they are the most relevant affected cells in the context of a relative sparing of other neuronal populations [28]. Also among MNs, specific subtypes of differently affected cells can be identified: oculomotor and Onuf's nucleus MNs proved to be much more resistant to the disease process [29]. Reasons accounting for the selective vulnerability of MN populations and, in general, for mechanisms of neurodegeneration remain poorly understood. Several pathogenetic mechanisms have been taken into consideration, including impaired RNA metabolism, aberrant proteic misfolding, mitochondrial alterations, defective axonal transport, excitotoxicity and local inflammation [30,31]. The discovery of causative genes has given new inputs to the field. After the first report of ALS causative mutations in the gene encoding the Cu/Zn-dependent antioxidant enzyme superoxide dismutase-1 (*SOD1*) [32], researchers have started to investigate non cell-autonomous mechanisms linked to the development of ALS disease (*i.e.*, the role of the oxidative damage). The identification of *C9ORF72* repeat expansion as the major factor responsible for ALS onset in the familial forms has focused attention on the causative role of alterations in RNA metabolism [33–35], a line of research supported also by the involvement of mutations in *TARDBP* and *FUS* genes (encoding DNA/RNA binding proteins) in ALS development [36].

The establishment of human cell platforms has allowed for the first time to test *in vitro* some of these pathogenetic hypotheses and to model and investigate early disease mechanisms. Eggan's group pioneered the field in 2008, when they investigated the potential of human MNs derived from embryonic stem cells (ESCs) to provide key data on ALS pathogenesis [37]. ESC-derived human MNs were cultured on primary cortical glia obtained from *SOD1* mutated mice. After 10 days in culture, a significant decrease in MN number could be observed in a time-dependent manner, thus suggesting a strong implication of non-cell autonomous mechanisms in ALS onset. Moreover, they tested if the same toxic glial effect could be detected with human interneurons and they found that the glia-induced toxicity is rather specific for MNs: interneurons treated for 20 days with *SOD1G93A* glia-conditioned medium appeared fully preserved. Complementary, MNs co-cultured with *SOD1G93A* mouse embryonic fibroblasts remained unaffected, thus indicating that the toxic effect is specifically related to the presence of astrocytes. Oligonucleotide arrays were exploited to identify genes differentially expressed in mutant glia. After these analyses, Di Giorgio and colleagues focused their investigation on the role of prostaglandin D2, which resulted responsible for a significant decrease of MN survival in culture. This work proved the advantages to use human cells for *in vitro* disease studies and provided the basis for further investigations on ALS pathogenesis.

The same research group proceeded beyond these results with a recent study aiming to elucidate pathways which are impaired by the expression of mutated *SOD1* in human MNs [26]. Kiskinis and colleagues derived iPSCs from skin fibroblasts of ALS patients; these cells harbored the patient-specific genetic combination, thus providing a precious tool to model the development of human pathology. Human iPSCs were differentiated towards MNs and compared with two healthy human iPSC lines. Diseased MN number decreased in culture in a time-dependent manner, a process that did not affect the non-motor neuronal cells present in the plate. Both control and *SOD1* iPSC lines presented a further reduced survival when co-cultured with *SOD1* glia, but this effect was much more amplified in the latter case implying the presence of a strong cell-autonomous component in ALS pathology. *SOD1* MNs presented also an unhealthy morphology with shorter processes and reduced soma, thus summarizing the changes observed in the human pathology. Importantly, ZFN-mediated gene correction of *SOD1* mutation resulted in the rescue of both altered morphology and reduced lifespan. Data from RNA-seq of *SOD1* MNs highlighted a strong down-regulation of genes related to mitochondria functions and protein translation. Further analyses showed impairment in mitochondria motility in addition to an enrichment of mitochondria number located in neuronal processes. A substrate of ER stress has been found in healthy human MNs, which could be related to the cell size; this result is in line with the well-known early degeneration of largest alpha MNs in ALS. A combination of oxidative and ER stress and the up-regulation of the unfolded protein response (UPR) have been shown and could be additive causative mechanisms of neuronal toxicity. Moreover, the electrical activity of MNs could be involved in the ER stress, a result which nicely correlates with the report of the intrinsic hyperexcitability displayed by iPSCs-derived MNs from ALS patients [38]. Finally, comparison between human-iPSCs derived *C9ORF72* and *SOD1* lines led to the discovery of common pathways downstream of these mutations related to enhanced oxidative stress response and decreased mitochondria activity.

C9ORF72 iPSC lines were obtained by Sareen *et al.* to investigate the pathological processes underlying the most common genetic form of ALS [39]. They investigated whether the toxicity linked to the repeat expansion in *C9ORF72* was due to either gain of function or loss of function or both mechanisms. To address this question, iPSCs lines were developed from different *C9ORF72* hexanucleotide expansion carriers affected by ALS and/or frontotemporal lobar degeneration (FTLD). Southern blot analyses were performed on derived MNs assessing the expansion and also highlighting differences among patients, which in some cases could be reflected in more severe forms of the disease. FISH analyses detected the presence of RNA foci within *C9ORF72*-ALS MNs (and also in the neuronal progenitors and astrocytes), in line with previous data from patients' tissues [40]. Observed RNA foci co-localized with Pur-alpha and hnRNAP1 but not with FUS or TDP43, responsible for other genetic forms of ALS. However, hnRNAP1 is known to interact with TDP43 [41] and its involvement in the disease process could suggest an indirect connection between *C9ORF72* and TDP43 ALS forms. This work provided data in the direction of a "gain of function" mechanism linked to *C9ORF72* hexanucleotide expansion. It has been shown that the mutated allele is usually transcribed and its downregulation using antisense oligonucleotides did not affect cell viability, but resulted in the correction of cell transcriptional profile. The specific pathogenetic role of the involvement of different RNA binding proteins interacting with RNA foci needs further investigations and could represent a common causative mechanism shared by different forms of ALS. Indeed, the aberrant cytoplasmatic aggregation of TDP43 represents a rather common pathological hallmark both in familial and sporadic ALS. Processes leading from the cytoplasmic aggregation to the selective MN loss appear to be exquisitely human and not easily detectable in animal models, where overexpression of TDP43 is ubiquitously provoked. Indeed, the majority of cell platforms and animal models considered in ALS pathogenesis studies relied on the overexpression of TDP43 in nonhuman or nonneuronal cells. Reason underlying the selective vulnerability of MNs to the disease process could be misled as well as the investigation of key molecular events that cause the human disease [40]. The establishment of human iPSC-derived platforms has allowed significant advances in the field. Bilican *et al.* generated iPSCs from a patient affected by ALS carrying the TDP43 M337V mutation and used them as a tool to investigate TDP43 pathology in human neuronal cells [42]. No differences in the differentiation and maturation towards a motor neuronal fate could be observed between TDP43-iPSCs and healthy controls. However, affected MNs presented reduced survival in culture and higher levels of soluble and detergent-resistant TDP43, probably due to an alteration in post-translational mechanisms. Interestingly, mutant MNs appeared to be vulnerable to PI3K inhibition, while they were not affected by inhibitors of other kinase pathways. This suggests also a specificity in the neuronal response to different neurotrophic factors involved in PI3K rather than MAPK pathways. The role of neurotrophines in the survival of TDP43 MNs is worthy of further investigation and this work opened up the path to the use of TDP43-ALS patients' iPSCs as a valid disease model.

Alami *et al.* proceeded beyond these data to elucidate the role of TDP43 in physiological conditions and its impairment in ALS related disease [43]. Using at first a Drosophila model, they discovered that TDP43 cytoplasmatic granules are motile and dynamically transported along axons. Further studies in murine cortical neurons showed that this transport is microtubule-dependent and resulted in impaired in TPD43 mutated neurons, where granules appeared more immotile and often reversed direction. Other forms of axonal transport, such as mitochondria movement, were unaffected, thus suggesting a selective function and, consequently, alteration of TDP43 granules. These granules were found to be directly involved in the transport of specific mRNAs, such as Neurofilament-L (NEFL) mRNA, along the axons. To avoid influences related to the overexpression of TDP43 in the animal models, these results needed to be validated in patients' iPSC-derived MNs. NEFL transport was analyzed in iPSC-MNs derived from patients carrying the same mutations studied in Drosophila and murine neurons (M337V and A315T) plus G298S. An impairment of the anterograde transport of NEFL granules was demonstrated together with an increase of retrograde movement. It is also important to highlight that TDP43 domain affected by the mutation is a prion-like domain known to be involved in the assembly of RNA granules. This study provided important data on a physiological function of TDP43 cytoplasmatic granules and how their impairment could significantly contribute to ALS pathology.

Neurofilament aggregation is a well-known pathological hallmark of ALS. Thanks to iPSC-based technology, Chen *et al.* could investigate the causative role of mutant *SOD1* in impairing neurofilament (NF) turnover within MNs [44]. To bypass concerns related to heterogeneity among individuals, they generated ALS patients' iPSCs and used transcription activator-like effector nucleases (TALEN) technology to correct the *D90ASOD1* mutation, thus obtaining isogenic controls. A modified differentiation protocol was applied to originate synchronized mature cells avoiding the generation of later-born MNs or glial cells.

Indeed, challenges that need to be overcome when producing iPSC-derived neurons involve both the generation of immature cells and significant differences in the time rate of differentiation among iPSC colonies. These issues could lead to the production of heterogonous populations in terms of neural differentiated phenotype. The optimization of differentiation protocols has allowed generating neural cell populations that are synchronized regarding their growth in culture, in order to properly observe and investigate all the phases of their development [42].

NF subunits in ALS-MNs appeared to be unbalanced and developed a tendency to aggregate leading to neurite degeneration, an effect that probably interests the early phases of the disease *in vivo* when patients present phenotypically asymptomatic or with very mild symptoms. This effect was due to the presence of mutated *SOD1*, as demonstrated by gain of function and loss of function experiments. Further analyses revealed that binding of *SOD1* to 3' UTR of NF-L mRNA could cause the alteration of NF structure, making them prone to aggregate. These events were selectively present in ALS-MNs and not in control cells or non-MNs. Moreover, human ALS MNs presented *in vitro* lower/normal levels of *SOD1* (and increased amount of NF) compared to control MNs, strongly contrasting data from animal models where mutant *SOD1* levels are much higher.

Overall, these results highlight the importance of validating data obtained from animal models in human cells and using them as a precious tool to elucidate mechanisms which are peculiar of human physiology and pathology. The identification of the mechanisms underlying the development of ALS is crucial for the discovery of new therapeutic compounds. Indeed, the elucidation of the role of misregulated neurofilament turnover [44], granular impaired trafficking [43] rather than the mitochondrial dysfunction [26], together with other recent discoveries [45], may be a key moment in the identification of specific molecular targets for the development of effective therapies. Most likely, an effective therapeutic approach should be as comprehensive as possible to counteract the multiple aspects of ALS multifactorial pathogenesis. Certainly, the use of human cells for disease modeling *in vitro* has provided crucial data for this purpose (Table 1). The optimization of iPSC-based platforms can also represent an effective tool for *in vitro* screening of potential therapeutic compounds previously identified [46]. Finally, it is worth mentioning that Kondo *et al.* reported very recently how local transplants of human iPSC-derived glial-rich neural progenitors (hiPSC-GRNPs) were able to reduce MN degeneration and increase lifespan in a murine model of mutant *SOD1* ALS [47]. ALS astrocytes are known to contribute to neuroinflammation and neuronal death within the spinal cord.

Table 1. iPSC-Based studies on amyotrophic lateral sclerosis/spinal muscular atrophy (ALS/SMA) pathogenesis.

Reference	Cells	Reprogramming Method	Differentiation Protocol	Mechanism
Di Giorgio *et al.* 2008 [37]	Human ESC-derived MNs	-	Human ESC media without FGF2 or plasmanate + RA (Sigma) (1 µM) and an agonist of the SHH signaling pathway (1 µM) in N2 media: 1:1 DMEM:F12 + Glutamate (Gibco), penicillin (10,000 units) and streptomycin (Gibco) (1 mg/mL), N2 Supplement (Gibco) (1%), AA (Sigma-Aldrich) (0.2 mM), D-(+)-Glucose (Sigma-Aldrich) (0.16%), BDNF (R&D) (10 ng/mL), for 14 days.	MNs co-cultured with *SOD1G93A* astrocytes undergo cell death. Prostaglandin D2 is responsible for the decrease in MN survival.
Kiskinis *et al.* 2014 [26]	Fibroblasts from *SOD1A4V* ALS patients → iPSC-derived MNs	Retroviral transduction (KLF4, SOX2, OCT4, and c-MYC)	DMEM/F12, KSR (15%) on days 1–4; DMEM/F12 with L-glutamine, NEAAs, HE (2 µg/mL), N2 supplement (Gibco) on days 5–24; SB431542 (Sigma) (10 µM) + DM (Segment) (1 µM) on days 1–6; BDNF (R&D) (10 ng/mL), AA (Sigma) (0.4 mg/mL), RA (Sigma) (1 µM) and SAG 1.3 (Calbiochem) (1 µM) on days 5–24.	*SOD1* iPSCs and MNs suffer a reduction in survival when co-cultured with *SOD1* glia. *SOD1* MNs exhibit shorter processes and reduced soma. Gene correction of *SOD1* mutation rescues both morphology and survival. *SOD1* MNs show a down-regulation of genes implied in mitochondria homeostasis. Oxidative and ER stress and the up-regulation of UPR may contribute to neuronal toxicity. *C9ORF72* and *SOD1* MNs share common disrupted pathways leading to enhanced oxidative stress response and decreased mitochondria activity.

Table 1. *Cont.*

Reference	Cells	Reprogramming Method	Differentiation Protocol	Mechanism
Sareen *et al.* 2013 [39]	Fibroblasts from *C9ORF72* ALS patients → iPSC-derived MNs	Episomal plasmid nucleofection (OCT4, SOX2, KLF4, L-MYC, LIN28, and p53 shRNA)	IMDM supplemented with B27-vitamin A (2%) and N2 (1%) on days 1–6; addition of all-trans RA (0.1 μM) on days 6–25; Neurobasal, B27 (2%) and N2 (1%) + RA (0.1 μM) and PMN (1 μM) on days 17–25; DMEM/F12, B27 (2%), RA (0.1 μM), PMN (1 μM), db-cAMP (1 μM), AA (200 ng/mL), BDNF (10 ng/mL), and GDNF (10 ng/mL) for a further 2–7 weeks; Chemically defined medium supplemented with SB431542 (Tocris) (10 μM), DM (Calbiochem) (2.5 μM), and NAC (Sigma) (0.5 μM) for 5–7 days; chemically defined medium with RA (Sigma) (0.1 μM) for 7–12 days;	RNA foci in *C9ORF72* MNs co-localize with hnRNAP1, suggesting an indirect connection between *C9ORF72* and TDP43 ALS forms. The toxicity linked to *C9ORF72* hexanucleotide expansion may be due to a "gain of function" mechanism. The downregulation of the mutated allele with antisense oligonucleotides corrects the cell transcriptional profile. TDP43 MNs present a reduced survival in culture and high levels of TDP43 due to aberrant post-translational mechanisms.
Bilican *et al.* 2012 [42]	Fibroblasts from TDP43 M337V ALS patients → iPSC-derived MNs	Retroviral transduction (KLF4, SOX2, OCT4, and c-MYC)	Neurobasal medium (Invitrogen), RA (0.1 μM), PMN (Calbiochem) (1 μM), N2 supplement (Invitrogen) (1%), NEAAs (Invitrogen) (1%), penicillin/streptomycin (Invitrogen) (1%), GlutaMAX (Invitrogen) (1%), and basic FGF (5 ng/mL) for 7–10 days; Neurobasal medium (Invitrogen), N2 supplement (Invitrogen) (0.5%), NBAAs (Invitrogen) (1%), penicillin/streptomycin (Invitrogen) (1%), GlutaMAX (Invitrogen) (0.5%), BDNF (PeproTech) (10 ng/mL), GDNF (PeproTech) (10 ng/mL), and F (Tocris) (10 μM) for 3–6 weeks.	Neuronal response to neurotrophic factors involved in PI3K pathways influences TDP43 MN survival.

Table 1. *Cont.*

Reference	Cells	Reprogramming Method	Differentiation Protocol	Mechanism
Alami *et al.* 2014 [43]	Fibroblasts from TDP43 A315T and TPD43 G298S ALS patients → iPSC-derived MNs	Retroviral transduction (OCT4, SOX2, and KLF4)	KSR medium (KO-DMEM (Life Technologies) supplemented with KSR (Life Technologies) (15%), 1 × Gibco GlutaMAX (Life Technologies) and NEAAs (100 μM) on days 0–10; N2 medium (Neurobasal (Life Technologies)) supplemented with 1 × N2 (Life Technologies), 1X Gibco GlutaMAX (Life Technologies) and NEAAs (100 μM) on days 4–14; SB431542 (Sigma) (10 μM) and LDN-193189 (Segment) (100 nM) on days 0–5; RA (Sigma) (1 μM), SAG (EMD Millipore) (1 μM), DAPT (EMD Millipore) (5 μM) and SU-5402 (Biovision) (4 μM) on days 2–14; murine glia-conditioned N2 medium supplemented with 1 × B-27 (Life Technologies), and BDNF (10 ng/mL), GDNF (10 ng/mL) and CNTF (R&D) (10 ng/mL).	The microtubule-dependent transport of NEFL mRNA granules along the axon is impaired in TDP43 MNs. TDP43 domain affected by the mutation is involved in the assembly of RNA granules.
Chen *et al.* 2014 [44]	Fibroblasts from *SOD1A4V* and *SOD1D90A* ALS patients → iPSC-derived MNs	Non-integrating Sendai virus transduction (OCT3/4, SOX2, KLF4, and c-MYC)	DMEM/F12, N2 supplement, NEAAs, SB431542 (2 μM), LDN193189 (300 nM), and CHIR99021 (3 μM, all from Stemgent, Cambridge, MA, USA) on days 1–7; addition of RA (0.1 μM) and PMN (0.5 μM) on days 8–14; DMEM/F12, N2 supplement, and NEAAs on days 14–21.	Binding of *SOD1* to 3' UTR of NF-L mRNA may be responsible for neurofilament tendency to aggregate leading to neurite degeneration. Unlike mice *SOD1* MNs, human *SOD1* MNs have lower or normal levels of *SOD1* compared to control MNs.

Table 1. *Cont.*

Reference	Cells	Reprogramming Method	Differentiation Protocol	Mechanism
Ebert *et al.* 2009 [48]	Fibroblasts from a *SMN1* SMA type I patient → iPSC-derived MNs	Lentiviral transduction (OCT4, SOX2, NANOG, and LIN28)	NIM (1:1 DMEM/F12 and N2 supplement (Gibco) (1%)) supplemented with RA (0.1 μM) for 1 week; addition of SHH (R&D) (100 ng/mL) for 1 week; RA and SHH medium supplemented with cAMP (1 mM), AA (200 ng/mL), BDNF and GDNF (both 10 ng/mL, PeproTech Inc., Rocky Hill, USA) for 2–6 weeks.	SMA iPSCs show reduced levels of SMN full-length transcripts, due to *SMN1* loss, and a few truncated transcripts lacking exon 7. After a robust production, SMA iPSC-derived MNs undergo a reduction in number and size compared to WT iPSC-derived MNs. MN ontogenesis in SMA is disrupted by post-development damage.
Sareen *et al.* 2012 [49]	Fibroblasts from a *SMN1* SMA type I patient → iPSC-derived MNs	Episomal plasmid nucleofection (OCT4, SOX2, NANOG, and LIN28)	Stemln Neural Expansion Media (Sigma) supplemented with EGF (100 g/mL), FGF-2 (100 ng/mL), and HE (5 μg/mL) for 3 weeks; NIM (1:1 DMEM/F12 and N2 (1%)) in the presence of all-trans RA (0.1 μM) for 1 week; addition of PMN (1 μM) or SHH (10 ng/mL) for 1–3 weeks	SMA MNs show increased levels of cleaved caspase-3 and caspase-8 and membrane-bound Fas ligand, suggesting that apoptosis is implied in MN dysfunction and loss in SMA. The administration of Anti Fas-Ab rescues MN survival in *in vitro* models of SMA.
Corti *et al.* 2012 [20]	Fibroblasts from *SMN1* SMA type I patients → iPSC-derived MNs	Episomal plasmid nucleofection (OCT4, SOX2, NANOG, LIN28, c-MYC, and KLF4)	DMEM/F12 (Gibco, Invitrogen), supplemented with MEM NEAAs solution, N2, and HE (Sigma-Aldrich) (2 mg/mL) for 10 days; addition of RA (Sigma-Aldrich) (0.1 μM) for 7 days; same medium with RA (0.1 μM) and SHH (R&D) (100–200 ng/mL) for 7 days; addition of BDNF, GDNF, and IGF-1 (PeproTech) (10 ng/mL) on day 24.	SMA MNs show a reduction in size, axonal elongation, neuromuscular junction production and overall decreased survival. SMA MNs exhibit a different splicing profile in a subset of genes encoding proteins involved in RNA metabolism, MN differentiation, axonal guidance and signal transduction. Gene correction of *SMN2* with antisense oligodeoxynucleotides rescues the cellular damage and the altered splicing profile secondary to *SMN1* deficiency *in vitro*.

Table 1. *Cont.*

Reference	Cells	Reprogramming Method	Differentiation Protocol	Mechanism
McGivern *et al.* 2013 [50]	Fibroblasts from *SMN1* SMA patients → iPSC-derived glia	Lentiviral transduction (OCT4, SOX2, NANOG, and LIN28); Episomal plasmid nucleofection (OCT4, SOX2, NANOG, LIN28)	Human neural progenitor growth medium (Stemline, Sigma-Aldrich) supplemented with basic FGF-2 (Chemicon) (100 ng/mL), EGF (Chemicon) (100 ng/mL), and HE (Sigma-Aldrich) (5 μg/mL); DMEM: Nutrient Mixture F12 (Invitrogen) supplemented with B27 (Invitrogen) (2%) with or without CNTF for 2–8 weeks.	SMA astrocytes show increased basal calcium levels with a minimal response to ATP and an activated state that precedes MN loss. The ERK apoptosis pathways of SMA MNs may be initiated by the defective calcium homeostasis and the deficiency of trophic factors.

AA = Ascorbic Acid; BDNF = Brain-Derived Neurotrophic Factor; cAMP = cyclic Adenosine MonoPhosphate; CNTF = Ciliary Neurotrophic Factor; DAPT = Difluorophenacetyl-Alanyl-Phenylglycine-T-butyl ester; DM = Dorsomorphin; DMEM = Dulbecco's Modified Eagle Medium; EGF = Epidermal Growth Factor; F = Forskolin; FGF-2 = Fibroblasts Growth Factor-2; GDNF = Glial cell line-Derived Neurotrophic Factor; HE = Heparin; IGF-1 = Insulin-like Growth Factor-1; IMDM = Iscove's Modified Dulbecco's Medium; KSR = Knock-out Serum Replacement; NAC = *N*-Acetyl-Cysteine; NEAAs = Non-Essential Amino Acids; NIM = Neural Induction Medium; PMN = Purmorphamine; RA = Retinoic Acid; SAG = Smoothened Agonist; SHH = Sonic Hedgehog.

HiPSC-GRNPs represent a renewable source of autologous cells able to give rise to healthy astrocytes, which can provide trophic support to endogenous diseased MNs. Kondo and colleagues observed an improvement of ALS pathology even when hiPSC-GRNPs were transplanted after the disease onset (the most probable clinical setting) thus providing evidence that glia cells could play a major role in ALS pathogenesis and, eventually, therapy.

3. Modeling and Studying Spinal Muscular Atrophy Using IPSCs

Ebert and Svendsen were the first authors to demonstrate that human iPSCs can be employed to recapitulate the specific pathology that underlies SMA [48]. Until then, the only models available for research purposes on the disease were provided by worms, flies and mice, which presented considerable limitations, including technical constraints like the necessity of performing complicated knockout strategies. Similarly, human fibroblasts did not prove to be suitable for the study of the disease mechanisms and the screening of new drug compounds, since the SMN protein presents features that are peculiar to neural line-belonging cells. Applying lentiviral infection methods, SMA iPSCs were generated from fibroblasts of a 3 years old boy affected by type I SMA. Wild-type (WT) iPSCs derived from fibroblasts of his unaffected mother served as controls. Through RT-PCR analysis, that was performed in both WT and SMA iPSCs and fibroblasts in order to assess SMN mRNA, WT-iPSCs turned out to have comparable levels of SMN to WT fibroblasts, while SMA iPSCs showed significantly reduced levels of SMN full-length transcripts, as a result of the loss of *SMN1* gene. RT-PCR analysis also detected a few truncated transcripts lacking exon 7, along with the full-length SMN transcripts, witnessing the maintenance of functional *SMN2* gene and its alternative splicing. Since lower alpha MNs are the main target of the pathological processes of SMA, iPSCs from SMA and WT fibroblasts were directed towards a motor neuronal and glial fate, in order to disclose in which phase of maturation the pathogenetic events occur. If in the early stages of the differentiation protocol a robust production of MNs was described and no significant difference was documented between the SMA- and WT-derived MNs, interestingly, around week 10 of the protocol, the SMA-derived MNs appeared to be decreased both from a quantitative and a qualitative point of view, as they were fewer and smaller compared to the WT-derived MNs. It was then speculated that the SMA phenotype hampers MN ontogenesis at later developmental time periods, either by inhibiting the generation of new cells or increasing the degeneration of those already matured. This was the first study to report that human iPSCs can be adopted as a reliable model of a genetically inherited disease, such as SMA, and serve as a powerful tool for a better understanding of its etiopathogenesis.

Sareen and Svendsen's group carried on the experiment for a more precise definition of the mechanisms that are responsible for the post-developmental damage that leads to cell death, as observed *in vitro* [49]. Sareen and colleagues generated two lines of iPSCs from two patients affected by SMA type I and one line of control iPSCs, and then differentiated them into MNs. The first results were consistent with the previous work: after a normal production of MNs at 4 weeks into the differentiation protocol, the cell population underwent a selective reduction in number and size compared to the control iPSC-derived MN cultures. The group ascribed this degeneration to the activation of apoptosis pathways, as suggested by the significantly high percentage of apoptotic cells after 7–10 weeks of differentiation. In particular, the assay of increased levels of apoptotic markers at 8 weeks of differentiation, namely cleaved caspase-3 and caspase-8, supported the assumption that apoptosis plays a crucial role in cell death in SMA iPSCs-derived MN cultures. The intracellular apoptotic signaling cascade is known to be initiated by caspase-8, triggered by the binding of Fas-ligands to their receptors (a TNF family transmembrane protein) [51]. This was confirmed by increased levels of membrane-bound Fas ligand in SMA MNs after 6 weeks of differentiation. The next step was to evaluate whether the inhibition of the Fas-receptor apoptotic pathway could rescue the degeneration of MNs in the SMA lines: the administration of a monoclonal antibody targeting the Fas-receptor (Anti Fas-Ab), starting from the second week of differentiation and for the whole duration of the differentiation process, proved to significantly increase the number of MNs in SMA lines at 8 weeks of differentiation, compared to the untreated cultures [49]. Taken together, these data suggest that an iPSCs-based model of SMA not only may provide new insights on the molecular and pathological processes behind neuronal dysfunction and loss in SMA, but may also represent an invaluable testing ground for the screening and development of new drug compounds, that may eventually be beneficial for patients.

Another contribution to the knowledge on the pathogenic mechanisms of SMA was given by Corti and colleagues [20]. Using a viral- and transgene-free method, they reprogrammed fibroblasts of two type I SMA patients into iPSCs by nucleofecting them with plasmids encoding pluripotency factors (OCT4, SOX2, NANOG, LIN28, c-Myc, and KLF4). A parallel experiment was conducted on a subpopulation of the obtained iPSCs that were treated, and therefore genetically corrected, with *SMN2* sequence-specific oligodeoxynucleotides. The correction of SMA iPSCs consisted in the exchange of a T to C at position +6 of exon 7, thus converting *SMN2* into *SMN1* through the inclusion of exon 7 in SMN2 transcripts. Subsequently, the model required the differentiation of SMA fibroblasts-derived iPSCs, both treated and untreated, into MNs, the cell-type majorly involved in SMA, in order to evaluate the effects of *SMN1* deficiency on these cells. At week 8 of the multistage differentiation protocol, based on the administration of Retinoic Acid and Sonic Hedgehog, they observed specific disease effects of the *SMN1* defect on untreated SMA iPSCs-derived MNs compared to the cultures treated with oligodeoxynucleotides. The statistically significant alterations included an overall reduction in cell soma size, axonal elongation and in the ability to form neuromuscular junctions, resulting in a decreased survival of MNs derived from untreated iPSCs. This experiment well demonstrates that a SMA model reproducing at least some aspects of the disease can be generated, and that MN dysfunction in SMA is the result of multiple neuropathological events likely occurring at a late differentiative state. Genetic correction of *SMN2* via oligodeoxynucleotides proved to rescue the cellular damage to the defective *SMN1* gene and to significantly increase the number of detectable gems, nuclear aggregates of SMN protein which correlate with the rate of translation of the full-length protein.

Given the recent hypothesis on the role of RNA and splicing abnormalities as a primary determinant of selective MN death in SMA [52,53], the experiment was then directed to the analysis of transcriptional changes in untreated SMA iPSC-derived MNs compared to heterozygous iPSC- and treated SMA iPSC-MNs. Gene expression and exon array analysis of RNA revealed a different splicing profile in a subset of genes encoding transcripts that are considered to play a crucial role in SMA pathogenesis, being involved in RNA metabolism, MN differentiation, axonal guidance and signal transduction. Remarkably, the molecular correction with oligodeoxynuleotides proved to shift most of the genes that are differentially expressed or spliced in SMA iPSC-derived MNs towards the heterozygous pattern, further supporting the data on the efficacy of this strategy in correcting the alterations secondary to *SMN1* deficiency.

Following the hypothesis that a cell population other than MNs may be implied in the activation of the apoptotic cascade, the attention was then focused on glial cells. Indeed, astrocytes had already proved to contribute to MN dysfunction in *SOD1* mutated models of ALS [54,55] and to play a key role as mediators of neurodegeneration in a variety of nosological conditions, including Parkinson's disease [56]. In order to examine morphologic and functional alterations in glial sub-populations, Ebert's group differentiated human SMA-derived iPSCs and WT iPSCs into astrocytes [50], the most abundant cell type in the central nervous system, that are supposed to be responsible for the maintenance of the perfect environment for neurons' homeostasis [57]. They described an activated phenotype of SMA astrocytes, as shown by the intense cytoplasmic staining of Glial Fibrillary Protein (GFAP) and Nestin, two components of intermediate filament proteins that are upregulated in reactive glial cells. The activation state was accompanied by significant changes in astrocyte morphology, as they displayed enlarged bodies and thick, short processes. The observation that such alterations occur in the early stages of the differentiation protocol of SMA-derived iPSCs into astrocytes was crucial to infer that the MN loss is preceded by the activation of glial cells, suggesting a causal relationship between the two events. The alterations in the phenotype of astrocytes turned out to be the epiphenomenon of their functional impairments, as ratiometric live-cell calcium imaging reported increased basal calcium levels with a minimal response to ATP in SMA astrocytes compared to WT iPSCs-derived astrocytes. The authors concluded that the defective calcium homeostasis may lead to the activation of apoptotic pathways triggered by the upregulation of pERK1/2 in SMA iPSCs-derived astrocytes, and the resulting increased expression of proinflammatory cytokines like TNF-alpha, IL-1 and IL-6. The ERK programmed cell death cascade was speculated to be initiated also by the deficiency of trophic factors, as witnessed by a decrease in the secretion of Growth Derived Neurotrophic Factor (GDNF), and the whole apoptotic process was attributed to a Fas-mediated mechanism.

Overall, the possibility to isolate cell types that are specifically damaged in the disease process, like MNs and glia cells in SMA, makes iPSCs an unprecedented tool to disclose pathogenetic mechanisms that have been inaccessible so far (Table 1). Moreover, the establishment of reliable disease models is a fundamental milestone in the process of testing novel therapeutic strategies and finally finding a definitive treatment for SMA [58].

4. Discussion

The pathogenesis of several MNDs is still obscure under multiple aspects, thus hampering the development of potential therapies [2]. Experimental studies conducted on animal models are crucial, but unfortunately results so far are insufficient [2]. Concerning ALS research, it has been found the overexpression of *SOD1* which characterizes mutant *SOD1* mice may influence observed molecular phenotypes [59]. With regard to SMA, mice physiologically lack the homologous *SMN2* gene, which plays a crucial role in determining clinical phenotypes [60]. As a consequence, data derived from pathogenetic studies need to be validated in human cellular models. Human ESCs have been largely employed for this purpose [37,61], but their use may be limited by ethical issues. Moreover, ESCs are not always available in substantial amount for large scale *in vitro* studies. On the other hand, the development of iPSC-based technology has allowed to generate human pluripotent cells in abundance to perform any *in vitro* study bypassing ethical constraints [22]. Furthermore, a great advantage of iPSCs is that they carry the genetic combination of an individual, thus permitting the study of patient-specific mutations. Issues concerning the heterogeneity of iPSC lines, which could provide misleading results, may be overcome by a careful experimental setting. This should be based on rigorous statistical analysis and standardized protocols. Moreover, the use of cutting-edge molecular methods allows correcting the mutation in patient-derived iPSCs, thus obtaining isogenic controls [44]. Another critical issue is represented by reprogramming techniques: reliable results could be obtained with the use of non-integrative methods or at least sparing the original cell genotype [20]. It is crucial to pay attention to the cellular subtypes obtained in culture with varying differentiation protocols in order to avoid misleading results: well established cellular markers need to be used to assess both the neuronal phenotype and the maturation state. In addition, several studies have highlighted the possibility that reprogrammed cells might maintain an epigenetic memory of the cell of origin, which could interfere with the expression of membrane markers [62]. Recently, advances in reprogramming methods have led to the possibility of directly differentiating mature cells (*i.e.*, fibroblasts or astrocytes) into relevant cell types (*i.e.*, induced neurons) [63]. These rather novel methods are quite efficient in reducing time in culture and speed up the differentiation protocol, but need further assessment. It also needs to be pointed out that pathogenesis studies benefit from long-term observation, from the cell pluripotent state to the mature phenotype, in order to speculate on the time-dependent disease alteration.

5. Conclusions

The development and optimization of iPSC-based platforms has allowed elucidating disease-specific mechanisms, which are exquisitely human (Figure 1). Further advances may finally open up the path to a full understanding of key pathogenetic events, leading to the development of effective treatments for ALS, SMA and other MNDs.

Acknowledgments

Cariplo grant to SC 2012-0513.
The support of Associazione Amici del Centro Dino Ferrari is gratefully acknowledged.

Author Contributions

We confirm that all authors have participated in the writing of the manuscript (Irene Faravelli and Emanuele Frattini conceived the idea, revised all the literature and contributed to all parts; Giulia Stuppia revised the literature regarding ALS, and Agnese Ramirez revised the literature regarding SMA; Monica Nizzardo and Stefania Corti supervised and critically revised the manuscript, contributed to the revision of online websites and editing).

Conflicts of Interest

The authors declare no conflict of interest.

References

1. McDermott, C.J.; Shaw, P.J. Diagnosis and management of motor neurone disease. *BMJ* **2008**, *336*, 658–662.
2. Gordon, P.H. Amyotrophic lateral sclerosis: An update for 2013 clinical features, pathophysiology, management and therapeutic trials. *Aging Dis.* **2013**, *4*, 295–310.
3. Patten, S.A.; Armstrong, G.A.; Lissouba, A.; Kabashi, E.; Parker, J.A.; Drapeau, P. Fishing for causes and cures of motor neuron disorders. *Dis. Model. Mech.* **2014**, *7*, 799–809.

4. Rafiq, M.K.; Proctor, A.R.; McDermott, C.J.; Shaw, P.J. Respiratory management of motor neurone disease: A review of current practice and new developments. *Pract. Neurol.* **2012**, *12*, 166–176.

5. Kiernan, M.C.; Vucic, S.; Cheah, B.C.; Turner, M.R.; Eisen, A.; Hardiman, O.; Burrell, J.R.; Zoing, M.C. Amyotrophic lateral sclerosis. *Lancet* **2011**, *377*, 942–955.

6. Finsterer, J.; Burgunder, J.M. Recent progress in the genetics of motor neuron disease. *Eur. J. Med. Genet.* **2014**, *57*, 103–112.

7. Logroscino, G.; Traynor, B.J.; Hardiman, O.; Chio, A.; Mitchell, D.; Swingler, R.J.; Millul, A.; Benn, E.; Beghi, E. Incidence of amyotrophic lateral sclerosis in europe. *J. Neurol. Neurosurg. Psychiatry* **2010**, *81*, 385–390.

8. Beghi, E.; Chio, A.; Couratier, P.; Esteban, J.; Hardiman, O.; Logroscino, G.; Millul, A.; Mitchell, D.; Preux, P.M.; Pupillo, E.; *et al.* The epidemiology and treatment of als: Focus on the heterogeneity of the disease and critical appraisal of therapeutic trials. *Amyotroph. Lateral Scler.* **2011**, *12*, 1–10.

9. Al-Chalabi, A.; Hardiman, O. The epidemiology of ALS: A conspiracy of genes, environment and time. *Nat. Rev. Neurol.* **2013**, *9*, 617–628.

10. Majounie, E.; Renton, A.E.; Mok, K.; Dopper, E.G.; Waite, A.; Rollinson, S.; Chio, A.; Restagno, G.; Nicolaou, N.; Simon-Sanchez, J.; *et al.* Frequency of the *C9ORF72* hexanucleotide repeat expansion in patients with amyotrophic lateral sclerosis and frontotemporal dementia: A cross-sectional study. *Lancet Neurol.* **2012**, *11*, 323–330.

11. Lorson, C.L.; Rindt, H.; Shababi, M. Spinal muscular atrophy: Mechanisms and therapeutic strategies. *Hum. Mol. Genet.* **2010**, *19*, doi:10.1093/hmg/ddq147.

12. Prior, T.W.; Snyder, P.J.; Rink, B.D.; Pearl, D.K.; Pyatt, R.E.; Mihal, D.C.; Conlan, T.; Schmalz, B.; Montgomery, L.; Ziegler, K.; *et al.* Newborn and carrier screening for spinal muscular atrophy. *Am. J. Med. Genet. A* **2010**, *152A*, 1608–1616.

13. Russman, B.S. Spinal muscular atrophy: Clinical classification and disease heterogeneity. *J. Child Neurol.* **2007**, *22*, 946–951.

14. Lefebvre, S.; Burlet, P.; Liu, Q.; Bertrandy, S.; Clermont, O.; Munnich, A.; Dreyfuss, G.; Melki, J. Correlation between severity and smn protein level in spinal muscular atrophy. *Nat. Genet.* **1997**, *16*, 265–269.

15. Monani, U.R.; Lorson, C.L.; Parsons, D.W.; Prior, T.W.; Androphy, E.J.; Burghes, A.H.; McPherson, J.D. A single nucleotide difference that alters splicing patterns distinguishes the SMA gene *SMN1* from the copy gene *SMN2*. *Hum. Mol. Genet.* **1999**, *8*, 1177–1183.

16. Vitte, J.; Fassier, C.; Tiziano, F.D.; Dalard, C.; Soave, S.; Roblot, N.; Brahe, C.; Saugier-Veber, P.; Bonnefont, J.P.; Melki, J.; *et al.* Refined characterization of the expression and stability of the smn gene products. *Am. J. Pathol.* **2007**, *171*, 1269–1280.

17. Wang, C.H.; Finkel, R.S.; Bertini, E.S.; Schroth, M.; Simonds, A.; Wong, B.; Aloysius, A.; Morrison, L.; Main, M.; Crawford, T.O.; *et al.* Consensus statement for standard of care in spinal muscular atrophy. *J. Child Neurol.* **2007**, *22*, 1027–1049.

18. Wee, C.D.; Kong, L.; Sumner, C.J. The genetics of spinal muscular atrophies. *Curr. Opin. Neurol.* **2010**, *23*, 450–458.

19. Takahashi, K.; Yamanaka, S. Induction of pluripotent stem cells from mouse embryonic and adult fibroblast cultures by defined factors. *Cell* **2006**, *126*, 663–676.

20. Corti, S.; Nizzardo, M.; Simone, C.; Falcone, M.; Nardini, M.; Ronchi, D.; Donadoni, C.; Salani, S.; Riboldi, G.; Magri, F.; *et al.* Genetic correction of human induced pluripotent stem cells from patients with spinal muscular atrophy. *Sci. Transl. Med.* **2012**, *4*, doi:10.1126/scitranslmed.3004108.

21. Chipman, P.H.; Toma, J.S.; Rafuse, V.F. Generation of motor neurons from pluripotent stem cells. *Prog. Brain Res.* **2012**, *201*, 313–331.

22. Sandoe, J.; Eggan, K. Opportunities and challenges of pluripotent stem cell neurodegenerative disease models. *Nat. Neurosci.* **2013**, *16*, 780–789.

23. Kondo, T.; Asai, M.; Tsukita, K.; Kutoku, Y.; Ohsawa, Y.; Sunada, Y.; Imamura, K.; Egawa, N.; Yahata, N.; Okita, K.; *et al.* Modeling alzheimer's disease with ipscs reveals stress phenotypes associated with intracellular abeta and differential drug responsiveness. *Cell Stem Cell* **2013**, *12*, 487–496.

24. Camnasio, S.; Delli Carri, A.; Lombardo, A.; Grad, I.; Mariotti, C.; Castucci, A.; Rozell, B.; Lo Riso, P.; Castiglioni, V.; Zuccato, C.; *et al.* The first reported generation of several induced pluripotent stem cell lines from homozygous and heterozygous huntington's disease patients demonstrates mutation related enhanced lysosomal activity. *Neurobiol. Dis.* **2012**, *46*, 41–51.

25. Chung, C.Y.; Khurana, V.; Auluck, P.K.; Tardiff, D.F.; Mazzulli, J.R.; Soldner, F.; Baru, V.; Lou, Y.; Freyzon, Y.; Cho, S.; *et al.* Identification and rescue of alpha-synuclein toxicity in parkinson patient-derived neurons. *Science* **2013**, *342*, 983–987.

26. Kiskinis, E.; Sandoe, J.; Williams, L.A.; Boulting, G.L.; Moccia, R.; Wainger, B.J.; Han, S.; Peng, T.; Thams, S.; Mikkilineni, S.; *et al.* Pathways disrupted in human ALS motor neurons identified through genetic correction of mutant *SOD1*. *Cell Stem Cell* **2014**, *14*, 781–795.

27. Miller, R.G.; Brooks, B.R.; Swain-Eng, R.J.; Basner, R.C.; Carter, G.T.; Casey, P.; Cohen, A.B.; Dubinsky, R.; Forshew, D.; Jackson, C.E.; *et al.* Quality improvement in neurology: Amyotrophic lateral sclerosis quality measures: Report of the quality measurement and reporting subcommittee of the american academy of neurology. *Neurology* **2013**, *81*, 2136–2140.

28. Tovar, Y.R.L.B.; Ramirez-Jarquin, U.N.; Lazo-Gomez, R.; Tapia, R. Trophic factors as modulators of motor neuron physiology and survival: Implications for ALS therapy. *Front. Cell. Neurosci.* **2014**, *8*, doi:10.3389/fncel.2014.00061.

29. Brockington, A.; Ning, K.; Heath, P.R.; Wood, E.; Kirby, J.; Fusi, N.; Lawrence, N.; Wharton, S.B.; Ince, P.G.; Shaw, P.J.; *et al.* Unravelling the enigma of selective vulnerability in neurodegeneration: Motor neurons resistant to degeneration in als show distinct gene expression characteristics and decreased susceptibility to excitotoxicity. *Acta Neuropathol.* **2013**, *125*, 95–109.

30. Sreedharan, J.; Brown, R.H., Jr. Amyotrophic lateral sclerosis: Problems and prospects. *Ann. Neurol.* **2013**, *74*, 309–316.

31. Vucic, S.; Rothstein, J.D.; Kiernan, M.C. Advances in treating amyotrophic lateral sclerosis: Insights from pathophysiological studies. *Trends Neurosci.* **2014**, *37*, 433–442.

32. Rosen, D.R.; Sapp, P.; O'Regan, J.; McKenna-Yasek, D.; Schlumpf, K.S.; Haines, J.L.; Gusella, J.F.; Horvitz, H.R.; Brown, R.H., Jr. Genetic linkage analysis of familial amyotrophic lateral sclerosis using human chromosome 21 microsatellite DNA markers. *Am. J. Med. Genet.* **1994**, *51*, 61–69.

33. DeJesus-Hernandez, M.; Mackenzie, I.R.; Boeve, B.F.; Boxer, A.L.; Baker, M.; Rutherford, N.J.; Nicholson, A.M.; Finch, N.A.; Flynn, H.; Adamson, J.; *et al.* Expanded GGGGCC hexanucleotide repeat in noncoding region of *C9ORF72* causes chromosome 9p-linked FTD and ALS. *Neuron* **2011**, *72*, 245–256.

34. Su, X.W.; Broach, J.R.; Connor, J.R.; Gerhard, G.S.; Simmons, Z. Genetic heterogeneity of amyotrophic lateral sclerosis: Implications for clinical practice and research. *Muscle Nerve* **2014**, *49*, 786–803.

35. Ling, S.C.; Polymenidou, M.; Cleveland, D.W. Converging mechanisms in ALS and FTD: Disrupted RNA and protein homeostasis. *Neuron* **2013**, *79*, 416–438.

36. Renton, A.E.; Chio, A.; Traynor, B.J. State of play in amyotrophic lateral sclerosis genetics. *Nat. Neurosci.* **2014**, *17*, 17–23.

37. Di Giorgio, F.P.; Boulting, G.L.; Bobrowicz, S.; Eggan, K.C. Human embryonic stem cell-derived motor neurons are sensitive to the toxic effect of glial cells carrying an ALS-causing mutation. *Cell Stem Cell* **2008**, *3*, 637–648.

38. Wainger, B.J.; Kiskinis, E.; Mellin, C.; Wiskow, O.; Han, S.S.; Sandoe, J.; Perez, N.P.; Williams, L.A.; Lee, S.; Boulting, G.; *et al.* Intrinsic membrane hyperexcitability of amyotrophic lateral sclerosis patient-derived motor neurons. *Cell Rep.* **2014**, *7*, 1–11.

39. Sareen, D.; O'Rourke, J.G.; Meera, P.; Muhammad, A.K.; Grant, S.; Simpkinson, M.; Bell, S.; Carmona, S.; Ornelas, L.; Sahabian, A.; *et al.* Targeting RNA foci in iPSC-derived motor neurons from ALS patients with a *C9ORF72* repeat expansion. *Sci. Transl. Med.* **2013**, *5*, doi:10.1126/scitranslmed.3007529.

40. Renton, A.E.; Majounie, E.; Waite, A.; Simon-Sanchez, J.; Rollinson, S.; Gibbs, J.R.; Schymick, J.C.; Laaksovirta, H.; van Swieten, J.C.; Myllykangas, L.; *et al.* A hexanucleotide repeat expansion in *C9ORF72* is the cause of chromosome 9p21-linked ALS-FTD. *Neuron* **2011**, *72*, 257–268.

41. Buratti, E.; Brindisi, A.; Giombi, M.; Tisminetzky, S.; Ayala, Y.M.; Baralle, F.E. TDP-43 binds heterogeneous nuclear ribonucleoprotein A/B through its C-terminal tail *J. Biol. Chem.* **2005**, *280*, 37572–37584.

42. Bilican, B.; Serio, A.; Barmada, S.J.; Nishimura, A.L.; Sullivan, G.J.; Carrasco, M.; Phatnani, H.P.; Puddifoot, C.A.; Story, D.; Fletcher, J.; *et al.* Mutant induced pluripotent stem cell lines recapitulate aspects of TDP-43 proteinopathies and reveal cell-specific vulnerability. *Proc. Natl. Acad. Sci. USA* **2012**, *109*, 5803–5808.

43. Alami, N.H.; Smith, R.B.; Carrasco, M.A.; Williams, L.A.; Winborn, C.S.; Han, S.S.; Kiskinis, E.; Winborn, B.; Freibaum, B.D.; Kanagaraj, A.; *et al.* Axonal transport of TDP-43 mRNA granules is impaired by ALS-causing mutations. *Neuron* **2014**, *81*, 536–543.

44. Chen, H.; Qian, K.; Du, Z.; Cao, J.; Petersen, A.; Liu, H.; Blackbourn, L.W., IV; Huang, C.L.; Errigo, A.; Yin, Y.; *et al.* Modeling als with ipscs reveals that mutant *SOD1* misregulates neurofilament balance in motor neurons. *Cell Stem Cell* **2014**, *14*, 796–809.

45. Poppe, L.; Rue, L.; Robberecht, W.; van Den Bosch, L. Translating biological findings into new treatment strategies for amyotrophic lateral sclerosis (ALS). *Exp. Neurol.* **2014**, doi:10.1016/j.expneurol.2014.07.001.

46. Egawa, N.; Kitaoka, S.; Tsukita, K.; Naitoh, M.; Takahashi, K.; Yamamoto, T.; Adachi, F.; Kondo, T.; Okita, K.; Asaka, I.; *et al.* Drug screening for ALS using patient-specific induced pluripotent stem cells. *Sci. Transl. Med.* **2012**, *4*, doi:10.1126/scitranslmed.3004052.

47. Kondo, T.; Funayama, M.; Tsukita, K.; Hotta, A.; Yasuda, A.; Nori, S.; Kaneko, S.; Nakamura, M.; Takahashi, R.; Okano, H.; *et al.* Focal transplantation of human iPSC-derived glial-rich neural progenitors improves lifespan of als mice. *Stem Cell Rep.* **2014**, *3*, 242–249.

48. Ebert, A.D.; Yu, J.; Rose, F.F., Jr.; Mattis, V.B.; Lorson, C.L.; Thomson, J.A.; Svendsen, C.N. Induced pluripotent stem cells from a spinal muscular atrophy patient. *Nature* **2009**, *457*, 277–280.

49. Sareen, D.; Ebert, A.D.; Heins, B.M.; McGivern, J.V.; Ornelas, L.; Svendsen, C.N. Inhibition of apoptosis blocks human motor neuron cell death in a stem cell model of spinal muscular atrophy. *PLoS ONE* **2012**, *7*, e39113.

50. McGivern, J.V.; Patitucci, T.N.; Nord, J.A.; Barabas, M.E.; Stucky, C.L.; Ebert, A.D. Spinal muscular atrophy astrocytes exhibit abnormal calcium regulation and reduced growth factor production. *Glia* **2013**, *61*, 1418–1428.

51. Lafont, E.; Milhas, D.; Teissie, J.; Therville, N.; Andrieu-Abadie, N.; Levade, T.; Benoist, H.; Segui, B. Caspase-10-dependent cell death in Fas/CD95 signalling is not abrogated by caspase inhibitor zVAD-fmk. *PLoS One* **2010**, *5*, e13638.

52. Zhang, Z.; Lotti, F.; Dittmar, K.; Younis, I.; Wan, L.; Kasim, M.; Dreyfuss, G. SMN deficiency causes tissue-specific perturbations in the repertoire of snRNAs and widespread defects in splicing. *Cell* **2008**, *133*, 585–600.

53. Baumer, D.; Lee, S.; Nicholson, G.; Davies, J.L.; Parkinson, N.J.; Murray, L.M.; Gillingwater, T.H.; Ansorge, O.; Davies, K.E.; Talbot, K.; *et al.* Alternative splicing events are a late feature of pathology in a mouse model of spinal muscular atrophy. *PLoS Genet.* **2009**, *5*, e1000773.

54. Brites, D.; Vaz, A.R. Microglia centered pathogenesis in als: Insights in cell interconnectivity. *Front. Cell. Neurosci.* **2014**, *8*, 117, doi:10.3389/fncel.2014.00117.

55. Benkler, C.; Ben-Zur, T.; Barhum, Y.; Offen, D. Altered astrocytic response to activation in *SOD1(G93A)* mice and its implications on amyotrophic lateral sclerosis pathogenesis. *Glia* **2013**, *61*, 312–326.

56. Hirsch, E.C.; Hunot, S.; Hartmann, A. Neuroinflammatory processes in parkinson's disease. *Park. Relat. Disord.* **2005**, *11* (Suppl. 1), 9–15.

57. Wang, D.D.; Bordey, A. The astrocyte odyssey. *Prog. Neurobiol.* **2008**, *86*, 342–367.

58. Garbes, L.; Heesen, L.; Holker, I.; Bauer, T.; Schreml, J.; Zimmermann, K.; Thoenes, M.; Walter, M.; Dimos, J.; Peitz, M.; *et al.* VPA response in sma is suppressed by the fatty acid translocase CD36. *Hum. Mol. Genet.* **2013**, *22*, 398–407.

59. Van Den Bosch, L. Genetic rodent models of amyotrophic lateral sclerosis. *J. Biomed. Biotechnol.* **2011**, *2011*, doi:10.1155/2011/348765.

60. Schmid, A.; DiDonato, C.J. Animal models of spinal muscular atrophy. *J. Child Neurol.* **2007**, *22*, 1004–1012.

61. Re, D.B.; Le Verche, V.; Yu, C.; Amoroso, M.W.; Politi, K.A.; Phani, S.; Ikiz, B.; Hoffmann, L.; Koolen, M.; Nagata, T.; *et al.* Necroptosis drives motor neuron death in models of both sporadic and familial ALS. *Neuron* **2014**, *81*, 1001–1008.

62. Vaskova, E.A.; Stekleneva, A.E.; Medvedev, S.P.; Zakian, S.M. "Epigenetic memory" phenomenon in induced pluripotent stem cells. *Acta Naturae* **2013**, *5*, 15–21.

63. Hermann, A.; Storch, A. Induced neural stem cells (iNSCs) in neurodegenerative diseases. *J. Neural Transm.* **2013**, *120* (Suppl. 1), 19–25.

Chapter 2:
Cardiac

Bioengineering and Stem Cell Technology in the Treatment of Congenital Heart Disease

Alexis Bosman, Michael J. Edel, Gillian Blue, Rodney J. Dilley, Richard P. Harvey and David S. Winlaw

Abstract: Congenital heart disease places a significant burden on the individual, family and community despite significant advances in our understanding of aetiology and treatment. Early research in ischaemic heart disease has paved the way for stem cell technology and bioengineering, which promises to improve both structural and functional aspects of disease. Stem cell therapy has demonstrated significant improvements in cardiac function in adults with ischaemic heart disease. This finding, together with promising case studies in the paediatric setting, demonstrates the potential for this treatment in congenital heart disease. Furthermore, induced pluripotent stems cell technology, provides a unique opportunity to address aetiological, as well as therapeutic, aspects of disease.

Reprinted from *J. Clin. Med.* Cite as: Bosman, A.; Edel, M.J.; Blue, G.; Dilley, R.J.; Harvey, R.P.; Winlaw, D.S. Bioengineering and Stem Cell Technology in the Treatment of Congenital Heart Disease. *J. Clin. Med.* **2015**, *4*, 768–781.

1. Clinical Consideration of Congenital Heart Disease

Treatment of congenital heart disease (CHD) occupies a unique place in the human history of cardiovascular medicine. This dates back to the pioneering development of early heart-lung machines in the early 1950s. Subsequent development of this technology allowed correction of simple heart defects in childhood that would have otherwise led to early death, with further evolution permitting routine adult cardiac surgery for ischaemic and valvular heart disease, now accepted as "everyday surgery".

In modern CHD clinical research, both patients and practitioners look forward to similar paradigm shifts in treatments to address some of the inadequacies of current management that continue to impact individuals, families and workplaces. There are now more adults with congenital heart disease than children in advanced societies [1] and whilst many are effectively "cured" with childhood intervention (such as closure of infant ventricular septal defects) others have an ongoing need for close medical management including those with single ventricle physiology [2] or who require repeated surgeries, for example, those who will need replacement of right ventricle to pulmonary artery conduits.

The burden of disease is significant and has physical, psychological and economic impacts [3]. CHD occurs in ~7–8 in 1000 live births [4,5]. A subset of CHD is invariably lethal around birth unless treated, and these cases present significant challenges with respect to surgical reconstruction, critical care patient management, long term follow up and the ethics of focusing major health resources onto few individuals. CHD successfully treated in childhood carries a strong likelihood of complications in later life and a life-long emotional and financial burden for affected families [6].

The dramatic reduction in mortality after surgical correction of CHD in recent years has been accompanied by increasing recognition of poor neurological outcomes in survivors of CHD, which may involve genetic factors, abnormal brain perfusion and development *in utero* and/or susceptibilities to hypoxia resulting from CHD, or other environmental parameters such as anesthesia [7,8]. A key bottleneck in patient care is the transition from childhood to adulthood, where patients may be lost to follow up.

Childhood treatment is very costly and paediatric cardiac surgery is the most common reason for admission to paediatric intensive care. Over the last three decades, surgery has become more complex and is generally performed earlier—often during the neonatal period—to gain better functional outcomes in the long term. A diagnosis of CHD is associated with important psychosocial dysfunction with many parents reporting symptoms equivalent to post-traumatic stress disorders, high levels of parental depression and ongoing anxiety with similar problems observed in adolescent and adult survivors [9].

Addressing causation of CHD has been a high priority over the last decades, particularly for the minority of cases that show familial inheritance. Classical linkage analysis has been the mainstay methodology underpinning these studies. Studies on the interaction between genetic and environmental factors have revealed clinically important perturbations of the highly conserved and tightly regulated developmental cardiogenic processes but only in a smaller number of patients with single gene disorders and associated syndromes [10]. In the new era of genetic research, genome wide association studies have identified areas of common chromosomal variation associated with the most common but simple form of CHD, secundum ASD [11], but with relatively low odds ratios and limited clinical application. Massively parallel sequencing of the whole exome [12] and its more targeted approaches [13] have dramatically accelerated the disease gene discovery pipeline, yielding answers for additional families. Polygenic contribution, variable penetrance and variation in phenotype present ongoing challenges.

On the horizon is a new era of stem cell-based therapies and bioengineering, and it is hoped that these approaches can help reduce the burden of CHD. In broad terms, stem cell and bioengineering approaches may make contributions to: (i) improving structural solutions in repair of malformed hearts; (ii) improving the function of repaired hearts and their circulation; and (iii) facilitating modelling of CHD to advance our understanding of its molecular underpinnings. These will be discussed further below.

1.1. Structural Solutions

In paediatric heart surgery, there is a need to address the current demands of the circulation as well as future growth. Many forms of advanced neonatal surgery involve utilisation of the existing ventriculo-arterial connection as the systemic outflow (usually through a large ventricular septal defect) and creation of an extra-anatomic right ventricle to pulmonary artery conduit. Repairs of pulmonary atresia with VSD, and truncus arteriosus are examples that utilise this approach. Usually either a human cadaveric allograft (homograft) is used for this purpose, or a bovine jugular venous conduit, combining a "tube" with a valve. A larger group of patients, those with tetralogy of

Fallot, may require pulmonary valve replacement, currently also utilising allograft or xenograft tissue valves.

Whilst effective in the short term, the long term functional outcomes of such approaches are poor, with all requiring replacement within 3 to 8 years depending on the size of the patient, patient growth, host response to the allograft or xenograft and other factors including the occasional development of endocarditis. Supplies of both types of conduit are limited and are associated with significant expense. Allosensitisation to donated human products can also be a problem if transplantation is later required. Percutaneous approaches are now available that are suitable for some patients, particularly in the adolescent group, but as xenoproducts they remain susceptible to immune mediated structural valve deterioration and infection.

Many biologic approaches have been attempted to improve longevity of the implanted valve, including decellularising and re-seeding allograft tissue with host endothelial cells [14]; however this approach has not yet been shown to produce meaningfully increased graft survival or somatic growth [15]. Generation of a vascularised matrix that can then be seeded and shaped [16] is emerging as an approach that avoids the need for allograft material but will require complex 3D construction to simulate tube and valve formation. Patients undergoing the Fontan operation as a final step in construction of a cavo-pulmonary connection have been managed with tissue engineered vascular grafts to convey the inferior vena caval blood to the pulmonary arteries [17]. This is valuable proof of principle work yielding understandings of optimal matrix construction, albeit that no significant growth is presently required of this connection using current surgical approaches [18]. Electrospinning and microfabrication techniques to engineer scaffolds that support the growth of valvular interstitial cells and mesenchymal stem cells [19] offer a way to customise the size and shape of the replacement tissue, perhaps guided by 3D imaging of the planned recipient. Repopulation with engineered patient-specific cells utilising adult stem cell or induced pluripotent stem cell technologies would seem logical for the future [20,21].

1.2. Stem Cells to Improve Cardiac Function

There is extensive and ongoing work to support the use of stem cells in recovery from myocardial infarction in adult populations, particularly using bone marrow derived cells, albeit that the rationale for such studies is under intense scrutiny [22]. Regeneration of scar tissue into functional myocardium and improved ventricular performance are the aims of such interventions with recent promise [23–25]. In paediatric cardiology the aim would be the optimisation of ventricular performance for children subjected to volume or pressure loads, usually after correction of the structural abnormalities that promote ventricular dysfunction. There is particular interest in the subpopulation of patients with a functional single ventricle, especially those who have undergone complex single ventricle surgery such as the Norwood operation for hypoplastic left heart (HLH) [26].

Typically HLH patients would be infants after the first two stages of surgery involving long periods of cardiopulmonary bypass and shorter periods of planned and "protected" myocardial ischaemia. An increased volume load related to the shunt providing pulmonary blood flow after the initial operation adds to the work that the single right ventricle must perform, which is already at an anatomic disadvantage being a morphologic right ventricle working against systemic vascular resistance. It is not uncommon for the function of such ventricles to deteriorate, particularly after second stage surgery, promoting atrioventricular valve regurgitation which positively reinforces the ventricular dysfunction. Relative coronary insufficiency [27] or a primary myocardial process may contribute. Structural abnormalities have been identified in single right ventricular tissue [28]. Ventricular performance is a major determinant of suitability for the last stage of the single ventricle pathway, Fontan completion (total cavo-pulmonary connection) as well as performance and survival with the Fontan circulation.

In parallel with studies in animal models [29,30], various approaches to ventricular support using stem cell technology are being trialled in CHD patients with differing donor cell origins and modes of administration, as outlined by Tarui *et al.* [31]. A number of stem cell populations have been described in the mammalian heart using cell surface markers and various functional assays including colony formation, and growth and differentiation potential *in vitro* and *in vivo* [22] Cardiosphere-derived cells are among the first populations to be trialled in humans for ischaemic heart disease in adults [32,33]. They are heterogeneous cell preparations derived from the 3D cellular clusters (cardiospheres) that can be readily established from heart biopsies, and which are thought to provide a harbour (niche) for cells with stem or progenitor cell properties during *in vitro* culture. Cells derived from atrial tissue and administered via the intracoronary route at cardiac catheterisation, have been trialled in patients with HLH in Phase I and Phase II clinical trials, with other groups utilising umbilical cord [34] and bone marrow derived cell fractions [31]. Phase 1 trials have indicated the safety of this approach with some improvement in right ventricular systolic function evident, and Phase 2 studies are underway. In the recently reported Phase 1 study of autologous cardiosphere-derived cells delivered via the intracoronary route [35], no safety concerns were raised and an improvement in right ventricular function was observed at 18 months compared to controls. The effect size is encouraging and clinically relevant (a 10% increase in right ventricular ejection fraction). The use of autologous cells represents a clear advantage in this environment. Similar approaches may be of benefit in paediatric heart failure presenting as dilated cardiomyopathy.

Uncertainty persists about the mechanism by which the stem cells might induce functional improvement. In ischaemic disease and cardiomyopathy, paracrine activation of local regenerative pathways may significantly contribute to the improvements in performance, while tissue replacement due to stem cell deployment does not seem to be a dominant feature in animal studies [36].

Cord blood stem cells have been shown to engraft and augment right ventricular function in an ovine model in the presence of increased workload [30]. A similar model of right ventricular overloading in rats demonstrated improved diastolic dysfunction and suppression of ventricular fibrosis following skeletal myoblast transplantation (Hoashi *et al.* 2009). Case reports demonstrate improvement in ventricular function following intracoronary delivery of bone marrow derived cells in children with terminal cardiomyopathy [37,38] as well as ventricular failure following surgery for HLH [39]. In HLH, adaptation of the right ventricle to increased work load may require cellular proliferation beyond the capability of the intrinisic regenerative systems. The capacity for autologous modified cells in CHD to influence cardiac performance or myocyte proliferation may be diminished by the persistence of genetic characteristics that caused or contributed to abnormal development during primary cardiogenesis. However, the development of refined cell therapy approaches may support the growth and development required.

2. Induced Pluripotent Stem Cells to Study Causation in Congenital Heart Disease

Induced pluripotent stem cells (iPSC) can be created from virtually any somatic cell, most commonly from dermal fibroblasts [40]. These pluripotent cell types are created by the reprogramming of adult cells to a pluripotent state, giving them the ability to differentiate into all cell types of the human body, including cardiomyocytes (see Figure 1) as well as smooth muscle, endothelial and epicardial cells, the highly specialised cell types of the heart. This makes iPSC an invaluable resource for the study of CHD. The technology offers the unique opportunity to create human models of disease and development in a patient-specific context that incorporates the individual clinical features of the disease. Additionally, iPSC provide material to study the earliest time points in development, previously difficult due to restrictions on the availability of primary human tissue for study.

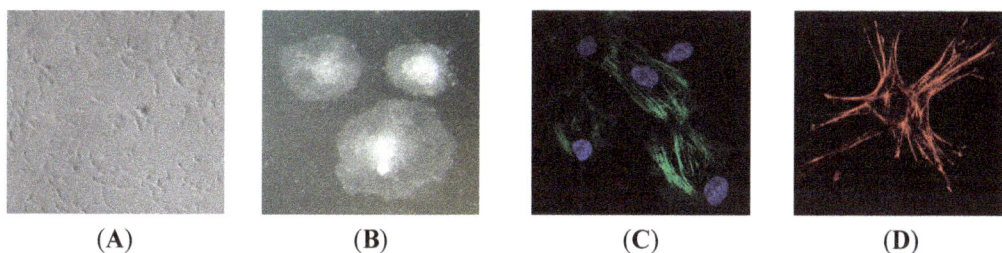

| (A) | (B) | (C) | (D) |

Figure 1. (A) Patient-derived fibroblasts generated from a skin biopsy; (B) Undifferentiated iPSC colonies derived from patient-derived fibroblasts; (C) Cardiomyocytes derived from iPSC stained for the sarcomeric protein, cardiac troponin T; (D) Smooth muscle cells derived from iPSC stained for the cell scaffolding protein, alpha smooth muscle actin.

iPSC are playing an increasing role in personalised medicine, specifically in disease profiling of both rare and common diseases, and in the design of personalised therapies. Due to the recent success of directed differentiation protocols [41–43], iPSC allow the provision of lineage-specific stem and progenitor cells, as well as differentiated specialised cell types, for disease research, cellular therapies and tissue engineering. However, before iPSC are used as a source of biologic material for clinical application, concerns regarding the oncogenic effect of retained transgenes [44] and trans-differentiation need to be addressed [45]. Until then, iPSC are being increasingly used as a test bed to study development and disease mechanism. In the cardiac area, iPSC approaches have been successful in assessing the functional disorder associated with LEOPARD Syndrome [46,47] and various arrhythmias and cardiomyopathies [48,49].

iPSC are playing an increasing role in personalised medicine, specifically in disease profiling of both rare and common diseases, and in the design of personalised therapies. Due to the recent success of directed differentiation protocols [41–43], iPSC allow the provision of lineage-specific stem and progenitor cells, as well as differentiated specialised cell types, for disease research, cellular therapies and tissue engineering. However, before iPSC are used as a source of biologic material for clinical application, concerns regarding the oncogenic effect of retained transgenes [44] and trans-differentiation need to be addressed [45]. Until then, iPSC are being increasingly used as a test bed to study development and disease mechanism. In the cardiac area, iPSC approaches have been successful in assessing the functional disorder associated with LEOPARD Syndrome [46,47] and various arrhythmias and cardiomyopathies [48,49].

The approach is applicable to CHD particularly for cell-autonomous genetic disorders affecting, for example, the development or function of cardiomyocytes that can be modelled in 2D cell cultures or 3D tissue constructs [50,51]. The approach has its obvious limitations with respect to modelling the complex tissue interactions necessary for organ structure, and the non-cell autonomous environmental or epigenetic influences on disease. However, rapid progress is being made on directed differentiation of highly complex organoids and tissue layers from pluripotent stem cells [52,53], opening up vast new potential for therapies and modelling disease in this system.

Using a patient-specific *in vitro* model of HLH is of particular interest to clinicians and scientists in the field attempting to reconcile the most common theory about the genesis of HLH—reduced transventricular flow and altered loading during development—with the heterogeneity in morphology as well as performance and decline observed in clinical cases [54,55]. An iPSC approach will complement the forward genetic approach being taken in mice [56]. While it has been suggested that HLH is essentially a severe form of valve malformation [56,57], some cases of HLH have a bulky LV and small but formed mitral and aortic valves, whilst others have barely a recognisable LV cavity. In combination these studies lead to speculation that a primary myocardial disorder is present in HLH, which likely predetermines the size and function of the ventricle and perhaps contributes to difficulties in later childhood in some with this condition. HLH is thought to have a high genetic component with complex inheritance, and is often associated with chromosomal abnormalities [58], which could impact on either valvular structures or ventricular cardiomyocyte growth and function, or both. Of the limited number of gene pathways implicated in HLH [58], the transcription factors NKX2-5 and NOTCH1 are known to be involved in both valvular and chamber development [59,60]. Both genes are also involved in aortic coarctation and bicuspid aortic valve, which exist within the spectrum of left-sided abnormalities that includes HLH at its most severe end [61–63].

Jiang and colleagues made iPSC from a single HLH patient and used them to derive cardiomyocytes by directed differentiation. They found a number of important primary cardiac defects including altered expression of key cardiac transcription factors, fewer beating clusters and reduced myofibrillar organisation, persistence of a fetal gene expression pattern as well as altered calcium transients and calcium handling [54]. Kobayashi *et al.* analysed single clones from three HLH patients, using a clone from a patient with bicuspid aortic valve and total anomalous pulmonary venous connection as a control [55]. They showed reduced expression of a number of cardiac transcription factors at late time points after induced cardiomyocyte differentiation, and associated changes in total chromatin marks—di-methylation on histone H3 lysine 4, tri-methylation on histone H3 lysine 27, and acetylation of histone H3. Whether the reported changes are common to all cases of HLH remains to be seen. Such molecular phenotypes in patient specific iPSC-derived cardiomyocytes raises the possibility that disease modelling using the iPSC platform can provide both molecular diagnosis, as has been utilised in other cardiovascular diseases [64] and cell therapy into the future.

Bioengineering Heart Muscle Using iPS Cells

Investigations into the creation of functional heart tissue *in vitro* by tissue engineering techniques using donor cardiomyocytes is still in its very early stages [65–68]. While there are no clinical applications of the method to date, cardiac tissue engineering has seen progress over the last twenty years in all four of the elements central to this method: generation of donor cardiomyocytes, development of scaffold materials and control of cell survival, engraftment and growth with bioactive molecules (see recent reviews [51,69,70]). The latest developments include *ex vivo* and *in vivo* approaches that promote the growth of vascular and structural elements of cardiac tissue [71,72]. Growing cells as sheets has made possible the insertion of iPSC-derived cardiomyocytes into the porcine heart for short term benefits [73]. Human embryonic stem cell-derived cardiomyocytes have been successfully engrafted in a non-human primate model of myocardial infarction [74]. This approach included development and application of mass culture techniques able to support production and delivery of a billion cells, selection of delivery techniques to optimise survival, such as a supportive hydrogel scaffold and application of a cocktail of preconditioning regimes. While this demonstrates potential for successful remuscularization of the human heart, issues with the incomplete maturation of cardiomyocytes, as well as arrhythmogenesis, need to be addressed. Contractile and vascularised human cardiac tissues have also been created from iPS cells [75,76] to provide long term survival and contractility, and 3D microtissues derived from iPSC also show promise for transplantation [77].

The ability to make whole functional hearts or bioengineered patches and conduits is challenging and has not been achieved for clinical use thus far. A form of bioengineered hearts have been configured using human iPSC-derived multipotential cardiovascular progenitors (MCP), which are likely similar to the earliest cardiac progenitors in heart development, by implanting them into a decellularized donor mouse heart [78]. The decellularized heart provides an excellent 3D structure for bioengineering whole organs or surgical implants as it utilises the natural extracellular matrix to promote cardiomyocyte proliferation, differentiation and function. The use of such native cardiac scaffold provides appropriate cues for engraftment, promotes rapid vascularisation and also avoids the biocompatibility problems of some artificial scaffold materials. MCP may offer an advantageous cell type for cardiac tissue bioengineering applications as they can potentially self-organise into structures containing cardiomyocytes, smooth muscle cells and endothelial cells, guided by extracellular matrix cues. However, before a whole heart can be bioengineered, a number of challenges remain, including safeguards surrounding the use of iPSC as discussed, as well as modulation of the immune response and, in CHD applications, finding ways that allow growth of the graft along with the patient's heart.

3. Conclusions

Emerging technology in stem cells and bio-engineering may address major issues in congenital heart disease that limit lifespan and reduce quality of life for a significant number of children and adults. iPSC technology offers an opportunity to provide both molecular diagnosis and, in the future, tissue based therapy for some of the more complex reconstructive tasks in congenital heart disease.

Author Contributions

Alexis Bosman wrote sections of manuscript and provided figures and experimental data; Michael J. Edel, Gillian Blue, Rodney J. Dilley and Richard P. Harvey wrote sections of manuscript and provided critical review; David S. Winlaw drafted the initial manuscript, coordinated co-author's efforts, and provided critical revision of manuscript and response to reviewers.

Conflicts of Interest

The authors declare no conflict of interest.

References

1. Go, A.S.; Mozaffarian, D.; Roger, V.L.; Benjamin, E.J.; Berry, J.D.; Blaha, M.J.; Dai, S.; Ford, E.S.; Fox, C.S.; Franco, S.; *et al.* Heart disease and stroke statistics—2014 update: A report from the American Heart Association. *Circulation* **2014**, *129*, e28–e292.
2. D'Udekem, Y.; Iyengar, A.J.; Galati, J.C.; Forsdick, V.; Weintraub, R.G.; Wheaton, G.R.; Bullock, A.; Justo, R.N.; Grigg, L.E.; Sholler, G.F.; *et al.* Redefining expectations of long-term survival after the Fontan procedure: Twenty-five years of follow-up from the entire population of Australia and New Zealand. *Circulation* **2014**, *130*, S32–S38.
3. Leggat, S. *Childhood Heart Disease in Australia: Current Practices and Future Needs*; HeartKids Australia: Pennant Hills, NSW, Australia, 2011; pp. 1–52.
4. Hoffman, J.I.E.; Kaplan, S. The incidence of congenital heart disease. *JAC* **2002**, *39*, 1890–1900.
5. Go, A.S.; Mozaffarian, D.; Roger, V.L.; Benjamin, E.J.; Berry, J.D.; Borden, W.B.; Bravata, D.M.; Dai, S.; Ford, E.S.; Fox, C.S.; *et al.* Heart disease and stroke statistics—2013 update: A report from the American Heart Association. *Circulation* **2013**, *127*, e6–e245.
6. Tutarel, O. Acquired heart conditions in adults with congenital heart disease: A growing problem. *Heart* **2014**, *100*, 1317–1321.
7. Gaynor, J.W. The encephalopathy of congenital heart disease. *J. Thorac. Cardiovasc. Surg.* **2014**, *148*, 1790–1791.

8. Masoller, N.; Martínez, J.M.; Gómez, O.; Bennasar, M.; Crispi, F.; Sanz-Cortés, M.; Egaña-Ugrinovic, G.; Bartrons, J.; Puerto, B.; Gratacós, E. Evidence of second-trimester changes in head biometry and brain perfusion in fetuses with congenital heart disease. *Ultrasound Obstet. Gynecol.* **2014**, *44*, 182–187.

9. Kasparian, N.A.; Fidock, B.; Sholler, G.F.; Camphausen, C.; Murphy, D.N.; Cooper, S.G.; Kaul, R.; Jones, O.; Winlaw, D.S.; Kirk, E.P.E. Parents' perceptions of genetics services for congenital heart disease: The role of demographic, clinical, and psychological factors in determining service attendance. *Genet. Med.* **2014**, *16*, 460–468.

10. Blue, G.M.; Kirk, E.P.; Sholler, G.F.; Harvey, R.P.; Winlaw, D.S. Congenital heart disease: Current knowledge about causes and inheritance. *Med. J. Aust.* **2012**, *197*, 155–159.

11. Cordell, H.J.; Bentham, J.; Topf, A.; Zelenika, D.; Heath, S.; Mamasoula, C.; Cosgrove, C.; Blue, G.; Granados-Riveron, J.; Setchfield, K.; *et al.* Genome-wide association study of multiple congenital heart disease phenotypes identifies a susceptibility locus for atrial septal defect at chromosome 4p16. *Nat. Genet.* **2013**, *45*, 822–824.

12. Zaidi, S.; Choi, M.; Wakimoto, H.; Ma, L.; Jiang, J.; Overton, J.D.; Romano-Adesman, A.; Bjornson, R.D.; Breitbart, R.E.; Brown, K.K.; *et al. De novo* mutations in histone-modifying genes in congenital heart disease. *Nature* **2013**, *498*, 220–223.

13. Blue, G.M.; Kirk, E.P.; Giannoulatou, E.; Dunwoodie, S.L.; Ho, J.W.K.; Hilton, D.C.K.; White, S.M.; Sholler, G.F.; Harvey, R.P.; Winlaw, D.S. Targeted next-generation sequencing identifies pathogenic variants in familial congenital heart disease. *J. Am. Coll. Cardiol.* **2014**, *64*, 2498–2506.

14. Cebotari, S.; Lichtenberg, A.; Tudorache, I.; Hilfiker, A.; Mertsching, H.; Leyh, R.; Breymann, T.; Kallenbach, K.; Maniuc, L.; Batrinac, A.; *et al.* Clinical application of tissue engineered human heart valves using autologous progenitor cells. *Circulation* **2006**, *114*, I132–I137.

15. Dijkman, P.E.; Driessen-Mol, A.; Frese, L.; Hoerstrup, S.P.; Baaijens, F.P.T. Decellularized homologous tissue-engineered heart valves as off-the-shelf alternatives to xeno- and homografts. *Biomaterials* **2012**, *33*, 4545–4554.

16. Andrée, B.; Bela, K.; Horvath, T.; Lux, M.; Ramm, R.; Venturini, L.; Ciubotaru, A.; Zweigerdt, R.; Haverich, A.; Hilfiker, A. Successful re-endothelialization of a perfusable biological vascularized matrix (BioVaM) for the generation of 3D artificial cardiac tissue. *Basic Res. Cardiol.* **2014**, *109*, doi:10.1007/s00395-014-0441-x.

17. Udelsman, B.V.; Maxfield, M.W.; Breuer, C.K. Tissue engineering of blood vessels in cardiovascular disease: Moving towards clinical translation. *Heart* **2013**, *99*, 454–460.

18. Kurobe, H.; Maxfield, M.W.; Breuer, C.K.; Shinoka, T. Concise review: Tissue-engineered vascular grafts for cardiac surgery: Past, present, and future. *Stem Cells Transl. Med.* **2012**, *1*, 566–571.

19. Masoumi, N.; Annabi, N.; Assmann, A.; Larson, B.L.; Hjortnaes, J.; Alemdar, N.; Kharaziha, M.; Manning, K.B.; Mayer, J.E.; Khademhosseini, A. Tri-layered elastomeric scaffolds for engineering heart valve leaflets. *Biomaterials* **2014**, *35*, 7774–7785.

20. Weber, B.; Emmert, M.; Hoerstrup, S. Stem cells for heart valve regeneration. *Swiss Med. Wkly.* **2012**, *142*, doi:10.4414/smw.2012.13622.

21. Simpson, D.L.; Wehman, B.; Galat, Y.; Sharma, S.; Mishra, R.; Galat, V.; Kaushal, S. Engineering patient-specific valves using stem cells generated from skin biopsy specimens. *Ann. Thorac. Surg.* **2014**, *98*, 947–954.

22. Chong, J.J.H.; Forte, E.; Harvey, R.P. Developmental origins and lineage descendants of endogenous adult cardiac progenitor cells. *Stem Cell Res.* **2014**, *13*, 592–614.

23. Malliaras, K.; Makkar, R.R.; Smith, R.R.; Cheng, K.; Wu, E.; Bonow, R.O.; Marbán, L.; Mendizabal, A.; Cingolani, E.; Johnston, P.V.; *et al.* Intracoronary cardiosphere-derived cells after myocardial infarction: Evidence of therapeutic regeneration in the final 1-year results of the CADUCEUS trial (CArdiosphere-Derived aUtologous stem CElls to reverse ventricUlar dySfunction). *JAC* **2014**, *63*, 110–122.

24. Piepoli, M.F.; Vallisa, D.; Arbasi, C.; Cavanna, L.; Cerri, L.; Mori, M.; Passerini, F.; Tommasi, L.; Rossi, A.; Capucci, A. Two year follow-up results of the CARDIAC (CARDIomyoplasty by Autologous intraCoronary bone marrow in acute myocardial infarction) randomised controlled trial. *Int. J. Cardiol.* **2013**, *168*, e132.

25. Vrtovec, B.; Poglajen, G.; Lezaic, L.; Sever, M.; Domanovic, D.; Cernelc, P.; Socan, A.; Schrepfer, S.; Torre-Amione, G.; Haddad, F.; *et al.* Effects of intracoronary CD34+ stem cell transplantation in nonischemic dilated cardiomyopathy patients: 5-year follow-up. *Circ. Res.* **2013**, *112*, 165–173.

26. Tchervenkov, C.I.; Jacobs, J.P.; Weinberg, P.M.; Aiello, V.D.; Béland, M.J.; Colan, S.D.; Elliott, M.J.; Franklin, R.C.G.; Gaynor, J.W.; Krogmann, O.N.; *et al.* The nomenclature, definition and classification of hypoplastic left heart syndrome. *CTY* **2006**, *16*, 339–368.

27. Donnelly, J.P.; Raffel, D.M.; Shulkin, B.L.; Corbett, J.R.; Bove, E.L.; Mosca, R.S.; Kulik, T.J. Resting coronary flow and coronary flow reserve in human infants after repair or palliation of congenital heart defects as measured by positron emission tomography. *J. Thorac. Cardiovasc. Surg.* **1998**, *115*, 103–110.

28. Salih, C.; McCarthy, K.P.; Ho, S.Y. The fibrous matrix of ventricular myocardium in hypoplastic left heart syndrome: A quantitative and qualitative analysis. *Ann. Thorac. Surg.* **2004**, *77*, 36–40.

29. Yerebakan, C.; Sandica, E.; Prietz, S.; Klopsch, C.; Ugurlucan, M.; Kaminski, A.; Abdija, S.; Lorenzen, B.; Boltze, J.; Nitzsche, B.; *et al.* Autologous umbilical cord blood mononuclear cell transplantation preserves right ventricular function in a novel model of chronic right ventricular volume overload. *Cell Transpl.* **2009**, *18*, 855–868.

30. Davies, B.; Elwood, N.J.; Li, S.; Cullinane, F.; Edwards, G.A.; Newgreen, D.F.; Brizard, C.P. Human cord blood stem cells enhance neonatal right ventricular function in an ovine model of right ventricular training. *Ann. Thorac. Surg.* **2010**, *89*, 585–593.

31. Tarui, S.; Sano, S.; Oh, H. Stem cell therapies in patients with single ventricle physiology. *Methodist Debakey Cardiovasc. J.* **2014**, *10*, 77–81.

32. Bolli, R.; Chugh, A.R.; D'Amario, D.; Loughran, J.H.; Stoddard, M.F.; Ikram, S.; Beache, G.M.; Wagner, S.G.; Leri, A.; Hosoda, T.; *et al.* Cardiac stem cells in patients with ischaemic cardiomyopathy (SCIPIO): Initial results of a randomised phase 1 trial. *Lancet* **2011**, *378*, 1847–1857.

33. Makkar, R.R.; Smith, R.R.; Cheng, K.; Malliaras, K.; Thomson, L.E.J.; Berman, D.; Czer, L.S.C.; Marbán, L.; Mendizabal, A.; Johnston, P.V.; *et al.* Intracoronary cardiosphere-derived cells for heart regeneration after myocardial infarction (CADUCEUS): A prospective, randomised phase 1 trial. *Lancet* **2012**, *379*, 895–904.

34. Burkhart, H.M.; Qureshi, M.Y.; Peral, S.C.; O'Leary, P.W.; Olson, T.M.; Cetta, F.; Nelson, T.J.; The Wanek Program Clinical Pipeline Group. Regenerative therapy for hypoplastic left heart syndrome: First report of intraoperative intramyocardial injection of autologous umbilical-cord blood-derived cells. *J. Thorac. Cardiovasc. Surg.* **2014**, *149*, e35–e37.

35. Ishigami, S.; Ohtsuki, S.; Tarui, S.; Ousaka, D.; Eitoku, T.; Kondo, M.; Okuyama, M.; Kobayashi, J.; Baba, K.; Arai, S.; *et al.* Intracoronary autologous cardiac progenitor cell transfer in patients with hypoplastic left heart syndrome: The TICAP prospective phase 1 controlled trial. *Circ. Res.* **2015**, *116*, 653–664.

36. Li, T.-S.; Cheng, K.; Malliaras, K.; Smith, R.R.; Zhang, Y.; Sun, B.; Matsushita, N.; Blusztajn, A.; Terrovitis, J.; Kusuoka, H.; *et al.* Direct comparison of different stem cell types and subpopulations reveals superior paracrine potency and myocardial repair efficacy with cardiosphere-derived cells. *J. Am. Coll. Cardiol.* **2012**, *59*, 942–953.

37. Rupp, S.; Jux, C.; Bönig, H.; Bauer, J.; Tonn, T.; Seifried, E.; Dimmeler, S.; Zeiher, A.M.; Schranz, D. Intracoronary bone marrow cell application for terminal heart failure in children. *CTY* **2012**, *22*, 558–563.

38. Rupp, S.; Bauer, J.; Tonn, T.; Schächinger, V.; Dimmeler, S.; Zeiher, A.M.; Schranz, D. Intracoronary administration of autologous bone marrow-derived progenitor cells in a critically ill two-yr-old child with dilated cardiomyopathy. *Pediatr. Transpl.* **2009**, *13*, 620–623.

39. Rupp, S.; Zeiher, A.M.; Dimmeler, S.; Tonn, T.; Bauer, J.; Jux, C.; Akintuerk, H.; Schranz, D. A regenerative strategy for heart failure in hypoplastic left heart syndrome: Intracoronary administration of autologous bone marrow-derived progenitor cells. *J. Heart Lung Transplant.* **2010**, *29*, 574–577.

40. Takahashi, K.; Tanabe, K.; Ohnuki, M.; Narita, M.; Ichisaka, T. Induction of pluripotent stem cells from adult human fibroblasts by defined factors. *Cell* **2007**, *131*, 861–872.

41. Lian, X.; Zhang, J.; Azarin, S.M.; Zhu, K.; Hazeltine, L.B.; Bao, X.; Hsiao, C.; Kamp, T.J.; Palecek, S.P. Directed cardiomyocyte differentiation from human pluripotent stem cells by modulating Wnt/β-catenin signaling under fully defined conditions. *Nat. Protoc.* **2013**, *8*, 162–175.

42. Kattman, S.J.; Witty, A.D.; Gagliardi, M.; Dubois, N.C.; Niapour, M.; Hotta, A.; Ellis, J.; Keller, G. Stage-specific optimization of activin/nodal and BMP signaling promotes cardiac differentiation of mouse and human pluripotent stem cell lines. *Cell Stem Cell* **2011**, *8*, 228–240.

43. Witty, A.D.; Mihic, A.; Tam, R.Y.; Fisher, S.A.; Mikryukov, A.; Shoichet, M.S.; Li, R.-K.; Kattman, S.J.; Keller, G. Generation of the epicardial lineage from human pluripotent stem cells. *Nat. Biotechnol.* **2014**, *32*, 1026–1035.

44. Martinez-Fernandez, A.; Nelson, T.J.; Reyes, S.; Alekseev, A.E.; Secreto, F.; Perez-Terzic, C.; Beraldi, R.; Sung, H.-K.; Nagy, A.; Terzic, A. iPS cell-derived cardiogenicity is hindered by sustained integration of reprogramming transgenes. *Circ. Cardiovasc. Genet* **2014**, *7*, 667–676.

45. Addis, R.C.; Epstein, J.A. Induced regeneration—the progress and promise of direct reprogramming for heart repair. *Nat. Publ. Group* **2013**, *19*, 829–836.

46. Lin, B.; Kim, J.; Li, Y.; Pan, H.; Carvajal-Vergara, X.; Salama, G.; Cheng, T.; Li, Y.; Lo, C.W.; Yang, L. High-purity enrichment of functional cardiovascular cells from human iPS cells. *Cardiovasc. Res.* **2012**, *95*, 327–335.

47. Carvajal-Vergara, X.; Sevilla, A.; D'Souza, S.L.; Ang, Y.-S.; Schaniel, C.; Lee, D.-F.; Yang, L.; Kaplan, A.D.; Adler, E.D.; Rozov, R.; *et al.* Patient-specific induced pluripotent stem-cell-derived models of LEOPARD syndrome. *Nature* **2010**, *465*, 808–812.

48. Vitale, A.M.; Wolvetang, E.; Mackay-Sim, A. Induced pluripotent stem cells: A new technology to study human diseases. *Int. J. Biochem. Cell Biol.* **2011**, *43*, 843–846.

49. Sharma, A.; Marceau, C.; Hamaguchi, R.; Burridge, P.W.; Rajarajan, K.; Churko, J.M.; Wu, H.; Sallam, K.I.; Matsa, E.; Sturzu, A.C.; *et al.* Human induced pluripotent stem cell-derived cardiomyocytes as an *in vitro* model for coxsackievirus B3-induced myocarditis and antiviral drug screening platform. *Circ. Res.* **2014**, *115*, 556–566.

50. Hirt, M.N.; Boeddinghaus, J.; Mitchell, A.; Schaaf, S.; Börnchen, C.; Müller, C.; Schulz, H.; Hubner, N.; Stenzig, J.; Stoehr, A.; *et al.* Functional improvement and maturation of rat and human engineered heart tissue by chronic electrical stimulation. *J. Mol. Cell. Cardiol.* **2014**, *74*, 151–161.

51. Hirt, M.N.; Hansen, A.; Eschenhagen, T. Cardiac tissue engineering: State of the art. *Circ. Res.* **2014**, *114*, 354–367.

52. Stern, J.; Temple, S. Stem cells for retinal repair. *Dev. Ophthalmol.* **2014**, *53*, 70–80.

53. Takasato, M.; Maier, B.; Little, M.H. Recreating kidney progenitors from pluripotent cells. *Pediatr. Nephrol.* **2014**, *29*, 543–552.

54. Jiang, Y.; Habibollah, S.; Tilgner, K.; Collin, J.; Barta, T.; Al-Aama, J.Y.; Tesarov, L.; Hussain, R.; Trafford, A.W.; Kirkwood, G.; *et al.* An induced pluripotent stem cell model of hypoplastic left heart syndrome (HLHS) reveals multiple expression and functional differences in HLHS-derived cardiac myocytes. *Stem Cells Transl. Med.* **2014**, *3*, 416–423.

55. Kobayashi, J.; Yoshida, M.; Tarui, S.; Hirata, M.; Nagai, Y.; Kasahara, S.; Naruse, K.; Ito, H.; Sano, S.; Oh, H. Directed differentiation of patient-specific induced pluripotent stem cells identifies the transcriptional repression and epigenetic modification of NKX2-5, HAND1, and NOTCH1 in hypoplastic left heart syndrome. *PLoS ONE* **2014**, *9*, e102796.

56. Liu, X.; Francis, R.; Kim, A.J.; Ramirez, R.; Chen, G.; Subramanian, R.; Anderton, S.; Kim, Y.; Wong, L.; Morgan, J.; *et al.* Interrogating congenital heart defects with noninvasive fetal echocardiography in a mouse forward genetic screen. *Circ. Cardiovasc. Imaging* **2014**, *7*, 31–42.

57. Feinstein, J.A.; Benson, D.W.; Dubin, A.M.; Cohen, M.S.; Maxey, D.M.; Mahle, W.T.; Pahl, E.; Villafañe, J.; Bhatt, A.B.; Peng, L.F.; *et al.* Hypoplastic left heart syndrome: Current considerations and expectations. *J. Am. Coll. Cardiol.* **2012**, *59*, S1–S42.

58. Hinton, R.B., Jr.; Martin, L.J.; Tabangin, M.E.; Mazwi, M.L.; Cripe, L.H.; Benson, D.W. Hypoplastic left heart syndrome is heritable. *J. Am. Coll. Cardiol.* **2007**, *50*, 1590–1595.

59. Elliott, D.A.; Kirk, E.P.; Yeoh, T.; Chandar, S.; McKenzie, F.; Taylor, P.; Grossfeld, P.; Fatkin, D.; Jones, O.; Hayes, P.; *et al.* Cardiac homeobox gene NKX2-5 mutations and congenital heart disease: Associations with atrial septal defect and hypoplastic left heart syndrome. *JAC* **2003**, *41*, 2072–2076.

60. Iascone, M.; Ciccone, R.; Galletti, L.; Marchetti, D.; Seddio, F.; Lincesso, A.R.; Pezzoli, L.; Vetro, A.; Barachetti, D.; Boni, L.; *et al.* Identification of *de novo* mutations and rare variants in hypoplastic left heart syndrome. *Clin. Genet.* **2012**, *81*, 542–554.

61. Freylikhman, O.; Tatarinova, T.; Smolina, N.; Zhuk, S.; Klyushina, A.; Kiselev, A.; Moiseeva, O.; Sjoberg, G.; Malashicheva, A.; Kostareva, A. Variants in the NOTCH1 gene in patients with aortic coarctation. *Congenit. Heart Dis.* **2014**, *9*, 391–396.

62. Garg, V.; Muth, A.N.; Ransom, J.F.; Schluterman, M.K.; Barnes, R.; King, I.N.; Grossfeld, P.D.; Srivastava, D. Mutations in NOTCH1 cause aortic valve disease. *Nature* **2005**, *437*, 270–274.

63. Hinton, R.B.; Martin, L.J.; Rame-Gowda, S.; Tabangin, M.E.; Cripe, L.H.; Benson, D.W. Hypoplastic left heart syndrome links to chromosomes 10q and 6q and is genetically related to bicuspid aortic valve. *J. Am. Coll. Cardiol.* **2009**, *53*, 1065–1071.

64. Kinnear, C.; Chang, W.Y.; Khattak, S.; Hinek, A.; Thompson, T.; de Carvalho Rodrigues, D.; Kennedy, K.; Mahmut, N.; Pasceri, P.; Stanford, W.L.; *et al.* Modeling and rescue of the vascular phenotype of Williams-Beuren syndrome in patient induced pluripotent stem cells. *Stem Cells Transl. Med.* **2013**, *2*, 2–15.

65. Carrier, R.L.; Papadaki, M.; Rupnick, M.; Schoen, F.J.; Bursac, N.; Langer, R.; Freed, L.E.; Vunjak-Novakovic, G. Cardiac tissue engineering: Cell seeding, cultivation parameters, and tissue construct characterization. *Biotechnol. Bioeng.* **1999**, *64*, 580–589.

66. Shimizu, T.; Yamato, M.; Akutsu, T.; Shibata, T.; Isoi, Y.; Kikuchi, A.; Umezu, M.; Okano, T. Electrically communicating three-dimensional cardiac tissue mimic fabricated by layered cultured cardiomyocyte sheets. *J. Biomed. Mater. Res.* **2002**, *60*, 110–117.

67. Zimmermann, W.-H.; Schneiderbanger, K.; Schubert, P.; Didié, M.; Münzel, F.; Heubach, J.F.; Kostin, S.; Neuhuber, W.L.; Eschenhagen, T. Tissue engineering of a differentiated cardiac muscle construct. *Circ. Res.* **2002**, *90*, 223–230.

68. Dar, A.; Shachar, M.; Leor, J.; Cohen, S. Optimization of cardiac cell seeding and distribution in 3D porous alginate scaffolds. *Biotechnol. Bioeng.* **2002**, *80*, 305–312.

69. Coulombe, K.L.K.; Bajpai, V.K.; Andreadis, S.T.; Murry, C.E. Heart regeneration with engineered myocardial tissue. *Annu. Rev. Biomed. Eng.* **2014**, *16*, 1–28.

70. Dilley, R.J.; Morrison, W.A. Vascularisation to improve translational potential of tissue engineering systems for cardiac repair. *Int. J. Biochem. Cell Biol.* **2014**, *56*, 38–46.

71. Ott, H.C.; Matthiesen, T.S.; Goh, S.K.; Black, L.D.; Kren, S.M.; Netoff, T.I.; Taylor, D.A. Perfusion-decellularized matrix: Using nature's platform to engineer a bioartificial heart. *Nat. Med.* **2008**, *14*, 213–221.

72. Morritt, A.N.; Bortolotto, S.K.; Dilley, R.J.; Han, X.; Kompa, A.R.; McCombe, D.; Wright, C.E.; Itescu, S.; Angus, J.A.; Morrison, W.A. Cardiac tissue engineering in an *in vivo* vascularized chamber. *Circulation* **2007**, *115*, 353–360.

73. Kawamura, M.; Miyagawa, S.; Miki, K.; Saito, A.; Fukushima, S.; Higuchi, T.; Kawamura, T.; Kuratani, T.; Daimon, T.; Shimizu, T.; *et al.* Feasibility, safety, and therapeutic efficacy of human induced pluripotent stem cell-derived cardiomyocyte sheets in a porcine ischemic cardiomyopathy model. *Circulation* **2012**, *126*, S29–S37.

74. Chong, J.J.H.; Yang, X.; Don, C.W.; Minami, E.; Liu, Y.-W.; Weyers, J.J.; Mahoney, W.M.; van Biber, B.; Cook, S.M.; Palpant, N.J.; *et al.* Human embryonic-stem-cell-derived cardiomyocytes regenerate non-human primate hearts. *Nature* **2014**, *510*, 273–277.

75. Lim, S.Y.; Sivakumaran, P.; Crombie, D.E.; Dusting, G.J.; Pébay, A.; Dilley, R.J. Trichostatin A enhances differentiation of human induced pluripotent stem cells to cardiogenic cells for cardiac tissue engineering. *Stem Cells Transl. Med.* **2013**, *2*, 715–725.

76. Kawamura, M.; Miyagawa, S.; Fukushima, S.; Saito, A.; Miki, K.; Ito, E.; Sougawa, N.; Kawamura, T.; Daimon, T.; Shimizu, T.; *et al.* Enhanced survival of transplanted human induced pluripotent stem cell-derived cardiomyocytes by the combination of cell sheets with the pedicled omental flap technique in a porcine heart. *Circulation* **2013**, *128*, S87–S94.

77. Emmert, M.Y.; Wolint, P.; Wickboldt, N.; Gemayel, G.; Weber, B.; Brokopp, C.E.; Boni, A.; Falk, V.; Bosman, A.; Jaconi, M.E.; *et al.* Human stem cell-based three-dimensional microtissues for advanced cardiac cell therapies. *Biomaterials* **2013**, *34*, 6339–6354.

78. Lu, T.-Y.; Lin, B.; Kim, J.; Sullivan, M.; Tobita, K.; Salama, G.; Yang, L. Repopulation of decellularized mouse heart with human induced pluripotent stem cell-derived cardiovascular progenitor cells. *Nat. Commun.* **2013**, *4*, 2307.

Scalable Electrophysiological Investigation of iPS Cell-Derived Cardiomyocytes Obtained by a Lentiviral Purification Strategy

Stephanie Friedrichs, Daniela Malan, Yvonne Voss and Philipp Sasse

Abstract: Disease-specific induced pluripotent stem (iPS) cells can be generated from patients and differentiated into functional cardiomyocytes for characterization of the disease and for drug screening. In order to obtain pure cardiomyocytes for automated electrophysiological investigation, we here report a novel non-clonal purification strategy by using lentiviral gene transfer of a puromycin resistance gene under the control of a cardiac-specific promoter. We have applied this method to our previous reported wild-type and long QT syndrome 3 (LQTS 3)-specific mouse iPS cells and obtained a pure cardiomyocyte population. These cells were investigated by action potential analysis with manual and automatic planar patch clamp technologies, as well as by recording extracellular field potentials using a microelectrode array system. Action potentials and field potentials showed the characteristic prolongation at low heart rates in LQTS 3-specific, but not in wild-type iPS cell-derived cardiomyocytes. Hence, LQTS 3-specific cardiomyocytes can be purified from iPS cells with a lentiviral strategy, maintain the hallmarks of the LQTS 3 disease and can be used for automated electrophysiological characterization and drug screening.

Reprinted from *J. Clin. Med.* Cite as: Friedrichs, S.; Malan, D.; Voss, Y.; Sasse, P. Scalable Electrophysiological Investigation of iPS Cell-Derived Cardiomyocytes Obtained by a Lentiviral Purification Strategy. *J. Clin. Med.* **2015**, *4*, 102–123.

1. Introduction

Long QT syndrome (LQTS) is an inherited cardiac disease caused by mutations of cardiac ion channels or accessory subunits, which leads to the loss of function of repolarizing currents or the gain of function of depolarizing currents. Clinically, this disease is characterized by abnormal prolonged QT intervals in the ECG, and the patients affected can develop Torsades de Pointes ventricular tachycardia, which causes syncope and sudden cardiac death [1]. One of the most common LQTS gain of function mutations in humans is the deletion of three amino acids (ΔKPQ) in the α-subunit of the cardiac sodium channel (SCN5A) [2], which is classified as LQTS Type 3 (LQTS 3). This mutation results in faster recovery from inactivation of the sodium current and enhanced late sodium currents, which both lead to prolonged action potentials (APs) and early afterdepolarizations (EADs). Because the impact of this mutation is strongest at a low heart rate, lethal cardiac events mostly occur at rest or during sleep [1].

In the past, LQTSs were studied on heterologous expression systems that lack the typical cell biological and physiological features of cardiomyocytes and that do not generate APs [3,4]. Recently, we have shown that LQTS 3-specific cardiomyocytes can be generated from mouse iPS cells carrying the human ΔKPQ mutation and recapitulated the disease-specific biophysical effects of the mutation, as well as prolonged APs and EADs at low heart rates [5]. Furthermore, other groups have successfully generated iPS cells from LQTS 1, 2 and 3 patients, and the cardiomyocytes differentiated from these cells recapitulated the typical characteristics of the respective disease [6–11]. Therefore, human iPS cell-derived cardiomyocytes are a great advance for the understanding of LQTS, especially because "real" cardiomyocytes provide a model that is close to the patient's heart cells.

The unlimited proliferation of personalized iPS cells and the differentiation into cardiomyocytes would allow disease- or even patient-specific drug testing. In order to find new drugs to treat LQTS, pharmaceutical compound libraries have to be screened with scalable automatic assays. Potential automatic electrophysiological screening methods are planar patch clamp systems [12] or microelectrode array technologies [13]. One big challenge for all automated assays is the generation of a pure cardiac population, because during iPS cell differentiation, also non-cardiomyocytes are generated.

To date, several purification methods have been used to enrich cardiac cells. Fluorescence-activated cell sorting of cardiomyocytes with cardiac-specific GFP expression or after labeling with mitochondrial dyes can be used, but these methods result only in low amounts of pure cardiac cells and are difficult to scale up [14,15]. Better yields are achieved with scalable antibiotic selection of cardiomyocytes, which express a resistance gene under a cardiac-specific promoter [16,17]. For antibiotic selection, cells must be genetically modified, and here, we report a highly efficient and straightforward lentiviral gene transfer for the selection of cardiomyocytes by an antibiotic resistance gene without a time-consuming screening of individual clones. We have applied this method to obtain pure populations of cardiomyocytes from LQTS 3-specific iPS cells with the human ΔKPQ mutation and wild-type controls. Furthermore, we proved that purified cardiomyocytes showed the typical features of LQTS 3 in manual patch clamp, automatic planar patch clamp and scalable microelectrode array recording technologies.

2. Experimental Section

2.1. Generation of the Lentiviral αPaG-RexNeo Plasmid and Lentivirus Production

The lentiviral αPaG-RexNeo plasmid is based on a pRRLSIN lentiviral backbone from pRRLSIN.cPPT.PGK-GFP.WPRE (kindly provided by Didier Trono through Addgene #12252). Multiple cloning steps according to standard procedures were used to create an insert containing a short version of the cardiac-specific alpha myosin heavy chain (α-MHC) promoter, a puromycin resistance gene, the green fluorescence protein (GFP) and a fragment with the Rex-1 promoter driving a neomycin resistance gene. The short α-MHC promoter was excised from the α-MHC-pBK plasmid (kindly provided by Jeffrey Robbins) and contained 1745 bp from the 3′ part of the full α-MHC promoter. Parallel expression of puromycin and GFP was achieved by the introduction of the 2A self-cleaving peptide sequence (APVKQTLNFDLLKLAGDVESNPGP) [18] that was generated by annealing and in-frame ligation of appropriate oligonucleotides (MWG-Biotech, Ebersberg, Germany). The Rex-1-neomycin sequence was cut from the α-MHC-puro Rex-neo plasmid (kindly provided by Mark Mercola through Addgene #21230). Successful cloning was confirmed by restriction enzyme digestion and DNA sequencing (MWG-Biotech, Ebersberg,

Germany). All enzymes for cloning were from Life Technologies (Darmstadt, Germany) and Thermo Scientific Fermentas. For the preparation of lentivirus, 40 µg of the αPaG-RexNeo plasmid, 8.5 µg of the pMD2.G plasmid (for the VSV-G envelope, Addgene #12259), 16 µg of the pMDLg/pRRE plasmid (for Gag/Pol expression, Addgene #12251) and 7 µg of the pRSV-Rev plasmid (for Rev expression, Addgene #12253, all kindly provided by Didier Trono through Addgene), were cotransfected into 7×10^6 HEK293FT cells (ATCC) in a T75 culture flask, as previously described [19]. After 24 h, the medium was changed with fresh HEK cell medium that consisted of Dulbecco's Modified Eagle Medium (DMEM), 15% fetal calf serum (FCS), 0.1 mmol/L MEM nonessential amino acids, 0.1 mmol/L 2-mercaptoethanol, 100 U/mL penicillin and 100 mg/mL streptomycin (all from Invitrogen/Bernardi). Virus-containing supernatants were collected at Days 3 and 4 after transfection, passed through a 0.45-µm filter (Sigma-Aldrich, Taufkirchen, Germany) and concentrated by ultracentrifugation at 19.400 rpm for 2 h at 17 °C using an Optima L-90K ultracentrifuge with an SW 32 Ti rotor (Beckman Coulter, Krefeld, Germany). The pellet was resuspended in 50 µL HBSS without Ca^{2+} and Mg^{2+} (Life Technologies, Darmstadt, Germany) and stored frozen at −80 °C.

2.2. Cell Culture and Lentiviral Gene Transfer of iPS Cells

The iPS cells were cultured as reported before [5] on irradiated mouse embryonic feeder (MEF) layers (PMEF-NL; Millipore, Schwalbach, Germany) in iPS cell medium containing DMEM, 15% FCS, 0.1 mmol/L nonessential amino acids, 0.1 mmol/L 2-mercaptoethanol, 100 U/mL penicillin, 100 mg/mL streptomycin (all from Invitrogen/Life Technologies), 1000 U/mL leukemia inhibitory factor (Chemicon/Millipore), 3 µmol/L CHIR99021 and 1 µmol/L PD184352 (Axon Medchem, Groningen, The Netherlands). Every 2 to 3 days, iPS cells were passaged and seeded at a density of 0.1 to 0.2×10^6 cells in a T75 culture flask.

For gene transfer of αPaG-RexNeo, 0.2×10^6 iPS cells were plated on a T25 culture flask on irradiated MEFs, and 24 h later, the αPaG-RexNeo lentivirus from the production described in section 2.1 was added in 5 mL of iPS cell medium in the presence of 6 µg/mL protamine sulfate (Sigma-Aldrich) to enhance infection. The next day, fresh iPS cell medium was applied, and the selection of iPS cells with lentivirus integration was initiated 24 h to 48 h later by the addition of 300 µg/mL neomycin (G418, Invitrogen/Life Technologies). The genetically-engineered wild-type and Scn5aΔ/+ iPS cells were further cultivated and passaged in iPS cell medium in the presence of 300 µg/mL neomycin to avoid lentivirus silencing.

2.3. Differentiation of iPS Cells and Purification of Cardiomyocytes

Cardiomyocyte differentiation was induced using embryoid body (EB) formation with the hanging drop method in combination with a suspension protocol, as previously described [16]. Briefly, EBs were generated by aggregation of 400 cells in 20 µL differentiation medium for 2 days and subsequently cultured in suspension in 10-cm bacteriological dishes on a horizontal shaker in differentiation medium containing Iscove's Modified Dulbecco's Medium, 20% FCS, 0.1 mmol/L MEM nonessential amino acids, 0.1 mmol/L 2-mercaptoethanol, 100 U/mL penicillin, 100 mg/mL streptomycin (all from Invitrogen/Life Technologies). EBs started to beat at day 10 to 12 of differentiation and 10 µg/mL puromycin (Sigma-Aldrich) was added at that time point to initiate the selection of cardiomyocytes. One day later, EBs were pooled, washed with PBS and dissociated with 1 mg/mL collagenase B (Roche Diagnostics, Mannheim, Germany) in 1.6 mL in a 50-mL falcon tube for 60 min at 37 °C under shaking condition. The enzymatic reaction was stopped with the addition of 30 mL of differentiation medium. In order to avoid a centrifugation step that was found to be lethal for the freshly-dissociated cardiomyocytes, a subsequent passive sedimentation step was performed for 60 min in the incubator. The supernatant was removed except ~10 mL, in which the cardiomyocytes were resuspended and collected. For further selection and cultivation, cells were seeded on 0.01% fibronectin-coated (Sigma-Aldrich) 10-cm cell culture dishes in differentiation medium supplemented with 2.5 to 5 µg/mL puromycin. To obtain a more mature stage for electrophysiological analysis, single purified cardiomyocytes were kept in culture for an additional 6 to 10 days, because we have shown that longer differentiation leads to more cells with functional Na^+ currents [5].

2.4. Immunocytochemistry

For immunostainings, cells were fixed with 4% paraformaldehyde for 30 min, permeabilized with 0.2% Triton X-100 for 10 min (both from Sigma-Aldrich) and blocked with 5% donkey or goat serum for 30 min (Jackson ImmunoResearch, Suffolk, England). The primary antibodies were diluted in 0.5% donkey or goat serum, and cells were incubated for 2 h. Colonies of iPS cells were stained against Oct3/4 (rabbit, 1:100; Santa Cruz Biotechnology, Heidelberg, Germany) and SSEA1 (mouse, 1:80; Developmental Studies Hybridoma Bank, Iowa, USA). Single cardiomyocytes were stained against α-actinin (mouse, 1:400; Sigma-Aldrich) and the cardiac Na^+ channel (Nav1.5, rabbit, 1:400; Alomone Labs, Jerusalem, Israel). The appropriate fluorescence-conjugated secondary antibodies, donkey anti-mouse Cy2-labeled, donkey anti-rabbit Cy3-labeled (both 1:400; Jackson ImmunoResearch) and goat anti-mouse Alexa647-labeled (1:500; Invitrogen/Life Technologies), were diluted in 1 µg/mL of Hoechst 33342 (Sigma-Aldrich) and applied for 1 h. Samples were embedded in polyvinyl alcohol mounting medium (FLUKA; Sigma-Aldrich) and analyzed using an AxioObserver Z1 microscope equipped with an ApoTome optical sectioning device and the AxioVision software (Zeiss, Jena, Germany).

To analyze the purity of iPS cell-derived cardiomyocytes, purified cells at Days 13 to 15 of differentiation from 4 to 5 independent biological replicates were stained against α-actinin. The ratio of α-actinin-positive cells to the total cell number analyzed by nucleus labeling was quantified from large overview pictures that were acquired with the MosaiX function of the AxioVision software (Zeiss).

2.5. Conventional Manual Patch Clamp Analysis

Purified wild-type and Scn5aΔ/+ cardiomyocytes were dissociated and replated for 48 to 72 h at low densities on fibronectin-coated (0.01%) coverslips. Patch clamp experiments were performed after 48 to 72 h using an EPC10 amplifier (HEKA Elektronik, Lambrecht, Germany) in the whole cell configuration and the current clamp mode, as reported earlier [5], with continuous superfusion with extracellular solution at 37 °C containing (in mmol/L) 140 NaCl, 5.4 KCl, 1.8 CaCl$_2$, 1.2 MgCl$_2$, 10 Hepes and 10 glucose, pH 7.4 (NaOH), and an internal solution containing (in mmol/L) 50 KCl, 80 K-aspartate, 1 MgCl$_2$, 3 MgATP, 10 EGTA and 10 HEPES, pH 7.2 (KOH) (all from Sigma-Aldrich). APs were elicited by 2.5 ms-long current injections, and the strength of the pulse was increased stepwise until a stable action potential with a peak over the 0 mV line was reached. The stimulation frequency and amplitude was controlled by an external stimulator (Model 2100, A–M Systems) attached to the EPC10 amplifier.

2.6. Automated Planar Patch Clamp Analysis

For automated planar patch clamp measurements, single dissociated cardiomyocytes are required in suspension without damage of the cell membrane or transmembrane ion channels. Therefore, purified wild-type and Scn5aΔ/+ cardiomyocytes in a 10-cm cell culture dish were washed with 5 mL PBS containing EDTA (2 mM) and stored for 10 min at 4 °C in order to facilitate the detachment of cells by subsequent incubation with 2 mL 0.05% Trypsin in 4 mM EDTA (Gibco/Life Technologies) for 3 to 8 min. Cells were collected in 10 mL of differentiation medium, gently centrifuged for 3 min at 500 rpm, resuspended in 200 to 500 μL external solution and incubated at room temperature for at least 2 h to recover from dissociation. Automated electrophysiological recording was performed with a planar patch clamp robot (Patchliner, Nanion Technologies, Munich, Germany) equipped with an EPC-10 quadro patch clamp amplifier (HEKA Elektronik) for parallel recording of 4 cardiomyocytes in the whole cell configuration. Single-use borosilicate glass chips with medium resistance (1.8 to 3 MΩ, NPC-16, Nanion Technologies) were used for all recordings. The PatchControlHT software (Nanion Technologies) in combination with the PatchMaster software (HEKA Elektronik) was used for cell capture, seal formation, whole-cell access and subsequent recording of voltage ramps, automated determination of AP stimulus thresholds and AP measurements at different stimulation frequencies. The internal solution used contained (in mmol/L) 50 KCl, 60 K-fluoride, 10 NaCl, 20 EGTA and 10 HEPES, pH 7.2 (KOH), and the external solution 140 NaCl, 4 KCl, 2 CaCl$_2$, 5 Glucose and 10 HEPES, pH 7.4 (NaOH) (all from Sigma-Aldrich). A seal enhancer solution containing (in mmol/L) 80 NaCl, 3 KCl, 10 MgCl$_2$, 35 CaCl$_2$ and 10 HEPES (Na$^+$ salt), pH 7.4 (HCl) (all from Sigma-Aldrich), was automatically applied to the extracellular channel after cell capture in order to achieve better GΩ-seals and replaced with external solution when the whole cell configuration was established.

In order to identify mature cardiomyocytes, depolarizing voltage ramps (−100 mV to +60 mV in 250 ms) were applied, and the responding current was analyzed to identify the fast spike of Na$^+$ currents. APs were recorded in current clamp mode and to avoid spontaneous activity, and to record APs from a stable resting potential, the membrane potential was adjusted to −70 mV by current injection using the low frequency voltage clamp circuit of the amplifier. Before each AP recording, the low frequency voltage clamp was switched off, and the actual current was continuously injected to maintain the resting membrane potential. To determine the current injection threshold for AP generation for each cell individually, an automated macro was programmed and executed. This generated a 2-ms current injection of stepwise (100 pA) increasing intensities and automatically monitored the voltage responses. Leak subtraction was used to subtract the passive capacitive responses to the stimulus. Once the stimulus generates voltage responses with an amplitude of >30 mV above the resting membrane potential, this value was used, and 80 pA was added for safety. Subsequently, APs were automatically evoked and recorded for 30 to 60 s at 0.5 Hz, 1 Hz and 2 Hz by a protocol in the Patchmaster software (HEKA Elektronik).

Data from both conventional and planar patch clamp were acquired with the Patchmaster software and analyzed offline using the Fitmaster (HEKA Elektronik) and the Labchart software (AD Instruments, Oxford, England). The action potential duration at 90% of repolarization (APD90) was analyzed with the peak analysis module of Labchart software (AD Instruments). To quantify the frequency-dependent AP duration, cardiomyocytes were stimulated at different pacing periods (0.5 to 6 s for manual patch clamp and 0.5 to 2 s for automatic patch clamp), and at each period, the average APD90 was determined. For each individual cell, the APD90 values were plotted against the period between stimulation (1/frequency), and a linear regression analysis was used to determine the slope of this relationship.

2.7. Microelectrode Array Analysis

For the microelectrode array (MEA) measurements, purified cardiomyocytes from wild-type and Scn5aΔ/+ iPS cells were detached with 0.05% Trypsin in 0.5 mM EDTA (Gibco/Life Technologies) for 5 min at 37 °C, centrifuged for 5 min at 1000 rpm and resuspended in differentiation medium. Then, 20,000 to 40,000 cells were plated in each well of a 6-well MEA (60-6wellMEA200/30iR-Ti-tcr, Multi Channel Systems, Reutlingen, Germany) coated with 0.01% fibronectin (Sigma-Aldrich). After 24 to 72 h, the medium was replaced with external solution (see Section 2.5), and field potentials were recorded at a sampling rate of 10 kHz with the MC-Rack software at room temperature (22 °C) and at 37 °C by switching on the TC02 2-channel temperature controller (both from Multi Channel Systems). Triggered field potentials were averaged over 50 s, and the mean of all 9 electrodes in one well was calculated (OriginPro8G, OriginLab) to obtain one averaged field potential for further analysis. The field potential duration was manually measured from the minimum of the sharp negative spike to the following maximum (Figure 6c, right).

2.8. Statistics

Data are expressed as the mean ± S.E.M. Statistical tests were performed using appropriate unpaired or paired Student's t-test with Welch's correction for data with unequal variance using Prism (GraphPad software). A p-value of <0.05 was considered significant and is indicated by an asterisk (*) in the figures. Because of high variations in temperature-induced frequency between Scn5aΔ/+ and wild-type cardiomyocytes using MEA recordings (Scn5aΔ/+: high 1.4–1.8 Hz, low 0.7–1.0 Hz; wild-type: high 1.6–4.7 Hz, low 1.0–3.5 Hz), in these experiments, only paired Student's t-tests within individual genotypes were performed (Figure 6d).

3. Results

3.1. Lentiviral Strategy for Purification of iPS Cell-Derived Cardiomyocytes

In order to obtain a pure cardiomyocyte population from iPS cell differentiation, we have modified a previously-reported antibiotic resistance strategy [16] and used high efficiency lentiviral gene transfer [17]. Therefore, we have generated a lentiviral plasmid (αPaG-RexNeo) for the expression of a puromycin resistance gene and the green fluorescent protein (GFP) reporter gene under the control of a short (1.7 kb) version of the cardiac-specific alpha myosin heavy chain (α-MHC) promoter (Figure 1a). In addition, the plasmid contained a fragment with a neomycin resistance gene expressed under the control of the pluripotency promoter Rex-1 [20]. After infection of cells with this lentiviral plasmid, undifferentiated stem cells with stable integration of the lentivirus can be selected by cultivation in the presence of neomycin [17]. Upon differentiation, cardiomyocytes can be purified by puromycin application and used for electrophysiological investigations (Figure 1b). To test this strategy for the investigation of a clinically relevant cardiac disease, we have purified LQTS 3-specific cardiomyocytes from previously-reported Scn5aΔ/+ iPS cells [5] with the human ΔKPQ mutation in the cardiac sodium channel.

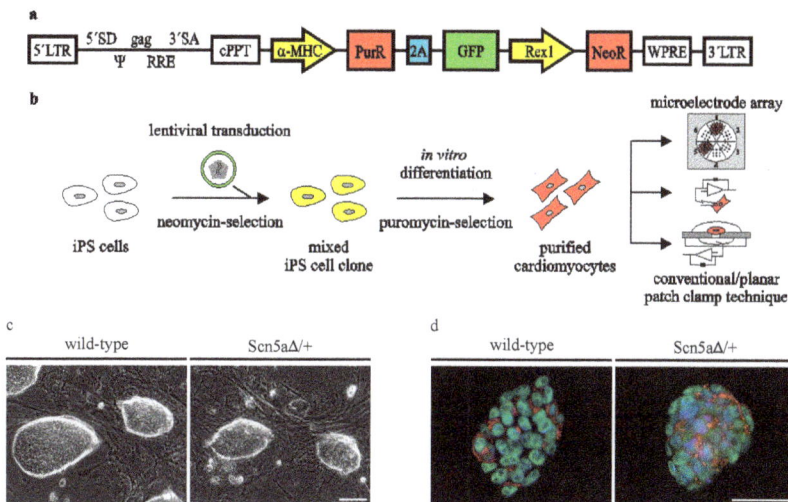

Figure 1. Lentiviral strategy for the purification of iPS cell-derived cardiomyocytes. (**a**) The lentiviral construct contains a puromycin resistance gene (*PurR*) and a GFP reporter gene separated by a 2A self-cleaving peptide sequence (2A) under the control of the cardiac α-MHC promoter, as well as a neomycin resistance gene (*NeoR*) under the control of the Rex1 promoter; (**b**) strategy of lentivirus gene transfer into iPS cells and purification of cardiomyocytes for electrophysiological analysis; (**c,d**) after lentiviral gene transfer and selection, wild-type and Scn5aΔ/+ iPS cell lines maintained the characteristic embryonic stem cell-like morphology (**c**) and expressed the embryonic stem cell-specific markers, Oct3/4 (**d**, green) and SSEA1 (**d**, red). Nuclei are shown in blue. Scale bars: 50 μm.

Therefore, a monolayer of undifferentiated Scn5aΔ/+ and wild-type iPS cells were infected with the αPaG-RexNeo lentivirus and further kept under neomycin selection for the isolation of cells with a stable integration. The surviving iPS cells were collected and pooled for each genotype. Although this non-clonal strategy results in a mixture of individual cell clones with uncontrolled variations in the number and location of lentiviral integrations, it does not require the very laborious picking and characterization of several individual clones. Importantly, after αPaG-RexNeo gene transfer and selection, we found that both wild-type and LQT 3-specific iPS cells maintained their characteristic embryonic stem cell morphology (Figure 1c) and expressed the stem cell-specific markers Oct3/4 and SSEA1 (Figure 1d).

3.2. Purification of αPaG-RexNeo iPS Cell-Derived Cardiomyocytes

In vitro differentiation of αPaG-RexNeo wild-type and Scn5aΔ/+ iPS cells was performed using the hanging drop method for embryoid body (EB) generation [21] followed by a mass culture protocol (Figure 2a) [16]. EBs showed spontaneously beating areas at Days 10 to 12 of differentiation with weak GFP signals. At this stage, cardiomyocyte selection was started by puromycin application for one day, and single cells were re-plated on fibronectin-coated culture dishes. Longer selection at the EB stage was inefficient, because dissociation of older and more compact EBs with enhanced extracellular matrix failed, resulting in a low number of single cardiomyocytes. Single dissociated cardiomyocytes were spontaneously beating and weakly GFP-positive (Figure 2b).

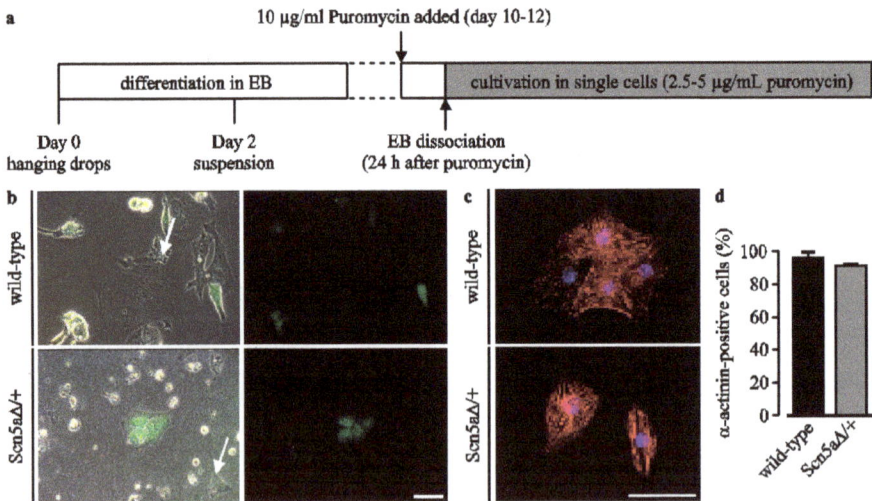

Figure 2. Purification of iPS cell-derived cardiomyocytes. (**a**) The cardiac differentiation protocol used in this study; (**b**) single dissociated cardiomyocytes were GFP-positive and beating, but some non-contracting and GFP-negative cells remained (arrows) after the puromycin selection for 24 h; (**c**) after further purification of single cells, mostly α-actinin-positive cardiomyocytes survived (red); (**d**) cell counting at Days 13 to 15 of differentiation showed the very high purity of wild-type and Scn5aΔ/+ cardiomyocytes. Scale bars: 50 μm. Error bars: S.E.M. EB, embryoid body.

Because cells without GFP expression or contractions were still present (Figure 2b, arrows), cultures were maintained under a low dose of puromycin selection, which led to further purification. Subsequently, the purity of cardiomyocytes was assessed by staining against cardiac α-actinin and cell nuclei (Figure 2c), and quantitative cell counting showed an almost pure population of cardiomyocytes (Figure 2d) from wild-type (92.8% ± 6.2%, n = 5) and Scn5aΔ/+ iPS cells (87.7% ± 9.7%, n = 4).

3.3. Phenotyping of Purified LQTS 3-Specific Cardiomyocytes from Scn5aΔ/+ iPS Cells

Purified cardiomyocytes from wild-type and Scn5aΔ/+ iPS cells showed no obvious difference in cardiac sodium channel distribution or sarcomeric structure (Figure 3a). To exclude that the lentivirus integration, the non-clonal strategy or the purification affect the LQTS 3-specific phenotype we characterized purified cardiomyocytes by classical manual patch clamp techniques.

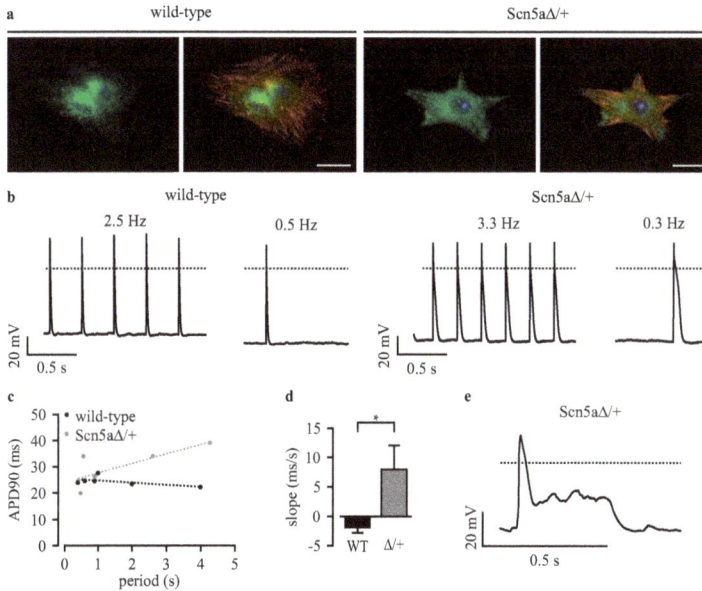

Figure 3. Patch clamp analysis of purified iPS-derived cardiomyocytes. (**a**) Cardiomyocytes from wild-type and Scn5aΔ/+ iPS cells showed a similar cardiac sodium channel distribution (green) and sarcomeric α-actinin pattern (red); (**b**) representative examples of action potentials (APs) from purified wild-type and Scn5aΔ/+ cardiomyocytes at high and low pacing frequencies; (**c**) relationship between action potential duration at 90% of repolarization (APD90) and pacing period from a representative wild-type and Scn5aΔ/+ cardiomyocyte with the analysis of the slope by linear fit (dashed lines); (**d**) statistical analysis of the slope of APD90 to the pacing period relationship from individual wild-type (WT) and Scn5aΔ/+ cardiomyocytes (Δ/+); (**e**) typical long QT syndrome 3 (LQTS 3)-specific early afterdepolarizations (EADs) observed in a Scn5aΔ/+ cardiomyocyte. Scale bar: 20 μm. Error bars: S.E.M. Dotted lines indicate 0 mV.

APs were evoked at various frequencies by current injection, and the frequency-dependent action potential duration at 90% repolarization (APD90) was analyzed. In Scn5aΔ/+ cardiomyocytes, but not in wild-type cells, we found a prolongation of APD90 at lower heart rates (Figure 3b, Table 1), which did not reach statistical significance because of the high variability of APD90 between individual cells. The high variability was not due to the non-clonal purification approach, because it was similarly observed in non-purified cardiomyocytes from the original iPS cell clones [5]. To compensate for this variability, we performed a longitudinal analysis for each individual cell and determined the slope of the relationship between APD90 and basic cycle length (APD restitution) using a linear fit (examples shown in Figure 3c), as reported before [5,22]. This analysis showed almost no influence of cycle length on APD90 in purified wild-type cardiomyocytes yielding flat slopes of APD restitution (-1.85 ± 0.73 ms/s, $n = 10$, Figure 3d). In contrast, purified Scn5aΔ/+ cardiomyocytes had a significant different positive slope (7.94 ± 4.05 ms/s, $n = 18$, Figure 3d) highlighting the prolongation of APD90 with a longer cycle length. This is the characteristic feature of LQTS 3 in patients [22] and is fully in line with previous reports on non-purified cardiomyocytes from Scn5aΔ/+ iPS cells [5], as well as on cardiomyocytes from the ΔKPQ LQTS 3 mouse model [23]. Importantly, these slope values are almost identical to those obtained from the non-purified original iPS cell clones (wild-type: -2.92 ± 1.27 ms/s; Scn5aΔ/+: 9.08 ± 3.60 ms/s; see Table 2 in Malan *et al.* [5]). Moreover, we detected EADs in some purified Scn5aΔ/+ cardiomyocytes (10.5%, $n = 19$, Figure 3e), but never in wild-type cells (0%, $n = 10$). Resting membrane potential, action potential amplitude and maximum upstroke velocity were not different between wild-type and Scn5aΔ/+ cardiomyocytes (Table 1).

Table 1. Action potential parameters determined by manual and automated planar patch clamp analysis. RMP, resting membrane potential; APA, action potential amplitude; Vmax, maximum upstroke velocity; APD90, APD at 90% of repolarization; Slope, slope of the linear relationship between APD90 and the pacing period. Values are the means ± S.E.M.

Method	Manual Patch Clamp			Automated Planar Patch Clamp		
Genotype	Wild-Type	Scn5aΔ/+	*p*-Value	Wild-Type	Scn5aΔ/+	*p*-Value
RMP at 1 Hz	-77.4 ± 4.9	-74.7 ± 3.5	0.6589	-69.4 ± 6.4	-78.2 ± 3.0	0.2040
(mV)	$n = 10$	$n = 17$		$n = 7$	$n = 9$	
APA 1 Hz	106.2 ± 5.7	103.3 ± 5.7	0.7207	81.1 ± 13.2	85.8 ± 10.1	0.7746
(mV)	$n = 10$	$n = 17$		$n = 7$	$n = 9$	
V max at 1 Hz	93.7 ± 11.1	71.6 ± 9.6	0.1484	56.6 ± 15.5	52.6 ± 10.2	0.8248
(V/s)	$n = 10$	$n = 17$		$n = 7$	$n = 9$	
APD90 at 2 Hz	36.2 ± 3.5	39.5 ± 5.1	0.6004	78.0 ± 28.7	64.9 ± 17.1	0.7019
(ms)	$n = 10$	$n = 14$		$n = 7$	$n = 7$	
APD90 at 1 Hz	35.5 ± 3.3	45.8 ± 6.8	0.1913	70.1 ± 26.6	76.7 ± 20.4	0.8454
(ms)	$n = 10$	$n = 15$		$n = 7$	$n = 9$	
APD90 at 0.2 Hz (manual) or 0.5 Hz (automated) (ms)	39.7 ± 2.2	46.8 ± 6.7	0.1761	69.6 ± 24.3	91.5 ± 25.0	0.5440
	$n = 5$	$n = 5$		$n = 7$	$n = 8$	
Slope	-1.85 ± 0.73	7.94 ± 4.05	0.0287	-5.39 ± 4.82	4.13 ± 1.20	0.0494
(ms/s)	$n = 10$	$n = 18$		$n = 7$	$n = 9$	

Importantly, we did not find differences in action potential parameters between early and late passages of the non-clonal iPS cell clones (Table 2).

Table 2. Action potential parameters at early (P12–P18) and late (P19–P35) passages determined by manual patch clamp recordings (the abbreviations are as in Table 1).

Genotype	Wild-Type			Scn5aΔ/+		
Passage	Early Passage	Late Passage	*p*-Value	Early Passage	Late Passage	*p*-Value
RMP at 1 Hz (mV)	−71.8 ± 2.3 $n = 4$	−68.3 ± 9.7 $n = 3$	0.7061	−71.5 ± 7.3 $n = 4$	−67.3 ± 5.6 $n = 7$	0.6593
APA 1 Hz (mV)	105.5 ± 6.9 $n = 4$	99.7 ± 16.5 $n = 3$	0.7312	97.3 ± 9.0 $n = 4$	91.3 ± 8.1 $n = 7$	0.6513
V max at 1 Hz (V/s)	98.8 ± 6.8 $n = 4$	88.3 ± 31.7 $n = 3$	0.7215	81.8 ± 15.6 $n = 4$	59.6 ± 17.6 $n = 7$	0.4230
APD90 at 1 Hz (ms)	33.1 ± 3.6 $n = 4$	27.7 ± 0.7 $n = 3$	0.2657	49.1 ± 15.7 $n = 4$	52.8 ± 11.3 $n = 7$	0.8499
Slope (ms/s)	−1.10 ± 0.32 $n = 4$	−1.10 ± 0.57 $n = 3$	1.00	14.75 ± 13.12 $n = 4$	8.94 ± 6.68 $n = 8$	0.7106

3.4. Automated Electrophysiological Investigation and AP Measurements of Purified Cardiomyocytes with a Planar Patch Clamp System

In order to implement the use of purified wild-type and Scn5aΔ/+ cardiomyocytes for automated screenings, we performed electrophysiological analysis with a planar patch clamp robot (Patchliner, Nanion Technologies). For this technique, freshly dissociated single cells in suspension are required. Therefore, a new and gentle dissociation procedure was used to minimize cell stress and to avoid partial digestion of ion channels, which are required for intact AP generation. Dissociation was facilitated by removal of Ca^{2+} and cooling of cells at 4 °C, which allowed subsequent dissociation with the very short application of Trypsin. After dissociation, cells were gently centrifuged and carefully resuspended in external solution. In order to let cardiomyocytes recover from the dissociation process, cells remained at least 2 h at room temperature before planar patch clamp experiments were performed. To verify the dissociation efficiency, single cells were counted, and the cell concentration was adjusted to 0.1 to 1×10^6 cells/mL to ensure a good catch rate by the planar patch clamp robot. For planar patch clamp measurements, 20 µL containing 2000 to 20,000 purified cardiomyocytes, was automatically pipetted into each recoding unit of the planar patch clamp chip. Once a cell was caught, a negative pressure was automatically applied and a seal enhancer was injected to form a good GΩ-seal for stable recording without leaks.

To estimate the quality of recording and the differentiation stage of cardiomyocytes, depolarizing voltage ramps were applied in the voltage clamp mode. This allowed determination of the intact seal without major leak conductance, as well as the detection of typical inward and outward currents of voltage-dependent ion channels (Figure 4a). Voltage ramps were also used to classify cardiomyocytes in immature cells with a slow inward Ca^{2+} current peak (Figure 4a, left, arrow) and in more mature cells with an additional fast Na^+ current component (Figure 4a, right, arrow). Because we wanted to characterize a disease based on a Na^+ channel mutation, only cardiomyocytes with a clear Na$^+$ current peak were subsequently used to record APs. APs were evoked by current injection in the current clamp mode (Figure 4c). To identify the minimal current required, a special protocol was executed by the PatchControlHT software (Nanion Technologies). Briefly, stepwise (100 pA steps) increasing 2 ms-long current stimuli were applied, and the voltage responses were analyzed (Figure 4b). As soon as the resulting amplitude was >30 mV above the resting membrane potential, the applied current was defined as the threshold-current and 80 pA was added for safety.

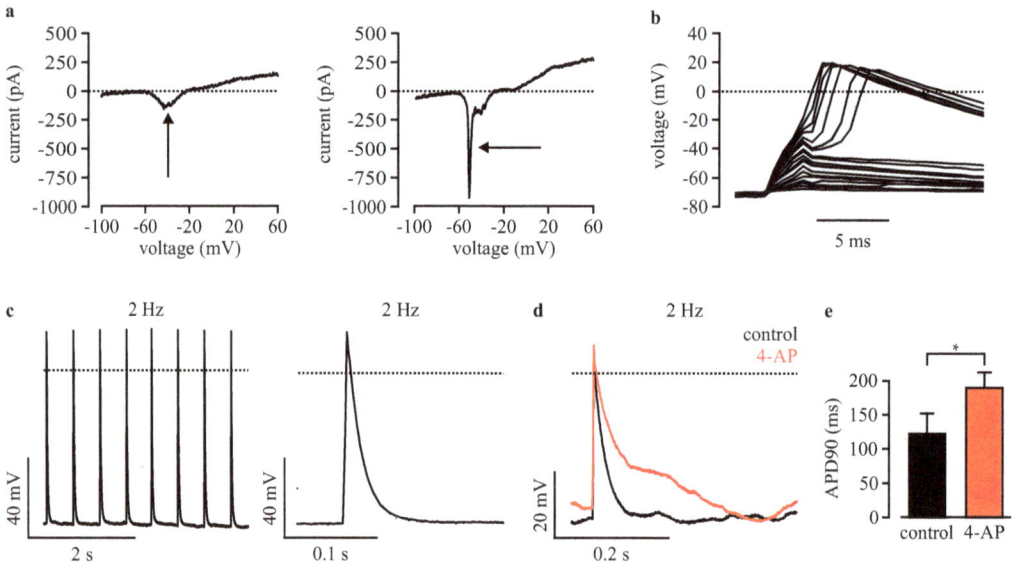

Figure 4. Automated planar patch clamp analysis of purified wild-type iPS-derived cardiomyocytes. (**a**) Examples of voltage ramps of an immature cardiomyocyte with Ca^{2+} current (left, arrow) and of a more mature cell with an additional fast Na$^+$ current (right, arrow); (**b**) Representative membrane potential changes in response to stepwise increasing current pulses during the protocol for finding the AP threshold; (**c**) Example of automated AP recording at fixed pacing rate (**left**) with magnification (**right**); (**d**) representative APs before (black) and after blocking of K$^+$ channels with automated application of 4-AP (red); (**e**) Statistical analysis of APD90 measured under control conditions and after 4-AP application. Error bars: S.E.M. Dotted lines indicate 0 mV or 0 pA.

To determine if AP recordings with a planar patch clamp system are useful to investigate LQTSs that mainly affects cardiac repolarization, we inhibited the repolarizing K$^+$ channels by automated application of 4-aminopyridine and measured the effect on APD90. As expected, we found AP prolongation in purified wild-type cardiomyocytes from 120.1 ± 30.5 ms to 188.9 ± 24.0 ms ($n = 4$, AP evoked at 2 Hz, Figure 4d,e).

3.5. Automated Phenotypic Characterization of LQTS 3-Specific Purified Cardiomyocytes from Scn5aΔ/+ iPS Cells with a Planar Patch Clamp Robot

To proof the feasibility to characterize LQTSs with automated electrophysiological analysis, we recorded APs from purified cardiomyocytes using the planar patch clamp system. Frequency dependence was determined with APs elicited at 2, 1 and 0.5 Hz pacing frequencies using the automatically determined current threshold (see the above Section 3.4). Similar to the results from manual patch clamp recordings (Figure 3), we found prolonged APs at low heart rates in Scn5aΔ/+ cardiomyocytes, but not in wild-type cells (Figure 5a,b). Furthermore, the longitudinal analysis of APD restitution in individual cells (examples shown in Figure 5c) showed a positive slope in Scn5aΔ/+ cardiomyocytes (4.13 ± 1.20 ms/s, n = 9) and a significant different negative slope in wild-type cells (−5.39 ± 4.82 ms/s, n = 7, Figure 5d, Table 1). Finally, we observed EADs in 30% of purified Scn5aΔ/+ cardiomyocytes (Figure 4e, n = 10), but none in wild-type cells (n = 7).

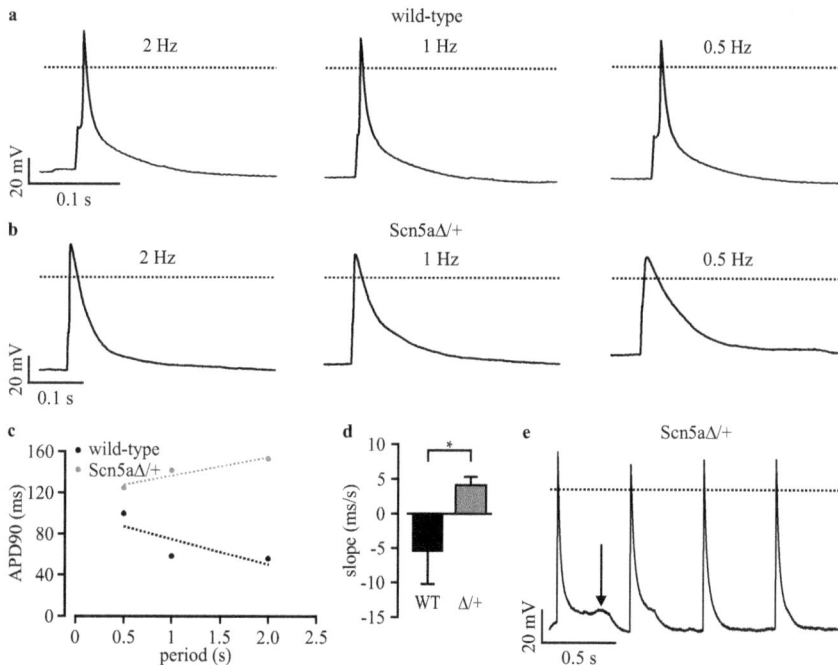

Figure 5. Automated characterization of LQTS 3-specific cardiomyocytes by planar patch clamp. (**a,b**) Representative traces of APs from wild-type (**a**) and Scn5aΔ/+ (**b**) cardiomyocytes at high and low pacing frequencies; (**c**) relationship between APD90 and the pacing period from a representative wild-type and a Scn5aΔ/+ cardiomyocyte with analysis of the slope by linear fit (dashed lines); (**d**) statistical analysis of the slope of APD90 to the pacing period relationship from individual wild-type (WT) and Scn5aΔ/+ cardiomyocytes (Δ/+); (**e**) typical LQTS 3-specific EADs observed in a Scn5aΔ/+ cardiomyocyte (arrow). Error bars: S.E.M. Dotted lines indicate 0 mV.

3.6. Analysis of Field Potentials from Purified iPS Cell-Derived Cardiomyocytes with Microelectrode Arrays

The duration of APs can not only be determined by patch clamp analysis, but can also be estimated indirectly from extracellular field potential recordings with microelectrode arrays, because of the good correlation of field potential duration to APD [24]. To prove the functionality of this technology for the characterization of LQTS 3, we plated purified cardiomyocytes obtained from wild-type and Scn5aΔ/+ iPS cells on six-well microelectrode arrays on which they formed a monolayer of synchronously beating cells (Figure 6a). This allowed recordings of field potentials from nine electrodes in six individual wells (example recording in Figure 6b). To determine frequency-dependent field potential duration, measurements were performed at 22 °C and at 37 °C, which accelerated the spontaneous beating frequency.

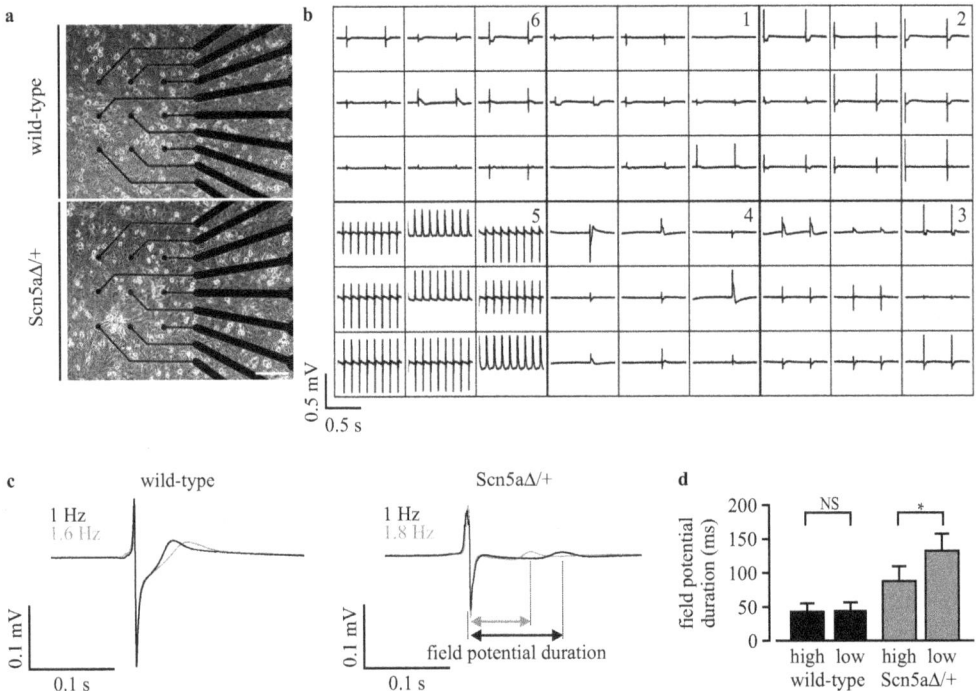

Figure 6. Field potential analysis with microelectrode arrays. (**a**) Image of the recording electrodes of a six-well microelectrode array with a monolayer of purified cardiomyocytes; (**b**) overview of field potential recordings from three wells with purified wild-type (**bottom**) and three wells with Scn5aΔ/+ cardiomyocytes (**top**); (**c**) examples of averaged field potentials with slow beating at 22 °C (black) and faster beating at 37 °C (grey) from purified wild-type and Scn5aΔ/+ cardiomyocytes. The analysis of the field potential duration is shown in the Scn5aΔ/+ recording; (**d**) statistical analysis of the field potential durations at low and high spontaneous beating frequencies from wild-type and Scn5aΔ/+ cardiomyocytes. Scale bar: 200 μm. Error bars: S.E.M. NS, not significant.

Field potential duration was analyzed after trigger-based averaging over 50 s and calculation of the mean field potential from all nine electrodes (for details, see Section 2.7), resulting in one averaged field potential for each well (examples in Figure 6c). Scn5aΔ/+ cardiomyocytes showed a significantly ($p = 0.011$) longer field potential duration at low frequencies (132.4 ± 25.2 ms, $n = 3$) compared to high frequencies (88.0 ± 22.6 ms, $n = 3$, Figure 6d). Importantly, such a frequency-dependent effect was not observed in wild-type cardiomyocytes (low frequency: 45.5 ± 9.5 ms, $n = 3$; high frequency: 42.1 ± 10.5 ms, $n = 3$; $p = 0.78$). Thus, also field potential analysis with a microelectrode array showed the disease-specific frequency dependence of prolonged AP durations in purified Scn5aΔ/+ cardiomyocytes.

4. Discussion

In this study, we present a novel, simple and fast lentiviral strategy for the purification of cardiomyocytes from iPS cells and show the feasibility of using these cells for automated electrophysiological investigations. The adverse effects of the random lentivirus integration, the non-clonal cell selection and the antibiotic purification on the pluripotency of iPS cells or the electrophysiological characteristics of cardiomyocytes were not detected. Importantly, purified cardiomyocytes had fast depolarizing Na$^+$ currents, AP generation and intact repolarization by K$^+$ currents and, therefore, were well suited to investigate LQTS in which these parameters are affected. We have proven this by showing the intact electrophysiological phenotype of purified LQTS 3-specific cardiomyocytes from previously published Scn5aΔ/+ iPS cells [5]. Furthermore, we have characterized purified cells with the automated planar patch clamp recordings and scalable microelectrode array analysis, which highlights the usefulness of these technologies for drug screening. Following, we discuss the achievements so far and the hurdles to overcome for large-scale purification and electrophysiological screening of cardiomyocytes.

4.1. Lentiviral Non-Clonal Gene Transfer Strategy

We have chosen cardiac-specific expression of an antibiotic resistance gene in order to kill all non-cardiomyocytes by antibiotic application. In contrast to low throughput single-cell sorting of labeled cardiomyocytes [14,15], this strategy enables the large-scale purification of cells. Because transfection of plasmid with common chemical, electroporation or lipofection methods suffers from poor efficiency in undifferentiated iPS cells, viral gene transfer methods are suitable alternatives [25,26]. We have used a lentivirus strategy that allows not only high efficient gene transfer, but also stable integration into the genome [25]. In addition to the cardiac-specific antibiotic resistance, we have employed a neomycin resistance gene under the control of the stem cell-specific promoter, Rex-1 [20], which was shown before to be useful for the selection of embryonic stem cell clones [17]. Thus, neomycin treatment allowed the selection of undifferentiated cells with stable lentivirus integration and without silencing or adverse positional effects of the surrounding host chromatin. One further advantage of using Rex-1-neomycin is that the continuous selection pressure at undifferentiated stages prevents iPS cell differentiation or lentiviral silencing at higher passages.

Usually, after classical or viral gene transfer into pluripotent stem cells, several single-cell clones are picked, propagated and characterized individually [16], a very time-consuming procedure and, therefore, an expensive task. In contrast to previous work, we decided to pool all iPS cells that survived the neomycin selection and generated one non-clonal iPS cell line for each genotype. This strategy harbors the risk that a single iPS cell clone with enhanced proliferation by lentivirus-induced mutations or chromosomal aberrations could overgrow the mixed population. However, the intact stem-cell morphology, the expression of stem cell markers, the normal proliferation of the mixed clones and the high similarity of all electrophysiological parameters in cardiomyocytes from early and late passages of the non-clonal iPS cell lines suggest no adverse effects of this strategy. Importantly, the phenotypical fingerprint of LQTS 3 (APD prolongation at slow rates) was only observed in Scn5aΔ/+ cardiomyocytes, both at early and late passages. Furthermore, the slope values of cardiomyocytes from the non-clonal iPS cells were almost identical to those from the original iPS cell clones [5].

The novel possibility to work with non-clonal iPS cells is also supported by a previous report on the successful generation of iPS cell clones in bulk culture without clone picking, which did not reveal differences with clonal selected iPS cell lines regarding pluripotency, gene expression profiles or differentiation potential [27]. Because a non-clonal strategy avoids manual clone picking and could be applied in 96-well or scalable formats, it enables the parallel generation and genetic modification of iPS cell lines from different patients at once. This would allow the purification of cardiomyocytes from many different patients for parallel and comparative electrophysiological screening.

The non-clonal lentiviral cardiomyocyte purification strategy might also have limitations and variations in efficacy because of uncontrolled variations in copy numbers and integration sites between iPS cells. High concentrations of neomycin could be used for selecting clones with the highest copy numbers, and this should be investigated in the future. Because lentiviruses have the tendency to integrate into euchromatin [28], infection at the stem cell level could lead to clones that are neomycin resistant at undifferentiated stages, but encounter lentiviral silencing upon differentiation and, therefore, fail to express puromycin for cardiomyocyte purification. Furthermore, the random integration of lentiviruses could cause insertional mutagenesis; however, this seems not to be frequent, because they tend to integrate away from promoters [29].

Recently, metabolic selection by the cultivation of stem-cell-derived cells in glucose-depleted medium containing only lactate as the energy source was described to be an efficient non-genetic method for the purification of cardiomyocytes [30]. Although the authors report a purity of 99% cardiomyocytes, this method seems to be highly dependent on the cell line used. In fact, although we have extensively tried to reproduce these purity values, we only obtained 45%–80% cardiomyocytes from mouse embryonic stem and human iPS cell lines using identical metabolic selection procedures [31].

4.2. Choice of a Cardiac-Specific Promoter

For cardiac-specific expression of the puromycin resistance gene, we have used the α-MHC promoter, which was shown to enable high efficient purification of cardiomyocytes from mouse and human iPS and embryonic stem cells [16,17,32,33]. Because of the size limitation for gene transfer using lentivirus (~9–10 kb between LTRs [27]), we had to use a short version (~1.7 kb) of the 3' end of the classical 6.5 kb-long α-MHC promoter. Although this fragment contained important gene expression regulatory elements (TATA box, MEF-1 MEF-2 and Nkx2.5 binding sites) [34], it is likely that unidentified enhancing elements were not present explaining the weak GFP expression. Nevertheless, purification of cardiomyocytes was unharmed, indicating sufficient expression of the puromycin resistance gene. This indicates a lower threshold for puromycin resistance than for GFP fluorescence, because the use of a 2A self-cleaving peptide should result in equimolar expression of both proteins [18].

In the future, the use of other promoters should be considered. Although the α-MHC promoter is labeling mature cardiomyocytes in mice, β-MHC is the predominant isoform in the human ventricle, and α-MHC is a marker rather for atrial or failing human cardiomyocytes [35]. Therefore, mature cardiomyocytes from human iPS cells should be selected with the β-MHC promoter. Furthermore, the choice of other subtype-specific promoters could be very useful to obtain the cardiomyocyte population of interest. For instance, LQTS could be best investigated in ventricular cardiomyocytes that have long AP durations and could be selected using the MLC2v promoter. Moreover, mutations inducing atrial fibrillation might be better investigated with atrial cell selection by the MLC2a promoter, and for studying inherited sick sinus syndromes, pacemaker cells could be purified with sinus node-specific HCN or Tbx promoters.

4.3. Automatable and Scalable Electrophysiological Screening

The use of screening procedures to analyze APs of iPS cell-derived cardiomyocytes is particularly important to identify drugs that induce LQTS or to screen compounds that could treat inherited LQTS. For the systematic screening of many compounds, the classical manual patch clamp is not suitable, and automated and scalable systems are mandatory. For instance, the planar patch clamp technique [12] or the microelectrode array system [24,36] allow the acquisition of more data points per day (planar patch clamp: 200–1000; microelectrode array: 500) than the conventional patch clamp (50 data points/day) [36].

The planar patch clamp system that we have used in this study allows the automated recording of up to eight cells in parallel, as well as the automated application of several compounds. Because cells must be measured in suspension, very gentle dissociation methods have to be further optimized to avoid digestion of transmembrane ion channels.

We found that most action potential parameters were similar between manual and planar patch clamp recordings; however, APD90 tends to be longer (statistically not significant) in the latter (Table 1). We speculate that when using the automated planar patch clamp method, the dissociation procedure or the suction process onto the small holes of the borosilicate glass chips could kill smaller atrial or pacemaker cells with shorter APD or might favor larger ventricular cells with longer APD. However, although absolute APD values seems to vary with the method, the phenotypical fingerprint of LQTS 3-specific cardiomyocytes (positive slopes in the longitudinal regression analysis) can be similarly detected with both patch clamp methods (Table 1).

Similar to the conventional patch clamp, also during automated planar patch clamp analysis, the intracellular milieu is dialyzed against the internal solution, which leads to the wash out of important intracellular components and, therefore, reduces the stability of long-term recordings. This limits the duration of electrophysiological recording of one cell and, therefore, also the number of different compounds and dosages. Thus, this technology seems to be not suited for real high throughput analysis of several thousands of compounds.

Although, here, we only performed six recordings on a microelectrode array in parallel, scalable and automatable systems were developed (QT screen Multi Channel Systems) for parallel field potential recording and compound testing on 96 channels. In contrast to conventional microelectrode measurements (500 data points/day), such systems allow the recoding of 6000 data points/day [36]. One remaining challenge is the almost impossible electrical stimulation of cardiomyocytes on microelectrode arrays for standardized recordings and to determine frequency-dependent effects. This could be solved by using optogenetic technology, which was shown to be effective for the stimulation of purified cardiomyocytes on microelectrode arrays [37].

5. Conclusions

The herein reported non-clonal lentiviral strategy for the purification of cardiomyocytes from iPS cells is simple, fast and cheap and could be applied to large numbers of different iPS cell lines at once. In contrast to the picking of classically-transfected iPS cell clones, this strategy would allow the parallel purification of cardiomyocytes from many different patients for comparative electrophysiological analysis. Because the disease-specific phenotype of purified iPS cell-derived cardiomyocytes was retained and could be analyzed with automated planar patch clamp and scalable microelectrode array technologies, these assay systems will be useful for patient-specific drug screening in the future.

Acknowledgments

We thank Frank Host (University Bonn) for technical assistance and Sonja Stoelzle-Feix (Nanion Technologies) for protocols and technical support on the planar patch clamp system. This work was supported by the German Research Foundation (SA 1785/5-1) and the "StemCellFactory" project, which is co-funded by the European Union (European Regional Development Fund-Investing in your future) and the German federal state, North Rhine-Westphalia (NRW).

Author Contributions

Stephanie Friedrichs and Daniela Malan contributed equally to the work. Stephanie Friedrichs, Daniela Malan and Yvonne Voss performed the experiments and analyzed the data. Stephanie Friedrichs, Daniela Malan and Philipp Sasse designed the study and wrote the manuscript.

Conflicts of Interest

The authors declare no conflict of interest.

References

1. Schwartz, P.J.; Priori, S.G.; Spazzolini, C.; Moss, A.J.; Vincent, G.M.; Napolitano, C.; Denjoy, I.; Guicheney, P.; Breithardt, G.; Keating, M.T.; *et al.* Genotype-phenotype correlation in the long-QT syndrome: Gene-specific triggers for life-threatening arrhythmias. *Circulation* **2001**, *103*, 89–95.
2. Bennett, P.B.; Yazawa, K.; Makita, N.; George, A.L., Jr. Molecular mechanism for an inherited cardiac arrhythmia. *Nature* **1995**, *376*, 683–685.
3. Chandra, R.; Starmer, C.F.; Grant, A.O. Multiple effects of KPQ deletion mutation on gating of human cardiac Na^+ channels expressed in mammalian cells. *Am. J. Physiol.* **1998**, *274*, H1643–H1654.
4. Charpentier, F.; Bourge, A.; Merot, J. Mouse models of SCN5A-related cardiac arrhythmias. *Prog. Biophys. Mol. Biol.* **2008**, *98*, 230–237.
5. Malan, D.; Friedrichs, S.; Fleischmann, B.K.; Sasse, P. Cardiomyocytes obtained from induced pluripotent stem cells with long-QT syndrome 3 recapitulate typical disease-specific features *in vitro. Circ. Res.* **2011**, *109*, 841–847.
6. Itzhaki, I.; Maizels, L.; Huber, I.; Zwi-Dantsis, L.; Caspi, O.; Winterstern, A.; Feldman, O.; Gepstein, A.; Arbel, G.; Hammerman, H.; *et al.* Modelling the long QT syndrome with induced pluripotent stem cells. *Nature* **2011**, *471*, 225–229.
7. Matsa, E.; Rajamohan, D.; Dick, E.; Young, L.; Mellor, I.; Staniforth, A.; Denning, C. Drug evaluation in cardiomyocytes derived from human induced pluripotent stem cells carrying a long qt syndrome type 2 mutation. *Eur. Heart J.* **2011**, *32*, 952–962.
8. Lahti, A.L.; Kujala, V.J.; Chapman, H.; Koivisto, A.P.; Pekkanen-Mattila, M.; Kerkela, E.; Hyttinen, J.; Kontula, K.; Swan, H.; Conklin, B.R.; *et al.* Model for long QT syndrome type 2 using human iPS cells demonstrates arrhythmogenic characteristics in cell culture. *Dis. Model. Mech.* **2012**, *5*, 220–230.
9. Davis, R.P.; Casini, S.; van den Berg, C.W.; Hoekstra, M.; Remme, C.A.; Dambrot, C.; Salvatori, D.; Oostwaard, D.W.; Wilde, A.A.; Bezzina, C.R.; *et al.* Cardiomyocytes derived from pluripotent stem cells recapitulate electrophysiological characteristics of an overlap syndrome of cardiac sodium channel disease. *Circulation* **2012**, *125*, 3079–3091.
10. Egashira, T.; Yuasa, S.; Suzuki, T.; Aizawa, Y.; Yamakawa, H.; Matsuhashi, T.; Ohno, Y.; Tohyama, S.; Okata, S.; Seki, T.; *et al.* Disease characterization using LQTS-specific induced pluripotent stem cells. *Cardiovasc. Res.* **2012**, *95*, 419–429.
11. Moretti, A.; Bellin, M.; Welling, A.; Jung, C.B.; Lam, J.T.; Bott-Flugel, L.; Dorn, T.; Goedel, A.; Hohnke, C.; Hofmann, F.; *et al.* Patient-specific induced pluripotent stem-cell models for long-QT syndrome. *N. Engl. J. Med.* **2010**, *363*, 1397–1409.

12. Stoelzle, S.; Haythornthwaite, A.; Kettenhofen, R.; Kolossov, E.; Bohlen, H.; George, M.; Bruggemann, A.; Fertig, N. Automated patch clamp on mesc-derived cardiomyocytes for cardiotoxicity prediction. *J. Biomol. Screen.* **2011**, *16*, 910–916.

13. Mauritz, C.; Schwanke, K.; Reppel, M.; Neef, S.; Katsirntaki, K.; Maier, L.S.; Nguemo, F.; Menke, S.; Haustein, M.; Hescheler, J.; *et al.* Generation of functional murine cardiac myocytes from induced pluripotent stem cells. *Circulation* **2008**, *118*, 507–517.

14. Huber, I.; Itzhaki, I.; Caspi, O.; Arbel, G.; Tzukerman, M.; Gepstein, A.; Habib, M.; Yankelson, L.; Kehat, I.; Gepstein, L. Identification and selection of cardiomyocytes during human embryonic stem cell differentiation. *FASEB J.* **2007**, *21*, 2551–2563.

15. Hattori, F.; Chen, H.; Yamashita, H.; Tohyama, S.; Satoh, Y.S.; Yuasa, S.; Li, W.; Yamakawa, H.; Tanaka, T.; Onitsuka, T.; *et al.* Nongenetic method for purifying stem cell-derived cardiomyocytes. *Nat. Methods* **2010**, *7*, 61–66.

16. Kolossov, E.; Bostani, T.; Roell, W.; Breitbach, M.; Pillekamp, F.; Nygren, J.M.; Sasse, P.; Rubenchik, O.; Fries, J.W.; Wenzel, D.; *et al.* Engraftment of engineered ES cell-derived cardiomyocytes but not bm cells restores contractile function to the infarcted myocardium. *J. Exp. Med.* **2006**, *203*, 2315–2327.

17. Kita-Matsuo, H.; Barcova, M.; Prigozhina, N.; Salomonis, N.; Wei, K.; Jacot, J.G.; Nelson, B.; Spiering, S.; Haverslag, R.; Kim, C.; *et al.* Lentiviral vectors and protocols for creation of stable hesc lines for fluorescent tracking and drug resistance selection of cardiomyocytes. *PLoS One* **2009**, *4*, e5046.

18. Fang, J.; Qian, J.J.; Yi, S.; Harding, T.C.; Tu, G.H.; VanRoey, M.; Jooss, K. Stable antibody expression at therapeutic levels using the 2A peptide. *Nat. Biotechnol.* **2005**, *23*, 584–590.

19. Pfeifer, A.; Hofmann, A. Lentiviral transgenesis. *Methods Mol. Biol.* **2009**, *530*, 391–405.

20. Hosler, B.A.; LaRosa, G.J.; Grippo, J.F.; Gudas, L.J. Expression of REX-1, a gene containing zinc finger motifs, is rapidly reduced by retinoic acid in F9 teratocarcinoma cells. *Mol. Cell. Biol.* **1989**, *9*, 5623–5629.

21. Wobus, A.M.; Wallukat, G.; Hescheler, J. Pluripotent mouse embryonic stem cells are able to differentiate into cardiomyocytes expressing chronotropic responses to adrenergic and cholinergic agents and Ca^{2+} channel blockers. *Differentiation* **1991**, *48*, 173–182.

22. Friedrichs, S.; Malan, D.; Sasse, P. Modeling long QT syndromes using induced pluripotent stem cells: Current progress and future challenges. *Trends Cardiovasc. Med.* **2013**, *23*, 91–98.

23. Nuyens, D.; Stengl, M.; Dugarmaa, S.; Rossenbacker, T.; Compernolle, V.; Rudy, Y.; Smits, J.F.; Flameng, W.; Clancy, C.E.; Moons, L.; *et al.* Abrupt rate accelerations or premature beats cause life-threatening arrhythmias in mice with long-QT3 syndrome. *Nat. Med.* **2001**, *7*, 1021–1027.

24. Halbach, M.; Egert, U.; Hescheler, J.; Banach, K. Estimation of action potential changes from field potential recordings in multicellular mouse cardiac myocyte cultures. *Cell. Physiol. Biochem.* **2003**, *13*, 271–284.

25. Ma, Y.; Ramezani, A.; Lewis, R.; Hawley, R.G.; Thomson, J.A. High-level sustained transgene expression in human embryonic stem cells using lentiviral vectors. *Stem Cells* **2003**, *21*, 111–117.

26. Fontes, A. Cloning technologies. *Methods Mol. Biol.* **2013**, *997*, 253–261.

27. Willmann, C.A.; Hemeda, H.; Pieper, L.A.; Lenz, M.; Qin, J.; Joussen, S.; Sontag, S.; Wanek, P.; Denecke, B.; Schuler, H.M.; *et al.* To clone or not to clone? Induced pluripotent stem cells can be generated in bulk culture. *PLoS One* **2013**, *8*, e65324.

28. Mitchell, R.S.; Beitzel, B.F.; Schroder, A.R.; Shinn, P.; Chen, H.; Berry, C.C.; Ecker, J.R.; Bushman, F.D. Retroviral DNA integration: ASLV, HIV, and MLV show distinct target site preferences. *PLoS Biol.* **2004**, *2*, e234.

29. Vannucci, L.; Lai, M.; Chiuppesi, F.; Ceccherini-Nelli, L.; Pistello, M. Viral vectors: A look back and ahead on gene transfer technology. *New Microbiol.* **2013**, *36*, 1–22.

30. Tohyama, S.; Hattori, F.; Sano, M.; Hishiki, T.; Nagahata, Y.; Matsuura, T.; Hashimoto, H.; Suzuki, T.; Yamashita, H.; Satoh, Y.; *et al.* Distinct metabolic flow enables large-scale purification of mouse and human pluripotent stem cell-derived cardiomyocytes. *Cell Stem Cell* **2013**, *12*, 127–137.

31. Malan, D.; Sasse, P. University of Bonn, Bonn, Germany. Unpublished work, 2014.

32. Zandstra, P.W.; Bauwens, C.; Yin, T.; Liu, Q.; Schiller, H.; Zweigerdt, R.; Pasumarthi, K.B.; Field, L.J. Scalable production of embryonic stem cell-derived cardiomyocytes. *Tissue Eng.* **2003**, *9*, 767–778.

33. Xu, X.Q.; Zweigerdt, R.; Soo, S.Y.; Ngoh, Z.X.; Tham, S.C.; Wang, S.T.; Graichen, R.; Davidson, B.; Colman, A.; Sun, W.; *et al.* Highly enriched cardiomyocytes from human embryonic stem cells. *Cytotherapy* **2008**, *10*, 376–389.

34. Jin, D.; Ni, T.T.; Hou, J.; Rellinger, E.; Zhong, T.P. Promoter analysis of ventricular myosin heavy chain (VMHC) in zebrafish embryos. *Dev. Dyn.* **2009**, *238*, 1760–1767.

35. Reiser, P.J.; Portman, M.A.; Ning, X.H.; Schomisch Moravec, C. Human cardiac myosin heavy chain isoforms in fetal and failing adult atria and ventricles. *Am. J. Physiol. Heart Circ. Physiol.* **2001**, *280*, H1814–H1820.

36. Meyer, T.; Leisgen, C.; Gonser, B.; Gunther, E. QT-screen: High-throughput cardiac safety pharmacology by extracellular electrophysiology on primary cardiac myocytes. *Assay Drug Dev. Technol.* **2004**, *2*, 507–514.

37. Bruegmann, T.; Malan, D.; Hesse, M.; Beiert, T.; Fuegemann, C.J.; Fleischmann, B.K.; Sasse, P. Optogenetic control of heart muscle *in vitro* and *in vivo*. *Nat. Methods* **2010**, *7*, 897–900.

Clinical Potentials of Cardiomyocytes Derived from Patient-Specific Induced Pluripotent Stem Cells

Kwong-Man Ng, Cheuk-Yiu Law and Hung-Fat Tse

Abstract: The lack of appropriate human cardiomyocyte-based experimental platform has largely hindered the study of cardiac diseases and the development of therapeutic strategies. To date, somatic cells isolated from human subjects can be reprogramed into induced pluripotent stem cells (iPSCs) and subsequently differentiated into functional cardiomyocytes. This powerful reprogramming technology provides a novel *in vitro* human cell-based platform for the study of human hereditary cardiac disorders. The clinical potential of using iPSCs derived from patients with inherited cardiac disorders for therapeutic studies have been increasingly highlighted. In this review, the standard procedures for generating patient-specific iPSCs and the latest commonly used cardiac differentiation protocols will be outlined. Furthermore, the progress and limitations of current applications of iPSCs and iPSCs-derived cardiomyocytes in cell replacement therapy, disease modeling, drug-testing and toxicology studies will be discussed in detail.

Reprinted from *J. Clin. Med.* Cite as: Ng, K.-M.; Law, C.-Y.; Tse, H.-F. Clinical Potentials of Cardiomyocytes Derived from Patient-Specific Induced Pluripotent Stem Cells. *J. Clin. Med.* **2014**, *3*, 1105–1123.

1. Introduction

Cardiomyocytes, or heart muscle cells, are fragile but important constituents of the myocardium. It is generally believed that humans are born with a fixed amount of cardiomyocytes; therefore, the death of these muscle cells may cause permanent damage to the heart. Recently, Bergmann and colleagues have evidenced a revolutionary notion of the *in vivo* regeneration and renewal of cardiomyocytes in humans [1]; nevertheless, the rate of cardiomyocyte turnover in their experiment appeared to be extremely slow. In fact, following myocardial injury, the heart usually repairs itself by cellular hypertrophy [2]. In case of a substantial loss of cardiomyocytes such as severe myocardial infarction, the damaged tissue is replaced with fibroblasts, rather than functional cardiomyocytes. To this end, the heart function is permanently impaired. Attempts of using adult stem cells or embryonic stem cells in replacing the damaged myocardium have been made, and several successful cases have been reported. Yet, such a replacement approach is impeded by various factors, for instance, the limiting sources of stem cells as well as the non-self rejection issues. In 2007, Yamanaka and colleagues demonstrated the first time that adult human fibroblasts could be reprogrammed into the pluripotent stem cells when supplemented with well-defined culturing factors [3]. Based on this revolutionary reprogramming approach, any fully differentiated cells obtained from patients should be theoretically able to be reprogrammed into induced pluripotent stem cells (iPSCs), and further differentiated into specialized cells of desired interest such as cardiac derivatives. The iPSCs obtained would be patient-specific; they not only provide a new source for regenerative medicine, but also offer a human cell based platform for the studies of modeling of inherited cardiac diseases and screening of potential cardiovascular drugs. In this review, the clinical potentials of patient-specific iPSCs in therapeutic treatments of cardiac disorders will be addressed in detail.

2. Patient-Specific iPSCs and Their Cardiac Derivatives

In 2006, Yamanaka and colleagues demonstrated for the first time that the exogenous expression of four transcription factors—Oct4, Klf-4, Sox-2 and c-Myc [4]—Initiated the reprogramming of terminally differentiated murine somatic cells (skin fibroblasts) into iPSCs, which were characterized with adequate pluripotency. Similar to embryonic stem cells, these iPSCs were able to self-renew, proliferate and differentiate into various cell types including neurons and cardiomyocytes [5,6]. The same research group at a later time showed that human somatic cells could also be reprogrammed into iPSCs [3,7]. These technological breakthroughs have made substantial impacts in cell replacement therapy, disease modeling and therapeutic discovery sectors. Although the cells from a patient with myocardial infarction can be reprogrammed and differentiated into functional cardiomyocytes, the replacement of the defective cells of a particular patient is still theoretical. Nevertheless, iPSCs generated from patients with inherited cardiac diseases, following *in vitro* cardiac differentiation, are still valuable tools for disease modeling and development of personalized medicine (Figure 1), as the iPSCs-derived cardiomyocytes possess the defective genes of the patients.

Figure 1. The clinical applications of the cardiomyocytes derived from patient-specific iPSCs.

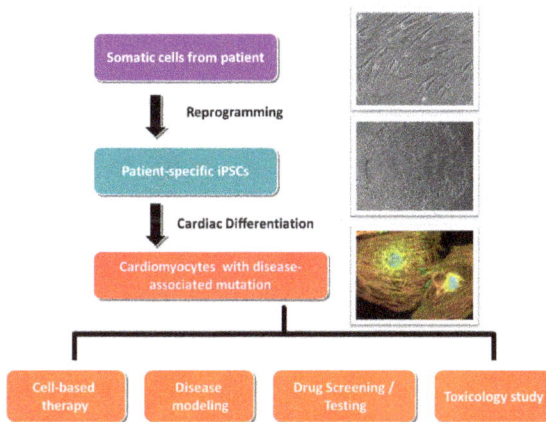

3. Standard Procedures in Generating Patient-Specific iPSCs and Their Cardiac Derivatives

In general, the generation of human iPSCs-derived cardiomyocytes involves three major steps: (i) collection of somatic tissues/cells; (ii) reprogramming; and (iii) cardiac differentiation.

3.1. Collection of Somatic Tissues/Cells

The protocol of Yamanaka and colleagues suggested the use of skin fibroblasts as the starting material of iPSCs generation. However, the invasive procedures of collecting skin biopsy actually caused many patients, especially pediatric subjects, to refuse donating tissue samples for iPSCs generation. In this regard, less invasive alternatives are obviously more preferable in clinical practices. It is now evidenced that apart from skin fibroblasts, many other cell types, such as hair follicle cells, peripheral blood cells as well as uro-epithelial cells, could also be reprogrammed into iPSCs [8–13]. Among these cells, the collection of uro-epithelial cells from urine accounts for the simplest and most convenient way. This non-invasive method eliminates pain or wound caused by skin biopsy collection; thus, is more likely to be accepted by patients. In fact, our laboratory is now routinely collecting urine samples from patients for iPSCs generation [14,15].

3.2. Reprogramming

The first generation of reprogramming method involved the use of retrovirus vectors in infecting four transcription factors (Oct4, Klf4, Sox2 and c-Myc) into cultured fibroblasts. This method is quite robust; for this reason, many laboratories, including ours, are routinely using this method for iPSCs generation. However, the reprogramming efficiency of this method is not high (about 0.0002%). Moreover, the use of retrovirus vectors is a big concern in clinical applications. Therefore, several alternative methods have been proposed. For example, Nanog and Lin28 are suggested as additional reprogramming factors in some protocols since the addition of these two factors increased the efficiency to about 0.05% for fetal fibroblasts [16]. As retrovirus only infects actively dividing cells, the use of lentivirus-based vectors may be a better option for the cell types that are non-actively dividing or less proliferative (e.g., cardiac fibroblasts). It is generally accepted that lentivirus-based vectors can transduce both dividing and non-dividing cells. On top of that, lentivirus-based vectors can accommodate much larger inserts. The four essential reprogramming factors Oct4, Klf4, Sox2 and c-Myc could be linked up within one single expression cassette [17] and simultaneously inserted into a single vector. This strategy eliminates the need for producing multiple transducing vectors; thus it avoids the possible stoichiometric and temporal interference among individual viruses [18].

Despite that retrovirus- and lentivirus-based vectors are widely used in iPSCs generation, the incorporation of viral sequences into the host genome is still an important concern in clinical applications, especially in the cell replacement therapy utilizing patient-specific iPSCs. For addressing this issue, the application of a Cre-loxP system in the lentivirus backbone has been suggested, so that the viral sequences could be eventually cleaved from the host genome upon the execution of Cre-recombinase [19,20]. Nevertheless, the use of non-integrative viruses appears to be a more acceptable method. For example, non-integrative viruses, such as adenovirus and Sendai virus, have been successfully used in some reprogramming protocols of human fibroblasts [21,22]. In addition, epigenetic reprogramming methods, such as transfection of mRNA, miRNA, minicircle vectors and episomal plasmids are regarded as the possible alternatives for footprint-free iPSCs reprogramming.

3.3. Cardiac Differentiation

In spontaneous differentiation, cardiomyocyte is one of the most easily identifiable cell types. Even in the absence of specific growth factors, spontaneous beating clusters could be observed when iPSCs are allowed to form aggregates (embryoid bodies) in a culturing suspension. However, the actual number of cardiomyocytes within a spontaneous beating embryoid body may comprise as low as merely 1% of the total cell population. It is obvious that spontaneous differentiation is not sufficient for the generation of iPSCs-derived cardiomyocytes in an adequate quantity for most experimental assays or applications. Early methods of directing cardiac differentiation involved the co-culture of iPSCs with END-2 endodermal cells. This END-2 co-culturing method has been used widely for cardiac differentiation of human embryonic stem cells and is relatively robust [23,24]. However, the difficulty in separating the cardiomyocytes from the feeder layers denotes a main drawback of this method. To date, many feeder-free cardiac differentiation protocols have been developed, so that problems associated with feeder layers can be eliminated. Most of these feeder-free methods involve the incubation with growth factors, such as the BMP4, Activin A, VEGF and DKK that regulate the pathways directing heart formation during fetal developments [6,25]. Recently, Palecek and colleagues reported a successful application of Wnt pathway inhibitors in directing cardiac differentiation of human iPSCs [26,27]. By modulating the Wnt/β-catenin signaling under fully defined conditions, monolayers of virtually pure cardiomyocytes (up to 98%) were obtained in merely 14 days.

4. Application of Patient-Specific iPSCs in Cell Replacement Therapy/Regenerative Medicine

Increasing evidences showed that the adult human heart possesses a certain degree of regenerating power. Following severe cardiac injury, cardiac hypertrophy and scarring are indeed the major repairing mechanisms to maintain minimum cardiac functions and prevent further damages. However, without the replacement of new cardiomyocytes, the ordinary repairing mechanisms usually result in the continual increase of cardiac workload that further worsens the injured condition and even leads to chronic heart failure of the patient. To this end, various studies have been converged on the use of pluripotent stem cells in cardiac recovery.

A previous study reported that the transplantation of human embryonic stem cells-derived cardiomyocytes into the infarcted myocardium of an immunodeficient rodent partially remuscularized myocardial infarcts and improved cardiac function [28,29]. At a later stage, Gaballa and colleagues demonstrated that cell sheets composed of rat or human cardiac progenitor cells, when transplanted into the infarcted heart, could proliferate and differentiate into functional cardiomyocytes, and rescue myocardial function [30].

Besides human embryonic stem cells, human iPSCs also possess the ability to differentiate into cardiac lineages. Since iPSCs can be derived from any individual, the use of human iPSCs in regenerative medicine can avoid the ethical issues arising from the use of embryonic materials. Furthermore, iPSCs can be produced from the same individual who is receiving the cell replacement therapy, so that immunological incompatibility should become less significant.

Recently, Watt and colleagues attempted to investigate the potential benefits of human iPSCs-derived progenitors. In their study, human iPSCs-derived cardiac progenitor cells were injected into the pre-infarct hearts of rats. The injected cells were able to differentiate into cardiomyocytes and smooth muscle fibers, and were retained in the rat hearts for at least 10 weeks after myocardial infarction. When comparing to the control group, the animals that received human-iPSCs-derived cardiac progenitor cells showed some improvement in the left ventricular ejection fraction [31].

It should be noted that although many studies have pointed out the beneficial effects of human embryonic stem cells and iPSCs against ischemic cardiac injuries, most of the studies only involved a relatively short follow-up period (see Table 1); thus, the long term efficacy of iPSCs-derived cardiac progenitors remains questionable.

Table 1. Examples of using iPSCs in cell replacement therapies.

Cell Type	Animal Model	Number of Cell	Delivery Method	Timing of the Delivery	Follow up Duration	Reference
iPSC	Mouse	50,000	IM	Immediately after MI induction	2 weeks	[30]
iPSC-derived cardiac progenitors	Rat	2×10^6	IM	10 min after MI induction	10 weeks	[31]
Cardiosphere	Rat	-	Cell sheet	Immediately after MI induction	3 weeks	[32]

5. Applications of iPSCs-Derived Cardiomyocytes in Modeling Genetic Cardiomyopathies

Cardiomyopathies are heterogeneous groups of diseases of cardiomyocytes. Pathologically, the diseases could be caused by non-genetic factors such as viral infection though genetic contributions are frequently observed [33]. To date, over 50 genes have been reported to be associated with various forms of cardiomyopathies; yet, the studies of the pathogenic mechanisms underlying specific genetic defects remain elusive due to the lack of appropriate experimental models.

Theoretically, the affected tissues obtained from patients with cardiomyopathies are the best options for pathophysiological studies; however, for cardiac diseases, the limitation in obtaining and maintaining cardiac biopsy samples highly hindered this strategy.

To compensate this limitation, transgenic animals are commonly used for modeling human genetic defects. Nonetheless, due to the substantial physiological differences between the hearts of human and those of mice [34–36], the use of transgenic mouse lines in modeling human genetic cardiomyopathies is of little practical value. For example, in terms of ion-channel physiology, transgenic mouse models, in most cases, only partly recapitulate the disease phenotypes [36,37]. The phenotypic differences between species accentuate the importance of a novel human cardiomyocyte-based model in the studies of heritable cardiac defects, and the cardiomyocytes derived from patient-specific iPSCs should be one of the most desirable options.

In general, if the mutation of the gene of interest does not interfere in cardiac differentiation, cardiomyocytes can be continually generated from patient-specific iPSCs. This continuous supply of cardiomyocytes indeed resembles the cardiac biopsy samples that could hardly be obtained from patients with specific inherited cardiac defects; thus these patient-specific iPSCs-derived cardiomyocytes provide a convenient and valuable platform for research purposes. In fact, various recent reports have demonstrated that the cardiomyocytes derived from patient-specific iPSCs were able to recapitulate disease phenotypes of various types of Long QT syndromes [38–40]. These data clearly evidenced the feasibility of utilizing the patient-specific iPSCs-derived cardiomyocytes in modeling heritable cardiomyopathies.

In 2010, Laugwitz and colleagues established the first patient-specific iPSCs based model for type 1 Long QT syndrome [41]. In their study, the skin fibroblasts from patients carrying an autosomal dominant missense mutation (R190Q) in the *KCNQ1* gene were effectively reprogrammed into iPSCs. The resultant iPSCs were further differentiated into atrial- and ventricular-like cardiomyocytes and subjected to patch-clamp analysis. When comparing to the control, the iPSCs-derived cardiomyocytes with the *KCNQ1* mutation showed a markedly prolonged duration of action potential, altered activation and deactivation properties of IKs, and an abnormal response to catecholamine stimulation. Immunostaining analysis demonstrated the failure of mutated $K_v7.1$ potassium channel protein in its trafficking to the plasma membrane; this finding may provide an explanation to the cellular pathogenic mechanism of the $KCNQ1_{R190Q}$ mutation. Undoubtedly, the use of iPSCs-derived cardiomyocytes in modeling inherited cardiac disorders is feasible.

In addition to Long QT syndromes, cardiomyocytes derived from patient-specific iPSCs have also been used in the modeling of some other genetic cardiac disorders (Table 2); examples are outlined as follows:

Table 2. Examples of using iPSCs-derived cardiomyocytes for modeling genetic cardiomyopathies.

Disorder	Gene Involved	Details of the Mutation	Ref.
Long QT syndrome, Type 1	*KCNQ1*	missense mutation (R190Q) leads to the production of a mutant protein	[41]
Long QT syndrome, Type 2	*KCNH2*	missense mutation (A614V) leads to the production of a mutant protein	[38]
Long QT syndrome, Type 2	*KCNH2*	missense mutation (G1618A) leads to the production of a mutant protein	[40]
Long QT syndrome, Type 2	*KCNH2*	missense mutation (R176W) leads to the production of mutant protein	[42]
Long QT syndrome, Type 3	*SCN5A*	Multiple mutations (G5287A; V1763M) leads the production of a mutant protein	[43]
Long QT syndrome, Type 8	*CACNA1C*	Missense mutation (G406R) leads to the production of a mutant protein	[44]
Catecholaminergic polymorphic ventricular tachycardia, Type 1	*RYR2*	Missense mutation (F2483I) leads to the production of a mutant protein with an altered FKBP12.6 binding domain	[45]
Catecholaminergic polymorphic ventricular tachycardia, Type 1	*RYR2*	Missense mutation (S406L) leads to the production of a mutant protein	[46]
Catecholaminergic polymorphic ventricular tachycardia, Type 2	*CASQ2*	Missense mutation (D307H) leads to the production of a mutant protein	[47]
Catecholaminergic polymorphic ventricular tachycardia, Type 2	*CASQ2*	Missense mutation (D307H) leads to the production of a mutant protein	[47]
Dilated cardiomyopathy	*TNNT2*	missense mutation (R173W) leads to the production of a mutant protein	[48]
Dilated cardiomyopathy	*DES*	missense mutation (A285V) leads to the production of a mutant protein	[49]
Hypertrophic cardiomyopathy	*MYH7*	Missense mutation (R663H) leads to the production of a mutant protein	[50]
Friedreich ataxia-associated hypertrophic cardiomyopathy	*FXN*	GAA repeat expansion in the first intron leads to the partial silencing of gene expression	[51]

5.1. Modeling Catecholaminergic Polymorphic Ventricular Tachycardia (CPVT)

Although inherited arrhythmogenic disorders are frequently associated with the mutations in the genes encoding the ion channel components, a special kind of inherited ventricular arrhythmia called catecholaminergic polymorphic ventricular tachycardia (CPVT) is caused by the mutations in genes encoding the proteins mediating intracellular calcium transient. In response to emotional or physical stress, CPVT patients may manifest ventricular premature beats and bidirectional or polymorphic ventricular tachycardia, which leads to episodic syncope, seizures and sudden death [52,53]. So far, two types of CPVT have been described based on their difference in the mode of inheritance. The autosomal dominant form that accounts for up to 50% of the cases has been linked to the mutations in the *RYR2* gene that encodes the cardiac ryanodine receptor [54], while a rare autosomal recessive form results from the mutations in the *CASQ2* gene that encodes the cardiac calsequestrin [55]. Functionally, ryanodine receptor and calsequestrin work together to mediate the release of calcium ions from the sarcoplasmic reticulum (SR) in the cardiac muscles during excitation-contraction coupling. As such, it is not surprising that mutations in the *RYR2* and *CASQ2* genes that result in functional derangements in intracellular calcium handling may result in arrhythmia. Since 2004, the pathophysiological roles of various *RYR2* and *CASQ2* mutations in driving the development of CPVT have been investigated in several transgenic animal or cell models [56–59]. Although most of the models were able to recapitulate the major CPVT phenotypes, such as SR calcium leak and catecholamine-induced delayed after-polarizations (DADs), the clinical significance of these models were limited by the substantial difference in the cardiac electrophysiology between rodents and human. Addressing this issue, the pathogenic effects of various CPVT associated mutations have been studied in patient-specific iPSCs models. These include the $RYR2_{F2483II}$, $RYR2_{S406L}$, $CASQ2_{D307H}$ mutations [45–47]. Similar to the rodent models, all these iPSCs-based models were able to recapitulate the CPVT phenotypes, and the results confirmed that the diastolic SR calcium leak contributes to generation of DADs [45–47]. Except for disease modeling, the iPSCs-based CPVT models also provided a human cardiomyocytes-based platform for drug testing and toxicology studies. For example, in a recent report, Laugwitz and colleagues demonstrated that dantrolene ameliorates the CPVT phenotypes caused by $RYR2_{S406L}$ mutation using the cardiomyocytes differentiated from the CPVT patient-specific iPSCs [46]. So far, only limited therapeutics, such as beta-blockers, are being used for treating CPVT. It is anticipated that the success in generating the CPVT-specific iPSCs may help facilitate the development of novel therapeutic approaches in treating CPVT.

5.2. Modeling Dilated Cardiomyopathy Associated with TNNT2 Mutation

Dilated cardiomyopathy (DCM) is the most common subtype of cardiomyopathy, and is characterized by the abnormal enlargement of ventricles, thinning of ventricular walls and the marked systolic dysfunction [33]. It has been estimated that about 50% of the cases are of genetic causes [60–63]. The pathological mechanisms associated with *TNNT2* gene mutations have been evaluated in a transgenic mouse model, in which the null mutation of this gene denoted an impaired contractile function of the heart [64,65]. Yet, how the specific *TNNT2* mutation contributes to the development of DCM phenotype in human remains ambiguous.

In 2012, Wu and colleagues generated iPSCs from DCM patients carrying a disease associated-mutation in the gene encoding cardiac troponin-T (*TNNT2*) [48]. Sequencing analysis showed that such mutation causes the 173rd amino acid residue of the cardiac troponin-T to change from an arginine (R) to a tryptophan (W). Clinically, patients with this mutation develop the typical DCM symptoms including left ventricle dilation and reduced ejection fraction. Skin biopsy samples were collected from affected and normal individuals of three generations of a single family for iPSCs generation. The resultant iPSCs were then differentiated into cardiomyocytes for functional analyses. When comparing to the control, the cardiomyocytes derived from the mutation containing-iPSCs showed abnormal sarcomeric alpha-actinin distribution. Functionally, the mutant cardiomyocytes exhibited impairments in contractility and reduction in calcium handling ability upon β-adrenergic stimulation. These observations indicated that the increased susceptibility to inotropic stress may be a signature characteristic of the *TNNT2*R173W mutation in DCM development.

5.3. Modeling Cardiomyopathy Associated with DES Mutation

The *DES* gene encodes the intermediate filament protein desmin, but the exact function of desmin is not well defined. Nevertheless, mutations in the *DES* gene are commonly observed in DCM patients [66]. Phenotypically, mutations leading to the loss of *DES* gene function usually give rise to a significant accumulation of desmin-positive aggregates in the cardiomyocytes of affected individuals.

Lately, by utilizing the whole-exome sequencing approach, our laboratory has identified a novel *DES* mutation in a patient with left ventricular dilation and impaired left ventricular ejection function [49]. In this *DES* mutation, we recognized a change of the alanine (A) residue to valine (V) at the 285th amino acid position. In the transgenic mouse model with complete desmin deficiency, phenotypes such as hypertrophic and dilated cardiomyopathy [67] were observed. Surprisingly, the patient with *DES*A285V mutation produced a mutant desmin possessing molecular weight and immunoreactivity comparable to the wild type desmin protein. To investigate the pathological significance of this novel *DES* mutation, we have generated skin fibroblasts-derived iPSCs from this *DES*A285V patient. These *DES*A285V iPSCs were subsequently differentiated into cardiomyocytes for structural and functional studies. When compared to the normal cardiomyocytes, the ones carrying the *DES* mutation exhibited abnormal protein aggregations in sarcomere and Z-disc streaming. In addition, contraction arrest was observed in the mutant cardiomyocytes upon isoproterenol stimulation. These observations not only provided an explanation to the pathogenic mechanism underlying the *DES*A285V mutation, but also validated the causal ion relationship between the *DES* mutation and the DCM phenotype observed in that patient [49].

5.4. Modeling Hypertrophic Cardiomyopathy Associated with MYH7 Mutation

Hypertrophic cardiomyopathy (HCM) is a heritable cardiac disorder characterized by the abnormal left ventricular thickening and diastolic dysfunction in the absence of an identifiable hemodynamic cause [68]. About 13 HCM-associated genes have been identified to date and most of them encode sarcomeric proteins [69]. Transgenic mouse and rabbit models have been established for studying the pathological mechanisms of HCM [70–72]; however, the mechanistic roles of altered contractile function in the development of HCM remain inconclusive. Very recently, Lan and colleagues generated an iPSCs-line from patients carrying one HCM-associated mutation in the

MYH7 gene. In their case, the 663rd residue of the β-myosin heavy chain is changed from an arginine to a histidine as a result of a missense mutation. The patient-specific iPSCs were differentiated into cardiomyocytes for functional analyses. The mutant-containing cardiomyocytes recapitulated the key features of HCM, including increased cell size and arrhythmia. The intracellular calcium transient profile indicated that the diseased cardiomyocytes showed a significant increase in the resting intracellular calcium level when comparing to the normal cardiac muscle fibers. Interestingly, pharmaceutical inhibition of calcium entry helped to prevent the development of HCM phenotypes in the mutant cardiomyocytes suggesting the *MYH7* mutation altered the calcium homeostasis dysfunction [50].

5.5. Modeling Friedreich Ataxia Associated Cardiomyopathy

Apart from sarcomeric proteins, abnormality in the mitochondrial proteins may also contribute to HCM development. For example, deficiency in the mitochondrial protein frataxin may lead to Friederich ataxia (FRDA), in which patients usually develop with HCM phenotype to varying degrees [73]. In FRDA, abnormal expansions of the GAA repeat within the first intron of the *FXN* gene may result in the silencing of the gene, which in turn reduces or completely abolishes the production of the frataxin protein.

Frataxin has been implicated in the mechanism of iron-sulfur cluster biosynthesis; however, the contribution of frataxin-deficiency to cardiomyopathy development has yet to be elucidated.

To test whether iron homeostasis deregulation accelerates the reduction in energy synthesis dynamics that contributes to impaired cardiac calcium homeostasis and contractile force, we have recently generated skin fibroblasts-derived iPSCs from a FRDA patient [51]. The *FXN* gene expression in that patient was endogenously silenced. Phenotypically, the FRDA iPSCs-derived cardiomyocytes exhibited a disorganization of the mitochondrial network complemented with mitochondrial DNA depletion. Consistent with the mitochondrial disorganization, the energy synthesis dynamics, in terms of ATP production rate, in the diseased cardiomyocytes was impaired. Interestingly, when the diseased cardiomyocytes were subjected to iron overloading, a significant impairment in the calcium handling property was observed. These results indicated that patient-specific iPSCs are useful tools for studying FRDA-associated cardiac defects.

6. Application of Patient-Specific iPSCs-Derived Cardiomyocytes in Efficacy Testing and Drug Screening

Owing to the limited sources of human cardiomyocytes for *in vitro* analyses, the effects of a putative cardiac drug have to be conventionally tested in the well-established rabbit or canine Purkinje fiber model before proceeding to clinical trials. Nevertheless, as the non-human based cellular models often give false-positive or inconsistent results [74–76], many drugs that have passed the animal tests ended up with failure in the clinical trials. Recent reports demonstrated that human embryonic stem cells-derived cardiomyocytes exhibited excellent pharmacological response to various known antiarrhythmic agents; thus they may be a potential alternative to animal cardiomyocytes [77,78]. However, due to the difference in genetic background, individuals with similar cardiac disorders could show quite different responses towards a particular drug. In this regard, the patient-specific iPSC-derived cardiomyocytes offer an exclusive platform for evaluating the efficacy of a particular drug or treatment strategy on a personal basis.

Based on the latest breakthrough in the cardiac differentiation protocol, a yield of more than 80% in cardiomyocyte differentiation has been achieved [27]. When these patient-specific iPSCs-derived cardiomyocytes are applied to a high throughput assay platform, such as multielectrode arrays analysis, the effects of a testing drug on cellular electrophysiology can be evaluated in a short period of time. Emerging evidences from our group and other investigators have pointed out that altered calcium handling could be an important pathogenic mechanism underlying cardiomyopathies [48,49,79,80]; drugs that affect calcium homeostasis should be of great therapeutic potential. Mercola and colleagues have recently developed a high throughput automated kinetic image cytometry system for the measurement of calcium ion dynamics. This system enabled the authors to simultaneously measure individual calcium transients from 100 human iPSCs-derived cardiomyocytes [81]. Taking advantage of such system, high throughput screenings of calcium handling-enhancing properties of known or novel drugs can be performed on patient-specific iPSCs-derived cardiomyocytes.

7. Application of Patient-Specific iPSCs-Derived Cardiomyocytes in Toxicology Test

In addition to pharmacological studies, the cardiomyocytes derived from iPSCs are of great potential in the toxicology tests. So far, isolated canine cardiomyocytes are the most popular *pre*-clinical model for cardiac safety testing of a developing drug. However, as mentioned in the last section, the reliability of such model remains questionable. As a matter of fact, many drugs that have passed the animal tests turned out to show unanticipated cardiac toxicity when administered to patients [82], thus, a more predictive and reliable human cardiomyocyte-based model for toxicology test is of immediate demand. Increasing evidences suggested that the pharmacological sensitivities of human ESCs and iPSCs-derived cardiomyocytes are much more advanced than any animal models [77,78], and they should be good detectors for any undesired proarrhythmic side effects of a developing drug.

Recently, Mendenius and colleagues proposed the possibility of using human ESCs and iPSCs-derived cardiomyocytes in the evaluation of drug-induced cardiac injury [83,84]. In their studies, the human ESCs- and iPSCs-derived cardiomyocytes were treated with doxorubicin, and the release of cardiac troponin T in culture medium was measured utilizing a Biocore-based system for the degree of cell injury. Compared to the conventional ELISA based assay, the surface plasmon resonance-based method not only provides superior sensitivity and specificity, but also allows simultaneous analysis of multiple samples. Consequently, the use of iPSCs-derived cardiomyocytes in toxicity predication appears to be feasible.

8. Limitations of iPSCs

The recent achievement in the patient-specific iPSC technology has created a new platform for regenerative medicine, disease modeling and personalized medication development. Yet, like many other technologies, the clinical applications of patient-specific iPSCs-derived cardiomyocytes are also hindered by various limitations. Though the latest advancement in cardiac differentiation protocol allows efficient generation of cardiomyocytes in a high yield, the human iPSCs-derived cardiomyocytes are actually less mature in terms of calcium homeostasis when compared to the human ESCs-derived cardiomyocytes as demonstrated earlier by our laboratory [85]. In other words, the patient-specific iPSCs-derived cardiomyocytes may not be suitable for modeling cardiac defects resulted from mutations of genes that regulate calcium transients, such as the mutations in the gene encoding the phospholamban.

Furthermore, it should be noted that a high yield of cardiac differentiation is not equivalent to high purity. In fact, iPSCs-derived cardiomyocytes are always grown in a mixed population of atrial, ventricular and nodal subtypes. These subtypes do possess different electrophysiology properties. So far, most transplantation studies were performed in rodent models [28,29]. As rodents have a much faster heart rate compared to humans, the injection of human cardiomyocytes into rodent hearts may not create significant arrhythmia problems. However, the injection of mismatched subtypes of cardiomyocytes into a patient's heart may lead to a medical emergency. Unfortunately, no efficient way is available to sort the subtypes of iPSCs-derived cardiomyocytes into pure populations. The direct application of patient-specific iPSCs cardiomyocytes in regenerative medicine, therefore, remains a theoretic foundation. Besides the issue of mixed subtypes, the immature phenotype of iPSCs-derived cardiomyocytes also limits its application in drug screening experiments. To this end, it is important to verify and validate the results obtained in the initial screening steps.

9. Conclusions

The cardiomyocytes derived from patients-specific iPSCs are of great potential in many clinical applications. This authentic human cardiomyocyte-based system is expected to compensate for the limitations of the current experimental animal models. This review provides detailed descriptions in the strategies and workflow of using the patient-specific iPSCs-derived cardiomyocytes in regenerative medicine, disease modeling and pharmacological applications. The examples illustrated in this review clearly evidenced the practical values of this novel technology. However, various limitations, such as the immaturities of iPSCs-derived cardiomyocytes, still need to be addressed, and future studies resolving these issues would be beneficial to the use of patient-specific iPSCs in clinical applications.

Acknowledgments

This work was supported by the Hong Kong Research Grant Council: General Research Fund (HKU 775613).

Author Contributions

Kwong-Man Ng and Cheuk-Yiu Law were responsible for the literature review and the writing of the manuscript. While Hung-Fat Tse was responsible for providing suggestions on the organization of the article and the editing of the final draft.

Conflicts of Interest

The authors declare no conflict of interest.

References

1. Bergmann, O.; Bhardwaj, R.D.; Bernard, S.; Zdunek, S.; Barnabe-Heider, F.; Walsh, S.; Zupicich, J.; Alkass, K.; Buchholz, B.A.; Druid, H.; *et al.* Evidence for cardiomyocyte renewal in humans. *Science* **2009**, *324*, 98–102.
2. Goktepe, S.; Abilez, O.J.; Parker, K.K.; Kuhl, E. A multiscale model for eccentric and concentric cardiac growth through sarcomerogenesis. *J. Theor. Biol.* **2010**, *265*, 433–442.
3. Takahashi, K.; Tanabe, K.; Ohnuki, M.; Narita, M.; Ichisaka, T.; Tomoda, K.; Yamanaka, S. Induction of pluripotent stem cells from adult human fibroblasts by defined factors. *Cell* **2007**, *131*, 861–872.
4. Takahashi, K.; Yamanaka, S. Induction of pluripotent stem cells from mouse embryonic and adult fibroblast cultures by defined factors. *Cell* **2006**, *126*, 663–676.
5. Kwon, J.; Lee, N.; Jeon, I.; Lee, H.J.; Do, J.T.; Lee, D.R.; Oh, S.H.; Shin, D.A.; Kim, A.; Song, J. Neuronal differentiation of a human induced pluripotent stem cell line (FS-1) derived from newborn foreskin fibroblasts. *Int. J. Stem. Cells* **2012**, *5*, 140–145.
6. Kattman, S.J.; Witty, A.D.; Gagliardi, M.; Dubois, N.C.; Niapour, M.; Hotta, A.; Ellis, J.; Keller, G. Stage-specific optimization of activin/nodal and BMP signaling promotes cardiac differentiation of mouse and human pluripotent stem cell lines. *Cell Stem Cell* **2011**, *8*, 228–240.
7. Nakagawa, M.; Koyanagi, M.; Tanabe, K.; Takahashi, K.; Ichisaka, T.; Aoi, T.; Okita, K.; Mochiduki, Y.; Takizawa, N.; Yamanaka, S. Generation of induced pluripotent stem cells without myc from mouse and human fibroblasts. *Nat. Biotechnol.* **2008**, *26*, 101–106.
8. Novak, A.; Shtrichman, R.; Germanguz, I.; Segev, H.; Zeevi-Levin, N.; Fishman, B.; Mandel, Y.E.; Barad, L.; Domev, H.; Kotton, D.; *et al.* Enhanced reprogramming and cardiac differentiation of human keratinocytes derived from plucked hair follicles, using a single excisable lentivirus. *Cell. Reprogram.* **2010**, *12*, 665–678.
9. Merling, R.K.; Sweeney, C.L.; Choi, U.; De Ravin, S.S.; Myers, T.G.; Otaizo-Carrasquero, F.; Pan, J.; Linton, G.; Chen, L.; Koontz, S.; *et al.* Transgene-free ipscs generated from small volume peripheral blood nonmobilized CD34+ cells. *Blood* **2013**, *121*, doi:10.1182/blood-2012-03-420273.
10. Churko, J.M.; Burridge, P.W.; Wu, J.C. Generation of human ipscs from human peripheral blood mononuclear cells using non-integrative sendai virus in chemically defined conditions. *Methods Mol. Biol.* **2013**, *1036*, 81–88.
11. Wang, Y.; Liu, J.; Tan, X.; Li, G.; Gao, Y.; Liu, X.; Zhang, L.; Li, Y. Induced pluripotent stem cells from human hair follicle mesenchymal stem cells. *Stem Cell Rev.* **2013**, *9*, 451–460.

12. DeRosa, B.A.; van Baaren, J.M.; Dubey, G.K.; Lee, J.M.; Cuccaro, M.L.; Vance, J.M.; Pericak-Vance, M.A.; Dykxhoorn, D.M. Derivation of autism spectrum disorder-specific induced pluripotent stem cells from peripheral blood mononuclear cells. *Neurosci. Lett.* **2012**, *516*, 9–14.

13. Gianotti-Sommer, A.; Rozelle, S.S.; Sullivan, S.; Mills, J.A.; Park, S.M.; Smith, B.W.; Iyer, A.M.; French, D.L.; Kotton, D.N.; Gadue, P.; *et al.* Generation of human induced pluripotent stem cells from peripheral blood using the stemcca lentiviral vector. *J. Vis. Exp.* **2008**, *68*, doi:10.3791/4327.

14. Zhou, T.; Benda, C.; Dunzinger, S.; Huang, Y.; Ho, J.C.; Yang, J.; Wang, Y.; Zhang, Y.; Zhuang, Q.; Li, Y.; *et al.* Generation of human induced pluripotent stem cells from urine samples. *Nat. Protoc.* **2012**, *7*, 2080–2089.

15. Li, W.; Wang, X.; Fan, W.; Zhao, P.; Chan, Y.C.; Chen, S.; Zhang, S.; Guo, X.; Zhang, Y.; Li, Y.; *et al.* Modeling abnormal early development with induced pluripotent stem cells from aneuploid syndromes. *Human Mol. Genet.* **2012**, *21*, 32–45.

16. Yu, J.; Vodyanik, M.A.; Smuga-Otto, K.; Antosiewicz-Bourget, J.; Frane, J.L.; Tian, S.; Nie, J.; Jonsdottir, G.A.; Ruotti, V.; Stewart, R.; *et al.* Induced pluripotent stem cell lines derived from human somatic cells. *Science* **2007**, *318*, 1917–1920.

17. Sommer, C.A.; Stadtfeld, M.; Murphy, G.J.; Hochedlinger, K.; Kotton, D.N.; Mostoslavsky, G. Induced pluripotent stem cell generation using a single lentiviral stem cell cassette. *Stem Cells* **2009**, *27*, 543–549.

18. Papapetrou, E.P.; Tomishima, M.J.; Chambers, S.M.; Mica, Y.; Reed, E.; Menon, J.; Tabar, V.; Mo, Q.; Studer, L.; Sadelain, M. Stoichiometric and temporal requirements of Oct4, Sox2, Klf4, and c-Myc expression for efficient human ipsc induction and differentiation. *Proc. Natl. Acad. Sci. USA* **2009**, *106*, 12759–12764.

19. Sommer, C.A.; Sommer, A.G.; Longmire, T.A.; Christodoulou, C.; Thomas, D.D.; Gostissa, M.; Alt, F.W.; Murphy, G.J.; Kotton, D.N.; Mostoslavsky, G. Excision of reprogramming transgenes improves the differentiation potential of iPS cells generated with a single excisable vector. *Stem Cells* **2010**, *28*, 64–74.

20. Somers, A.; Jean, J.C.; Sommer, C.A.; Omari, A.; Ford, C.C.; Mills, J.A.; Ying, L.; Sommer, A.G.; Jean, J.M.; Smith, B.W.; *et al.* Generation of transgene-free lung disease-specific human induced pluripotent stem cells using a single excisable lentiviral stem cell cassette. *Stem Cells* **2010**, *28*, 1728–1740.

21. Zhou, W.; Freed, C.R. Adenoviral gene delivery can reprogram human fibroblasts to induced pluripotent stem cells. *Stem Cells* **2009**, *27*, 2667–2674.

22. Fusaki, N.; Ban, H.; Nishiyama, A.; Saeki, K.; Hasegawa, M. Efficient induction of transgene-free human pluripotent stem cells using a vector based on sendai virus, an rna virus that does not integrate into the host genome. *Phys. Biol. Sci.* **2009**, *85*, 348–362.

23. Mummery, C.; Ward, D.; van den Brink, C.E.; Bird, S.D.; Doevendans, P.A.; Opthof, T.; Brutel de la Riviere, A.; Tertoolen, L.; van der Heyden, M.; Pera, M. Cardiomyocyte differentiation of mouse and human embryonic stem cells. *J. Anat.* **2002**, *200*, 233–242.

24. Passier, R.; Oostwaard, D.W.; Snapper, J.; Kloots, J.; Hassink, R.J.; Kuijk, E.; Roelen, B.; de la Riviere, A.B.; Mummery, C. Increased cardiomyocyte differentiation from human embryonic stem cells in serum-free cultures. *Stem Cells* **2005**, *23*, 772–780.

25. Yang, L.; Soonpaa, M.H.; Adler, E.D.; Roepke, T.K.; Kattman, S.J.; Kennedy, M.; Henckaerts, E.; Bonham, K.; Abbott, G.W.; Linden, R.M.; *et al.* Human cardiovascular progenitor cells develop from a Kdr+ embryonic-stem-cell-derived population. *Nature* **2008**, *453*, 524–528.

26. Lian, X.; Hsiao, C.; Wilson, G.; Zhu, K.; Hazeltine, L.B.; Azarin, S.M.; Raval, K.K.; Zhang, J.; Kamp, T.J.; Palecek, S.P. Robust cardiomyocyte differentiation from human pluripotent stem cells via temporal modulation of canonical wnt signaling. In Proceeding of the National Academy of Sciences of the United States of America, Cambridge, MA, USA, 2012.

27. Lian, X.; Zhang, J.; Azarin, S.M.; Zhu, K.; Hazeltine, L.B.; Bao, X.; Hsiao, C.; Kamp, T.J.; Palecek, S.P. Directed cardiomyocyte differentiation from human pluripotent stem cells by modulating Wnt/beta-catenin signaling under fully defined conditions. *Nat. Protoc.* **2013**, *8*, 162–175.

28. Laflamme, M.A.; Chen, K.Y.; Naumova, A.V.; Muskheli, V.; Fugate, J.A.; Dupras, S.K.; Reinecke, H.; Xu, C.; Hassanipour, M.; Police, S.; *et al.* Cardiomyocytes derived from human embryonic stem cells in *pro*-survival factors enhance function of infarcted rat hearts. *Nat. Biotechnol.* **2007**, *25*, 1015–1024.

29. Van Laake, L.W.; Passier, R.; Monshouwer-Kloots, J.; Verkleij, A.J.; Lips, D.J.; Freund, C.; den Ouden, K.; Ward-van Oostwaard, D.; Korving, J.; Tertoolen, L.G.; *et al.* Human embryonic stem cell-derived cardiomyocytes survive and mature in the mouse heart and transiently improve function after myocardial infarction. *Stem Cell Res.* **2007**, *1*, 9–24.

30. Zakharova, L.; Mastroeni, D.; Mutlu, N.; Molina, M.; Goldman, S.; Diethrich, E.; Gaballa, M.A. Transplantation of cardiac progenitor cell sheet onto infarcted heart promotes cardiogenesis and improves function. *Cardiovasc. Res.* **2010**, *87*, 40–49.

31. Carpenter, L.; Carr, C.; Yang, C.T.; Stuckey, D.J.; Clarke, K.; Watt, S.M. Efficient differentiation of human induced pluripotent stem cells generates cardiac cells that provide protection following myocardial infarction in the rat. *Stem Cells Dev.* **2012**, *21*, 977–986.

32. Yan, B.; Abdelli, L.S.; Singla, D.K. Transplanted induced pluripotent stem cells improve cardiac function and induce neovascularization in the infarcted hearts of db/db mice. *Mol. Pharm.* **2011**, *8*, 1602–1610.

33. Maron, B.J.; Towbin, J.A.; Thiene, G.; Antzelevitch, C.; Corrado, D.; Arnett, D.; Moss, A.J.; Seidman, C.E.; Young, J.B.; American Heart, A.; *et al.* Contemporary definitions and classification of the cardiomyopathies. *Circulation* **2006**, *113*, 1807–1816.

34. Splawski, I.; Timothy, K.W.; Sharpe, L.M.; Decher, N.; Kumar, P.; Bloise, R.; Napolitano, C.; Schwartz, P.J.; Joseph, R.M.; Condouris, K.; *et al.* Ca(v)1.2 calcium channel dysfunction causes a multisystem disorder including arrhythmia and autism. *Cell* **2004**, *119*, 19–31.

35. Thiel, W.H.; Chen, B.; Hund, T.J.; Koval, O.M.; Purohit, A.; Song, L.S.; Mohler, P.J.; Anderson, M.E. Proarrhythmic defects in timothy syndrome require calmodulin kinase ii. *Circulation* **2008**, *118*, 2225–2234.

36. Cheng, E.P.; Yuan, C.; Navedo, M.F.; Dixon, R.E.; Nieves-Cintron, M.; Scott, J.D.; Santana, L.F. Restoration of normal l-type Ca2+ channel function during timothy syndrome by ablation of an anchoring protein. *Circ. Res.* **2011**, *109*, 255–261.

37. Bader, P.L.; Faizi, M.; Kim, L.H.; Owen, S.F.; Tadross, M.R.; Alfa, R.W.; Bett, G.C.; Tsien, R.W.; Rasmusson, R.L.; Shamloo, M. Mouse model of timothy syndrome recapitulates triad of autistic traits. *Proc. Natl. Acad. Sci. USA* **2011**, *108*, 15432–15437.

38. Itzhaki, I.; Maizels, L.; Huber, I.; Zwi-Dantsis, L.; Caspi, O.; Winterstern, A.; Feldman, O.; Gepstein, A.; Arbel, G.; Hammerman, H.; *et al.* Modelling the long qt syndrome with induced pluripotent stem cells. *Nature* **2011**, *471*, 225–229.

39. Yazawa, M.; Dolmetsch, R.E. Modeling timothy syndrome with iPS cells. *J. Cardiovasc. Transl. Res.* **2013**, *6*, 1–9.

40. Matsa, E.; Rajamohan, D.; Dick, E.; Young, L.; Mellor, I.; Staniforth, A.; Denning, C. Drug evaluation in cardiomyocytes derived from human induced pluripotent stem cells carrying a long QT syndrome type 2 mutation. *Eur. Heart J.* **2011**, *32*, 952–962.

41. Moretti, A.; Bellin, M.; Welling, A.; Jung, C.B.; Lam, J.T.; Bott-Flugel, L.; Dorn, T.; Goedel, A.; Hohnke, C.; Hofmann, F.; *et al.* Patient-specific induced pluripotent stem-cell models for long-QT syndrome. *N. Engl. J. Med.* **2010**, *363*, 1397–1409.

42. Lahti, A.L.; Kujala, V.J.; Chapman, H.; Koivisto, A.P.; Pekkanen-Mattila, M.; Kerkela, E.; Hyttinen, J.; Kontula, K.; Swan, H.; Conklin, B.R.; *et al.* Model for long QT syndrome type 2 using human iPS cells demonstrates arrhythmogenic characteristics in cell culture. *Dis. Model. Mech.* **2012**, *5*, 220–230.

43. Ma, D.; Wei, H.; Zhao, Y.; Lu, J.; Li, G.; Sahib, N.B.; Tan, T.H.; Wong, K.Y.; Shim, W.; Wong, P.; *et al.* Modeling type 3 long QT syndrome with cardiomyocytes derived from patient-specific induced pluripotent stem cells. *Int. J. Cardiol.* **2013**, *168*, 5277–5286.

44. Yazawa, M.; Hsueh, B.; Jia, X.; Pasca, A.M.; Bernstein, J.A.; Hallmayer, J.; Dolmetsch, R.E. Using induced pluripotent stem cells to investigate cardiac phenotypes in timothy syndrome. *Nature* **2011**, *471*, 230–234.

45. Fatima, A.; Xu, G.; Shao, K.; Papadopoulos, S.; Lehmann, M.; Arnaiz-Cot, J.J.; Rosa, A.O.; Nguemo, F.; Matzkies, M.; Dittmann, S.; *et al.* In vitro modeling of ryanodine receptor 2 dysfunction using human induced pluripotent stem cells. *Cell. Physiol. Biochem.* **2011**, *28*, 579–592.

46. Jung, C.B.; Moretti, A.; Mederos y Schnitzler, M.; Iop, L.; Storch, U.; Bellin, M.; Dorn, T.; Ruppenthal, S.; Pfeiffer, S.; Goedel, A.; *et al.* Dantrolene rescues arrhythmogenic RYR2 defect in a patient-specific stem cell model of catecholaminergic polymorphic ventricular tachycardia. *EMBO Mol. Med.* **2012**, *4*, 180–191.

47. Novak, A.; Barad, L.; Zeevi-Levin, N.; Shick, R.; Shtrichman, R.; Lorber, A.; Itskovitz-Eldor, J.; Binah, O. Cardiomyocytes generated from CPVTD307H patients are arrhythmogenic in response to beta-adrenergic stimulation. *J. Cell. Mol. Med.* **2012**, *16*, 468–482.

48. Sun, N.; Yazawa, M.; Liu, J.; Han, L.; Sanchez-Freire, V.; Abilez, O.J.; Navarrete, E.G.; Hu, S.; Wang, L.; Lee, A.; *et al.* Patient-specific induced pluripotent stem cells as a model for familial dilated cardiomyopathy. *Sci. Transl. Med.* **2012**, *4*, 130–147.

49. Tse, H.F.; Ho, J.C.; Choi, S.W.; Lee, Y.K.; Butler, A.W.; Ng, K.M.; Siu, C.W.; Simpson, M.A.; Lai, W.H.; Chan, Y.C.; *et al.* Patient-specific induced-pluripotent stem cells-derived cardiomyocytes recapitulate the pathogenic phenotypes of dilated cardiomyopathy due to a novel DES mutation identified by whole exome sequencing. *Human Mol. Genet.* **2013**, *22*, 1395–1403.

50. Lan, F.; Lee, A.S.; Liang, P.; Sanchez-Freire, V.; Nguyen, P.K.; Wang, L.; Han, L.; Yen, M.; Wang, Y.; Sun, N.; *et al.* Abnormal calcium handling properties underlie familial hypertrophic cardiomyopathy pathology in patient-specific induced pluripotent stem cells. *Cell Stem Cell* **2013**, *12*, 101–113.

51. Lee, Y.K.; Ho, P.W.; Schick, R.; Lau, Y.M.; Lai, W.H.; Zhou, T.; Li, Y.; Ng, K.M.; Ho, S.L.; Esteban, M.A.; *et al.* Modeling of friedreich ataxia-related iron overloading cardiomyopathy using patient-specific-induced pluripotent stem cells. *Pflug. Arch.: Eur. J. Physiol.* **2013**, *466*, 1831–1844.

52. Kontula, K.; Laitinen, P.J.; Lehtonen, A.; Toivonen, L.; Viitasalo, M.; Swan, H. Catecholaminergic polymorphic ventricular tachycardia: Recent mechanistic insights. *Cardiovasc. Res.* **2005**, *67*, 379–387.

53. Liu, N.; Ruan, Y.; Priori, S.G. Catecholaminergic polymorphic ventricular tachycardia. *Prog. Cardiovasc. Dis.* **2008**, *51*, 23–30.

54. Priori, S.G.; Napolitano, C.; Tiso, N.; Memmi, M.; Vignati, G.; Bloise, R.; Sorrentino, V.; Danieli, G.A. Mutations in the cardiac ryanodine receptor gene (*hRyR2*) underlie catecholaminergic polymorphic ventricular tachycardia. *Circulation* **2001**, *103*, 196–200.

55. Lahat, H.; Pras, E.; Olender, T.; Avidan, N.; Ben-Asher, E.; Man, O.; Levy-Nissenbaum, E.; Khoury, A.; Lorber, A.; Goldman, B.; *et al.* A missense mutation in a highly conserved region of CASQ2 is associated with autosomal recessive catecholamine-induced polymorphic ventricular tachycardia in bedouin families from israel. *Am. J. Human Genet.* **2001**, *69*, 1378–1384.

56. Viatchenko-Karpinski, S.; Terentyev, D.; Gyorke, I.; Terentyeva, R.; Volpe, P.; Priori, S.G.; Napolitano, C.; Nori, A.; Williams, S.C.; Gyorke, S. Abnormal calcium signaling and sudden cardiac death associated with mutation of calsequestrin. *Circ. Res.* **2004**, *94*, 471–477.

57. Terentyev, D.; Nori, A.; Santoro, M.; Viatchenko-Karpinski, S.; Kubalova, Z.; Gyorke, I.; Terentyeva, R.; Vedamoorthyrao, S.; Blom, N.A.; Valle, G.; *et al.* Abnormal interactions of calsequestrin with the ryanodine receptor calcium release channel complex linked to exercise-induced sudden cardiac death. *Circ. Res.* **2006**, *98*, 1151–1158.

58. Di Barletta, M.R.; Viatchenko-Karpinski, S.; Nori, A.; Memmi, M.; Terentyev, D.; Turcato, F.; Valle, G.; Rizzi, N.; Napolitano, C.; Gyorke, S.; *et al.* Clinical phenotype and functional characterization of CASQ2 mutations associated with catecholaminergic polymorphic ventricular tachycardia. *Circulation* **2006**, *114*, 1012–1019.

59. Cerrone, M.; Colombi, B.; Santoro, M.; di Barletta, M.R.; Scelsi, M.; Villani, L.; Napolitano, C.; Priori, S.G. Bidirectional ventricular tachycardia and fibrillation elicited in a knock-in mouse model carrier of a mutation in the cardiac ryanodine receptor. *Circ. Res.* **2005**, *96*, doi:10.1161/01.RES.0000169067.51055.72.

60. Burkett, E.L.; Hershberger, R.E. Clinical and genetic issues in familial dilated cardiomyopathy. *J. Am. Coll. Cardiol.* **2005**, *45*, 969–981.

61. Grunig, E.; Tasman, J.A.; Kucherer, H.; Franz, W.; Kubler, W.; Katus, H.A. Frequency and phenotypes of familial dilated cardiomyopathy. *J. Am. Coll. Cardiol.* **1998**, *31*, 186–194.

62. Goerss, J.B.; Michels, V.V.; Burnett, J.; Driscoll, D.J.; Miller, F.; Rodeheffer, R.; Tajik, A.J.; Schaid, D. Frequency of familial dilated cardiomyopathy. *Eur. Heart J.* **1995**, *16* (Suppl. O), 2–4.

63. Mahon, N.G.; Murphy, R.T.; MacRae, C.A.; Caforio, A.L.; Elliott, P.M.; McKenna, W.J. Echocardiographic evaluation in asymptomatic relatives of patients with dilated cardiomyopathy reveals preclinical disease. *Ann. Intern. Med.* **2005**, *143*, 108–115.

64. Ahmad, F.; Banerjee, S.K.; Lage, M.L.; Huang, X.N.; Smith, S.H.; Saba, S.; Rager, J.; Conner, D.A.; Janczewski, A.M.; Tobita, K.; *et al.* The role of cardiac troponin t quantity and function in cardiac development and dilated cardiomyopathy. *PLoS One* **2008**, *3*, e2642.

65. Lombardi, R.; Bell, A.; Senthil, V.; Sidhu, J.; Noseda, M.; Roberts, R.; Marian, A.J. Differential interactions of thin filament proteins in two cardiac troponin T mouse models of hypertrophic and dilated cardiomyopathies. *Cardiovasc. Res.* **2008**, *79*, 109–117.

66. Gudkova, A.; Kostareva, A.; Sjoberg, G.; Smolina, N.; Turalchuk, M.; Kuznetsova, I.; Rybakova, M.; Edstrom, L.; Shlyakhto, E.; Sejersen, T. Diagnostic challenge in desmin cardiomyopathy with transformation of clinical phenotypes. *Pediatr. Cardiol.* **2013**, *34*, 467–470.

67. Milner, D.J.; Taffet, G.E.; Wang, X.; Pham, T.; Tamura, T.; Hartley, C.; Gerdes, A.M.; Capetanaki, Y. The absence of desmin leads to cardiomyocyte hypertrophy and cardiac dilation with compromised systolic function. *J. Mol. Cell. Cardiol.* **1999**, *31*, 2063–2076.

68. Ghosh, N.; Haddad, H. Recent progress in the genetics of cardiomyopathy and its role in the clinical evaluation of patients with cardiomyopathy. *Curr. Opin. Cardiol.* **2011**, *26*, 155–164.

69. Keren, A.; Syrris, P.; McKenna, W.J. Hypertrophic cardiomyopathy: The genetic determinants of clinical disease expression. *Nat. Clin. Pract. Cardiovasc. Med.* **2008**, *5*, 158–168.

70. Geisterfer-Lowrance, A.A.; Christe, M.; Conner, D.A.; Ingwall, J.S.; Schoen, F.J.; Seidman, C.E.; Seidman, J.G. A mouse model of familial hypertrophic cardiomyopathy. *Science* **1996**, *272*, 731–734.

71. Marian, A.J.; Wu, Y.; Lim, D.S.; McCluggage, M.; Youker, K.; Yu, Q.T.; Brugada, R.; DeMayo, F.; Quinones, M.; Roberts, R. A transgenic rabbit model for human hypertrophic cardiomyopathy. *J. Clin. Investig.* **1999**, *104*, 1683–1692.

72. Tardiff, J.C.; Hewett, T.E.; Palmer, B.M.; Olsson, C.; Factor, S.M.; Moore, R.L.; Robbins, J.; Leinwand, L.A. Cardiac troponin T mutations result in allele-specific phenotypes in a mouse model for hypertrophic cardiomyopathy. *J. Clin. Investig.* **1999**, *104*, 469–481.

73. Gucev, Z.; Tasic, V.; Jancevska, A.; Popjordanova, N.; Koceva, S.; Kuturec, M.; Sabolic, V. Friedreich ataxia (FA) associated with diabetes mellitus type 1 and hyperthrophic cardiomyopathy. *Bosn. J. Basic. Med. Sci.* **2009**, *9*, 107–110.

74. Redfern, W.S.; Carlsson, L.; Davis, A.S.; Lynch, W.G.; MacKenzie, I.; Palethorpe, S.; Siegl, P.K.; Strang, I.; Sullivan, A.T.; Wallis, R.; *et al.* Relationships between preclinical cardiac electrophysiology, clinical QT interval prolongation and torsade de pointes for a broad range of drugs: Evidence for a provisional safety margin in drug development. *Cardiovasc. Res.* **2003**, *58*, 32–45.

75. Gintant, G.A.; Su, Z.; Martin, R.L.; Cox, B.F. Utility of herg assays as surrogate markers of delayed cardiac repolarization and QT safety. *Toxicol. Pathol.* **2006**, *34*, 81–90.

76. Dumotier, B.M.; Deurinck, M.; Yang, Y.; Traebert, M.; Suter, W. Relevance of *in vitro* screenit results for drug-induced QT interval prolongation *in vivo*: A database review and analysis. *Pharmacol. Ther.* **2008**, *119*, 152–159.

77. Yokoo, N.; Baba, S.; Kaichi, S.; Niwa, A.; Mima, T.; Doi, H.; Yamanaka, S.; Nakahata, T.; Heike, T. The effects of cardioactive drugs on cardiomyocytes derived from human induced pluripotent stem cells. *Biochem. Biophys. Res. Commun.* **2009**, *387*, 482–488.

78. Peng, S.; Lacerda, A.E.; Kirsch, G.E.; Brown, A.M.; Bruening-Wright, A. The action potential and comparative pharmacology of stem cell-derived human cardiomyocytes. *J. Pharmacol. Toxicol. Methods* **2010**, *61*, 277–286.

79. Reuter, H.; Schwinger, R.H. Calcium handling in human heart failure—Abnormalities and target for therapy. *Wien. Med. Wochenschr.* **2012**, *162*, 297–301.

80. Lou, Q.; Janardhan, A.; Efimov, I.R. Remodeling of calcium handling in human heart failure. *Adv. Exp. Med. Biol.* **2012**, *740*, 1145–1174.

81. Cerignoli, F.; Charlot, D.; Whittaker, R.; Ingermanson, R.; Gehalot, P.; Savchenko, A.; Gallacher, D.J.; Towart, R.; Price, J.H.; McDonough, P.M.; *et al.* High throughput measurement of Ca(2)(+) dynamics for drug risk assessment in human stem cell-derived cardiomyocytes by kinetic image cytometry. *J. Pharmacol. Toxicol. Methods* **2012**, *66*, 246–256.

82. Kola, I.; Landis, J. Can the pharmaceutical industry reduce attrition rates? *Nat. Rev. Drug Discov.* **2004**, *3*, 711–715.

83. Andersson, H.; Steel, D.; Asp, J.; Dahlenborg, K.; Jonsson, M.; Jeppsson, A.; Lindahl, A.; Kagedal, B.; Sartipy, P.; Mandenius, C.F. Assaying cardiac biomarkers for toxicity testing using biosensing and cardiomyocytes derived from human embryonic stem cells. *J. Biotechnol.* **2010**, *150*, 175–181.

84. Mandenius, C.F.; Steel, D.; Noor, F.; Meyer, T.; Heinzle, E.; Asp, J.; Arain, S.; Kraushaar, U.; Bremer, S.; Class, R.; *et al.* Cardiotoxicity testing using pluripotent stem cell-derived human cardiomyocytes and state-of-the-art bioanalytics: A review. *J. Appl. Toxicol.* **2011**, *31*, 191–205.

85. Lee, Y.K.; Ng, K.M.; Lai, W.H.; Chan, Y.C.; Lau, Y.M.; Lian, Q.; Tse, H.F.; Siu, C.W. Calcium homeostasis in human induced pluripotent stem cell-derived cardiomyocytes. *Stem Cell Rev.* **2011**, *7*, 976–986.

Chapter 3:
Eye

iPS Cells for Modelling and Treatment of Retinal Diseases

Fred K. Chen, Samuel McLenachan, Michael Edel, Lyndon Da Cruz, Peter J. Coffey and David A. Mackey

Abstract: For many decades, we have relied on immortalised retinal cell lines, histology of enucleated human eyes, animal models, clinical observation, genetic studies and human clinical trials to learn more about the pathogenesis of retinal diseases and explore treatment options. The recent availability of patient-specific induced pluripotent stem cells (iPSC) for deriving retinal lineages has added a powerful alternative tool for discovering new disease-causing mutations, studying genotype-phenotype relationships, performing therapeutics-toxicity screening and developing personalised cell therapy. This review article provides a clinical perspective on the current and potential benefits of iPSC for managing the most common blinding diseases of the eye: inherited retinal diseases and age-related macular degeneration.

Reprinted from *J. Clin. Med.* Cite as: Chen, F.K.; McLenachan, S.; Edel, M.; Cruz, L.D.; Coffey, P.J.; Mackey, D.A. iPS Cells for Modelling and Treatment of Retinal Diseases. *J. Clin. Med.* **2014**, *3*, 1511–1541.

1. Introduction

The ability to convert a differentiated somatic cell from a patient into a pluripotent stem cell has provided new tools for studying organ development and genotype-phenotype relationships. Three-dimensional tissue structures and cells derived from these induced pluripotent stem cells (iPSCs) are now being used to screen and test the therapeutic and toxic effects of potential pharmacologic agents and gene therapies. More importantly, iPSCs could also be used to provide an easily accessible source of tissue for autologous cellular therapy. To date, the greatest potential benefit of iPSC technology is in the treatment of retinal diseases.

The retina is a complex neurovascular tissue within the eye. It contains a network of neurons nourished by the retinal and choroidal circulations. Specialised neuronal cells, called rod and cone photoreceptors, capture light that enters into the eye. Through phototransduction within the photoreceptors and downstream neural processing by the bipolar, amacrine, horizontal and ganglion cells within the retina, light signals are transmitted to the primary and secondary visual cortex of the brain to enable visual sensation. The functions of these specialised neuronal cells are supported by the Muller glial cells and the retinal pigment epithelium (RPE). The ease of visualising retinal neurons and assessing the structure-function correlation in detail using readily available imaging devices will facilitate the *in vivo* clinical translation of iPSC technology in the diagnosis and treatment of retinal diseases (Figure 1).

Among hundreds of human retinal diseases, the most significant are age-related macular degeneration (AMD) and the inherited retinal diseases (IRDs). Both AMD and IRDs are neither preventable nor curable, and they remain the most significant causes of irreversible blindness. The underlying processes leading to retinal cell death range from cell-autonomous mechanisms related to single gene mutations to complex gene-metabolic-environment interaction, resulting in extracellular remodelling, abnormal angiogenesis, chronic inflammation, defective lipid metabolism and oxidative injury, as proposed in AMD [1]. The discovery of the pathological basis of these diseases was made possible through clinical observation using detailed retinal imaging techniques, human genetic studies, histology of post-mortem, enucleated or aborted foetal eyes, immortalised cell line culture systems and animal models of retinal diseases. However, in routine clinical practice, retinal diagnosis is rarely based on retinal histology because of the significant morbidity associated with retinal biopsy and the ease in making a diagnosis, because the retina is easily visualised. The availability of iPSC technology provides an opportunity to obtain retinal tissue without retinal biopsy. There are now several examples in which iPSC-derived retinal cells are used to confirm the clinical and genetic diagnosis of IRDs [2,3], understand the molecular mechanisms of developmental anomalies of the eye [4] and explore the cellular mechanisms of specific genetic mutations [5–8]. In addition to improving diagnostic capability, the use of iPSCs in clinical practice could also lead to new treatments for retinal diseases (Figure 2).

Figure 1. An example of high-resolution retinal images from a patient with hydroxychloroquine toxicity. (**A**) Wide-field colour photography; (**B**) Zoomed-in colour image highlighted by the yellow box in (**A**) of the macular region showing no obvious abnormality; (**C**) Near-infrared reflectance image of the macula showing no obvious abnormality; (**D**) Adaptive optics retinal image highlighted by the yellow box in (**C**) showing the loss of wave-guiding cone outer segments in the perifoveal region; (**E**) Microperimetry showing reduced sensitivity to light in the macular region; (**F**) Zoomed-in image of the perifoveal region showing reduced sensitivity (<25 dB is abnormal); (**G**) Corresponding optical coherence tomography through the fovea showing no obvious loss of the ellipsoid zone of the photoreceptors (yellow arrow).

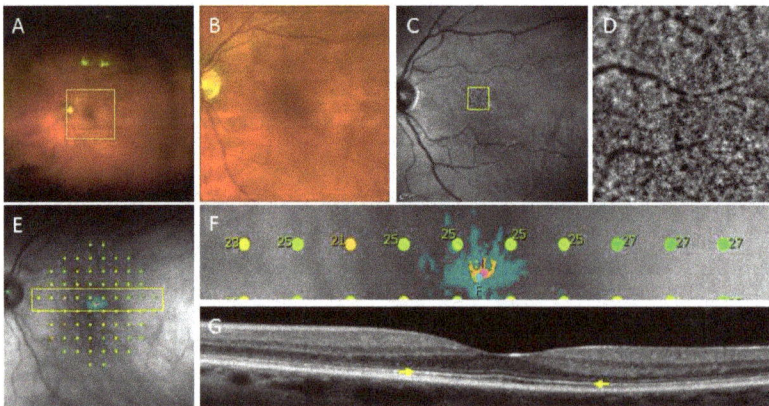

Central to most blinding retinal diseases is the loss of cone photoreceptors. Strategies to preserve or replace cone cells are under intense investigation. Cones can be preserved by: (1) anti-oxidant therapy; (2) pharmacological therapy that provides neuroprotection; (3) gene correction therapy; and (4) cell-based therapy to provide support to cone cells (e.g., RPE or rod cell transplantation). Lost cone cells can be replaced by: (1) transplantation of patient-specific or allogeneic photoreceptor precursors (along with supporting cells); (2) recruitment of endogenous cells to differentiate into new photoreceptor or to become light-responsive cells (optogenetics); or (3) implantation of *epi*-retinal, *sub*-retinal, suprachoroidal or optic nerve visual prostheses [9–11]. Some of these treatment modalities have been investigated in cell culture systems and animal models, and many of these have also been tested in phase I/II clinical trials [12–15]. A major limitation of clinical therapeutics trial in IRDs is the vast heterogeneity of the underlying genetic mutation. Many of the approaches to preserve cones may only be suitable for one genetic variant, but not another, despite a similar clinical phenotype. Given the rarity of many IRDs, randomised clinical trials are not feasible. As an alternative, iPSC-derived retinal tissue from many patients with IRDs can now be tested *in vitro*, simultaneously, in a pre-clinical study, for the potential dose-therapeutic effect response and toxicity of various pharmacologic agents or gene therapies. As genomic editing techniques are emerging and iPSCs are being used as a cell source for replacing lost retinal cells, we now also have the capability of eliminating specific mutations prior to retinal differentiation, thus providing the option of autologous transplantation even to patients with IRDs [16].

Figure 2. A somatic cell from the patient is used to derive induced pluripotent stem cells (iPSCs). The iPSC colonies are characterised to ensure pluripotency markers are present, they form teratoma or embryoid body and they have stable chromosomes. It may take up to three months to derive and validate iPSC lines. The validated iPSC colonies are differentiated to form optic vesicle structures, which contain retinal pigment epithelium and neural retinal cells. Mature retinal cells can be used for confirming the pathogenicity of newly-discovered genetic variants, modelling of developmental or degenerative retinal disease, testing of pharmacologic agents or gene therapy and autologous cellular therapy.

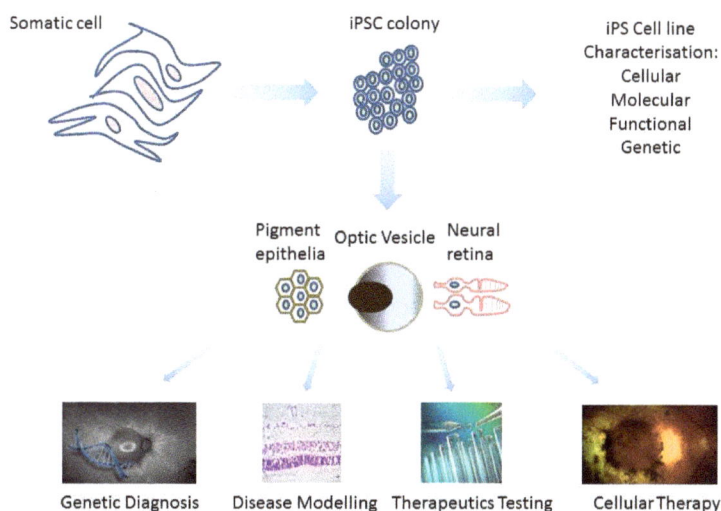

There are several excellent reviews on the use of human iPSCs in the study of retinogenesis, modelling retinal disease, screening of therapeutics and cell replacement therapy in both AMD and IRDs [17–22]. The purpose of this review is to provide an update, from a clinical perspective, on the potential for using iPSC technology in routine clinical care of patients with retinal diseases. It will expand on clinically relevant issues related to laboratory techniques to derive clinical grade iPSC-retina and illustrate examples in which iPSC technology has translated into patient care.

2. Derivation of Patient-Specific Retinal Cells from iPSC for Clinical Use

The availability of human retinal tissue and pure populations of specific types of retinal cells is critical to our ability to diagnose and treat retinal diseases. Allogeneic sources of retinal tissue and cells can be obtained from donor eyes or cell lines. However, these are not clinically useful for confirming genetic diagnosis of a patient or for autologous cellular therapy. Access to patient-specific retinal tissue requires an intraocular procedure, called a vitrectomy, followed by detachment of the retina, retinectomy, laser retinopexy and a vitreous substitute to provide a temporary tamponade. Although this type of procedure is rarely performed for obtaining retinal tissue for the diagnosis of vitreoretinal lymphoma, there are significant blinding complications, such as retinal detachment, and the harvested retinal tissue will not be of adequate quantity or quality for disease modelling, retinal regenerative therapy or screening new therapeutics. Therefore, there is a clinical need for obtaining patient-specific retinal cells without the need to perform retinal biopsy.

2.1. Creating iPSC from Patients

2.1.1. Using Pluripotent Stem Cells

An alternative method to obtain patient-specific retinal cells is to use patient-derived adult stem cells for differentiation into retinal lineages. Retinal neural and pigment epithelial progenitor cells [23,24] have been found in the adult retina, but access to these cells is also limited, as they will require vitrectomy surgery, making them equally unsuitable for clinical use in testing therapeutics and administering personalised cell therapy. Multipotent neural stem cells capable of generating retinal lineages have also been found in the ciliary margin zone and corneoscleral limbus [25–28]. The former source is located adjacent to the lens within the eye, and it is even more difficult to access than the retina. In contrast, limbal tissue is routinely harvested by corneal surgeons for autologous limbal transplantation. Despite the ease of limbal cell harvesting and the long-term safety of the limbal graft donor site [29,30], its use for retinal regeneration and disease modelling has not yet been explored due to limited data on the ability for *in vitro* expansion and the potential for differentiation into all retinal cell types.

Unlike adult stem cells that are multipotent or unipotent, *i.e.*, committed to specific cell types, pluripotent stem cells (PSCs) have a capacity for unlimited self-renewal (hence, large quantities of cells) and differentiation into any somatic cell type, including all classes of retinal cells. One source of PSC is the embryonic stem cells (ESCs), harvested from the inner cell mass of the blastocyst, from which each of the three germ layers—the endoderm, ectoderm and mesoderm—can be derived. However, ESCs are derived from discarded surplus embryos, and this is not patient-specific. Human ESC-derived RPE is currently being used in several clinical trials, but recipients are being immunosuppressed, because of the potential risk of graft rejection [12].

More recently, PSCs can also be generated by dedifferentiating a terminally differentiated patient-specific adult somatic cell, such as a fibroblast, into a pluripotent state by nuclear reprogramming. There are three established methods to induce pluripotency: (1) transfer of the nucleus of a differentiated cell into an enucleated oocyte (nucleus removed), so that pluripotency genes within the somatic cell genome are activated by the regulators within the oocyte cytoplasm (nuclear transfer) [31]; (2) fusion of a somatic cell with an ESC to create a hybrid or heterokaryon in which pluripotency regulators override cell differentiation regulators (cell fusion) [32]; and (3) induced overexpression of specific pluripotency transcriptional factors through transfection of an adult somatic cell with integrating virus, non-integrating virus, plasmids, mRNA or even exposure to protein or small molecules (induced pluripotent stem cell (iPSC) reprogramming) [33].

2.1.2. Induced Pluripotent Stem Cells

Since the original description of the iPSC protocol by Yamanaka [34], there has been significant development in the reprogramming approach, and many types of somatic cells have been successfully induced into a pluripotent state. Conceptually, this is a two-step process of (1) nuclear reprogramming of a chosen somatic cell into several clones of iPSC and (2) validation of the pluripotency of the various clones of iPSC to select the most suitable clone for the specific purpose that iPSCs will be used, for diagnostics or therapeutics. The time lag from biopsy to obtain patient's somatic cells to full validation of the best iPSC clone may take 2–3 months. Several factors will influence the choice of somatic cell for deriving iPSC.

For therapeutic purposes, such as autologous cell replacement therapy, the ideal iPSC clone should be derived from an easily accessible somatic cell type in facilities that comply with good manufacturing practice guidelines related to cell therapy. Both adult stem cells and differentiated cells have been used to derive good quality iPSC lines. Although adult stem cells may already express some of the pluripotency-related genes, their expression is significantly lower than that seen in ESC or iPSC. Therefore, the same protocol for deriving iPSC is generally required for adult stem cells as for differentiated cells. Cells that proliferate well also reprogram well. However, there is significant variability in genetic and epigenetic patterns and the degree of reprogramming, even between iPSC clones from the same cell source. Hu *et al.* showed that iPSCs derived from RPE retain a "memory" of cellular origin with respect to the propensity for differentiation back to RPE [35]. However, it will not be feasible to use patients' RPE as a source for deriving iPSC, due to surgical complications associated with tissue harvest. Furthermore, even without "memory" in source cells, RPE and neuroretinal cells have been generated readily from iPSC derived from cells of diverse background, such as cord blood cell, lymphocyte, keratinocyte, adipocyte and fibroblast [2,4,36–38]. Another easily accessible source of somatic cells is the ocular surface. The potential to generate iPSC from cells on the ocular surface (corneal epithelium and limbal niche) warrants further investigation, as they can potentially be reprogrammed to pluripotency without the introduction of transcriptional factors, as shown in rodent limbal-derived neurospheres [39,40]. In contrast to autologous transplantation of iPSC-derived retinal cells, special consideration needs to be given to the ease of transport and storage of somatic cells for deriving iPSC for the purpose of genetic diagnosis, disease modelling and high throughput drug screening. In this situation, blood-derived cells (activated T lymphocytes and endothelial progenitor cells) may be preferable, as they are easily collected, transported, isolated and stored [41–43].

The reprogramming protocol should preferably avoid the use of viruses, such as retroviruses, that were used to create the first human iPSC [34,44]. Non-integrating viral vectors, DNA plasmids, modified RNA, protein and small molecules have all been reported to induce a pluripotent state in a somatic cell [45–50]. There is no one perfect methodology for creating iPSC for all types of clinical use. The main trade-off for the potential mutagenesis by integrating virus is the lower efficiency and higher cost associated with non-integrating methods. There have also been variations on the transcriptional factors used for reprogramming since the original description by Yamanaka (OCT4, SOX2, KLF4 and c-MYC) and Thomson (OCT4, SOX2, NANOG and LIN28) (Figure 3) [34,44]. Some protocols also use additional small molecules, such as 5-aza-deoxycytidine, valproic acid or ascorbic acid, to modify the epigenetic environment and enhance the efficiency and accuracy of nuclear reprogramming. Ultimately, these protocol modifications will also have an impact on the cost and quality of the human iPSC line and the suitability for clinical application, such as autologous transplantation. Regardless of the cell source and reprogramming protocol, successful generation of retinal tissue from iPSCs will depend on the skills of the operator in identifying the "right" iPSC clones for retinal differentiation.

Figure 3. Retrovirus vector for induced pluripotent stem cell (iPSC) reprogramming. (**A**) Map of polycistronic retroviral vector. Human fibroblasts two days after infection with polycistronic GFP Oct4/Sox2/Klf4/cMyc; (**B**) iPSC after four weeks post infection negative for GFP indicating that the transgene is silenced in iPSC clone.

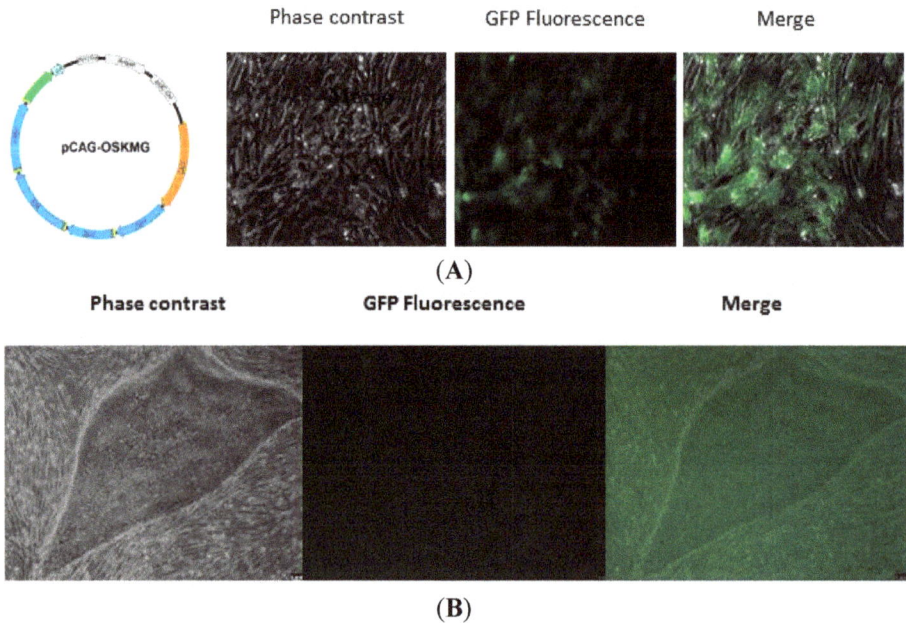

(**A**)

(**B**)

2.1.3. Validation of Human iPSC Lines

The key defining features of iPSC are the self-renewal capacity and the ability to produce all three germ layers. Not all iPSC clones generated from the same somatic cell line from the same patient will be fully reprogrammed or truly pluripotent, and the efficiency of various protocols in generating iPSC clones can vary from 1:100 to 1:10,000. Screening to distinguish partially and fully reprogrammed colonies may add further delay and cost to the generation of patient-specific iPSC lines, and the thoroughness of this process depends on the clinical reasons for deriving the iPSC. It has been suggested that between five and 10 clones may need to be isolated for characterisation and future differentiation, because not all clones will have the same propensity for retinal lineage derivation, despite their potential [6,7,51,52].

Four techniques are used for characterising and subsequently selecting iPSC clones: cellular, molecular, functional and genetic (Table 1). The extent of characterisation required will again depend on the purpose of generating iPSC. Less rigorous criteria may be sufficient for genetic diagnosis and disease modelling compared to drug screening and cellular therapy. However, a minimum set of criteria for establishing putative iPSC has been recommended by the European Consortium of stem cell research (the ESTOOLS project).

The unpredictable variability between clones may be related to the somatic origin of iPSC, the reprogramming technique or the intrinsic clonal variability within the individual. Furthermore, equal performance of iPSC clones against the same "pluripotency" tests does not translate to equal propensity for retinal lineage derivation. Further investigation is required to establish a selection screen and criteria for reducing clonal variation and identifying iPSC clones that have optimal retinal differentiation propensity. It can be envisaged that different criteria for establishing pluripotency may emerge for diagnostic and therapeutic use of iPSC.

2.2. Creating Retinal Tissue from iPSC

2.2.1. Derivation of Retina Lineages

The fundamental principles for differentiating iPSC into retinal progeny have been laid down by previous work on mouse and human ESCs. However, the different propensity between iPSC and ESC for retinal differentiation brings into question the validity of the various protocols proposed. Most of these protocols rely on the initial spontaneous induction of retinal differentiation, but there is variability between cell lines. The lack of reproducibility by other laboratories also raises concern regarding their utility in the clinical setting. Nevertheless, there are two broad approaches: one by default differentiation of iPSC into neuroectodermal lineages (upon withdrawal of FGF2) and the other through directed differentiation by the addition of extrinsic molecules, such as growth and transcription factors.

A common approach in deriving retinal cells is to allow human iPSCs to overgrow as adherent layers. With the use of specific extracellular matrix in addition to certain inducing factors and proteins, iPSCs may be preferentially differentiated into RPE or photoreceptor phenotypes. For example, Tucker et al. described the formation of two-dimensional eyecup-like structures in a synthetic xeno-free culture substrate when skin keratinocyte-derived iPSCs were used [2]. After formation of small pigmented foci at around 45 days, these clumps expanded over 150 days. In some of these clumps, neural cells fill the centre, whilst in other colonies, pigmented cells wraps around in a C-shape around neural rosettes resembling a cross-section of an optic cup [2].

Similar two-dimensional eye-cup structures have also been reported by Jin *et al.* [53] and Reichman *et al.* [54].

Table 1. Characterisation of induced pluripotent stem cells, photoreceptor cells and retinal pigment epithelium.

Techniques of Characterisation	Induced Pluripotent Stem Cells	Photoreceptor Cells	Retinal Pigment Epithelium
Morphology (light microscopy)	Flat colonies; small and round cells; high nuclear to cytoplasmic ratio	Located in outer nuclear layer; cell bodies with processes; inner and outer segments	Monolayer; pigmentation; hexagonal
Morphology (electron microscopy)	N/A	Outer segment discs, myoid and ellipsoid segments, connecting cilia, basal body	Apical microvilli, basal infoldings, tight-junctional complexes, pigment granules
Cellular markers (pluripotency)	Surface: SSEA-3, TRA-1-60, TRA-1-81; Others: NANOG, SOX2, OCT4	Loss of OCT3/4, SOX2, NANOG	Loss of OCT3/4, SOX2, NANOG
Cellular markers (progenitors/precursors)	N/A	PAX6, CHX10, CRX, OTX2, NRL	PAX6, MITF
Cellular markers (differentiated/mature)	N/A	Phototransduction: recoverin, transducing, cGMP phosphodiesterase, retinal guanylate cyclase, cyclic-nucleotide gated channel, rhodopsin, cone opsins (S or L/M), arrestin; visual cycle	Visual cycle: RPE65, RLBP1, CRALBP; phagocytosis: FAK, MERTK; pigmentation: tyrosinase; growth factor: VEGF, PEDF, PDGF; membrane: Na/K ATPase, ZO-1, BEST1
Molecular	RT-PCR, bisulphite sequence analysis	RT-PCR	RT-PCR
Functional (*in vitro*)	Embryoid body formation	Patch recordings; response to white flash	Phagocytosis assay/rhodopsin clearance; fluid transport, polarised secretion of growth factors (PEGF/VEGF); transepithelial resistance
Functional (*in vivo*)	Teratoma assay in animal to identify all three germ layers	Cell transplantation to demonstrate rescue of visual function	Cell transplantation (RCS rat) to demonstrate rescue of visual function
Genetic	Karyotyping sequencing to look for new mutations	Sequencing to check no new mutations	Sequencing to check no new mutations

RT-PCR, Reverse transcription polymerase chain reaction; RCS, Royal College of Surgeons.

An alternative approach is to culture iPSCs as suspended aggregates to enable the formation of three-dimensional cellular structures. Recapitulation of ocular organogenesis through the formation of an optic cup structure using a serum-free suspension culture system was first demonstrated using murine ESC by Eiraku *et al.* and then human ESC by Nakano *et al.* [55,56]. More recently, Meyer *et al.* described human iPSC-derived cell aggregates with vesicle-like and non-vesicular configurations after 20 days of culture using successive media changes from embryoid body medium (four days) to neural induction medium (seven days) and, finally, to retinal differentiation medium [6,51]. The vesicle-like structures expressed CHX10, a marker of retinal progenitor cells, whereas the non-vesicular spheres expressed ISLET-1, a homeodomain protein involved in early forebrain development. Upon further differentiation, photoreceptor-like cells and RPE were derived from the vesicle-like structures. Similar optic vesicle-like structures have also been generated from lymphocyte-iPSC [4,36]. Zhong *et al.* recently reported three-dimensional laminated retinal cups generated from human iPSC with distinct populations of neural retinal cells interacting through synaptic junctions and photoreceptor cells capable of forming outer segment discs and responding to light [57]. However, it is important to note that efficiency in generating PAX6+ neuroectodermal cells amongst different iPSC clones can vary from 5% to 56% of the total cell population using the same protocol, highlighting the need for further investigation into the methods and screening criteria to identify the most suitable iPSC clone for retinal differentiation [51].

Irrespective of the protocol used for inducing retinal differentiation, the timing of the derivation of specific retinal cell types generally reflects the timeline of embryological development. This temporal recapitulation of embryogenesis by iPSC differentiation supports the notion that derivation of retinal cells is not directed, but rather the outcome of subcloning and culture in a permissive microenvironment. During the first month of embryonic development, the forebrain portion of the primitive anterior neuroepithelium gives rise to cells expressing markers specific for the eye field. Optic vesicles then develop from the eye fields at the end of the first month with cells expressing PAX6 and MITF. Retinal progenitors destined to become RPE preferentially express MITF, whereas those becoming neuronal cells downregulate MITF in response to increased CHX10 expression. Then, there is a 1–2 month(s) lag in the expression of *CRX* and opsin genes in neural retinal cells after the formation of RPE. Hence, the time to generate RPE from iPSC is typically around 4–6 weeks, whereas differentiation of photoreceptor precursors occurs at 2–3 months after retinal induction. Formation of outer segments and the development of light response was reported by Zhong *et al.* at six months after retinal induction [57]. Recently, Reichman *et al.* described a floating culture system for generating neuroretinal-RPE containing retinal progenitor cells within two weeks, which bypassed embryoid body formation and obviated the need for exogenous molecules, coating or Matrigel [54].

The ability to recapitulate retinogenesis using iPSC has tremendous potential for studying diseases that interfere with retinal development and non-cell autonomous mechanisms, in addition to those that cause post-natal cell autonomous retinal degeneration. On a practical level, there are still significant barriers to routine clinical use of this technology, since the generation of patient-specific retinal cells may take 4–6 months from the time of biopsy, and there is significant overhead infrastructure cost to maintain an iPSC laboratory. Future advancement in three-dimensional culture and differentiation techniques may one day enable iPSCs to differentiate into other structures of the eye, such as the choroid and sclera, thus expanding the use of iPSC in understanding complex retinal diseases, such as AMD and myopia.

2.2.2. iPSC to Photoreceptor Cells

Hirami *et al.* described deriving photoreceptor cells using human iPSC from dermal fibroblast, serum-free embryoid body culture system, defined factors (Wnt and Nodal inhibitors) and subsequent plating of aggregates onto poly-D-lysine, laminin and fibronectin to generate retinal progenitors expressing *RX*, *PAX6* and *MITF* [58]. From Day 90, the application of retinoic acid and taurine to the culture system induced the expression of the photoreceptor marker, recoverin, in a quarter of the colonies by Day 120 (four months). Half of these recoverin-positive cells were also immune-positive for rhodopsin. Notably, only two of three iPSC lines could be differentiated into the retinal lineage, and functional assays of putative photoreceptor cells were not performed. Osakada *et al.* from the same group, at the RikenCenter for Developmental Biology, also reported a modified protocol using small molecules (casein kinase I inhibitor CKI-7, Rho-associated kinase inhibitor Y-27632 and ALK4 inhibitor SB-431542) to block Wnt and Nodal pathways to induce retinal progenitors [59]. This method has been used in generating photoreceptor cells from patients with *RP1*, *RP9*, *PRPH-2* and *RHO* mutations [7,53].

Meyer *et al.* [51] described a different culture system using embryonic stem cell medium without FGF2, then chemically-defined neural induction medium with N2 supplement followed by another chemically-defined retinal differentiation medium supplemented with B27. Rosettes were picked and selected for neurosphere culture and generation of optic vesicle-like structures. By Day 80, 14%

of the neurospheres expressed rod- and cone-specific transcription factor Crx, within which 65% of the cells were expressing Crx. However, only 8% of the cells within Crx+ spheres expressed recoverin and/or opsin. This protocol was modified by Zhong *et al.* to generate photoreceptor cells (within laminated retinal cup structure) that express synaptic junction proteins, phototransduction molecules, to form outer segments and to respond to light stimulus [57]. The optic vesicle-like system was used to study the effect of *CHX10* mutation [4].

Several other groups have also described the derivation of photoreceptor cells from human iPSC (Table 2). There are many morphological, cellular, molecular, functional and genetic assays for the characterisation of iPSC-derived photoreceptors and their precursors, but there is no consensus on the minimum criteria (Table 1). Lamba *et al.* used their protocol for ESC [60] to derive photoreceptor cells from human iPSCs [52]. Although, they did not test the function of these cells, they demonstrated integration into mouse retina following sub-retinal transplantation. Mellough *et al.* combined the techniques described by Lamba *et al.* and Osakada *et al.* for deriving retinal cells from ESC and added activin A, Shh and T3 to enhance photoreceptor differentiation from human iPSCs [60–62]. Their three-step differentiation protocol involved inducing a neural lineage, then retinal progenitors and, finally, photoreceptor cells expressing blue, red and green opsin. For iPSC-derived photoreceptor cells to be used in human transplantation, animal-derived products should be avoided where possible. Tucker *et al.* and Sridhar *et al.* recently reported the generation of photoreceptor cells from iPSCs using a xeno-free system, where a synthetic culture surface (Synthemax cell culture surface) is used for iPSC derivation and retinal differentiation [37,63].

Table 2. Derivation of retinal photoreceptor (precursor) cells from human induced pluripotent stem cells.

Reference	Source of iPSC	Duration	Markers to Confirm Photoreceptor Lineage	Tests to Suggest Photoreceptor Cell Function	Transplant	Disease Modelling	Therapeutics Screening
Hirami *et al.* [58]	Human fibroblast	120 days	CRX, RCVRN, RHO	No	No	No	No
Osakada *et al.* [59]	Human fibroblast	120–140 days	CRX, PDC, PDE6b, PDE6c, RHO, GRK1, SAG, RCVRN	Molecules required for photo-transduction	No	No	No
Jin *et al.* [7]	Patient fibroblast	120 days	CRX, RCVRN, RHO, OPN1SW, OPN1LW	Patch clamp to detect voltage dependent channels 8-OHdG, caspase-3, acrolein, BiP, CHOP	No	Yes	Yes
Jin *et al.* [53]	Patient fibroblast *	120–150 days	CRX, RCVRN	BiP, CHOP	No	Yes	No
Meyer *et al.* [51]	Human fibroblast	80 days	CRX, RCVRN, Opsin	No	No	No	No
Meyer *et al.* [6]	Patient fibroblast	80 days	CRX, RCVRN	No	No	No	No
Phillips *et al.* [36]	Patient T-cells	108 days	CRX, RCVRN, S-OPSIN, RHO, CX36, SNAP-25, VGLUT1	Molecules required for synaptic function	No	No	No
Phillips *et al.* [4]	Patient T-cells	80 days	CRX, RCVRN, NRL, OPN1SW, PED6B	Molecules required for photo-transduction	No	Yes	No
Tucker *et al.* [3]	Patient fibroblast	33 days	RCVRN	No	No	Yes	No
Tucker *et al.* [2]	Patient keratinocyte	60 days	CRX, NRL, RCVRN, RHO, Acy Tubulin, OPN1SW, OPN1LW	GRP78, GRP94	Yes	Yes	No
Burnight *et al.* [64]	Patient fibroblast	90 days	CRX, RHO, OPN1SW, RCVRN, ROM1	No	No	No	Yes

Table 2. *Cont.*

Reference	Source of iPSC	Duration	Markers to Confirm Photoreceptor Lineage	Tests to Suggest Photoreceptor Cell Function	Transplant	Disease Modelling	Therapeutics Screening
Tucker *et al.* [37]	Patient fibroblast, Human keratinocyte and IPE *,†	90 days	CRX, NRL, RCVRN, RHO	No	No	No	No
Sridhar *et al.* [63]	Human fibroblast	60 days	CRX, RCVRN	No	No	No	No
Mellough *et al.* [62]	Human fibroblast	60 days	CRX, OPN1SW, OPN1LW, RHO, RCVRN, ARRESTIN 3	No	No	No	No
Reichman *et al.* [54]	Human fibroblast	49–112 days	CRX, NRL, RHO, R/G/B OPSIN, ARRESTIN 3, RECVRN	No	No	No	No
Zhong *et al.* [57]	Human fibroblast	175 days	CRX, OPN1SW, OPN1LW, RHO, PDE6α/β, Gtα, CNGA1/B1, RetGC1	Patch clamp-light induced response; outer segment disc formation on EM; molecules required for photo-transduction	No	No	No
Lambda *et al.* [52]	Human fibroblast	28 days	CRX, OTX2, NRL, RECVRN, AIPL-1, RHO, S-Opsin, Arrestin, PAX6, Blimp1	Molecules required for photo-transduction	No	No	No
Yoshida *et al.* [8]	Patient fibroblast	35 days	NRL promoter, recoverin	BiP, CHOP, BID, NOXA LC3, ATG5, ATG7	No	Yes	No

8-OHdG, 8-Hydroxy-2'-deoxyguanosine (oxidative stress marker); BiP, Binding immunoglobulin protein; CHOP, C/BEP-homologous protein/DNA-damage-inducible transcript 3; RCVRN, Recoverin; * iPSC derived from integration-free iPSC; † iPSC derived from xeno-free culture.

2.2.3. iPSC to Retinal Pigmented Epithelial Cells

Although the embryoid body culture system can generate RPE from iPSC, adherent culture has been favoured if RPE is the only cell that is required. Hirami *et al.* and Meyer *et al.* showed RPE differentiation occurs earlier than neural retinal progeny derivation [51,58]. Carr *et al.* and Buchholz *et al.* demonstrated that RPE differentiation from human iPSC can be achieved within four weeks, and these cells demonstrated morphological and molecular signatures of RPE, as well as *in vitro* and *in vivo* functional characteristics [65,66]. Morphologically, RPE derived from iPSCs is indistinguishable from RPE in post-mortem eye or human ESC-derived RPE (Figure 4).

Characterisation of iPSC-RPE involves morphological, cellular, molecular, functional and genetic assays (Table 1). Key morphological features include pigmentation, monolayer of hexagonal cells and electron microscopic features of apical microvilli, tight junctions, basal infoldings and cytoplasmic melanosomes. The molecular signature of RPE cells reflects their eye field origin (PAX6 and MITF) and function: RPE65 and CRALBP (retinoid cycle), MERTK (phagocytosis), bestrophin (modulating calcium flux in endoplasmic reticulum) and ZO-1 (tight junctions). *In vitro* functional assessment includes transepithelial resistance measurement, vascular endothelial growth factor (VEGF), platelet-derived growth factor (PDGF) and pigment epithelium-derived factor (PEDF) secretion, extracellular matrix production (laminin and type IV collagen) and phagocytosis assay using photoreceptor outer segments. *In vivo* functional assessment requires subretinal transplantation in an animal model of RPE or retinal dystrophy, such as the Royal College of Surgeons (RCS) rat, to assess the rescue of visual function [65,67–69]. Gene expression comparing human iPSC-RPE to adult and foetal RPE and other controls through microarray and hierarchical clustering analysis needs to be performed to verify similarity to target tissue [70].

Figure 4. Morphology of the retinal pigment epithelium monolayer. (**A**) Hexagonal pigmented monolayer of retinal pigment epithelium derived from induced pluripotent stem cells; (**B**) Comparison of the morphology of retinal pigment epithelial stem cells derived from human embryonic stem cells (HESC), post-mortem (PM) eyes and induced pluripotent stem (iPS) cells.

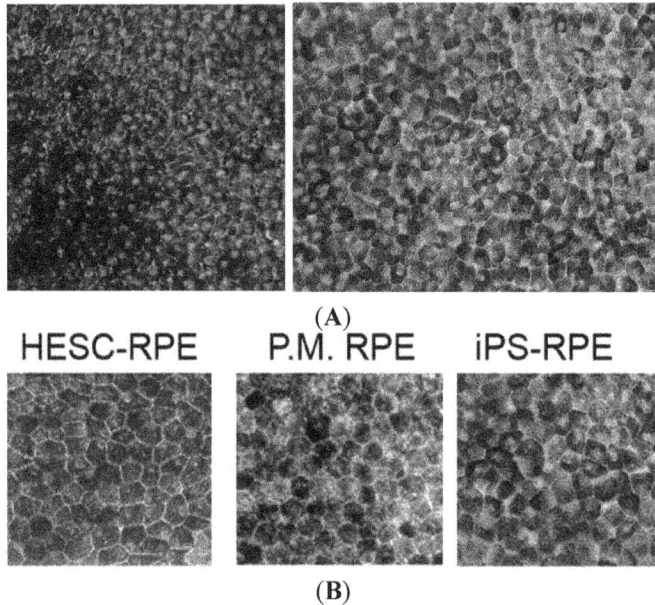

For autologous transplantation of iPSC-RPE, immunogenicity, cell survival and tumourigenicity studies are also required. These have been addressed for iPSC-RPE specifically by Kamao *et al.* and Kanemura *et al.* [70,71] as part of a pre-clinical study in preparation for human iPSC-RPE autologous transplantation. The generation of patient-specific iPSC-RPE has also been performed in gyrate atrophy and Best disease (BD) [5,6]. The following section will illustrate clinical examples of the use of iPSC-derived retinal cells in genetic diagnosis, discovery of genotype/phenotype relationship, screening of pharmaco- and gene therapies and as a source of autologous cell therapy.

3. Clinical Use of Patient-Specific iPSC-Derived Retinal Cells

The ability to generate patient-specific retinal tissue and cells offers the opportunity to study the relationship between genetic variants and disease phenotypes. This technology is particularly useful in modelling IRDs, as there are around 200 genes with over 4200 known and many other unknown mutations causing disease phenotype in IRDs [72]. One in 2000–3000 individual are affected by IRDs, and these, collectively, are the most common cause of blindness in children and young adults. Given that emerging therapies for IRDs are likely to be mutation specific, it is important to identify pathogenic mutation(s) in every affected individual [73–75].

Many IRDs have a poor genotype-phenotype correlation; defects in a single gene may lead to a variety of disease phenotypes, while, on the other hand, a particular disease phenotype may be caused by mutations in a large number of different genes. Adding to the challenge of identifying causative mutations is the relatively common occurrence of X-linked and *de novo* autosomal dominant variants. Although Sanger sequencing of selected genes followed by targeted next-generation sequencing (NGS) can identify known pathogenic mutation in many individuals, exome or whole genome NGS combined with genetic linkage studies are required for the identification of novel mutations. Traditionally, these rare mutations (<1%) have been validated through functional modelling, mouse and zebrafish studies and replication of genotyping in large patient and relevant control cohorts. More recently, iPSC technology has also been used to confirm the pathogenicity of genetic variants and to unravel the molecular mechanism of disease phenotype through the *in vitro* study of cellular function and the histogenesis of iPSC-derived retinal tissue.

3.1. IPSC for Genetic Diagnosis and Modelling

3.1.1. Confirming Pathogenicity of Mutation

Patient-specific iPSC has been used to confirm the pathogenicity of new rare genetic variants. For example, using NGS, single-strand conformation polymorphism screening and Sanger sequencing of a large validation cohort, Tucker *et al.* [3] identified a new mutation (Alu element insertion) in the male germ cell-associated kinase (*MAK*) gene causing rod-cone dystrophy. This was confirmed by examining and comparing the transcripts of *MAK* between iPSC and iPSC-derived photoreceptors from the patient and his unaffected sibling. The proband had no family history of retinal dystrophy, and the affected individual was heterozygous for pathogenic variants in *ABCA4* and *USH2A*. Using iPSC, they discovered a previously unrecognized exon 12 of the *MAK* gene that is expressed in cells differentiated into retinal precursors, but not in undifferentiated cells. This observation confirmed that the homozygous Alu element insertion in exon 9 is pathogenic by affecting the developmental switch from *MAK* bearing only exon 9 to a retina-specific transcript bearing both exons 9 and 12. The insertion of a 353-bp Alu repeat between codons 428 and 429 in exon 9 results in the insertion of 31 incorrect amino acids followed by a premature termination. In another study, Tucker *et al.* [2] reported the discovery of a new pathogenic variant of *USH2A* in another patient with rod-cone dystrophy who was presumed heterozygous for a pathogenic variant in *ABCA4* and *USH2A*. The second possibly disease-causing variant was found in intron 40 of *USH2A*, and this was confirmed by real-time PCR of patient-specific iPSC-derived photoreceptor precursor cells. A pseudoexon (IVS40) was formed by the intronic splice site mutation in the intervening sequence 40 of *USH2A*, and this caused a translation frameshift and a premature stop codon.

Lustremant *et al.* [76] examined the transcriptomics of human iPSC-derived neural stem cells and RPE from two patients with Leber congenital amaurosis (LCA). Although the pathogenic mutation was not known, they showed changes in the expression of 21 genes when compared to wild-type controls. Amongst these, three downregulated genes—*TRIM61*, *ZNF558* and *GSSTT1*—were related to the LCA disease process through protein degradation, altered transcription regulation and oxidation. With better understanding of the interactions between molecular pathways, detection of altered transcriptomics may help to narrow down candidate genes in this patient with LCA.

3.1.2. Modelling Developmental Diseases of the Retina

The impact of known mutations on retinogenesis and cellular function has also been explored. The transcription factor CHX10 (*Caenorhabditis elegans* Ceh-10 homeo-domain-containing homolog 10), also known as VSX2 (visual system homeobox 2), has a critical role in the development of the retina. The very rare mutation in *VSX2* leads to severe malformation of the eye. Although animal models of this disease (the *VSX2*$^{-/-}$ and (R200Q) *VSX2* mice) have contributed greatly to our understanding of the importance of *VSX2* in repressing MITF, production of the bipolar cell and maturation of the photoreceptors, it was not possible to confirm that the same mechanism occurs in humans. Phillips *et al.* [4] used iPSCs from a patient with a (R200Q) *VSX2* mutation to generate an embryoid body and then vesicles that recapitulated retinogenesis [6,36]. They confirmed previous observations in animal models and went a step further, using lentiviral *VSX2* overexpression to examine the reversibility of the developmental defect *in vitro*. Although suppression of MITF and enhanced photoreceptor maturation was achieved, bipolar cell markers were not restored by wild-type lenti-*VSX2*. Transcriptome analysis at Day 20 and 30 cells demonstrated overall upregulation of genes. Most of these were related to the WNT and TGFb signalling pathways that promote RPE differentiation. In contrast, the FGF pathway, which promotes neuroretinal differentiation, was downregulated.

The process of deriving retinal cells from iPSCs provides an opportunity for studying retinal development and developmental anomalies due to specific mutations that cause ocular and retinal dysgenesis (e.g., *MITF*, *PAX6*, *VSX2*, *CRB1*, etc.). However, terminally differentiated retinal cells from iPSCs can also be tested for altered cell function to understand degenerative diseases of the retina (see below). IRDs that have an earlier onset may be expected to demonstrate abnormality earlier in the differentiation protocol, whilst late onset IRDs (e.g., BD, pattern dystrophy, Sorsby fundus dystrophy and Doyne honeycomb retinal dystrophy) may not manifest altered cellular physiology unless the cells are aged and stressed *in vitro* to recapitulate senescence.

3.1.3. Modelling Degenerative Diseases of the Retina

Both RPE and photoreceptor disease models have been created using patient-specific iPSCs. AMD (Figure 5) and two types of RPE dystrophies have been modelled: Best disease and gyrate atrophy.

Figure 5. Clinical images of early age-related macular degeneration and its variants. (**A**) Colour photograph of the macula of a 72-year-old male showing soft drusen; (**B**) Optical coherence tomography (OCT) shows a sub-retinal pigment epithelial (RPE) deposit, which did not significantly alter fundus autofluorescence (**C**); (**D**) Colour photograph of the macula of a 78-year-old female showing reticular pseudo-drusen; (**E**) OCT shows deposits above the RPE, resulting in subtle hypo autofluorescent lesions (**F**); (**G**) Colour photograph of the macula of a 57-year-old female showing basal laminar drusen; (**H**) OCT shows a compact sub-RPE deposit forming a saw-tooth pattern, and these lesions were mildly hyper autofluorescent (**I**); (**J**) Colour photograph of the macula of an 83-year-old female showing dominant drusen or Doyne honeycomb retinal dystrophy; (**K**) OCT shows outer retinal layer loss; (**L**) The fovea was hypo autofluorescent due to RPE loss, and the linear radial drusen are seen as hyper autofluorescent streaks.

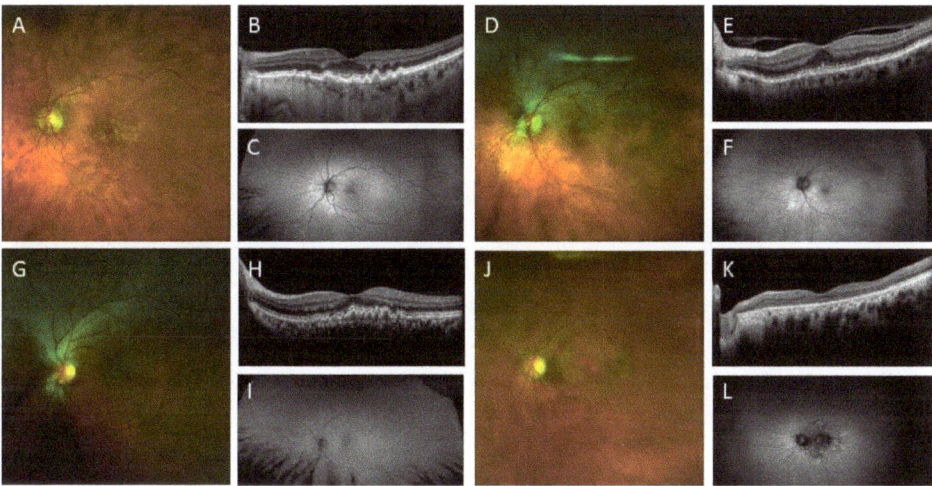

Chang *et al.* reported reduced ZO-1 and RPE65 staining in iPSC-RPE generated from five atrophic AMD patients compared to two controls [38]. There was also increased accumulation of reactive oxygen species following exposure to H_2O_2 compared to controls. Furthermore, expressions of antioxidant genes (*HO-1*, *SOD2* and *GPX1*) were lower, whilst PDGF, VEGF and IGFBP-2 expressions were higher compared to controls. There were no details regarding the age of the two control subjects, and the AMD risk allele profiles for all seven subjects were not reported. Further studies are needed to replicate these findings by controlling other potential confounders. It is particular important that control subjects are age matched when iPSC is used to model late-onset degeneration as AMD. This is because AMD cannot be diagnosed until drusen is visualised, usually after the age of 50 years. Although the presence of risk alleles and family history increases the risk of developing AMD, these biomarkers are not 100% predictive. Therefore, somatic cells from young healthy individual cannot be used as controls, because it is not possible at this stage to predict if this subject will or will not develop AMD later in life.

Heterozygous, compound heterozygous and homozygous mutation of the *BEST1* gene (bestrophin protein) can cause ocular disease characterised by abnormal RPE function, accumulation of debris between RPE and photoreceptors and a variable amount of retinal degeneration and ocular dysgenesis (Figure 6). There are over 100 mutations in *BEST1*, and the pathogenicity and molecular mechanism of RPE dysfunction arising from these mutations is not well understood. The traditional approach to study the effects of *BEST1* mutation is based on transfection of mutant *BEST1* gene into the human foetal RPE or Madin Darby canine kidney (MDCK II) epithelium cell lines. Sing *et al.* described the use of RPE derived from patient-specific iPSCs to study the impact of two mutations in the *BEST1* gene, (A146K and N296H) on RPE function. They demonstrated increased intracellular accumulation of autofluorescent materials compared to controls after long-term (3.5 months) feeding of the BD hiPSC-RPE with bovine photoreceptor outer segments (POS, 50/cell) and decreased net fluid transport. Conflicting data at 4 and 24 hours were shown regarding delayed degradation of POS when overfed with FITC-POS (50 *vs.* 20 POS per cell). As expected, there was no significant difference in the RPE differentiation potential of BD hiPSC compared to controls. BD hiPSC-RPE also had a similar transepithelial resistance, level of *BEST1* mRNA and localisation pattern of the mutant bestrophin compared to controls. The dysfunction in mutant bestrophin was found to be associated with altered endoplasmic reticulum (ER)-mediated calcium homeostasis. Furthermore, there was increased expression of genes involved in regulating oxidative stress (*GPX1*, *SOD2*) and iron homeostasis (*TRF*, *TRFR*) after long-term (3.5 months) POS feeding [5]. In this study, the genetic background between the cell lines was not controlled by genomic editing of the *BEST1* mutation into the control iPSC or out of the BD hiPSC (see below). Nevertheless, this is a good example where early onset disease with a well-characterised clinical disease phenotype can be recapitulated *in vitro*. It is not known if similar cellular abnormalities can also be detected in iPSC-RPE from patients with the much commoner late-onset vitelliform macular dystrophy due to other types of *BEST1* mutations. Phagocytosis assay may be a better readout for iPSC-RPE generated from patients with a known genetic defect that impairs phagocytosis, such as *MERTK* or *REP-1* mutation (choroideremia).

In a very different RPE dystrophy, gyrate atrophy, homozygous mutation in the ornithine-δ-aminotransferase gene (*OAT*) leads to RPE damage and loss, leading to severe peripheral and central vision loss. RPE has been successfully generated from iPSCs derived from the fibroblasts of a patient with *OAT* mutation (A226V). Enzyme activity of OAT within the iPSC-RPE can be measured [6]. Correction of the *OAT* mutation by bacterial artificial chromosome-mediated homologous recombination restored the enzymatic activity [77]. There are other RPE dystrophies resulting from mutations affecting visual cycle enzymes or regulators (e.g., the acyltransferase, LRAT, the isomerohydrolase, RPE65, the dehydrogenase, RDH12, and RPGR and RLBP1). Deriving iPSC-RPE from patients with various genetic mutations in these enzymes or regulators may also provide opportunities to understand genotype-phenotype molecular mechanisms and variability.

Figure 6. Clinical images of various types of inherited retinal diseases. (**A**) Colour photograph of the macula of a 10-year-old boy showing multifocal vitelliform lesions resulting from homozygous deletion of exon 2–6 of the *BEST1* gene; (**B**) Optical coherence tomography (OCT) shows intraretinal cystic change with sub-retinal fluid and vitelliform deposits; (**C**) Increased fundus autofluorescence was noted in the area of vitelliform deposits; (**D**) Colour photograph of the macula of a 57-year-old male showing yellow deposits due to pattern dystrophy of the retinal pigment epithelium (RPE); (**E**) OCT shows deposits above and below the RPE; (**F**) Multifocal hyper autofluorescent lesions are seen; (**G**) Colour photograph of the macula of a 56-year-old female showing extensive macular atrophy with cone-rod dystrophy due to two missense mutations in the *ABCA4* gene (c.2915 C > A and c.3041 T > G); (**H**) OCT shows severe retinal and choroidal atrophy with pigment migration into the fovea; (**I**) Extensive RPE loss resulting in wide-spread hypo autofluorescent lesions; (**J**) Colour photograph of the macula of a 32-year-old male showing retinal flecks with mild cone dysfunction due to two pathogenic mutations in the *ABCA4* gene (c.4139 C > T and c.6079 C > T); (**K**) OCT shows outer retinal layer loss to retinal atrophy; (**L**) Retinal flecks were hyper autofluorescent.

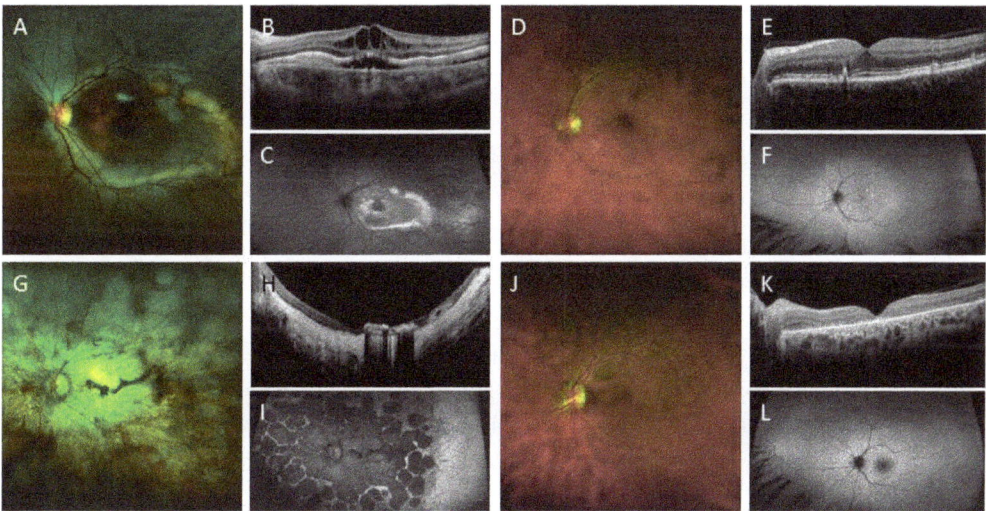

Many genes are involved in photoreceptor cell degeneration. Clinically, there are two broad classes of disease phenotypes based on electrophysiology: macular dystrophy, which is limited to the macular region, and retinal dystrophy, where the entire population of photoreceptors (central and peripheral) is affected. Generalised retinal dystrophy can affect cones or rods predominantly. Different mutations in one gene, such as *ABCA4*, can have varied disease phenotypes, including macular dystrophy, cone dystrophy, cone-rod dystrophy or rod-cone dystrophy (Figure 6). The overlap between various disease phenotypes and causative mutation reinforces the importance to understand the molecular mechanisms of genotype-phenotype relationships.

Amongst the genes causing rod-cone dystrophy, the molecular effect of mutations in *RHO*, *RP1*, *RP9*, *PRPH-2* and *USH2A* have been studied using iPSCs. Jin *et al.* [7] used iPSCs from patients with *RHO*, *RP1*, *RP9* and *PRPH-2* to generate rod photoreceptor precursors. They demonstrated reduced rod cell number at Day 120 in iPSC-rod precursors derived from patients with *RP9* mutation (early-onset retinal degeneration). This effect was seen in *RHO*, *RP1* and *RHO* mutation at Day 150, whereas no rods were detectable for the iPSC line carrying the *RP9* mutation. They also showed that the *RP9* mutant iPSC-rod precursors had increased oxidative stress. In contrast, the *RHO* mutant iPSC-rod precursors had mislocalisation of the rhodopsin protein and increased expression of ER stress markers, which might be explained by the accumulation of unfolded rhodopsin [7,53]. Tucker *et al.* also examined the impact of *USH2A* mutation on photoreceptor precursor cells. They described increased expression of *GRP78* and *GRP94* in iPSC-derived photoreceptor precursor cells, indicative of ER stress related to protein misfolding. It is important to note that controls used in these reports were not genetically matched, *i.e.*, the mutation was not removed by genomic editing.

A major limitation of these genotype-phenotype studies is the choice of controls. For metabolic syndromes or disease with early manifestation (ocular dysgenesis or early degeneration), healthy related or unrelated controls will be adequate, because of the robust and rapid cellular manifestation of the phenotype. However, controls used for studying diseases with delayed onset will need to be genetically matched to avoid the cofounding effect of the (1) genetic background, (2) retinal cell differentiation process and (3) genetic alteration introduced during the process of iPSC reprograming. Yoshida *et al.* confirmed the effect of *RHO* mutation (E18K) on rod precursor cell ER stress responses, apoptosis markers and autophagy activation by repairing and introducing the mutation in the affected and control (provided by Yamanka laboratory) cell lines, respectively, using a helper-dependent adenoviral vector gene transfer [8]. Similar genetic control was also reported for gyrate atrophy-iPSC-RPE, where restoration of the *OAT* gene in the iPSC using bacterial artificial chromosome-mediated homologous recombination resulted in normalisation of *OAT* enzyme activity in iPSC-RPE [6,77].

Once the clinically-relevant cellular phenotype and readouts can be defined for the specific genetic variant and mutation, high throughput analysis will need to be developed to enable a large number of therapeutics to be screened across the potential thousands of genetic variant cell lines from patients with IRDs. Although this is not yet possible, there are several examples where this has been reported on a smaller scale (see below). Further investigations are needed to determine if late-onset retinal or macular degeneration, such as reticular pseudodrusen (Figure 5), basal laminar drusen (Figure 5), pattern dystrophy of the RPE, vitelliform macular dystrophy and mutations arising from *EFEMP-1* (Doyne honeycomb retinal dystrophy, Figure 5), *TIMP-3* (Sorsby fundus dystrophy) or *CTRP5* (late-onset retinal degeneration), can also be modelled through derivation of retinal cells from iPSCs. The readout or functional assay for each of these diseases may differ significantly because of variable environmental contribution to the disease phenotype and diverse molecular pathogenic mechanisms. For example: Sorsby fundus dystrophy may be caused by deposition of abnormal extracellular protein (TIMP-3); Doyne honeycomb retinal dystrophy may be related to activation of unfolded protein response due to misfolded fibulin-3 (EFEMP-1); and late-onset retina degeneration may be associated with abnormal intracellular protein aggregates, as well as extracellular deposition [78–81]. There are also many IRDs that affect retinal cells downstream from the photoreceptors, such as congenital stationery night blindness and X-linked retinoschisis [82]. Patient-specific iPSC-derived laminated retinal structures may be ideal for the study of pathophysiology of these inner retinal IRDs, since many of the genes involved in these diseases (e.g., *NYX, CACNA1F, GRM6, TRPM1, CABP4, CACNA2D4* and *RS1*) are involved in the extracellular matrix of neural retina and the synaptic interaction between photoreceptor and bipolar cells [83].

3.2. IPSC for Therapeutics Development and Treatment

3.2.1. IPSC for Drug Screening

Current therapeutic modalities in IRDs are aiming to preserve residual cells or replace missing cells. Because gene therapies and many pharmacotherapies will need to be tailored for individual genetic variants or mutations, iPSCs provide an ideal platform for pre-clinical therapeutic and toxicology testing. There are several examples in both AMD and IRDs, where pharmaco- and gene therapies are tested using iPSC.

Chang *et al.* tested the protective effect of curcumin on iPSC-RPE derived from AMD patients [38]. They showed that curcumin had a beneficial effect on H_2O_2-induced cell death and reactive oxygen specifies generation in both control and AMD iPSC-RPE. Exposure of curcumin also increased the expression of *HO1, SOD2* and *GPX1* and decreased the expression of *PDGF, VEGF* and *IGFBP-2* in AMD iPSC-RPE. Whether this also occurred in control iPSC-RPE was not reported.

OAT deficiency in the RPE leads to a buildup of ornithine and a reduction in high-energy creatine phosphate. In some patients, the *OAT* enzymatic activity can be reversed by a high dose pyridoxine (vitamin B6) supplement, because of the effect of *OAT* mutation on the binding affinity to pyridoxine. Clinically, vitamin B6 responsiveness is tested in patient fibroblasts. Although based on the fibroblast assay, A226V *OAT* mutation is not responsive to vitamin B6, Meyer *et al.* has demonstrated that iPSC-RPE from this patient is, in fact, responsive to vitamin B6 based on an *in vitro* dose titration experiment. Therefore, this patient has directly benefited from iPSC disease modelling and pharmacotherapy screening.

Jin *et al.* [7] demonstrated the benefit of α-tocopherol (vitamin E) on improving the survival of iPSC-rod precursor cells in the *RP9* mutation. They also confirmed no toxic effect from 1.6 μM of ascorbic acid (vitamin C) and β-carotene (vitamin A) on iPSC-rod precursors affected by *RP1, RP9, PRPH-2* and *RHO* mutations. In addition to vitamins, modulators of signal pathways have also been screened using iPSC. Yoshida *et al.* showed that inhibition of mTOR (using rapamycin or PP242), activation of AMP kinase (using AICAR), inhibition of apoptosis signal-regulating kinase (using NQDI-1) and inhibition of protein synthesis (using salubrinal to inhibit eukaryotic translation initiation factor 2 subunit α phosphatase) can reverse the increased ER stress and apoptosis and autophagy marker expression seen in *RHO* mutant iPSC-rod precursor cells [8].

3.2.2. IPSC for Testing Gene Therapy

In addition to screening prospective pharmacological agents, iPSC has also been used to test the efficacy of gene therapy approaches in LCA and choroideremia, which aim to deliver the *CEP290* and *REP-1* genes, respectively, to retinal cells. CEP290 is a centrosomal protein involved in ciliogenesis and ciliary trafficking. Mutation in CEP290 leads to abnormality of the inner and outer segments of cone cells, resulting in early-onset severe visual loss. Previous ocular gene therapy used adeno-associated viral (AAV) vectors for delivery of the *RPE65* gene. However, the large size of CEP290 precludes the use of AAV, and therefore, lentivirus is necessary for gene delivery. Burnight *et al.* [64] described the method to package full-length human CEP290 into a lentiviral vector and demonstrated restoration of a ciliogenesis defect in LCA patient-derived fibroblasts. Although they also demonstrated expression of wild-type CEP290 after lentiviral transduction of the iPSC-photoreceptor precursor cells, they did not examine the impact of this on cone development and the formation of inner or outer segments. In contrast, Vasireddy *et al.* [84] showed successful transfection of AAV2 carrying full-length human *REP-1* cDNA into iPSCs rather than transfection into differentiated retinal cells, the presumed target cell primarily affected in choroideremia. They used a prenylation assay to confirm restoration of *REP-1* function following AAV2. *REP-1* infection of the iPSC. There was also improved trafficking of RAB27 in iPSCs, because of prenylation by viral-derived REP-1. The efficiency and toxicity of iPSC transduction was compared to patients' fibroblasts, but not patient-derived iPSC-RPE. These two examples demonstrate the potential of iPSC in pre-clinical studies of patient-specific gene therapy.

3.2.3. iPSC for Cellular Therapy

Cell therapy for retinal disease aims to replace (1) photoreceptors and/or (2) supporting cells that provide trophic and metabolic support to prevent further degeneration of remaining photoreceptors. The main challenges in establishing clinically acceptable cell therapy for retinal disease are: patient selection, surgical technique, carrier system and choice of cell source. Each of these questions has its complexity in several dimensions. However, the use of iPSCs as a source for retinal cell transplantation is one of the most exciting, but also complex and challenging, issues facing scientists, clinicians, pharmaceutical companies and regulatory authorities.

In comparison to human ESC, the use of iPSC-derived cells for cell therapy has the additional requirement of quality control associated with the surgical procedure in harvesting patient somatic cells, isolation of a single cell type from the tissue biopsy, reprogramming vectors and techniques, methods of genomic editing in the case of IRDs and techniques of hiPSC clone selection and storage. Some of these steps have been defined in standard operating procedures for the production of clinical-grade iPSCs from retrovirus reprogramming. However, this is yet to be established for the numerous published non-integrating reprogramming methods.

Derivation of clinical-grade retinal cells from hESC has been conducted in GMP facilities, and it is currently being used in phase I/II clinical trials as hESC-RPE suspension for Stargardt disease, geographic atrophy due to AMD and myopic atrophic macular degeneration (Clinical Trial: NCT01469832, NCT01345006, NCT01344993, NCT02122159) and hESC-RPE patch graft for wet

AMD (NCT01691261). There is only one human trial using iPSC-RPE, at the RIKEN Center for Developmental Biology (CDB), Japan. In the CDB trial, a monolayer of iPSC-RPE without substrate is used to treat neovascular AMD after a course of ranibizumab injections. One patient, in her 70s with wet AMD, has already received her own iPSC-RPE as a 1.3 × 3.0-mm cell patch at Kobe City Medical Center General Hospital in September [85]. This group has published data to support the *in vitro* and *in vivo* function of the iPSC-RPE in performing the visual cycle [68]. They also demonstrated suppression of the tumour-forming potential of iPSC by iPSC-RPE following subcutaneous transplantation in NOD/Shi-*scid*/IL-2Rγ^{null} (NOG) mice. They postulated that pigment epithelium-derived factor secreted from iPSC-RPE or RPE of host tissue can cause apoptotic cell death of iPSC [86]. Following from this, the tumourigenicity of iPSC-RPE was also tested in nude, severe combined immune deficiency (SCID), non-obese diabetic (NOD)-SCID and NOG mice in the subretinal and subcutaneous location. They observed no tumour formation at 6–12 months following transplant [71]. Immune reaction to autologous iPSCs has not been studied, but Kamao *et al.* [70] demonstrated a lack of immune response after one year when nonhuman primate iPSC-RPE was transplanted as an autograft into the subretinal space. This study also confirmed no evidence of tumour formation following monkey iPSC-RPE autograft [70]. The RIKEN CDB has already enrolled patients with neovascular AMD for iPSC-RPE transplantation after the disease is stabilised with anti-VEGF therapy. Although the functionality of the graft seems to be well characterised, significant work still needs to be done in developing the optimal surgical instrumentation, technique and approach in resurfacing the RPE in the submacular space and patient selection for optimal visual and anatomical outcome. It is not known if iPSC-RPE survive, as multiple small patches of epithelial monolayer are superior to cell suspension and not inferior to a single large sheet of epithelial-substrate complex that can cover the entire macular region. The importance of restoring damaged Bruch's membrane during iPSC-RPE replacement therapy in AMD cannot be underestimated, as this is considered as an important aspect of the pathophysiology of AMD [87].

In vitro genomic editing or mutation repair of harvested somatic cells, iPSCs or iPSC-derived retinal cells will provide patients with IRDs the opportunity to receive autologous cell therapy. For some IRDs that develop late-onset degeneration, genetic mutation correction in the patient-specific iPSCs may not be necessary [2]. This is relevant in the situation where the strategy is to transplant (1) iPSC-derived retinal supporting cells that are not affected by the mutation (e.g., RPE cells for ABCA4 retinopathy); or (2) iPSC-derived retinal cells affected by the mutation, but it has delayed non-cell autonomous effects due to reduced trophic factor release (e.g., rod precursor cells for the cone preservation function through the release of rod-derived cone viability factor) [88]. For replacement of cone photoreceptor cells in cone dystrophy or RPE in RPE dystrophy, *in vitro* genomic editing may be required to allow iPSCs to differentiate into mature photoreceptors or the RPE phenotype and to ensure long-term survival of the autograft. Examples of *in vitro* gene therapy testing have been described in the previous section. Future strategies may include site-specific transcription activator-like effector nucleases (TALEN) or clustered regularly interspaced short palindromic repeats (CRISPR) based genome editing techniques, where the mutation is edited through a double-strand break (DSB) and off-target mutagenesis minimised by single-guide RNA.

Following induction and subsequent homology-directed repair (HDR), the corrected gene will remain under the normal endogenous expression control elements.

4. Conclusions

Since the description of iPSCs in 2006, there has been an exponential increase in the translation of this technology towards understanding disease mechanisms and the discovery of therapeutics. The full potential is yet to be realised because of the complexity and variations in reprograming technology and retinal differentiation protocols. The relationship between the clinical disease phenotype and the molecular and cellular features of specific genetic variants in iPSC-derived retinal cells is still poorly understood. These issues will need to be resolved for iPSC-derived retinal tissue to become clinically relevant and useful in modelling retinal dysgenesis and degeneration. Standardisation and development of high throughput technology to interrogate specific retinal progeny derived from iPSCs will facilitate screening of genetic mutation and testing of pharmacologic and gene therapy in rare IRDs. Early data from several publications show that this may have a direct benefit to the patient [2,3,64,84]. iPSCs as a source of autologous cells are an attractive option, but there is a significant barrier to overcome for this to become scalable to treat large numbers of patients. However, progress in cell culture automation and refinements of reprogramming methods will undoubtedly facilitate the translation of iPSC-derived tissue into clinically applicable personalized cell therapy. Despite the mountain of challenge, the escalating costs of biologic therapy for treating neovascular and atrophic AMD and the suffering from irreversible childhood blindness due to IRDs, further ophthalmic translational research in iPSCs is worthy of the costly investment.

Acknowledgments

The authors would like to thank Lori Bonertz for proof reading the manuscript.

Author Contributions

Fred K. Chen, Samuel McLenachan, Michael Edel, Lyndon Da Cruz, Peter J. Coffey and David A. Mackey contributed reagents/materials/analysis tools; Fred K. Chen wrote the paper; Samuel McLenachan, Michael Edel, Lyndon Da Cruz, Peter J. Coffey and David A. Mackey proof read and made amendments to the paper.

Conflicts of Interest

The authors declare no conflict of interest.

References

1. Ding, X.; Patel, M.; Chan, C.C. Molecular pathology of age-related macular degeneration. *Prog. Retin. Eye Res.* **2009**, *28*, 1–18.

2. Tucker, B.A.; Mullins, R.F.; Streb, L.M.; Anfinson, K.; Eyestone, M.E.; Kaalberg, E.; Riker, M.J.; Drack, A.V.; Braun, T.A.; Stone, E.M. Patient-specific iPSC-derived photoreceptor precursor cells as a means to investigate retinitis pigmentosa. *eLife* **2013**, *2*, e00824.

3. Tucker, B.A.; Scheetz, T.E.; Mullins, R.F.; DeLuca, A.P.; Hoffmann, J.M.; Johnston, R.M.; Jacobson, S.G.; Sheffield, V.C.; Stone, E.M. Exome sequencing and analysis of induced pluripotent stem cells identify the cilia-related gene male germ cell-associated kinase (MAK) as a cause of retinitis pigmentosa. *Proc. Natl. Acad. Sci. USA* **2011**, *108*, doi:10.1073/pnas.1108918108.

4. Phillips, M.J.; Perez, E.T.; Martin, J.M.; Reshel, S.T.; Wallace, K.A.; Capowski, E.E.; Singh, R.; Wright, L.S.; Clark, E.M.; Barney, P.M.; *et al.* Modeling human retinal development with patient-specific induced pluripotent stem cells reveals multiple roles for visual system homeobox 2. *Stem Cells* **2014**, *32*, 1480–1492.

5. Singh, R.; Shen, W.; Kuai, D.; Martin, J.M.; Guo, X.; Smith, M.A.; Perez, E.T.; Phillips, M.J.; Simonett, J.M.; Wallace, K.A.; *et al.* IPS cell modeling of Best disease: Insights into the pathophysiology of an inherited macular degeneration. *Hum. Mol. Genet.* **2013**, *22*, 593–607.

6. Meyer, J.S.; Howden, S.E.; Wallace, K.A.; Verhoeven, A.D.; Wright, L.S.; Capowski, E.E.; Pinilla, I.; Martin, J.M.; Tian, S.; Stewart, R.; *et al.* Optic vesicle-like structures derived from human pluripotent stem cells facilitate a customized approach to retinal disease treatment. *Stem Cells* **2011**, *29*, 1206–1218.

7. Jin, Z.B.; Okamoto, S.; Osakada, F.; Homma, K.; Assawachananont, J.; Hirami, Y.; Iwata, T.; Takahashi, M. Modeling retinal degeneration using patient-specific induced pluripotent stem cells. *PLoS One* **2011**, *6*, e17084.

8. Yoshida, T.; Ozawa, Y.; Suzuki, K.; Yuki, K.; Ohyama, M.; Akamatsu, W.; Matsuzaki, Y.; Shimmura, S.; Mitani, K.; Tsubota, K.; *et al.* The use of induced pluripotent stem cells to reveal pathogenic gene mutations and explore treatments for retinitis pigmentosa. *Mol. Brain* **2014**, *7*, doi:10.1186/1756-6606-7-45.

9. Da Cruz, L.; Coley, B.F.; Dorn, J.; Merlini, F.; Filley, E.; Christopher, P.; Chen, F.K.; Wuyyuru, V.; Sahel, J.; Stanga, P.; *et al.* The Argus II epiretinal prosthesis system allows letter and word reading and long-term function in patients with profound vision loss. *Br. J. Ophthalmol.* **2013**, *97*, 632–636.

10. Zrenner, E.; Bartz-Schmidt, K.U.; Benav, H.; Besch, D.; Bruckmann, A.; Gabel, V.P.; Gekeler, F.; Greppmaier, U.; Harscher, A.; Kibbel, S.; *et al.* Subretinal electronic chips allow blind patients to read letters and combine them to words. *Proc. Biol. Sci. R. Soc.* **2011**, *278*, 1489–1497.

11. Villalobos, J.; Nayagam, D.A.; Allen, P.J.; McKelvie, P.; Luu, C.D.; Ayton, L.N.; Freemantle, A.L.; McPhedran, M.; Basa, M.; McGowan, C.C.; *et al.* A wide-field suprachoroidal retinal prosthesis is stable and well tolerated following chronic implantation. *Investig. Ophthalmol. Vis. Sci.* **2013**, *54*, 3751–3762.

12. Schwartz, S.D.; Hubschman, J.P.; Heilwell, G.; Franco-Cardenas, V.; Pan, C.K.; Ostrick, R.M.; Mickunas, E.; Gay, R.; Klimanskaya, I.; Lanza, R. Embryonic stem cell trials for macular degeneration: A preliminary report. *Lancet* **2012**, *379*, 713–720.

13. Kauper, K.; McGovern, C.; Sherman, S.; Heatherton, P.; Rapoza, R.; Stabila, P.; Dean, B.; Lee, A.; Borges, S.; Bouchard, B.; *et al.* Two-year intraocular delivery of ciliary neurotrophic factor by encapsulated cell technology implants in patients with chronic retinal degenerative diseases. *Investig. Ophthalmol. Vis. Sci.* **2012**, *53*, 7484–7491.

14. Carvalho, L.S.; Vandenberghe, L.H. Promising and delivering gene therapies for vision loss. *Vis. Res.* **2014**, doi:10.1016/j.visres.2014.07.013.

15. Marc, R.; Pfeiffer, R.; Jones, B. Retinal Prosthetics, Optogenetics, and Chemical Photoswitches. *ACS Chem. Neurosci.* **2014**, *5*, 895–901.

16. Mali, P.; Yang, L.; Esvelt, K.M.; Aach, J.; Guell, M.; DiCarlo, J.E.; Norville, J.E.; Church, G.M. RNA-Guided human genome engineering via Cas9. *Science* **2013**, *339*, 823–826.

17. Tucker, B.A.; Mullins, R.F.; Stone, E.M. Stem cells for investigation and treatment of inherited retinal disease. *Hum. Mol. Genet.* **2014**, *23*, doi:10.1093/hmg/ddu124.

18. Wright, L.S.; Phillips, M.J.; Pinilla, I.; Hei, D.; Gamm, D.M. Induced pluripotent stem cells as custom therapeutics for retinal repair: Progress and rationale. *Exp. Eye Res.* **2014**, *123*, 161–172.

19. Al-Shamekh, S.; Goldberg, J.L. Retinal repair with induced pluripotent stem cells. *Trans. Res. J. Lab. Clin. Med.* **2014**, *163*, 377–386.

20. Borooah, S.; Phillips, M.J.; Bilican, B.; Wright, A.F.; Wilmut, I.; Chandran, S.; Gamm, D.; Dhillon, B. Using human induced pluripotent stem cells to treat retinal disease. *Prog. Retin. Eye Res.* **2013**, *37*, 163–181.

21. Davidson, K.C.; Guymer, R.H.; Pera, M.F.; Pebay, A. Human pluripotent stem cell strategies for age-related macular degeneration. *Optom. Vis. Sci.* **2014**, *91*, 887–893.

22. Gamm, D.M.; Phillips, M.J.; Singh, R. Modeling retinal degenerative diseases with human iPS-derived cells: Current status and future implications. *Exp. Rev. Ophthalmol.* **2013**, *8*, 213–216.

23. Salero, E.; Blenkinsop, T.A.; Corneo, B.; Harris, A.; Rabin, D.; Stern, J.H.; Temple, S. Adult human RPE can be activated into a multipotent stem cell that produces mesenchymal derivatives. *Cell Stem Cell* **2012**, *10*, 88–95.

24. Moshiri, A.; Close, J.; Reh, T.A. Retinal stem cells and regeneration. *Int. J. Dev. Biol.* **2004**, *48*, 1003–1014.

25. Chen, X.; Thomson, H.; Hossain, P.; Lotery, A. Characterisation of mouse limbal neurosphere cells: A potential cell source of functional neurons. *Br. J. Ophthalmol.* **2012**, *96*, 1431–1437.

26. Zhao, X.; Das, A.V.; Bhattacharya, S.; Thoreson, W.B.; Sierra, J.R.; Mallya, K.B.; Ahmad, I. Derivation of neurons with functional properties from adult limbal epithelium: Implications in autologous cell therapy for photoreceptor degeneration. *Stem Cells* **2008**, *26*, 939–949.

27. Zhao, X.; Das, A.V.; Thoreson, W.B.; James, J.; Wattnem, T.E.; Rodriguez-Sierra, J.; Ahmad, I. Adult corneal limbal epithelium: A model for studying neural potential of non-neural stem cells/progenitors. *Dev. Biol.* **2002**, *250*, 317–331.

28. Yip, H.K. Retinal stem cells and regeneration of vision system. *Anat. Rec.* **2014**, *297*, 137–160.

29. Pellegrini, G.; Rama, P.; di Rocco, A.; Panaras, A.; de Luca, M. Concise review: Hurdles in a successful example of limbal stem cell-based regenerative medicine. *Stem Cells* **2014**, *32*, 26–34.

30. Miri, A.; Said, D.G.; Dua, H.S. Donor site complications in autolimbal and living-related allolimbal transplantation. *Ophthalmology* **2011**, *118*, 1265–1271.

31. Wilmut, I.; Schnieke, A.E.; McWhir, J.; Kind, A.J.; Campbell, K.H. Viable offspring derived from fetal and adult mammalian cells. *Nature* **1997**, *385*, 810–813.

32. Cowan, C.A.; Atienza, J.; Melton, D.A.; Eggan, K. Nuclear reprogramming of somatic cells after fusion with human embryonic stem cells. *Science* **2005**, *309*, 1369–1373.

33. Yamanaka, S.; Blau, H.M. Nuclear reprogramming to a pluripotent state by three approaches. *Nature* **2010**, *465*, 704–712.

34. Takahashi, K.; Tanabe, K.; Ohnuki, M.; Narita, M.; Ichisaka, T.; Tomoda, K.; Yamanaka, S. Induction of pluripotent stem cells from adult human fibroblasts by defined factors. *Cell* **2007**, *131*, 861–872.

35. Hu, Q.; Friedrich, A.M.; Johnson, L.V.; Clegg, D.O. Memory in induced pluripotent stem cells: Reprogrammed human retinal-pigmented epithelial cells show tendency for spontaneous redifferentiation. *Stem Cells* **2010**, *28*, 1981–1991.

36. Phillips, M.J.; Wallace, K.A.; Dickerson, S.J.; Miller, M.J.; Verhoeven, A.D.; Martin, J.M.; Wright, L.S.; Shen, W.; Capowski, E.E.; Percin, E.F.; *et al.* Blood-derived human iPS cells generate optic vesicle-like structures with the capacity to form retinal laminae and develop synapses. *Investig. Ophthalmol. Vis. Sci.* **2012**, *53*, 2007–2019.

37. Tucker, B.A.; Anfinson, K.R.; Mullins, R.F.; Stone, E.M.; Young, M.J. Use of a synthetic xeno-free culture substrate for induced pluripotent stem cell induction and retinal differentiation. *Stem Cells Trans. Med.* **2013**, *2*, 16–24.

38. Chang, Y.C.; Chang, W.C.; Hung, K.H.; Yang, D.M.; Cheng, Y.H.; Liao, Y.W.; Woung, L.C.; Tsai, C.Y.; Hsu, C.C.; Lin, T.C.; *et al.* The generation of induced pluripotent stem cells for macular degeneration as a drug screening platform: Identification of curcumin as a protective agent for retinal pigment epithelial cells against oxidative stress. *Front. Aging Neurosci.* **2014**, *6*, doi:10.3389/fnagi.2014.00191.

39. Balasubramanian, S.; Babai, N.; Chaudhuri, A.; Qiu, F.; Bhattacharya, S.; Dave, B.J.; Parameswaran, S.; Carson, S.D.; Thoreson, W.B.; Sharp, J.G.; *et al.* Non cell-autonomous reprogramming of adult ocular progenitors: Generation of pluripotent stem cells without exogenous transcription factors. *Stem Cells* **2009**, *27*, 3053–3062.

40. Sareen, D.; Saghizadeh, M.; Ornelas, L.; Winkler, M.A.; Narwani, K.; Sahabian, A.; Funari, V.A.; Tang, J.; Spurka, L.; Punj, V.; *et al.* Differentiation of Human Limbal-Derived Induced Pluripotent Stem Cells Into Limbal-Like Epithelium. *Stem Cells Trans. Med.* **2014**, *3*, 1002–1012.

41. Geti, I.; Ormiston, M.L.; Rouhani, F.; Toshner, M.; Movassagh, M.; Nichols, J.; Mansfield, W.; Southwood, M.; Bradley, A.; Rana, A.A.; *et al.* A practical and efficient cellular substrate for the generation of induced pluripotent stem cells from adults: Blood-derived endothelial progenitor cells. *Stem Cells Trans. Med.* **2012**, *1*, 855–865.

42. Seki, T.; Yuasa, S.; Fukuda, K. Generation of induced pluripotent stem cells from a small amount of human peripheral blood using a combination of activated T cells and Sendai virus. *Nat. Protocols* **2012**, *7*, 718–728.

43. Brown, M.E.; Rondon, E.; Rajesh, D.; Mack, A.; Lewis, R.; Feng, X.; Zitur, L.J.; Learish, R.D.; Nuwaysir, E.F. Derivation of induced pluripotent stem cells from human peripheral blood T lymphocytes. *PLoS One* **2010**, *5*, e11373.

44. Yu, J.; Vodyanik, M.A.; Smuga-Otto, K.; Antosiewicz-Bourget, J.; Frane, J.L.; Tian, S.; Nie, J.; Jonsdottir, G.A.; Ruotti, V.; Stewart, R.; *et al.* Induced pluripotent stem cell lines derived from human somatic cells. *Science* **2007**, *318*, 1917–1920.

45. Fusaki, N.; Ban, H.; Nishiyama, A.; Saeki, K.; Hasegawa, M. Efficient induction of transgene-free human pluripotent stem cells using a vector based on Sendai virus, an RNA virus that does not integrate into the host genome. *Proc. Jpn. Acad. Ser. B Phys. Biol. Sci.* **2009**, *85*, 348–362.

46. Yu, J.; Hu, K.; Smuga-Otto, K.; Tian, S.; Stewart, R.; Slukvin, I.I.; Thomson, J.A. Human induced pluripotent stem cells free of vector and transgene sequences. *Science* **2009**, *324*, 797–801.

47. Yu, J.; Chau, K.F.; Vodyanik, M.A.; Jiang, J.; Jiang, Y. Efficient feeder-free episomal reprogramming with small molecules. *PLoS One* **2011**, *6*, e17557.

48. Warren, L.; Manos, P.D.; Ahfeldt, T.; Loh, Y.H.; Li, H.; Lau, F.; Ebina, W.; Mandal, P.K.; Smith, Z.D.; Meissner, A.; *et al.* Highly efficient reprogramming to pluripotency and directed differentiation of human cells with synthetic modified mRNA. *Cell Stem Cell* **2010**, *7*, 618–630.

49. Kim, D.; Kim, C.H.; Moon, J.I.; Chung, Y.G.; Chang, M.Y.; Han, B.S.; Ko, S.; Yang, E.; Cha, K.Y.; Lanza, R.; *et al.* Generation of human induced pluripotent stem cells by direct delivery of reprogramming proteins. *Cell Stem Cell* **2009**, *4*, 472–476.

50. Lin, T.; Ambasudhan, R.; Yuan, X.; Li, W.; Hilcove, S.; Abujarour, R.; Lin, X.; Hahm, H.S.; Hao, E.; Hayek, A.; *et al.* A chemical platform for improved induction of human iPSCs. *Nat. Methods* **2009**, *6*, 805–808.

51. Meyer, J.S.; Shearer, R.L.; Capowski, E.E.; Wright, L.S.; Wallace, K.A.; McMillan, E.L.; Zhang, S.C.; Gamm, D.M. Modeling early retinal development with human embryonic and induced pluripotent stem cells. *Proc. Natl. Acad. Sci. USA* **2009**, *106*, 16698–16703.

52. Lamba, D.A.; McUsic, A.; Hirata, R.K.; Wang, P.R.; Russell, D.; Reh, T.A. Generation, purification and transplantation of photoreceptors derived from human induced pluripotent stem cells. *PLoS One* **2010**, *5*, e8763.

53. Jin, Z.B.; Okamoto, S.; Xiang, P.; Takahashi, M. Integration-free induced pluripotent stem cells derived from retinitis pigmentosa patient for disease modeling. *Stem Cells Trans. Med.* **2012**, *1*, 503–509.

54. Reichman, S.; Terray, A.; Slembrouck, A.; Nanteau, C.; Orieux, G.; Habeler, W.; Nandrot, E.F.; Sahel, J.A.; Monville, C.; Goureau, O. From confluent human iPS cells to self-forming neural retina and retinal pigmented epithelium. *Proc. Natl. Acad. Sci. USA.* **2014**, *111*, 8518–8523.

55. Nakano, T.; Ando, S.; Takata, N.; Kawada, M.; Muguruma, K.; Sekiguchi, K.; Saito, K.; Yonemura, S.; Eiraku, M.; Sasai, Y. Self-formation of optic cups and storable stratified neural retina from human ESCs. *Cell Stem Cell* **2012**, *10*, 771–785.

56. Eiraku, M.; Watanabe, K.; Matsuo-Takasaki, M.; Kawada, M.; Yonemura, S.; Matsumura, M.; Wataya, T.; Nishiyama, A.; Muguruma, K.; Sasai, Y. Self-organized formation of polarized cortical tissues from ESCs and its active manipulation by extrinsic signals. *Cell Stem Cell* **2008**, *3*, 519–532.

57. Zhong, X.; Gutierrez, C.; Xue, T.; Hampton, C.; Vergara, M.N.; Cao, L.H.; Peters, A.; Park, T.S.; Zambidis, E.T.; Meyer, J.S.; *et al.* Generation of three-dimensional retinal tissue with functional photoreceptors from human iPSCs. *Nat. Commun.* **2014**, *5*, doi:10.1038/ncomms5047.

58. Hirami, Y.; Osakada, F.; Takahashi, K.; Okita, K.; Yamanaka, S.; Ikeda, H.; Yoshimura, N.; Takahashi, M. Generation of retinal cells from mouse and human induced pluripotent stem cells. *Neurosci. Lett.* **2009**, *458*, 126–131.

59. Osakada, F.; Jin, Z.B.; Hirami, Y.; Ikeda, H.; Danjyo, T.; Watanabe, K.; Sasai, Y.; Takahashi, M. *In vitro* differentiation of retinal cells from human pluripotent stem cells by small-molecule induction. *J. Cell Sci.* **2009**, *122*, 3169–3179.

60. Lamba, D.A.; Karl, M.O.; Ware, C.B.; Reh, T.A. Efficient generation of retinal progenitor cells from human embryonic stem cells. *Proc. Natl. Acad. Sci. USA.* **2006**, *103*, 12769–12774.

61. Osakada, F.; Ikeda, H.; Mandai, M.; Wataya, T.; Watanabe, K.; Yoshimura, N.; Akaike, A.; Sasai, Y.; Takahashi, M. Toward the generation of rod and cone photoreceptors from mouse, monkey and human embryonic stem cells. *Nat. Biotechnol.* **2008**, *26*, 215–224.

62. Mellough, C.B.; Sernagor, E.; Moreno-Gimeno, I.; Steel, D.H.; Lako, M. Efficient stage-specific differentiation of human pluripotent stem cells toward retinal photoreceptor cells. *Stem Cells* **2012**, *30*, 673–686.

63. Sridhar, A.; Steward, M.M.; Meyer, J.S. Nonxenogeneic growth and retinal differentiation of human induced pluripotent stem cells. *Stem Cells Trans. Med.* **2013**, *2*, 255–264.

64. Burnight, E.R.; Wiley, L.A.; Drack, A.V.; Braun, T.A.; Anfinson, K.R.; Kaalberg, E.E.; Halder, J.A.; Affatigato, L.M.; Mullins, R.F.; Stone, E.M.; *et al.* CEP290 gene transfer rescues Leber congenital amaurosis cellular phenotype. *Gene Ther.* **2014**, *21*, 662–672.

65. Carr, A.J.; Vugler, A.A.; Hikita, S.T.; Lawrence, J.M.; Gias, C.; Chen, L.L.; Buchholz, D.E.; Ahmado, A.; Semo, M.; Smart, M.J.; *et al.* Protective effects of human iPS-derived retinal pigment epithelium cell transplantation in the retinal dystrophic rat. *PLoS One* **2009**, *4*, e8152.

66. Buchholz, D.E.; Hikita, S.T.; Rowland, T.J.; Friedrich, A.M.; Hinman, C.R.; Johnson, L.V.; Clegg, D.O. Derivation of functional retinal pigmented epithelium from induced pluripotent stem cells. *Stem Cells* **2009**, *27*, 2427–2434.

67. Maruotti, J.; Wahlin, K.; Gorrell, D.; Bhutto, I.; Lutty, G.; Zack, D.J. A simple and scalable process for the differentiation of retinal pigment epithelium from human pluripotent stem cells. *Stem Cells Trans. Med.* **2013**, *2*, 341–354.

68. Maeda, T.; Lee, M.J.; Palczewska, G.; Marsili, S.; Tesar, P.J.; Palczewski, K.; Takahashi, M.; Maeda, A. Retinal pigmented epithelial cells obtained from human induced pluripotent stem cells possess functional visual cycle enzymes *in vitro* and *in vivo*. *J. Biol. Chem.* **2013**, *288*, 34484–34493.

69. Li, Y.; Tsai, Y.T.; Hsu, C.W.; Erol, D.; Yang, J.; Wu, W.H.; Davis, R.J.; Egli, D.; Tsang, S.H. Long-term safety and efficacy of human-induced pluripotent stem cell (iPS) grafts in a preclinical model of retinitis pigmentosa. *Mol. Med.* **2012**, *18*, 1312–1319.

70. Kamao, H.; Mandai, M.; Okamoto, S.; Sakai, N.; Suga, A.; Sugita, S.; Kiryu, J.; Takahashi, M. Characterization of human induced pluripotent stem cell-derived retinal pigment epithelium cell sheets aiming for clinical application. *Stem Cell Rep.* **2014**, *2*, 205–218.

71. Kanemura, H.; Go, M.J.; Shikamura, M.; Nishishita, N.; Sakai, N.; Kamao, H.; Mandai, M.; Morinaga, C.; Takahashi, M.; Kawamata, S. Tumorigenicity studies of induced pluripotent stem cell (iPSC)-derived retinal pigment epithelium (RPE) for the treatment of age-related macular degeneration. *PLoS One* **2014**, *9*, e85336.

72. Ran, X.; Cai, W.J.; Huang, X.F.; Liu, Q.; Lu, F.; Qu, J.; Wu, J.; Jin, Z.B. "RetinoGenetics": A comprehensive mutation database for genes related to inherited retinal degeneration. *Database J. Biol. Databases Curation* **2014**, *2014*, doi:10.1093/database/bau047.

73. Bainbridge, J.W.; Smith, A.J.; Barker, S.S.; Robbie, S.; Henderson, R.; Balaggan, K.; Viswanathan, A.; Holder, G.E.; Stockman, A.; Tyler, N.; *et al.* Effect of gene therapy on visual function in Leber's congenital amaurosis. *N. Engl. J. Med.* **2008**, *358*, 2231–2239.

74. Maguire, A.M.; High, K.A.; Auricchio, A.; Wright, J.F.; Pierce, E.A.; Testa, F.; Mingozzi, F.; Bennicelli, J.L.; Ying, G.S.; Rossi, S.; *et al.* Age-dependent effects of *RPE65* gene therapy for Leber's congenital amaurosis: A phase 1 dose-escalation trial. *Lancet* **2009**, *374*, 1597–1605.

75. MacLaren, R.E.; Groppe, M.; Barnard, A.R.; Cottriall, C.L.; Tolmachova, T.; Seymour, L.; Clark, K.R.; During, M.J.; Cremers, F.P.; Black, G.C.; *et al.* Retinal gene therapy in patients with choroideremia: Initial findings from a phase 1/2 clinical trial. *Lancet* **2014**, *383*, 1129–1137.

76. Lustremant, C.; Habeler, W.; Plancheron, A.; Goureau, O.; Grenot, L.; de la Grange, P.; Audo, I.; Nandrot, E.F.; Monville, C. Human induced pluripotent stem cells as a tool to model a form of Leber congenital amaurosis. *Cell. Reprogram.* **2013**, *15*, 233–246.

77. Howden, S.E.; Gore, A.; Li, Z.; Fung, H.L.; Nisler, B.S.; Nie, J.; Chen, G.; McIntosh, B.E.; Gulbranson, D.R.; Diol, N.R.; *et al.* Genetic correction and analysis of induced pluripotent stem cells from a patient with gyrate atrophy. *Proc. Natl. Acad. Sci. USA.* **2011**, *108*, 6537–6542.

78. Chong, N.H.; Alexander, R.A.; Gin, T.; Bird, A.C.; Luthert, P.J. TIMP-3, collagen, and elastin immunohistochemistry and histopathology of Sorsby's fundus dystrophy. *Investig. Ophthalmol. Vis. Sci.* **2000**, *41*, 898–902.

79. Chong, N.H.; Kvanta, A.; Seregard, S.; Bird, A.C.; Luthert, P.J.; Steen, B. TIMP-3 mRNA is not overexpressed in Sorsby fundus dystrophy. *Am. J. Ophthalmol.* **2003**, *136*, 954–955.

80. Roybal, C.N.; Marmorstein, L.Y.; Vander Jagt, D.L.; Abcouwer, S.F. Aberrant accumulation of fibulin-3 in the endoplasmic reticulum leads to activation of the unfolded protein response and *VEGF* expression. *Investig. Ophthalmol. Vis. Sci.* **2005**, *46*, 3973–3979.

81. Hayward, C.; Shu, X.; Cideciyan, A.V.; Lennon, A.; Barran, P.; Zareparsi, S.; Sawyer, L.; Hendry, G.; Dhillon, B.; Milam, A.H.; *et al.* Mutation in a short-chain collagen gene, *CTRP5*, results in extracellular deposit formation in late-onset retinal degeneration: A genetic model for age-related macular degeneration. *Hum. Mol. Genet.* **2003**, *12*, 2657–2667.

82. Audo, I.; Robson, A.G.; Holder, G.E.; Moore, A.T. The negative ERG: Clinical phenotypes and disease mechanisms of inner retinal dysfunction. *Surv. Ophthalmol.* **2008**, *53*, 16–40.

83. Audo, I.; Kohl, S.; Leroy, B.P.; Munier, F.L.; Guillonneau, X.; Mohand-Said, S.; Bujakowska, K.; Nandrot, E.F.; Lorenz, B.; Preising, M.; *et al.* TRPM1 is mutated in patients with autosomal-recessive complete congenital stationary night blindness. *Am. J. Hum. Genet.* **2009**, *85*, 720–729.

84. Vasireddy, V.; Mills, J.A.; Gaddameedi, R.; Basner-Tschakarjan, E.; Kohnke, M.; Black, A.D.; Alexandrov, K.; Zhou, S.; Maguire, A.M.; Chung, D.C.; *et al.* AAV-mediated gene therapy for choroideremia: Preclinical studies in personalized models. *PLoS One* **2013**, *8*, e61396.

85. Cyranoski, D. Japanese woman is first recipient of next-generation stem cells. *Nature* **2014**, doi:10.1038/nature15915.

86. Kanemura, H.; Go, M.J.; Nishishita, N.; Sakai, N.; Kamao, H.; Sato, Y.; Takahashi, M.; Kawamata, S. Pigment epithelium-derived factor secreted from retinal pigment epithelium facilitates apoptotic cell death of iPSC. *Sci. Rep.* **2013**, *3*, doi:10.1038/srep02334.

87. Heller, J.P.; Martin, K.R. Enhancing RPE Cell-Based Therapy Outcomes for AMD: The Role of Bruch's Membrane. *Trans. Vis. Sci. Technol.* **2014**, *3*, doi:10.1167/tvst.3.4.4.

88. Leveillard, T.; Fridlich, R.; Clerin, E.; Ait-Ali, N.; Millet-Puel, G.; Jaillard, C.; Yang, Y.; Zack, D.; van-Dorsselaer, A.; Sahel, J.A. Therapeutic strategy for handling inherited retinal degenerations in a gene-independent manner using rod-derived cone viability factors. *C. R. Biol.* **2014**, *337*, 207–213.

Patient-Specific iPSC-Derived RPE for Modeling of Retinal Diseases

Huy V. Nguyen, Yao Li and Stephen H. Tsang

Abstract: Inherited retinal diseases, such as age-related macular degeneration and retinitis pigmentosa, are the leading cause of blindness in the developed world. Currently, treatments for these conditions are limited. Recently, considerable attention has been given to the possibility of using patient-specific induced pluripotent stem cells (iPSCs) as a treatment for these conditions. iPSCs reprogrammed from adult somatic cells offer the possibility of generating patient-specific cell lines *in vitro*. In this review, we will discuss the current literature pertaining to iPSC modeling of retinal disease, gene therapy of iPSC-derived retinal pigmented epithelium (RPE) cells, and retinal transplantation. We will focus on the use of iPSCs created from patients with inherited eye diseases for testing the efficacy of gene or drug-based therapies, elucidating previously unknown mechanisms and pathways of disease, and as a source of autologous cells for cell replacement.

Reprinted from *J. Clin. Med.* Cite as: Nguyen, H.V.; Li, Y.; Tsang, S.H. Patient-Specific iPSC-Derived RPE for Modeling of Retinal Diseases. *J. Clin. Med.* **2015**, *4*, 567–578.

1. Introduction

Human vision is vital for nearly every major activity of daily living, and degeneration of one of the responsible cell types, the retinal pigmented epithelium (RPE), leads to severe visual impairment and blindness. RPE cells exist as a monolayer located at the back of the eye between the retina and Bruch's membrane and is essential for photoreceptor function and survival. Retinal diseases such as age-related macular degeneration (AMD) and retinitis pigmentosa (RP) result in clinical pathophysiology characterized by progressive loss of RPE. The adult retina does not intrinsically regenerate, so RPE degeneration may ultimately lead to blindness. Anti-vascular endothelial growth factor (VEGF) therapy has been shown to slow the rate of vision loss, but it has no more than a 10% rate of effectiveness in all AMD cases [1]. There are no other treatments currently established for RPE degenerative diseases, so the disease burden of these conditions are expected to continue to rise. AMD and RP are both leading causes of blindness in the developed world, affecting up to one third of people over the age of 75. Among the elderly, blindness is feared more than any other illness outside of cancer. Currently, nine million Americans have been diagnosed with AMD, and its incidence is expected to double within a decade, affecting 20% of Americans between the ages of 65 and 75 years [2].

Cell transplantation into the human retina has the potential to restore vision and provide treatment in diseases like AMD and RP with significant RPE loss. Since these diseases spare the inner retina and optic nerve, retinal transplantation has focused on replacement of the photoreceptors and RPE. Retinal stem cells have been shown to be efficient at integrating into the degenerative host retina [3]. Replacement of damaged RPE in patients with AMD is now being offered [4]. In 2011, the U.S.

Food and Drug Administration advanced the treatment of macular degenerations by approving clinical trials using embryonic stem (ES) cell-derived RPE transplants [5].

Induced pluripotent stem (iPS) cells reprogrammed from adult somatic cells offer the possibility of generating patient-specific cell lines *in vitro*. As a platform to study patient-specific targeted disease cells, iPS cells (iPSC) have exciting potential in regenerative medicine and human disease modeling. As one example, after human embryonic stem cells were shown to be able to produce 3-D optic vesicle-like structures displaying a precise apical-basal orientation [6], human iPS cells were used to also create optic vesicle-like structures which self-assembled into rudimentary, multilayered retinal tissue [7]. Similarly, human iPSCs have been used to model primary open-angle glaucoma (POAG). The optineurin E50K mutation is a mutation currently affirmed as causative for POAG, and human iPSCs have been created with the E50K mutation to study the molecular and cellular characterization of POAG onset [8]. hiPSC modeling has also suggested that normal-tension glaucoma via TBK1 gene duplication is due increased levels of LC3-II, a key marker of autophagy [9].

Specifically, iPS-based therapies holds great promise for treating retinal degenerative diseases, given the advantage of ocular immune privilege and the ease of ocular non-invasive imaging. Moreover, iPS cell technology facilitates investigations of pathophysiological mechanisms of genetic mutations and testing of gene therapy vectors on RPE-based disease models. Indeed, iPS-derived RPE (iPS-RPE) can be reproducibly isolated and closely monitored both morphologically and functionally before experiments, effectively minimizing variability in the timing of differentiation. In addition, RPE, unlike many other human cell types, has a well-described culture standard, which ensures proper controls [4,10].

The *in vitro* phenotypes of disease-specific iPS-derived cells can be used to bridge the gap between the clinical phenotype and molecular or cellular mechanisms, creating new strategies for drug screening, and developing novel therapeutic agents [11]. Human iPS cell-based disease models can prove that a disease is caused by a genetic mutation, hypothesize potential treatment options before using more expensive animal models [12], and assist in the development of novel treatments for clinical trials [13–15].

2. iPSC Disease Modeling

2.1. Use of iPS-Derived RPE Cells for Cell Therapy

The eye is an ideal site for stem cell therapies. First, it is considered an immune privileged organ since the inflammatory responses of the eye differ significantly from those in other tissues. Second, the eye allows for easy accessibility for monitoring and imaging. Third, in the case of serious complications, the eye as a unit can be removed, due to its relative isolation from other body systems. Stem cells in turn are an appealing option for retinal cell replacement due to their pluripotency and potentially unlimited capacity for self-renewal. Currently, there are two leading options for stem cells in retinal transplantation: (i) embryonic stem cells (ESCs), which can be isolated from developing embryos four to five days after fertilization; and (ii) induced pluripotent stem cells (iPSCs), which can be created from adult cells by the viral transduction of transcription factors [16].

However, due to the ethical and technical concerns with using ESCs, iPSCs have largely been favored for retinal transplantation.

iPSCs in particular offer a compelling alternative approach for stem cell therapy. When derived from the transplant recipient, autologous iPS-derived cells reduce the risk of post-transplant rejection and obviate the need for immunosuppression after transplantation. The well-described iPSC culture standards also aid in the development of functional testing and optimization studies. Likewise, RPE transplantation into the retina poses fewer challenges than other kinds of cell transplantation since routine culture of RPE cells has been well described [17,18]. RPE monolayers exist in an easily identifiable hexagonal structure and can be isolated and transferred to a variety of substrates without the need for synaptic integration. Subsequently, studies on RPE replacement therapies using pluripotent stem cells have progressed rapidly. A multicenter trial focusing on the treatment of dry macular degeneration and Stargardt macular dystrophy showed that purified human ESC-derived RPE can be subretinally injected into patients with good results [5]. This is also possible since the retina normally enjoys relative immune privilege, due to the blood-retinal barrier. This barrier consists of non-fenestrated retinal vasculature ensheathed by pericyte and astrocyte processes on the inner aspect and by tight junctions between RPE on the outer aspect. In a healthy state, this blood-retinal barrier provides protection to transplanted cells beneath the retina from the systemic immune system. However, in a diseased RPE state, the monolayer is disrupted due to faulty tight junctions and the retina may also become much more pro-inflammatory [19,20]. Therefore, cells transplanted into a diseased retina are likely to be at a higher risk for rejection, so autologous iPSC transplantation represents the best stem cell approach for curing degenerative retinal diseases. In fact, hiPSC-derived RPE has recently been approved in Japan for use in patient safety trials for treatment of AMD [21].

Currently, human iPS-derived RPE (iPS-RPE) experiments are largely confined to animal models. In 2009, Carr *et al.* performed subretinal injections of dissociated human iPS-RPE into Royal College of Surgeons (RCS) rats and observed restoration of RPE phagocytotic function, as measured by intracellular RHO staining, and long-term preservation of visual function, as measured by optokinetic head-tracking [22]. Another model is the RPE-specific protein 65 kDA (RPE65) mutant mouse model, which is used to study Leber congenital amaurosis (LCA) and RP since the RPE 65 defect leads to a faulty isomerase which can no longer convert the chromophore necessary for rhodopsin to detect light [23]. In 2012, Li *et al.* injected dissociated human iPS-RPE into the subretinal space of the RPE65 mutant mouse model and showed integration of the transplant with host RPE, as well as a modest improvement of visual function as measured by electroretinogram (ERG) [10]. The $Mfrp^{rd6}/Mfrp^{rd6}$ (rd6) mouse, which has a deletion in the Membrane Frizzled-Related Protein (*Mfrp*) gene, is another widely used model. The resulting MFRP protein, an RPE-specific membrane receptor of unknown function, is abnormal and the mice exhibit progressive retinal degeneration, making the model a preclinical and progressive model of RP [24]. In a recent study, subretinal injections of AAV-packaged wild-type *Mfrp* into rd6 mice showed improvement in visual function and RPE cell layer thickness [25].

The most advantageous aspect of iPSC based therapy is the potential of autologous transplantation, which intends to address the problem of immune rejection. Despite the assumption that these autologous cells should not provoke an immune response in the recipient from whom the cells were derived, there have been conflicting reports that raise some concern of the immunogenicity of iPSCs. In a recent study, teratomas originating from subcutaneous injection of murine derived iPSCs were found to have abnormal gene expression in some cells, which elicited a T-cell dependent immune response in syngeneic mice [26]. However, when Guha *et al.* transplanted various types of murine iPS-derived cells to a site under the kidney capsule of B6 mice, they found no evidence of immune response to the iPSCs, no increased T cell proliferation *in vitro*, no rejection of syngeneic iPSC-derived cells after transplantation, and no antigen-specific secondary immune response [27]. Findings by Liu *et al.* in 2013 suggests that iPSC immunogenicity increases with *in vivo* differentiation, as the authors observed immune responses after transplantation of differentiated iPS-derived cardiomyocytes but no response when transplanting undifferentiated iPSCs [28]. In contrast, Morizane *et al.* performed a direct comparison between autologous and allogeneic transplantation of iPS-derived neural cells in brains of non-human primates and found that the autologous transplantation of iPS-derived neurons caused only a minimal immune response in the brain, while the allografts elicited an acquired immune response [29]. Moreover, a higher number of dopaminergic neurons survived in autografted iPS-derived cells, which further support their use. Taken together, these findings reveals that different cell types derived from iPSCs might have distinctive immunogenicities in their syngeneic hosts. For the development of human iPS-based cell therapy, there remains still a challenge to evaluate the immunogenicity of human iPS-derived cells in an autologous human immune system.

2.2. Progress of RPE Disease Modeling Using iPSCs

Human iPS cells are useful for modeling RPE disorders since they can be isolated, expanded, re-seeded, and closely monitored both morphologically and functionally prior to testing [30]. Phenotypes of patient-specific iPS cells may differ from those from a mouse model with the same mutation [25], underscoring the necessity for multiple models of human genetic diseases. Since differences in phenotypic expression can be observed among species with the same genetic mutation, it is important to study patient-specific cell lines as a complement to mouse models.

The first retinal disease modeled with patient-specific iPS cells is Best vitelliform macular dystrophy (BVMD) [13]. Caused by a defect in the RPE gene BEST1, which results in the subretinal accumulation of photoreceptor waste products, BVMD is characterized by central vision loss due to photoreceptor death. Singh *et al.* created iPS-RPE from affected patients and compared them with those created from unaffected siblings. From their model, they concluded that the pathophysiology of the disease included delayed rhodopsin degradation after photoreceptor outer segment feeding, as evidenced by disrupted fluid flux and increased accumulation of autofluorescent material [13]. This hiPSC model of BVMD possessed functional deficiencies consistent with the clinical features of the disease and was used to characterize clinically relevant disease phenotypes for BVMD.

iPS-derived RPE cells have also recently been used to model and study the pathophysiology of AMD. While genome-wide association studies (GWAS) have identified risk alleles for the disease, such as the ARMS2 and HTRA1 genes, how these alleles lead to pathology is still unclear. There is currently a lack of appropriate models for AMD; autopsy eyes from end-stage patients already possess terminal changes and cannot be used to determine how abnormal gene expression can lead to RPE pathology, and mice do not have maculae. To bypass these obstacles, Yang *et al.* created a model for AMD by obtaining patient-specific iPS-derived RPE and pharmacologically accelerating the aging process with treatment of bisretinoid N-retinylidine-N-ethanolamine (A2E) and blue light [12]. From a proteome screen of multiple A2E-aged patient-specific iPS-RPE lines, impaired superoxide dismutase 2 (SOD2) function was identified as a high risk factor for developing AMD. Using their iPS model, the researchers concluded that the ARMS2/HTRA1 risk alleles decreased SOD2 defense, making RPE more susceptible to oxidative damage and thus contributing to AMD pathogenesis.

3. Personalized Medicine: Patient-Specific iPSC-Based Therapy

3.1. Development of Gene Therapy on Patient-Specific iPSCs

Gene-corrected patient specific iPSCs offer a unique approach to autologous therapies, which have the potential to treat a wide range of acquired and inherited diseases. However, gene targeting in human pluripotent stem cells has been exceedingly difficult [31]. One approach is using recombinant adeno-associated virus (AAV) as a gene transfer vector to carry the missing gene into affected cells. Vasireddy *et al.* published the first study which successfully transduced iPSCs developed from a patient with choroideremia with AAV subtype 2 (AAV2) [32]. Choroideremia is an inherited disorder due to loss of the *CHM* gene and the resulting Rab Escort Protein 1 (REP-1), which leading to degeneration of the choroid and retina and blindness by the 2nd decade of life. Research moving towards clinical trials has been stymied due to a lack of an animal model with similar functional and morphological features as the human retina, since the knockout of the murine *Chm* is lethal. The authors developed a preclinical model of choroideremia using iPSCs and successfully transduced wildtype human *Chm* cDNA into these cells using AAV2 mediated therapy. They observed a functional restoration of REP-1 enzymatic activity and protein trafficking, showing that their gene therapy was successful and that iPSCs can be used as a preclinical model for choroideremia [32].

The development of genome editing tools such as zinc finger nucleases (ZFNs), transcription activator-like effector nucleases (TALENs), and the clustered regularly interspaced short palindromic repeats (CRISPR)-Cas system have facilitated gene targeting in human iPSCs [33]. These tools use double strand break induction and subsequent homology-directed repair to edit the mutations in the patients' genomic DNA, so that the corrected gene will remain under the normal endogenous promoters and enhancers. Thus, compared to conventional viral-mediated gene replacement, gene editing using ZFNs, TALENs, or the CRISPR system can avoid genetic expression in inappropriate cell types as well as incorrect levels of expression [34].

The CRISPR-Cas system has several advantages over ZFNs and TALENs for enhancing gene targeting efficiency. Most CRISPR-Cas subtypes target DNA directly, suggesting the possibility of engineered, RNA-directed gene editing systems. This usage of easily generated RNA guides avoid the need for repeated protein design, which sets CRISPR-Cas apart from ZFNs and TALENs, which use protein-based DNA targeting motifs. Using the CRISPR-Cas9 system, Mali *et al.* targeted the endogenous AAVS1 locus in human iPSCs to achieve homology-directed repair of fibroblast-derived iPSCs [35]. Recently, Hou *et al.* developed a CRISPR-Cas system from *N. meningitides* to generate accurately targeted clones in human iPSCs with increased efficiency as compared to TALENs [36]. There several concerns with CRISPR-Cas technology in human genome editing, primarily off-target DNA cleavage [37]. However, recent experiments showed that "nickases", or enzymes that cleave only a single strand of DNA in DNA repair, can increase the specificity and safety of the CRISPR-Cas9 system [38].

3.2. Gene Therapy on Patient-Specific iPSC-Derived RPE Cells

With the aim of correcting genetic defects, gene therapy has been attempted not only on patient-specific iPS cells, but also RPE cells derived from these cell lines. A proof of concept study was performed by Cereso *et al.* which used a hybrid vector comprised of AAV2 and AAV5 (AAV2/5) to mediate gene therapy to the RPE derived from iPS created from a choroideremia patient [39]. The authors successfully developed a human iPS-derived retinal cell model of choroideremia, performed gene therapy on the iPS-RPE, and showed that AAV2/5-mediated therapy could potentially restore RPE phenotype. Working with MFRP, Li *et al.* also showed that patient-specific iPS-RPE could be a recipient for gene therapy [25]. The researchers applied the AAV8 vector expressing human MFRP to iPS-RPE from patients with MFRP mutations and confirmed that gene therapy led to restoration of RPE phenotype, specifically with regards to actin organization. These studies suggest that gene therapy using AAV vectors can be applied to RPE created from patient-specific iPS for retinal diseases without previous models, and that these diseases may be potential targets for additional gene therapy trials.

3.3. Transplantation of iPSC-Derived RPE Cells

Considerable attention has been paid to the potential of human iPSCs as a source for regenerative medicine, disease modeling, and drug testing. In particular, the limitations in existing treatments for AMD have led to attention being given to alternative approaches in which damaged RPE is replaced by healthy RPE. In a recent landmark trial in Japan, patient specific iPSC-derived RPE cells were transplanted for the first time into a human patient with AMD. Clearance for a human trial was given after Takahashi *et al.* showed that transplantation of iPSC-derived RPE did not provoke an immune reaction nor lead to tumor growth in monkeys or mice [40]. Autologous iPSCs were created from the patient's skin cells and then differentiated into RPE so that they would grow in a monolayer without the use of synthetic scaffolds or matrices. To achieve this, iPSC-RPE were seeded onto type I collagen gel on a Transwell insert. After the RPE reached confluence, collagenase was applied to dissolve the collagen gel and leave a sheet of RPE. A 1.3 millimeter by 3.0 millimeter cut of this sheet was then grafted into the patient's retina following excision of her existing damaged RPE.

This marks the first clinical trial on humans using iPSCs. The safety and feasibility of using iPSCs from patients to treat their blindness is still being established, but this trial holds great potential for the advancement of translational medicine in retinal disease.

4. Future Directions

Patient-specific iPSCs have been shown to not only complement animal models of human disease, but also function as an excellent model in their own right. Patient-specific cell lines created from somatic cells from patients with inherited eye diseases can: (i) provide a window for testing the efficacy of gene or drug-based therapies; (ii) elucidate previously unknown mechanisms and pathways of disease; (iii) demonstrate the pathogenicity of unusual mutations in individual patients; and (iv) enable researchers to optimize parameters for successful cell replacement therapy *in vitro*. Skin-derived iPSCs can be used to investigate the function or dysfunction of a mutant gene product in tissues such as retina that are inaccessible to molecular analysis in living patients [41]. Finally, gene therapy tools such as ZFNs, TALENs, and the CRISPR-Cas system are rapidly improving the prospects of restoring the function of diseased RPE from patients with inherited retinal diseases. These patient-specific iPS-RPE, after undergoing gene therapy, can be optimized to become transplantable retinal cells, with the goal of restoring sight to patients with no other therapeutic options.

However, despite these advances, improvements still must be made in reprogramming, differentiation, and cell characterization protocols before employing this technology in clinical transplantation trials. In moving from animal models to human trials, potential safety issues must be carefully addressed. The use of potent oncogenic transgenes such as c-myc and Klf4 in the reprogramming process as outlined by Yamanaka is one area of concern [16]. If these transgenes are not silenced or are reactivated after reprogramming, genomic instability may result and not only confound results of disease modeling studies but also cause tumor formation after transplantation. To this end, iPS reprogramming protocols are still being optimized. An alternative reprogramming protocol by Yu *et al.* obviates the use of oncogenic transgenes by using a combination of Oct4, Sox2, Nanog, and Lin28 [42]. The methodology for generating iPSCs has markedly improved and now integration-free iPSCs, without transgene insertion in the host genome, can be obtained using plasmid vectors, RNA viruses, or mature microRNAs [43–47]. Integration-free iPSCs appear ideal since exogenous genes integrated in the host genome may affect the genetic properties of the iPSCs generated and thus modify the resulting cellular phenotypes of differentiated progeny. Additional studies are also required to ensure that the risk of rejection is significantly reduced in patient-specific iPSCs, given that immune rejection when certain tissues derived from iPSCs were transplanted into syngeneic murine hosts have been reported [26].

ESCs are still the gold standard for *in vitro* pluripotency. A significant concern of using iPSCs in development of therapies is still whether they are truly equivalent to ESCs. For example, key differences between iPSCs and ESCs in transcribed genes, epigenetic landscape, differentiation potential, mutational load, and premature senescence has been described [48]. If iPSCs cannot closely replicate ESCs, the results from studies using iPSCs must be interpreted with this in mind. Significant differences between iPSCs and ESCs may hinder the translation of study results from an *in vitro* iPSC-based disease model to human disease.

A further step likely to accelerate the integration of iPS technology in regenerative medicine is the development of industry and biotechnology collaboration in order to develop large-scale stem cell production [49]. In this way, availability of iPS-based technology will increase, making them more widespread in investigative and translational studies in the future. Patient-specific iPS-derived cells offer the hope of slowing progression or improving visual function for patients with currently untreatable retinal diseases. In addition to curing blindness, stem cell transplantation in the eye can also be seen as a model system for investigating cell-based treatments for other degenerative disorders of the CNS.

5. Conclusions

Stem cells have revolutionized the field of human cell culture because they provide an immortal population of pluripotent cells which can theoretically differentiate into any cell type in the body. This technology, when applied to retinal cells, has the promise to make significant contributions to our understanding of the most pressing blinding diseases of our time. Stem cells also allow for the development of therapies for exceedingly rare retinal conditions which currently have little to no funding for research. In particular, patient-specific iPSCs represent an excellent tool for modeling retinal disease since they can be generated from adult somatic cells, thus avoiding the ethical considerations involved with using embryonic stem cells. iPSCs will continue to be a sustainable method to model disease as gene therapies, drug therapies, and transplantable retinal cells continue to be developed for inherited retinal disorders.

Acknowledgments

Stephen H. Tsang is a member of the RD-CURE Consortium and is supported by Tistou and Charlotte Kerstan Foundation, NIH R01EY018213, the Research to Prevent Blindness Physician-Scientist Award, the Schneeweiss Stem Cell Fund, New York State (N09G-302 and N13G-275), and the Foundation Fighting Blindness New York Regional Research Center Grant (C-NY05-0705-0312), the Joel Hoffman Fund, Gale and Richard Siegel Stem Cell Fund, Charles Culpeper Scholarship, Laszlo Bito and Olivia Carino Foundation, Irma T. Hirschl Charitable Trust, Bernard and Anne Spitzer Stem Cell Fund, Gertrude Rothschild Stem Cell Foundation, and Gebroe Family Foundation. Huy V. Nguyen is supported by the RPB Medical Student Fellowship.

Author Contributions

Huy V. Nguyen, Yao Li and Stephen H. Tsang performed research and wrote the paper.

Conflicts of Interest

The authors declare no conflict of interest.

References

1. Rosenfeld, P.J.; Brown, D.M.; Heier, J.S.; Boyer, D.S.; Kaiser, P.K.; Chung, C.Y.; Kim, R.Y. Ranibizumab for neovascular age-related macular degeneration. *N. Engl. J. Med.* **2006**, *355*, 1419–1431.

2. Phillips, C.O.; Higginbotham, E.J. Multivitamin supplements, ageing, and loss of vision: Seeing through the shadows. *Arch. Intern. Med.* **2009**, *169*, 1180–1182.

3. Zhang, Y.; Klassen, H.J.; Tucker, B.A.; Perez, M.T.-R.; Young, M.J. CNS progenitor cells promote a permissive environment for neurite outgrowth via a matrix metalloproteinase-2-dependent mechanism. *J. Neurosci.* **2007**, *27*, 4499–4506.

4. Wang, N.-K.; Tosi, J.; Kasanuki, J.M.; Chou, C.L.; Jian, K.; Parmalee, N. Transplantation of reprogrammed embryonic stem cells improves visual function in a mouse model for retinitis pigmentosa. *Transplantation* **2010**, *89*, 911–919.

5. Schwartz, S.D.; Hubschman, J.-P.; Heilwell, G.; Franco-Cardenas, V.; Pan, C.K.; Ostrick, R.M.; Mickunas, E.; Gay, R.; Klimanskaya, I.; Lanza, R. Embryonic stem cell trials for macular degeneration: A preliminary report. *Lancet* **2012**, *379*, 713–720.

6. Nakano, T.; Ando, S.; Takata, N.; Kawada, M.; Muguruma, K.; Sekiguchi, K.; Saito, K.; Yonemura, S.; Eiraku, M.; Sasai, Y. Self-formation of optic cups and storable stratified neural retina from human ESCs. *Cell Stem Cell* **2012**, *10*, 771–785.

7. Phillips, M.J.; Wallace, K.A.; Dickerson, S.J.; Miller, M.J.; Verhoeven, A.D.; Martin, J.M.; Wright, L.S.; Shen, W.; Capowski, E.E.; Percin, E.F.; *et al.* Blood-derived human iPS cells generate optic vesicle-like structures with the capacity to form retinal laminae and develop synapses. *Investig. Ophthalmol. Vis. Sci.* **2012**, *53*, 2007–2019.

8. Minegishi, Y.; Iejima, D.; Kobayashi, H.; Chi, Z.-L.; Kawase, K.; Yamamoto, T.; Seki, T.; Yuasa, S.; Fukuda, K.; Iwata, T. Enhanced optineurin E50K-TBK1 interaction evokes protein insolubility and initiates familial primary open-angle glaucoma. *Hum. Mol. Genet.* **2013**, *22*, 3559–3567.

9. Tucker, B.A.; Solivan-Timpe, F.; Roos, B.R.; Anfinson, K.R.; Robin, A.L.; Wiley, L.A.; Mullins, R.F.; Fingert, J.H. Duplication of TBK1 Stimulates Autophagy in iPSC-derived Retinal Cells from a Patient with Normal Tension Glaucoma. *J. Stem Cell Res. Ther.* **2014**, *3*, doi:10.4172/2157-7633.1000161.

10. Li, Y.; Tsai, Y.T.; Hsu, C.W.; Erol, D.; Yang, J.; Wu, W.H.; Davis, R.J.; Egli, D.; Tsang, S.H. Long-term safety and efficacy of human-induced pluripotent stem cell (iPS) grafts in a preclinical model of retinitis pigmentosa. *Mol. Med.* **2012**, *18*, 1312–1319.

11. Tsuji, O.; Miura, K.; Okada, Y.; Fujiyoshi, K.; Mukaino, M.; Nagoshi, N.; Kitamur, K.; Kumagai, G.; Nishino, M.; Tomisato, S.; *et al.* Therapeutic potential of appropriately evaluated safe-induced pluripotent stem cells for spinal cord injury. *Proc. Natl. Acad. Sci. USA* **2010**, *107*, 12704–12709.

12. Yang, J.; Li, Y.; Chan, L.; Tsai, Y.T.; Wu, W.H.; Nguyen, H.V.; Hsu, C.W.; Li, X.; Brown, L.M.; Egli, D.; *et al.* Validation of genome-wide association study (GWAS)-identified disease risk alleles with patient-specific stem cell lines. *Hum. Mol. Genet.* **2014**, *23*, 3445–3455.

13. Singh, R.; Shen, W.; Kuai, D.; Martin, J.M.; Guo, X.; Smith, M.A.; Perez, E.T.; Phillips, M.J.; Simonett, J.M.; Wallace, K.A.; *et al.* iPS cell modeling of Best disease: Insights into the pathophysiology of an inherited macular degeneration. *Hum. Mol. Genet.* **2013**, *22*, 593–607.

14. Jin, Z.-B.; Okamoto, S.; Osakada, F.; Homma, K.; Assawachananont, J.; Hirami, Y.; Iwata, T.; Takahashi, M. Modeling retinal degeneration using patient-specific induced pluripotent stem cells. *PLoS ONE* **2011**, *6*, e17084.

15. Lustremant, C.; Habeler, W.; Plancheron, A.; Goureau, O.; Grenot, L.; de la Grange, P.; Audo, I.; Nandrot, E.F.; Monville, C. Human induced pluripotent stem cells as a tool to model a form of Leber congenital amaurosis. *Cell. Reprogram.* **2013**, *15*, 233–246.

16. Takahashi, K.; Tanabe, K.; Ohnuki, M.; Ohnuki, M.; Narita, M.; Ichisaka, T.; Tomoda, K.; Yamanaka, S. Induction of pluripotent stem cells from adult human fibroblasts by defined factors. *Cell* **2007**, *131*, 861–872.

17. Idelson, M.; Alper, R.; Obolensky, A.; Ben-Shushan, E.; Hemo, I.; Yachimovich-Cohen, N.; Khaner, H.; Smith, Y.; Wiser, O.; Gropp, M.; *et al.* Directed differentiation of human embryonic stem cells into functional retinal pigment epithelium cells. *Cell Stem Cell* **2009**, *5*, 396–408.

18. Sonoda, S.; Spee, C.; Barron, E.; Ryan, S.J.; Kannan, R.; Hinton, D.R. A protocol for the culture and differentiation of highly polarized human retinal pigment epithelial cells. *Nat. Protoc.* **2009**, *4*, 662–673.

19. Rutar, M.; Provis, J.M.; Valter, K. Brief exposure to damaging light causes focal recruitment of macrophages, and long-term destabilization of photoreceptors in the albino rat retina. *Curr. Eye Res.* **2010**, *35*, 631–643.

20. Chinnery, H.R.; McLenachan, S.; Humphries, T.; Kezic, J.M.; Chen, X.; Ruitenberg, M.J.; McMenamin, P.G. Accumulation of murine subretinal macrophages: Effects of age, pigmentation and CX3CR1. *Neurobiol. Aging* **2012**, *33*, 1769–1776.

21. Cyranoski, D. Stem cells cruise to clinic. *Nature* **2013**, *494*, 413.

22. Carr, A.-J.; Vugler, A.A.; Hikita, S.T.; Lawrence, J.M.; Gias, C.; Chen, L.L.; Buchholz, D.E.; Ahmado, A.; Semo, M.; Smart, M.J.K.; *et al.* Protective effects of human iPS-derived retinal pigment epithelium cell transplantation in the retinal dystrophic rat. *PLoS ONE* **2009**, *4*, e8152.

23. Jin, M.; Li, S.; Moghrabi, W.N.; Sun, H.; Travis, G.H. Rpe65 is the retinoid isomerase in bovine retinal pigment epithelium. *Cell* **2005**, *122*, 449–459.

24. Kameya, S.; Hawes, N.L.; Chang, B.; Heckenlively, J.R.; Naggert, J.K.; Nishina, P.M. Mfrp, a gene encoding a frizzled related protein, is mutated in the mouse retinal degeneration 6. *Hum. Mol. Genet.* **2002**, *11*, 1879–1886.

25. Li, Y.; Wu, W.-H.; Hsu, C.-W.; Nguyen, H.V.; Tsai, Y.T.; Chan, L.; Nagasaki, T.; Maumenee, I.H.; Yannuzzi, L.A.; Hoang, Q.V.; *et al.* Gene Therapy in Patient-specific Stem Cell Lines and a Preclinical Model of Retinitis Pigmentosa With Membrane Frizzled-related Protein Defects. *Mol Ther.* **2014**, *22*, 1688–1697.

26. Zhao, T.; Zhang, Z.-N.; Rong, Z.; Xu, Y. Immunogenicity of induced pluripotent stem cells. *Nature* **2011**, *474*, 212–215.

27. Guha, P.; Morgan, J.W.; Mostoslavsky, G.; Rodrigues, N.P.; Boyd, A.S. Lack of immune response to differentiated cells derived from syngeneic induced pluripotent stem cells. *Cell Stem Cell* **2013**, *12*, 407–412.

28. Liu, Z.; Wen, X.; Wang, H.; Zhou, J.; Zhao, M.; Lin, Q.; Wang, Y.; Li, J.; Li, D.; Du, Z.; *et al.* Molecular imaging of induced pluripotent stem cell immunogenicity with *in vivo* development in ischemic myocardium. *PLoS ONE* **2013**, *8*, e66369.

29. Morizane, A.; Doi, D.; Kikuchi, T.; Okita, K.; Hotta, A.; Kawasaki, T.; Hayashi, T.; Onoe, H.; Shiina, T.; Yamanaka, S.; *et al.* Direct comparison of autologous and allogeneic transplantation of iPSC-derived neural cells in the brain of a non-human primate. *Stem Cell Rep.* **2013**, *1*, 283–292.

30. Okamoto, S.; Takahashi, M. Induction of retinal pigment epithelial cells from monkey iPS cells. *Investig. Ophthalmol. Vis. Sci.* **2011**, *52*, 8785–8790.

31. Zwaka, T.P.; Thomson, J.A. Homologous Recombination in Human Embryonic Stem Cells. *Nat. Biotechnol.* **2003**, *21*, 319–321.

32. Vasireddy, V.; Mills, J.A.; Gaddameedi, R.; Basner-Tschakarjan, E.; Kohnke, M.; Black, A.D.; Alexandrov, K.; Zhou, S.; Maguire, A.M.; Chung, D.C.; *et al.* AAV-mediated gene therapy for choroideremia: Preclinical studies in personalized models. *PLoS ONE* **2013**, *8*, e61396.

33. Zou, J.; Maeder, M.L.; Mali, P.; Pruett-Miller, S.M.; Thibodeau-Beganny, S.; Chou, B.K.; Chen, G.; Ye, Z.; Park, I.H.; Daley, G.Q.; *et al.* Gene targeting of a disease-related gene in human induced pluripotent stem and embryonic stem cells. *Cell Stem Cell* **2009**, *5*, 97–110.

34. Tucker, B.A.; Mullins, R.F.; Stone, E.M. Stem cells for investigation and treatment of inherited retinal disease. *Hum. Mol. Genet.* **2014**, *23*, R9–R16.

35. Mali, P.; Yang, L.; Esvelt, K.M.; JAach; Guell, M.; DiCarlo, J.E.; Norville, J.E.; Church, G.M. RNA-guided human genome engineering via Cas9. *Science* **2013**, *339*, 823–826.

36. Hou, Z.; Zhang, Y.; Propson, N.E.; Howden, S.E.; Chu, L.-F.; Sontheimer, E.J.; Thomson, J.A. Efficient genome engineering in human pluripotent stem cells using Cas9 from Neisseria meningitidis. *Proc. Natl. Acad. Sci. USA* **2013**, *110*, 15644–15649.

37. Fu, Y.; Foden, J.A.; Khayter, C.; Maeder, M.L.; Reyon, D.; Joung, J.K.; Sander, J.D. High-frequency off-target mutagenesis induced by CRISPR-Cas nucleases in human cells. *Nat. Biotechnol.* **2013**, *31*, 822–826.

38. Ran, F.A.; Hsu, P.D.; Lin, C.-Y.; Gootenberg, J.S.; Konermann, S.; Trevino, A.E.; Scott, D.A.; Inoue, A.; Matoba, S.; Zhang, Y.; *et al.* Double nicking by RNA-guided CRISPR Cas9 for enhanced genome editing specificity. *Cell* **2013**, *154*, 1380–1389.

39. Cereso, N.; Pequignot, M.O.; Robert, L.; Becker, F.; de Luca, V.; Nabholz, N.; Rigau, V.; de Vos, J.; Hamel, C.P.; Kalatzis, V. Proof of concept for AAV2/5-mediated gene therapy in iPSC-derived retinal pigment epithelium of a choroideremia patient. *Mol. Ther. Methods Clin. Dev.* **2014**, *1*, doi:10.1038/mtm.2014.11.

40. Kamao, H.; Mandai, M.; Okamoto, S.; Sakai, N.; Suga, A.; Sugita, S.; Kiryu, J.; Takahashi, M. Characterization of human induced pluripotent stem cell-derived retinal pigment epithelium cell sheets aiming for clinical application. *Stem Cell Rep.* **2014**, *2*, 205–218.

41. Tucker, B.A.; Scheetz, T.E.; Mullins, R.F.; DeLuca, A.P.; Hoffmann, J.M.; Johnston, R.M.; Jacobson, S.G.; Sheffield, V.C.; Stone, E.M. Exome sequencing and analysis of induced pluripotent stem cells identify the cilia-related gene male germ cell-associated kinase (MAK) as a cause of retinitis pigmentosa. *Proc. Natl. Acad. Sci. USA* **2011**, *108*, E569–E576.

42. Yu, J.; Vodyanik, M.A.; Smuga-Otto, K.; Antosiewicz-Bourget, J.; Frane, J.L.; Tian, S.; Nie, J.; Jonsdottir, G.A.; Ruotti, V.; Stewart, R.; *et al.* Induced pluripotent stem cell lines derived from human somatic cells. *Science* **2007**, *318*, 1917–1920.

43. Ban, H.; Nishishita, N.; Fusaki, N.; Tabata, T.; Saeki, K.; Shikamura, M.; Takada, N.; Inoue, M.; Hasegawa, M.; Kawamata, S.; *et al.* Efficient generation of transgene-free human induced pluripotent stem cells (iPSCs) by temperature-sensitive Sendai virus vectors. *Proc. Natl. Acad. Sci. USA* **2011**, *108*, 14234–14239.

44. Warren, L.; Manos, P.D.; Ahfeldt, T.; Loh, Y.H.; Li, H.; Lau, F.; Ebina, W.; Mandal, P.K.; Smith, Z.D.; Meissner, A.; *et al.* Highly efficient reprogramming to pluripotency and directed differentiation of human cells with synthetic modified mRNA. *Cell Stem Cell* **2010**, *7*, 618–630.

45. Yu, J.; Hu, K.; Smuga-Otto, K.; Tian, S.; Stewart, R.; Slukvin, I.I.; Thomson, J.A. Human induced pluripotent stem cells free of vector and transgene sequences. *Science* **2009**, *324*, 797–801.

46. Miyoshi, N.; Ishii, H.; Nagano, H.; Haraguchi, N.; Dewi, D.L.; Kano, Y.; Nishikawa, S.; Tanemura, M.; Mimori, K.; Tanaka, F.; *et al.* Reprogramming of mouse and human cells to pluripotency using mature microRNAs. *Cell Stem Cell* **2011**, *8*, 633–638.

47. Kim, D.; Kim, C.-H.; Moon, J.-I.; Chung, Y.-G.; Chang, M.-Y.; Han, B.-S.; Ko, S.; Yang, E.; Cha, K.Y.; Lanza, R.; *et al.* Generation of human induced pluripotent stem cells by direct delivery of reprogramming proteins. *Cell Stem Cell* **2009**, *4*, 472–476.

48. Bilic, J.; Izpisua Belmonte, J.C. Concise review: Induced pluripotent stem cells *versus* embryonic stem cells: Close enough or yet too far apart? *Stem Cells* **2012**, *30*, 33–41.

49. Borooah, S.; Phillips, M.J.; Bilican, B.; Wright, A.F.; Wilmut, I.; Chandran, S.; Gamm, D.; Dhillon, B. Using human induced pluripotent stem cells to treat retinal disease. *Prog. Retin. Eye Res.* **2013**, *37*, 163–181.

Potential Role of Induced Pluripotent Stem Cells (IPSCs) for Cell-Based Therapy of the Ocular Surface

Ricardo P. Casaroli-Marano, Núria Nieto-Nicolau, Eva M. Martínez-Conesa, Michael Edel and Ana B. Álvarez-Palomo

Abstract: The integrity and normal function of the corneal epithelium are crucial for maintaining the cornea's transparency and vision. The existence of a cell population with progenitor characteristics in the limbus maintains a dynamic of constant epithelial repair and renewal. Currently, cell-based therapies for bio replacement—cultured limbal epithelial transplantation (CLET) and cultured oral mucosal epithelial transplantation (COMET)—present very encouraging clinical results for treating limbal stem cell deficiency (LSCD) and restoring vision. Another emerging therapeutic approach consists of obtaining and implementing human progenitor cells of different origins in association with tissue engineering methods. The development of cell-based therapies using stem cells, such as human adult mesenchymal or induced pluripotent stem cells (IPSCs), represent a significant breakthrough in the treatment of certain eye diseases, offering a more rational, less invasive, and better physiological treatment option in regenerative medicine for the ocular surface. This review will focus on the main concepts of cell-based therapies for the ocular surface and the future use of IPSCs to treat LSCD.

Reprinted from *J. Clin. Med.* Cite as: Casaroli-Marano, R.P.; Nieto-Nicolau, N.; Martínez-Conesa, E.M.; Edel, M.; Álvarez-Palomo, A.B. Potential Role of Induced Pluripotent Stem Cells (IPSCs) for Cell-Based Therapy of the Ocular Surface. *J. Clin. Med.* **2015**, *4*, 318–342.

1. Introduction

The ocular surface is mainly composed of the cornea and the conjunctiva with their epithelia. The cornea is the primary refractive element at the anterior surface of the eye that is responsible for approximately two-thirds of its total optical power. Basically, the cornea is composed of five well-defined layers (Figure 1). It consists of an outermost stratified, squamous and non-keratinized epithelial layer (corneal epithelium) limited posteriorly by Bowman's layer. The underlying stroma, which accounts for about 90% of the middle thickness of the cornea, comprises aligned arrays of collagen fibrils interspersed with cellular components (keratocytes) and it is this highly organized arrangement of lamellae that is responsible for the cornea's transparency. The stroma is separated from the endothelial layer (corneal endothelium) by Descemet's membrane, which acts as a basement membrane for these endothelial cells. The corneal endothelium is a single cuboidal layer of metabolically active cells that are in direct contact with the aqueous humor in the anterior chamber. These cells help to maintain corneal transparency by actively pumping water out of the stroma [1]. The corneal epithelium has a key role in keeping the cornea transparent and free of blood vessels and, to this end, presents permanent repair phenomena essential for the conservation of the cornea's physiology [1–3]. The homeostasis of the corneal epithelium is crucial to maintaining the structural integrity of the ocular surface, the transparency of the cornea and visual function.

1.1. Limbal Stem Cells

It has been observed that progenitor cells responsible for the continual renewal of the corneal epithelium are located in the basal layers of the sclerocorneal limbus. The human limbus—the circumferential anatomic area (approximately 1.5 mm wide) that separates the clear cornea from the opaque sclera, which is covered by conjunctiva—serves as the "reservoir" for the stem cells and also provides a barrier to the overgrowth of conjunctival epithelial cells and its blood vessels onto the cornea [1–3] (Figure 1). Due to their particularities, the *limbal stem cells* (LSCs) have a crucial role in maintaining the integrity and in the renewal events of corneal epithelium. Their main features are highlighted: it is their behavior as oligopotent progenitor cells, with high nuclear-cytoplasmic ratio a slow cell cycle, and a high proliferative potential that adds its great capacity for self-renewal by asymmetric division [3–5]. In the limbus, it is possible to identify several cell subpopulations of different progenies (typical progenitors and amplifying cells at different stages of differentiation), melanocytes, antigen-presenting and mesenchymal cells, vascular elements and nerve endings that form a specialized and unique environment called *niche*. This particular microenvironment is considered responsible for the proliferative and self-renewal cellular characteristics of the limbal region [2,3,6]. The LSC niche is an anatomically defined area that is thought to provide a variety of factors, such as physical protection, survival factors and cytokines and is deemed essential to the maintenance of the "stemness" of the stem cell population while preventing entry into differentiation [2,6]. Within the niche, LSCs maintenance and function are controlled in a particular environment by several elements, including extracellular matrix components, cell adhesion molecules, and growth and survival factors secreted by stromal fibroblasts, mesenchymal stem cells and blood capillaries [6]. To date, four limbal anatomic structures have been proposed as the corneal stem cell niche [2,6], Palisades of Vogt, limbal epithelial crypts [7], limbal crypts and focal stromal projections [8].

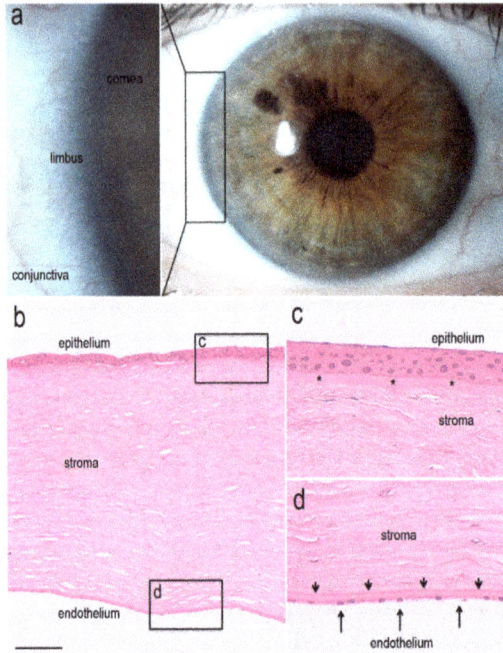

Figure 1. The corneal limbus is the circumferential anatomic area, approximately 1.5 mm wide, which separates the clear cornea from the opaque sclera (**a**); The limbal region represents the "reservoir" for LSCs in the ocular surface. In a cross-section of the human cornea stained with hematoxylin-eosin, (**b**) to (**d**), details of its main layers can be observed. The cornea is composed of a stratified non-keratinized squamous epithelial layer (epithelium), the stroma and an endothelial cuboidal layer (endothelium) (**b**); The corneal epithelium (48 to 55 μm thick) consists of the outermost layer, which presents five to seven stratified cell layers (**c**), limited posteriorly by Bowman's layer (10 to 12 μm thick; c, asterisk). The stroma (480 to 510 μm thick; b), composed of compacted collagen lamellae and keratocytes (c and d), offers transparency and scaffolding to maintain the shape of the cornea in its middle portion. The stroma is separated from the endothelium (about 5 μm thick; d, large arrows) by Descemet's membrane (8 to 10 μm thick; d, narrow arrows), which acts as a basement membrane for the corneal endothelial cells (**d**). Bar = 150 μm for b; Bar = 25 μm for c and d.

1.2. Renewal of Corneal Epithelium

It has been shown that cell subpopulations with progenitor features, located in the deeper basal layers of the corneal epithelium, have the capacity to differentiate into post-mitotic cell populations located in the outermost epithelial layers. This continuous centripetal movement (the XYZ hypothesis)—from the peripheral deeper epithelial layers to the more central outermost layers—ensures constant renewal of the corneal epithelium and maintains its integrity [1–6,9]. The X component represents the anterior migration from cells of the basal epithelium of the limbal region, the Y component represents the centripetal migration of cells from the limbus, and the Z component represents the desquamation from the surface of corneal epithelium. However, this XYZ theory has recently been challenged by evidence in the mouse and other mammals suggesting that uninjured cells in the central cornea can generate holoclones with characteristics of stem cells, presenting regenerative epithelial capabilities, which may also be responsible for the maintenance of the corneal epithelium [10]. Also, in support of these controversial findings, the presence of central islands of normal corneal epithelial cells has been described in patients with apparently complete clinical absence of LSCs [11]. These interesting observations may have the following interpretation: the central basal epithelial cells of the surviving corneal epithelium present the capability to regenerate, or some LSCs remain and contribute to the maintenance of the central epithelium.

1.3. Limbal Stem Cell Multipotency

An *in vitro* study of the clonogenic capacity of epithelial cells located in the ocular limbal region revealed a progenitor cell system stratified into levels (cellular stages or "compartments") [2,6,12]. Undifferentiated small cells presenting progenitor cell features with high self-renewal capacity are found in the first compartment but they lose these characteristics as they migrate through the following compartments. Lastly, the final level contains a cell population with terminal differentiation features associated with little or no self-renewal capability. The latter cells, once their epithelial differentiation events are completed, lose their ability to self-renew and are incorporated as corneal epithelial cells on the surface of the central cornea. In this regard, some studies [12,13] concluded that epithelial cells of the limbal region can form holoclones with higher clonogenic potential, in contrast to epithelial cells from the central cornea. In addition, epithelial cells isolated from basal layers in the limbal region exhibit a high proliferative potential *in vitro* during expansion or in response to corneal injury [14], and show an undifferentiated phenotype lacking the expression of differentiated corneal cell markers such as cytokeratins 3 and 12 [15]. They have also been shown to retain labeled precursors of DNA for an extended time, in contrast to more differentiated cells that quickly lose them due a higher division rate [16]. This lack of differentiation and slow cell cycling are characteristics of the quiescent state of stem cells.

2. Limbal Stem Cell Deficiency (LSCD)

The disappearance, reduction or functional impairment of LSCs may produce a clinical state (limbal stem cell deficiency, LSCD) that can give rise to significant changes in the ocular surface. These changes include the occurrence of persistent corneal defects, epithelial keratinization, conjunctivalization phenomena with the development of newly formed vessels in the corneal tissue, and scarring. All this compromises the corneal physiology, reducing transparency and decreasing vision [1–5]. The presence of a complete loss of the corneal-limbal epithelium leads to a reactive reepithelialization by conjunctival cells, which have a high proliferative capacity. This event is followed by neovascularization, chronic inflammation with scarring of corneal stroma, causing a pronounced decrease in vision and severe discomfort (Figure 2). Furthermore, the chronic inflammatory condition not only leads to the death of more LSCs but also leaves the surviving epithelial cells unable to function properly, explaining the worsening of clinical symptoms and features over time [17–24]. In patients with severe lacrimal dysfunction syndrome (dry eye) suffering from LSCD, the conjunctival epithelium that replaced the corneal epithelium (conjunctivalization) becomes partially or totally keratinized [18,21,22,24]. Several processes and diseases (Table 1) may lead to unilateral or bilateral LSCD, and depending on its extent, the disorder can be classified as either partial or total. Chemical burns (alkalis and acids) are, however, the most frequent cause of limbal ischemia and epithelial destruction causing the loss and/or impairment of LSCs function, and are the main indication for cell-based therapy approaches [18–24].

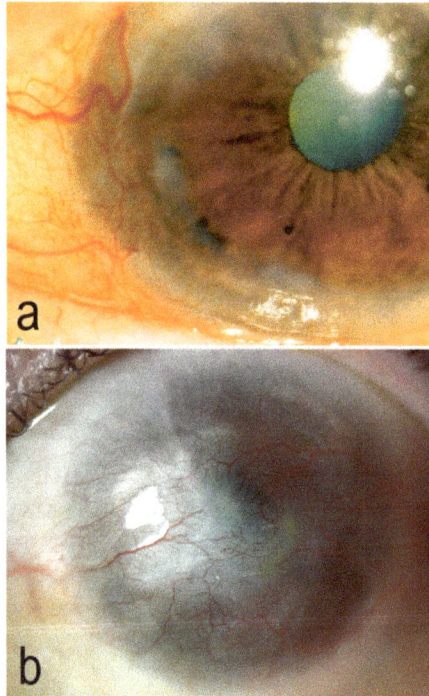

Figure 2. Clinical findings related to Limbal Stem Cell Deficiency (LSCD). Limbal deficiency secondary to ocular cicatricial pemphigoid with the presence of peripheral newly formed vessels leading to a loss of corneal transparency (**a**); Limbal deficiency, secondary to a chemical burn (bleach) of the ocular surface leads to a corneal conjuntivalization and neovascularization with loss of transparency (**b**). LSCD can be treated with cell therapy techniques such as cultured limbal epithelial transplantation (CLET) or cultured oral mucosal epithelial transplantation (COMET).

Table 1. Main etiologies and pathological conditions for primary and secondary Limbal Stem Cell Deficiency (LSCD).

Etiology	Ocular Pathology
Idiopathic	-
Hereditary	Aniridia
	Autosomal dominant keratitis
	Gelatinous drop-like corneal dystrophy
	Iris coloboma
	Xeroderma pigmentosa
	Epidermolysis bullosa
	Dyskeratosis congenita
	Ectodermic dysplasia
	Multiple endocrine neoplasia
	Polyglandular autoimmune syndromes
Neoplasic	Intraepithelial neoplasia
	Conjuntival tumors (melanoma)
	Limbal dermoid
Degenerative	Recurrent pterygium
	Salzmann nodular corneal dystrophy
Infections	Severe infeccious keratitis
	Chlamydia conjunctivitis
Mechanical	Alkali, acid, thermal burns
	Bullous keratopathy
	Tumor excision
	Cryotherapy, radioterapy
	Systemic and local chemotherapy (MMC, 5FU)
	UV radition
	Phototherapeutic keratectomy
Anoxic	Contact lenses misuse or prolonged use
Trophic	Neurotrophic keratopathy
Inflammation	Superior limbic keratoconjunctivitis
	Collagen diseases related ulcers
	Mooren ulcer
	Atopic keratoconjunctivitis
	Ocular pemphigoid
	Ocular rosacea
	Stevens-Johnson syndrome
	Graft-versus-host disease
	Vitamin A deficiency

MMC, mitomycin-C; 5FU, 5-fluorouracil; UV, ultra-violet.

2.1. Cell-Based Treatments for LSCD

The concept of ocular surface reconstruction was introduced with the application of autologous conjunctiva for unilateral ocular chemical alkali burns [25]. Since then, several surgical approaches have been developed with the aim of restoring the corneal epithelium on the diseased ocular surface. In recent decades, limbal transplantation techniques using auto or allografts have been introduced as bio-replacement approaches for limbal tissues to improve and reconstruct the altered ocular surface [5]. Building on previous experience treating patients with large surface areas of burned skin, the epithelial cells of the ocular surface have been obtained by cell culture techniques for *ex vivo* expansion. Subsequently, the ocular surface was successfully reconstructed by using LSCs in patients with severe unilateral ocular surface pathology [17]. Since then, various translational approaches have been developed and optimized, with satisfactory long-term clinical results [18–23].

Treatment approaches for LSCD can be divided into three main categories [4,5,23,24]: (a) transplants and bio-replacement of tissue; (b) cell-based therapy by *ex vivo* cell culture expansion; and (c) symptomatic and alternative treatment: keratoprosthesis implantation, provisional debridement of conjunctival corneal tissue, therapeutic contact lenses and drug (steroids, anti-angiogenic drugs, tear substitutes, autologous serum) therapy [5].

Ex vivo expansion of LSCs is the most innovative approach for ocular surface bio-replacement (CLET: cultured limbal epithelial transplantation). From a minimally invasive biopsy (1–2 mm^2) of the healthy limbal region (the same or the contralateral eye), an explant culture technique can be applied on a suitable substrate (such as the amniotic membrane) or by separating the epithelial layer from the fragment obtained by enzymatic treatment [19,21,22,26–29]. In the latter approach, the cells obtained are *in vitro* co-cultured on feeder-layers (3T3 murine fibroblasts growth arrested by irradiation or mitomycin-C). Once cell growth is achieved, the cell suspensions are transferred to suitable substrates, such as fibrin, collagen or biocompatible polymers. The bio-replacement is carried out after removal of most of the diseased tissue from the ocular surface [17–21]. This methodology has many advantages over the tissue transplantation techniques used to date: essentially, it requires a substantially smaller limbal biopsy, which reduces the risk of limbal deficiency in healthy donor tissue. Its other advantages include a final high cell population that is more efficiently selected, homogeneous and, theoretically, more enriched with progenitor characteristic cells [26–29]. However, enzymatic techniques involve a more complex approach, with additional manipulation of the tissue and the need for xenoproducts at different stages of cell culture production. For its part, the explant technique has certain advantages—among them its technical simplicity, the lack of xenoproducts and its cost-effectiveness, despite the heterogeneity of the cell population cultured (sclera fibroblasts, antigen presenting cells, melanocytes, conjunctival epithelium cells and others) [21,22,26–29]. It is always desirable to use autologous cells for *ex vivo* expansion to avoid the risk of immune response. However, in the presence of severe bilateral ocular pathology, the use of heterologous epithelial cells (from cadaveric or related living donor corneas) is acceptable [18–21]. Autologous oral mucosal epithelia expanded *ex vivo* have also been successfully used as an alternative source of epithelial cells (COMET: cultured oral mucosal epithelial transplantation) [30,31].

The mechanism by which cultured LSCs may restore the ocular surface is still poorly understood. Cells may replace the progenitor population, and/or "reactivate" nonfunctioning host progenitor cells by providing stimuli for growth, or change niche behavior. It has been speculated that there may be "dormant" stem cells despite clinical features of LSCD [11].

Currently, *ex vivo* expansion methods applied in cell-based therapy for clinical application are based mostly on the use of xenogeneic or allogeneic products such as murine cells for feeder layer approaches, fetal calf or bovine serum in culture media, supplements of non-human origin for cell growth and maintenance and the human amniotic membrane as a cell carrier. These products potentially carry a risk for transmitting diseases; they may induce tumorigenesis or precipitate an immunological response in the host [18,20–23,28,29]. They also show idiosyncratic biological variability that may adversely affect the quality of cultured grafts and also the final results after transplantation. Thus, there is currently a special need to investigate options for replacing potentially hazardous xenobiotic materials with others of human origin or xeno-free chemically defined media.

2.2. Alternative Cell Sources for LSCD Treatment

Corneal transplantation (penetrating keratoplasty) is considered the conventional therapy to restore the corneal tissue. However, this technique is not a viable strategy for patients suffering LSCD because it does not replace the LSCs population [32]. Cell-based therapy is the most rational approach for ocular surface bio-replacement, and the ideal cells for corneal reconstruction are autologous corneal LSCs using CLET approach. Minimally invasive biopsy of the limbal tissue from the same patient's healthy eye (unilateral disease) is the preferred method, although this source of progenitor cells is not always available. If both eyes present serious surface damage, the source of healthy LSCs will be lost; COMET is among the current therapeutic alternatives. In fact, therapy for LSCD is also rapidly evolving to include alternative cell types (of autologous or heterologous origin) and clinical approaches as treatment modalities. As a consequence, other strategies, such as the use of mesenchymal stem cells from adult tissue (bone marrow mesenchymal stromal cells or adipose derived stromal cells, among others) for cell regenerative therapy in corneal injuries, are gaining prominence at present. Other sources of cells or stem cells have been tested with regenerative aims in the ocular surface, and may be useful in situations where both eyes are affected although many of them, still without clinical use at present, but which have great translational potential (Table 2).

Table 2. Cell sources for *ex vivo* expansion cell-based therapy to treat Limbal Stem Cell Deficiency (LSCD).

Cell Sources	Application	References
Cultured Limbal Epithelial Cells (CLET)	Clinical application	[17–21]
Cultured Oral Mucosal Epithelial Cells (COMET)	Clinical application	[30,31,33–37]
Cultured Conjunctival Epithelial Cells	Clinical application	[38–41]
Cultured Embryonic Stem Cells	Mice model	[42–45]
Cultured Adult Epidermal Stem Cells	Goat model	[46–48]
Cultured Bone-Marrow Derived Mesenchymal Stem Cells	Rat and rabbit models	[49–53]
Cultured Adipose Derived Mesenchymal Stem Cells	*In vitro* model	[54,55]
Cultured Orbital Fat Mesenchymal Progenitor Cells	Mice model; *in vitro* model	[56–58]
Cultured Immature Dental Pulp Stem Cells	Rabbit model	[59,60]
Cultured Hair Follicle-Derived Stem Cells	Mice model	[61,62]
Cultured Umbilical Cord Stem Cells	Rabbit model	[63,64]

Nevertheless, the application of CLET using human amniotic membrane (hAM) or fibrin gel as a scaffold has been clinically validated and today is the most frequently used cell-based therapy applied at clinical level in ophthalmology [18–21]. Since its introduction [17], it has been used with long-term clinical follow-up periods. Despite many differences between studies regarding inclusion/exclusion criteria, the culture methods applied, transplantation techniques, and clinical outcome measures, the overall success rate of this procedure is around 70% [18,21,23]. On the other hand, oral mucosa has also been shown to be an attractive autologous epithelial cell source for cases of severe bilateral LSCD. COMET has already been used in clinical settings, offering promising long-term results with improved vision in over half of treated patients [30–35]. However, peripheral corneal neovascularization is commonly found with this approach since oral mucosal cells have greater angiogenic potential than limbal epithelial cells [65,66]. It has been suggested that these new-formed vessels may regress following local anti-angiogenic therapy [33–35]. Further studies are needed in this regard to assess the long-term efficacy of COMET technique. In the past five years, several clinical trials have been conducted to test, compare or consolidate the application of other approaches and other sources of progenitor cells for the treatment of LSCD (Table 3).

Table 3. Current cell-based therapy clinical trials for the treatment of Limbal Stem Cell Deficiency (LSCD).

Clinical Trial	Identifier	Phase	Study Characteristics	Cell Source	Situation
Corneal Epithelium Repair and Therapy Using Autologous Limbal Stem Cell Transplantation.	NCT02148016	Phase 1, Phase 2	Open label, Interventional Non-randomized, SGA	Autologous LSCs	Currently recruiting
Multicenter Study of CAOMECS Transplantation to Patients With Total Limbal Stem Cell Deficiency.	NCT01489501	Phase 3	Open label, Interventional Non-randomized, SGA	Autologous OMC	Not yet open
The Improvement of Limbal Epithelial Culture Technique by Using Collagenase to Isolate Limbal Stem Cells.	NCT02202642	Phase 1	Open label, Interventional Non-randomized, SGA	Autologous LSCs	Currently recruiting
Autologous Transplantation of Cultivated Limbal Stem Cells on Amniotic Membrane in Limbal Stem Cell Deficiency (LSD) Patients.	NCT00736307	Phase 1, Phase 2	Open label, Interventional Non-randomized, SGA	Autologous LSCs	Completed

Table 3. *Cont.*

Clinical Trial	Identifier	Phase	Study Characteristics	Cell Source	Situation
Clinical Trial on the Effect of Autologous Oral Mucosal Epithelial Sheet Transplantation.	NCT02149732	Phase 1, Phase 2	Open label, Interventional Non-randomized, SGA	Autologous OMEC	Currently recruiting
Cultivated Stem Cell Transplantation for the Treatment of Limbal Stem Cell Deficiency (LECT).	NCT00845117	Phase 1, Phase 2	Open label, Interventional Non-randomized, SGA	Autologous LSCs	Ongoing, but not recruiting
Limbal Epithelial Stem Cell Transplantation: a Phase II Multicenter Trial (MLEC)	NCT02318485	Phase 2	Open label, Interventional Non-randomized, SGA	Allogenic or autologous LSCs	Not yet open
Cell Therapy in Failure Syndromes in Limbal Stem Cells (TC181).	NCT01619189	Phase 2	Single blind, Interventional Non-randomized, SGA	Allogenic or autologous LSCs	Currently recruiting
Autologous Cultured Corneal Epithelium (CECA) for the Treatment of Limbal Stem Cell Deficiency.	NCT01756365	Phase 1, Phase 2	Open label, Interventional Non-randomized, SGA	Autologous cultured corneal epithelium	Enrolling by invitation
Ocular Surface Reconstruction With Cultivated Autologus Mucosal Epithelial Transplantation.	NCT01942421	Phase 2, Phase 3	Open label, Interventional Non-randomized, SGA	Autologous OMEC	Ongoing, but not recruiting
Efficacy of Cultivated Corneal Epithelial Stem Cell for Ocular Surface Reconstruction.	NCT01237600	Phase 2, Phase 3	Open label, Interventional Non-randomized, SGA	Allogenic or autologous LSCs	Completed
Safety Study of Stem Cell Transplant to Treat Limbus Insufficiency Syndrome.	NCT01562002	Phase 1, Phase 2	Double blind, Interventional Randomized, Parallel assignment	Allogenic LSCs *vs.* BM-MSCs	Ongoing, but not recruiting

Table 3. Current cell-based therapy clinical trials for the treatment of Limbal Stem Cell Deficiency (LSCD).

Clinical Trial	Identifier	Phase	Study Characteristics	Cell Source	Situation
Corneal Epithelium Repair and Therapy Using Autologous Limbal Stem Cell Transplantation.	NCT02148016	Phase 1, Phase 2	Open label, Interventional Non-randomized, SGA	Autologous LSCs	Currently recruiting
Multicenter Study of CAOMECS Transplantation to Patients With Total Limbal Stem Cell Deficiency.	NCT01489501	Phase 3	Open label, Interventional Non-randomized, SGA	Autologous OMC	Not yet open
The Improvement of Limbal Epithelial Culture Technique by Using Collagenase to Isolate Limbal Stem Cells.	NCT02202642	Phase 1	Open label, Interventional Non-randomized, SGA	Autologous LSCs	Currently recruiting
Autologous Transplantation of Cultivated Limbal Stem Cells on Amniotic Membrane in Limbal Stem Cell Deficiency (LSD) Patients.	NCT00736307	Phase 1, Phase 2	Open label, Interventional Non-randomized, SGA	Autologous LSCs	Completed

3. IPSCs and Corneal Epithelial Differentiation

As discussed above, adult stem cells make it possible to repair and regenerate damaged epithelial tissue. In general, these cells reside in the basal layer of the epithelium, are able to self-renew continuously, and produce transient amplifying cells (TACs) that differentiate terminally after a brief period of proliferation [68–72]. However, there are limitations to LSCs transplantation therapies. On one hand, for unilateral LSCD, taking biopsies from the healthy eye carries along the risk of damaging the donor eye. On the other hand, for bilateral LSCD, allogenic transplantation presents the risk of immune rejection by the patient. In this sense, induced pluripotent stem cells (IPSCs) can be obtained from minimally invasive sources from the patient himself and be differentiated into LSCs, avoiding immune rejection problems and cell availability. The discovery of IPSCs has been one of the most significant advances in regenerative medicine in the last decade. Overexpression of a specific set of transcription factors (e.g., Oct4, Sox2, c-Myc, and Klf4; or Oct4, Sox2, Lin28 and Nanog) in adult differentiated cells can reprogram cell fate and IPSCs [68–70]. These can be differentiated into various cell types, a property that has opened up a wide range of possibilities for the investigation of cell states, the mechanisms of differentiation, pluripotency and other related cellular identities and behaviors. Contrary to embryonic stem cells, IPSCs can be created from easy access differentiated cells, such as fibroblast or keratinocytes, and allow the creation of autologous sources of different cell types for regenerative therapies or disease modeling.

More recently, direct reprogramming of cells into different states (either pluripotent or somatic) offers one of the most promising approaches in the field of regenerative medicine, with enormous potential for examining clinical and therapeutic applications in more depth [71]. The "direct reprogramming" is characterized by a process wherein mature, fully differentiated somatic cells, can be induced to other cell types without necessarily going through a pluripotent state [71]. To this end, cells can be reprogrammed by transient overexpression of transcriptional factors for a relatively short time interval. The cells in this state are called IPS-partial cells; they respond to different signal environments (e.g., growth factors, cytokines, inductors agents, *etc.*) and have the ability to direct cell fate decisions in reprogramming [71]. For corneal repair direct reprogramming would be of great advantage by not only eliminating the pluripotent stages (potentially carcinogenic) but also avoiding the lengthy production and characterization of IPSC lines. As very few cells are needed for ocular surface cell therapy, the limited expansion capacity of IPSCs is not a limiting factor as well as the production time, which would be much shorter with an easier methodology. However, there are still very limited references to the LSCs production by transdifferentiation from easily accessible adult somatic cells. Rat adult stem cells from the bulge of hair follicle were transdifferentiated into corneal epithelial-like cells by culturing with corneal limbus soluble factors and forced overexpression of the transcripton factor Pax6 [73]. More recently, Sainchanma and colleagues [74] described a method to obtain corneal epithelial-like cells from human skin-derived precursor cells—which present some multipotency markers—by culturing them with three specific growth factors: epidermal growth factor (EGF), keratinocyte growth factor (KGF) and hepatocyte growth factor (HGF) [74]. These are encouraging results to open the way for new sources of LSCs autologous supply. However further work is necessary to refine the protocol to obtain final cells that are closer to LSCs in their marker profiling and their functionality in restoring corneal epithelium should be tested.

3.1. Application of IPSCs for Ocular Pathology

Regarding the application of IPSCs in the field of cell therapy for ocular pathology, IPSCs have shown great promise in treating certain degenerative retinal diseases, particularly those that affect the functionality of the retinal pigment epithelium (RPE) due to its dysfunction or loss. In this context—dry age-related macular degeneration (geographic atrophy)—cell-based therapy may be a rational and effective therapeutic alternative for certain forms of retinitis pigmentosa and gyrate atrophy [75].

The use of stem cell therapy for eye diseases presents many advantages, for a variety of reasons: (a) the intraocular environment benefits from a state of immune privilege; (b) the target tissue to be treated has certain individual anatomical and functional characteristics (defined subretinal space and specialized single stratified epithelium); (c) the intraocular space is small and limited, as is required by the treatment given the low number of cells involved; and (d) the intraocular space is easily controllable by sophisticated diagnostic imaging systems in ophthalmology that allow convenient monitoring with satisfactory clinical follow up—for example, by injection of cells under the subretinal space or into the vitreous body—which permits the visualization of the therapeutic effect and possible complications. For this reason, several recent research studies are being carried out [75–77].

The regeneration of the ocular surface and restoration of corneal transparency following injury is one of the fields where IPSCs may also be applicable. The first attempt to obtain LSC-like cells from pluripotent cells were carried out by Notara and colleagues [78]. Using mouse ESCs treated with conditioned media from limbal fibroblasts they obtained cells with cobblestone morphology that expressed cytokeratin (CK) 12 and ΔNp63α, opening the door for the study of pluripotent cells-derived cells in the regeneration of corneal epithelium. Yu and co-researchers [79] also obtained about 13% of conversion of mouse IPSCs to corneal epithelium-like cells by co-culture of IPSCs with corneal limbal stroma in the presence of additional growth factors related to corneal development: basic fibroblast growth factor (bFGF), EGF and nerve growth factor (NGF). Moving toward human cells, Hayashi and colleagues [80] aimed to establish IPSCs derived from human LSCs and to examine the ability of both limbal-derived and human dermal fibroblast-derived IPSCs to differentiate into corneal epithelial cells. Corneal epithelial cells were then successfully induced by the stromal cell-derived inducing activity (SDIA) differentiation method, after prolonged differentiation culture (12 weeks or later) in both, limbal (with higher corneal epithelial differentiation efficiency) and fibroblastic IPSCs. This study was the first to demonstrate a strategy for corneal epithelial cell differentiation from human IPSCs, and further suggested that an epigenomic status related to DNA methylation in specific epithelium-related genes—CK3, CK12 and Pax6—was associated with the propensity of IPSCs to differentiate into corneal epithelial cells and could be used as a criteria to choose IPSCs source for LSCs differentiation However, this protocol is lengthy and the efficiency is low, as the population obtained after the differentiation protocol is mixed with other cell types, such as RPE or lens epithelium. Ljubimov's group [81] recently successfully generated IPSCs from human primary LSCs to re-differentiate these IPSCs back into the limbal corneal epithelium, maintaining them on natural substrate that mimicked the native LSC niche, including denuded hAM and de-epithelialized corneas. This choice of parent cells represented an improvement for limbal cell differentiation by partial retention of parental epigenetic signatures in IPSCs. The authors observed that when the gene methylation patterns were compared in IPSCs to parental LSCs, limbal-derived IPSCs presented fewer unique methylation changes than fibroblast-derived IPSCs, suggesting the retention of epigenetic memory (genes promoting methylation) during reprogramming. Interestingly, limbal-derived IPSCs cultured for two weeks on hAM induced markedly higher expression of LSC markers (ABCG2, ΔNp63, CK14, CK15, CK17, N-cadherin, and TrkA) than fibroblast-derived IPSCs. On hAM, the methylation profiles of select limbal-derived IPSC genes became closer to the parental cells, but fibroblast-derived IPSCs remained closer to parental fibroblasts. On denuded air-lifted corneas, limbal-derived IPSCs even upregulated differentiated corneal CK3 and CK12. Taking all the data together, the authors emphasize the importance of the natural niche and the limbal tissue of origin in generating IPSCs as LSCs for clinical aims [81]. Compared to the previous work of Hayashi and colleagues [80], this method presents two interesting improvements. The differentiation medium is serum free and contains defined growth supplements, allowing for a more standardized protocol and bringing it closer to a clinical application. Also, differentiating the IPSCs on hAM provides an advantage for the success of future transplantation [21]. Both research [80,81] lead to the conclusion that the initial cell type from which IPSCs are derived is important for the quality of the final LSC-like cells obtained. However, for clinical applications easily accessible donor cell types should be identified to create IPSCs-LSCs. Other than fibroblasts, adult progenitor cells like bone-marrow or hair follicle -derived mesenchymal stem cells should be also tested.

In an elegant approach applying a directed two-stage differentiation protocol without the use of feeder cells or serum in the culture medium, researchers generated relatively pure populations of corneal epithelial-like progenitor cells capable of terminal differentiation toward mature corneal epithelial-like cells [82]. Early developmental mechanisms could be reproduced *in vitro* by blocking the transforming growth factor β (TGF-β) and Wnt-signaling pathways with small molecule inhibitors and activating bFGF signaling. IPSCs were cultured onto collagen IV substrate in specific corneal epithelial cell growth media which differentiated them into LSCs. Cells expressed typical LSC markers such as cytokeratins (CK3, CK12 and CK15) as well as Pax6, ABCG2 and ΔNp63 after five weeks of differentiation [82]. Interestingly, the differentiation protocol described by the authors, using growth factors and small molecules inhibitors, can be performed totally in xeno-free, feeder-free and serum-free conditions, allowing for a reproducible and clinical grade production of the IPSCs-LSCs ready to be used in the clinical setting. To bring one more step closer into the clinic, Wu's team [83] described a IPSCs-LSCs transplantation system that introduces a 3D scaffolding in which IPSCs are seeded, differentiated and grafted into an acellular porcine matrix scaffold. This bioengineering system is aimed to overcome the gradual loss of viability over time of LSC grafted cells and the limitations of amniotic membrane. The method improved the outcome in rabbit experimental models [83].

In conclusion, even if several adult stem cells types have been used for regeneration of corneal epithelium, LSCs themselves have shown superior results and are the cells of choice for LSCD treatment. Since IPSCs grow indefinitely, IPSC-derived LSCs are an unlimited source of autologous LSCs for patients with bilateral LSCD—and therefore no LSCs left—and to avoid the risks of surgical intervention in unilateral LSCD. Moreover, the idea of creating IPSCs banks to provide HLA matched (immune-compatible) tissues is being strongly considered by the scientific community [84]. This would provide a ready-to-go source of material for LSCs derivation avoiding the high cost of personalized IPSCs development.

3.2. Molecular Mechanisms of Corneal Epithelial Reprogramming

Molecular mechanisms of epithelial reprogramming have been analyzed, and ΔNp63 has emerged as a central protein in IPSC reprogramming routes. ΔNp63 has been found to enhance IPSCs generating efficiency, as the loss of function of this protein decreased the mesenchymal-epithelial transition (MET) and pluripotency genes [85]. Accordingly, in cell oncogenic transformation (a process that may share similarities with IPSCs reprogramming at signaling level) it was found that Oct4 upregulation could enhance the expression of ΔNp63 while repressing p53 [86]. APR-246/ PRIMA-1^{met} (a small compound which restores the functionality of mutant p53 in human tumor cells that target mutant forms of ΔNp63) was found to reverse corneal epithelial lineage commitment and to reinstate a normal p63-related signaling pathway [87]. In this study [87], the authors designed a unique cellular model that recapitulated major embryonic defects related to ectrodactyly ectodermal dysplasia cleft (lip/palate) syndrome (EEC syndrome), which is caused by single point mutations in the *p63* gene. Fibroblasts from healthy donors and from EEC patients carrying two different point mutations in the DNA binding domain of p63 were reprogrammed into IPSC lines. Phenotypic defects in EEC syndrome include skin defects and LSCD, with loss of corneal transparency. In this interesting *in vitro* model, EEC-derived IPSCs failed to terminal differentiate into CK14 cells (epidermis and LSCs) or CK3/CK12 cells (corneal epithelial cells) [87]. This research team also described previously the possible roles of specific miRs in corneal development using IPSC corneal differentiation methods [88]. Similarly, IPSC epithelial somatic differentiation seems to recapitulate the molecular steps during embryonic development, in which ΔNp63 is a master regulator of epithelial differentiation. Moreover, during IPSCs generation it is widely accepted that MET is needed [89]. Blocking MET during cell reprogramming (using TGF-β or Snail1) prevents IPSCs induction. In this change of cell state, the inverse of MET occurs during embryonic development, in which epithelial-mesenchymal transition (EMT) pointing out the parallelism between embryonic development and cell reprogramming [89]. Another interesting signaling pathway that may be involved in the IPSC differentiation into epithelial cells is the Pax6/β-catenin pathway [90]. During the embryonic development of the chicken eye, eye specification seems to be established by the inhibition of the canonical Wnt pathway and TGF-β, which induces the upregulation of Pax6 in the lens ectoderm [87]. In support of this theory, the trans-differentiation of multipotent hair follicle stem cells into corneal epithelial-like cells is mediated by the upregulation of Pax6 and the inhibition of the canonical Wnt-signaling pathway [73]. Thus, further investigation is needed to clarify whether this mechanism really affects the differentiation of IPSCs into corneal epithelial cells.

3.3. Restoration of Corneal Stromal Transparency

The restoration of corneal transparency after stromal or endothelial damage is another field of interest in which IPSCs generation and differentiation may have an impact. The production of corneal keratocytes from pluripotent cells also has significant implications for cell-based therapy and tissue engineering for treatment of corneal diseases. At present, however, there are very few studies of the use of IPSCs as an effective and conclusive approach for cell therapy applications for recovery corneal stroma, and the results are very preliminary.

Funderburgh's group [91] developed a methodology for inducing the differentiation of human embryonic stem cells (hESCs) into cells with a gene-expression phenotype similar to that of adult human corneal keratocytes. The transparency of the cornea depends on the unique molecular composition and organization of the extracellular matrix of the stroma (collagen fibrils), which is a product of keratocytes—specialized neural crest (NC)-derived mesenchymal cells. In Funderburgh's study, neural differentiation of the hESC cell line was induced by co-culture with mouse PA6 fibroblasts as a feeder-layer. After a few days in co-culture, hESCs acquired the ability to express cell-surface nerve growth factor receptor (NGFR, p75NTR) of low affinity. These cells were then isolated from co-cultures by immunoaffinity adsorption and cultured further as a monolayer. Corneal keratocyte phenotype was induced in serum-free medium containing ascorbate and was independent of the substratum for cultivation. Interestingly, hESC co-cultures upregulated the expression of some specific *NC* genes, and when NGFR-expressing cells were expanded as a monolayer, mRNAs typifying adult stromal stem cells were detected. Further, when these cells were cultured as substratum-free pellets, several corneal keratocyte markers were upregulated, among them keratocan, a corneal stroma-specific proteoglycan. The analysis of culture medium obtained from the pellets also contained high concentrations of keratocan modified with keratan sulfate, considered a unique molecular component of corneal stroma. This study showed the possibility to differentiate keratocytes *in vitro*. The authors also hypothesized that IPSCs derived from adult somatic cells could be used in place of hESCs for both, to provide autologous material for bioengineered corneal matrix or for direct stromal cell-based therapy [91].

Human corneal keratocytes could also be reprogrammed into IPSCs exhibiting pluripotent properties. To prevent feeder cell contamination and to improve the clinical utility of reprogrammed IPSCs, Chien and colleagues [92] developed a feeder-free (without MEF, mouse embryonic fibroblasts cells) and serum-free method to stably expand human IPSCs *in vitro*. This approach allows cells to remain stable through 30 passages, maintaining ESC-like pluripotent properties. Furthermore, to improve IPSCs delivery and engraftment, a biocompatible injectable nanogel (thermo-gelling carboxymethyl-hexanoyl chitosan; CHC) was developed. The authors also evaluated whether the viability and pluripotent properties of human corneal keratocyte-derived IPSCs can be retained in a CHC hydrogel system, and explored the therapeutic potential of these cells on corneal impairment using CHC hydrogel as delivery vehicle in a rat model of corneal damage induced by either chemical burns or surgical ablation. They concluded that the IPSC/CHC system enhanced corneal regeneration by downregulating oxidative stress and recruiting endogenous epithelial cells to restore corneal epithelial thickness, and also reconstructing the corneal microenvironment niche [92].

Very recently, Fukuta and co-researchers [93] developed an efficient induction protocol using chemically defined culture medium containing inhibitors for TGF-β signaling and inhibitors for Wnt-signaling pathway (GSK3β). This approach allow differentiate human neural crest cells (hNCC) from human pluripotent cells, with the same efficiency (70%–80%), independent of the parental cell type (ESCs or IPSCs), or method of generation (viral-integrated or plasmid-episomal). Furthermore, cells have been kept under feeder-free and xeno-free culture systems. Interestingly, generated hNCCs could be differentiated into corneal endothelial cells, among other complex cell types, such as peripheral neurons, glial cells and melanocytes. Endothelial cells of the cornea have been differentiated culturing hNCCs in corneal endothelial cell conditioned medium supplemented with selective ROCK inhibitor (Y-27632). After two weeks of induction, cells changed their morphology into that of polygonal corneal endothelial-like cells and started to express ZO-1, type IV and type VIII collagens, which are recognized corneal endothelial cell markers [93]. These results also open new and promising perspectives for possible clinic applications in corneal pathologies where the endothelium is primarily affected.

3.4. Future Trends for IPSC Technology

The ideal source of cells for ocular clinical application needs to meet certain criteria: (a) easy accessibility and minimal risks for patients; (b) availability in sufficient quantities for bio-replacement; and (c) a high likelihood of successful reprogramming [72]. However, present evidence confirms that the methods involving IPSCs production should be considered with caution before immediate clinical application. An example is exome sequencing of several human IPSC lines, identified over a hundred point mutations in the generated cells but not in the parental cells. Many missense mutations associated with the function of different proteins and other point mutations in genes related to cancers have been observed [94]. In this sense, a better understanding of the molecular mechanisms for differentiation into various cell types associated with more directed protocols for the reprogramming, without the need to induce complete states of non-differentiation, could contribute to mitigate possible aberrations in the genome of produced cell populations.

4. Conclusions

In recent years there have been significant developments in the use of cell-based cultures combined with biomaterials or biocompatible substrates for corneal epithelial tissue engineering bio-replacement. Current approaches for improving these therapeutic strategies include standardization of culture conditions and development of xenobiotic free culture systems, evaluation of novel bio-functional scaffolds to enhance stem cell expansion and transplantation efficacy, and exploration of alternative autologous progenitor cell sources. To date, the search for innovative strategies and approaches in the field of ocular surface reconstruction has produced some encouraging results. Several new strategies have emerged for future therapies for LSCD, although the best cell source and the ideal technique still need to be established. One of the key elements is the role of the cellular microenvironment or niche. The limbal stem cell niche contains stem cells that promote proliferation and migration and have immunosuppressive mechanisms to protect them from immunological reactions. The current findings suggest that the CLET and COMET approaches using autologous epithelial progenitor cells are the most widely accepted clinical techniques for treating LSCD.

One emerging alternative cell source for treating the ocular surface is the use of adult stem cells, which provide high proliferative potential, differentiated capability and lower immunogenicity; they are non-tumorigenic and can be obtained by minimally invasive methodologies. They represent a more physiological, more rational, and less invasive treatment. Meanwhile, stem cells from adult tissue, as in the case of mesenchymal stem cells, although they have showed an intrinsic potential for a possible epithelial differentiation, this has not yet been achieved. Also, the prospects for therapies derived from autologous mesenchymal and IPSCs that may yield a multitude of engineered tissue types are exciting. Although IPSCs are yet to be used for ocular surface reconstruction, a recent study has shown successful corneal epithelial cell generation. The search for alternative sources of stem cells in the treatment of ocular surface diseases represents a challenge. IPSCs represent a very promising option for obtaining corneal epithelial cells to apply in cell-based therapy for the ocular surface. In the future, a deeper understanding of the behavioral characteristics of the LSC niche as well as of proliferation and differentiation pathway events should help to expand and develop the use of IPSCs in ocular surface regenerative medicine.

Acknowledgments

Part of this work was funded by Fondo de Investigaciones Sanitarias del Instituto de Salud Carlos III (FIS09-PI040654), Dirección General de Terapias Avanzadas y Trasplantes del Ministerio de Sanidad y Política Social (TRA-072), and Fundació Marató TV3 (120630).

Author Contributions

Núria Nieto-Nicolau and Eva M. Martínez-Conesa performed the literature searches and bibliography, and contributed to the writing of the manuscript. Michael Edel contributed to draft the manuscript. Ana B. Álvarez-Palomo contributed to perform literature searches and bibliography compilations, to draft and revise the final manuscript. Ricardo P. Casaroli-Marano drafted, formatted and wrote the manuscript, prepared the figures and tables, performed literature searches and bibliography compilations, and edited and revised the final manuscript.

Conflicts of Interest

The authors have no proprietary or financial interest in any materials, methods or subject matter discussed in this article.

References

1. Notara, M.; Alatza, A.; Gilfillan, J.; Harris, A.R.; Levis, H.J.; Schrader, S.; Vernon, A.; Daniels, J.T. In sickness and in health: Corneal epithelial stem cell biology, pathology and therapy. *Exp. Eye Res.* **2010**, *90*, 188–195.
2. Osei-Bempong, C.; Figueiredo, F.C.; Lako, M. The limbal epithelium of the eye—A review of limbal stem cell biology, disease and treatment. *Bioessays* **2013**, *35*, 211–219.
3. Casaroli-Marano, R.P.; Nieto-Nicolau, N.; Martínez-Conesa, E.M. Progenitor cells for ocular surface regenerative therapy. *Ophthalmic Res.* **2013**, *49*, 115–121.
4. Ahmad, S.; Kolli, S.; Lako, M.; Figueiredo, F.C.; Daniels, J.T. Stem cell therapies for ocular surface disease. *Drug Discov. Today* **2010**, *15*, 306–313.
5. Utheim, T.P. Limbal epithelial cell therapy: Past, present, and future. *Methods Mol. Biol.* **2013**, *1014*, 3–43.
6. Li, W.; Hayashida, Y.; Chen, Y.T.; Tseng, S.C. Niche regulation of corneal epithelial stem cells at the limbus. *Cell Res.* **2007**, *17*, 26–36.
7. Dua, H.S.; Shanmuganathan, V.A.; Powell-Richards, A.O.; Tighe, P.J.; Joseph, A. Limbal epithelial crypts: A novel anatomical structure and a putative limbal stem cell niche. *Br. J. Ophthalmol.* **2005**, *89*, 529–532.

8. Shortt, A.J.; Secker, G.A.; Munro, P.M.; Khaw, P.T.; Tuft, S.J.; Daniels, J.T. Characterization of the limbal epithelial stem cell niche: Novel imaging techniques permit *in vivo* observation and targeted biopsy of limbal epithelial stem cells. *Stem Cells* **2007**, *25*, 1402–1409.

9. Thoft, R.A.; Friend, J. The X, Y, Z hypothesis of corneal epithelial maintenance. *Invest. Ophthalmol. Vis. Sci.* **1987**, *24*, 1442–1443.

10. Majo, F.; Rochat, A.; Nicolas, M.; Jaoude, G.A.; Barrandon, Y. Oligopotent stem cells are distributed throughout the mammalian ocular surface. *Nature* **2008**, *456*, 250–254.

11. Dua, H.S.; Miri, A.; Alomar, T.; Yeung, A.M.; Said, D.G. The role of limbal stem cells in corneal epithelial maintenance: Testing the dogma. *Ophthalmology* **2009**, *116*, 856–863.

12. Pellegrini, G.; Golisano, O.; Paterna, P.; Lambiase, A.; Bonini, S.; Rama, P.; De Luca, M. Location and clonal analysis of stem cells and their differentiated progeny in the human ocular surface. *J. Cell Biol.* **1999**, *145*, 769–782.

13. Lindberg, K.; Brown, M.E.; Chaves, H.V.; Kenyon, K.R.; Rheinwald, J.G. *In vitro* propagation of human ocular surface epithelial cells for transplantation. *Invest. Ophthalmol. Vis. Sci.* **1993**, *34*, 2672–2679.

14. Kruse, F.E. Stem cells and corneal epithelial regeneration. *Eye* **1994**, *8*, 170–183.

15. Kiritoshi, A.; Sundar-Raj, N.; Thoft, R.A. Differentiation in cultured limbal epithelium as defined by keratin expression. *Invest. Ophthalmol. Vis. Sci.* **1991**, *32*, 3073–3077.

16. Cotsarelis, G.; Cheng, S.Z.; Dong, G.; Sun, T.T.; Lavker, R.M. Existence of slow-cycling limbal epithelial basal cells that can be preferentially stimulated to proliferate: Implications on epithelial stem cells. *Cell* **1989**, *57*, 201–209.

17. Pellegrini, G.; Traverso, C.E.; Franzi, A.T.; Zingirian, M.; Cancedda, R.; de Luca, M. Long-term restoration of damaged corneal surfaces with autologous cultivated corneal epithelium. *Lancet* **1997**, *349*, 990–993.

18. Shortt, A.J.; Secker, G.A.; Notara, M.D.; Limb, G.A.; Khaw, P.T.; Tuft, S.J.; Daniels, J.T. Transplatation of *ex vivo* cultured limbal epitehlial stem cells: A review of techniques and clinical results. *Surv. Ophthalmol.* **2007**, *52*, 483–502.

19. Rama, P.; Matuska, S.; Paganoni, G.; Spinelli, A.; de Luca, M.; Pellegrini, G. Limbal stem-cell therapy and long-term corneal regeneration. *N. Engl. J. Med.* **2010**, *363*, 147–155.

20. Sangwan, V.S.; Basu, S.; Vemuganti, G.K.; Sejpal, K.; Subramaniam, S.V.; Bandyopadhyay, S.; Krishnaiah, S.; Gaddipati, S.; Tiwari, S.; Balasubramanian, D. Clinical outcomes of xeno-free autologous cultivated limbal epithelial transplantation: A 10-year study. *Br. J. Ophthalmol.* **2011**, *95*, 1525–1529.

21. Baylis, O.; Figueiredo, F.; Henein, C.; Lako, M.; Ahmad, S. 13 years of cultured limbal epithelial cell therapy: A review of the outcomes. *J. Cell Biochem.* **2011**, *112*, 993–1002.

22. Pellegrini, G.; Rama, P.; di Rocco, A.; Panaras, A.; de Luca, M. Concise review: Hurdles in a successful example of limbal stem cell-based regenerative medicine. *Stem Cells* **2014**, *32*, 26–34.

23. Menzel-Severing, J.; Kruse, F.E.; Schlötzer-Schrehardt, U. Stem cell-based therapy for corneal epithelial reconstruction: Present and future. *Can. J. Ophthalmol.* **2013**, *48*, 13–21.

24. Ahmad, S. Concise review: Limbal stem cell deficiency, dysfunction, and distress. *Stem Cells Transl. Med.* **2012**, *1*, 110–115.

25. Mönks, T.; Busin, M. Modified technique of autologous conjunctival transplantation after corneal chemical burn. *Klin. Monbl. Augenheilkd.* **1994**, *204*, 121–125.

26. Ahmad, S.; Osei-Bempong, C.; Dana, R.; Jurkunas, U. The culture and transplantation of human limbal stem cells. *J. Cell Physiol.* **2010**, *225*, 15–19.

27. Tseng, S.C.; Chen, S.Y.; Shen, Y.C.; Chen, W.L.; Hu, F.R. Critical appraisal of *ex vivo* expansion of human limbal epitelial stem cells. *Curr. Mol. Med.* **2010**, *10*, 841–850.

28. Di Iorio, E.; Ferrari, S.; Fasolo, A.; Böhm, E.; Ponzin, D.; Barbaro, V. Techniques for culture and assessment of limbal stem cell grafts. *Ocul. Surf.* **2010**, *8*, 146–153.

29. O'Callaghan, A.R.; Daniels, J.T. Limbal epithelial stem cell therapy: Controversies and challenges. *Stem Cells* **2011**, *29*, 1923–1932.

30. Nishida, K.; Yamato, M.; Hayashida, Y.; Watanabe, K.; Yamamoto, K.; Adachi, E.; Nagai, S.; Kikuchi, A.; Maeda, N.; Watanabe, H.; *et al.* Corneal reconstruction with tissue engineered cell sheets composed of autologous oral mucosal epithelium. *N. Engl. J. Med.* **2004**, *351*, 1187–1196.

31. Kolli, S.; Ahmad, S.; Mudhar, H.S.; Meeny, A.; Lako, M.; Figueiredo, F.C. Successful application of *ex vivo* expanded human autologous oral mucosal epithelium for the treatment of total bilateral limbal stem cell deficiency. *Stem Cells* **2014**, *32*, 2135–2146.

32. Vemuganti, G.K.; Fatima, A.; Madhira, S.L.; Basti, S.; Sangwan, V.S. Limbal stem cells: Application in ocular biomedicine. *Int. Rev. Cell Mol. Biol.* **2009**, *275*, 133–181.

33. Priya, C.G.; Arpitha, P.; Vaishali, S.; Prajna, N.V.; Usha, K.; Sheetal, K.; Muthukkaruppan, V. Adult human buccal epithelial stem cells: Identification, *ex-vivo* expansion, and transplantation for corneal surface reconstruction. *Eye* **2011**, *25*, 1641–1649.

34. Nakamura, T.; Takeda, K.; Inatomi, T.; Sotozono, C.; Kinoshita, S. Long-term results of autologous cultivated oral mucosal epithelial transplantation in the scar phase of severe ocular surface disorders. *Br. J. Ophthalmol.* **2011**, *95*, 942–946.

35. Liu, J.; Sheha, H.; Fu, Y.; Giegengack, M.; Tseng, S.C. Oral mucosal graft with amniotic membrane transplantation for total limbal stem cell deficiency. *Am. J. Ophthalmol.* **2011**, *152*, 739–747.

36. Inatomi, T.; Nakamura, T.; Kojyo, M.; Koizumi, N.; Sotozono, C.; Kinoshita, S. Ocular surface reconstruction with combination of cultivated autologous oral mucosal epithelial transplantation and penetrating keratoplasty. *Am. J. Ophthalmol.* **2006**, *142*, 757–764.

37. Takeda, K.; Nakamura, T.; Inatomi, T.; Sotozono, C.; Watanabe, A.; Kinoshita, S. Ocular surface reconstruction using the combination of autologous cultivated oral mucosal epithelial transplantation and eyelid surgery for severe ocular surface disease. *Am. J. Ophthalmol.* **2011**, *152*, 195–201.

38. Sangwan, V.S.; Vemuganti, G.K.; Iftekhar, G.; Bansal, A.K.; Rao, G.N. Use of autologous cultured limbal and conjunctival epithelium in a patient with severe bilateral ocular surface disease induced by acid injury: A case report of unique application. *Cornea* **2003**, *22*, 478–481.

39. Tan, D.T.; Ang, L.P.; Beuerman, R.W. Reconstruction of the ocular surface by transplantation of a serum-free derived cultivated conjunctival epithelial equivalent. *Transplantation* **2004**, *77*, 1729–1734.

40. Ang, L.P.; Tanioka, H.; Kawasaki, S.; Ang, L.P.; Yamasaki, K.; Do, T.P.; Thein, Z.M.; Koizumi, N.; Nakamura, T.; Yokoi, N.; *et al.* Cultivated human conjunctival epithelial transplantation for total limbal stem cell deficiency. *Invest. Ophthalmol. Vis. Sci.* **2010**, *51*, 758–764.

41. Subramaniam, S.V.; Sejpal, K.; Fatima, A.; Gaddipati, S.; Vemuganti, G.K.; Sangwan, V.S. Coculture of autologous limbal and conjunctival epithelial cells to treat severe ocular surface disorders: Long-term survival analysis. *Indian J. Ophthalmol.* **2013**, *61*, 202–207.

42. Homma, R.; Yoshikawa, H.; Takeno, M.; Kurokawa, M.S.; Masuda, C.; Takada, E.; Tsubota, K.; Ueno, S.; Suzuki, N. Induction of epithelial progenitors *in vitro* from mouse embryonic stem cells and application for reconstruction of damaged cornea in mice. *Invest. Ophthalmol. Vis. Sci.* **2004**, *45*, 4320–4326.

43. Ueno, H.; Kurokawa, M.S.; Kayama, M.; Homma, R.; Kumagai, Y.; Masuda, C.; Takada, E.; Tsubota, K.; Ueno, S.; Suzuki, N. Experimental transplantation of corneal epithelium-like cells induced by *Pax6* gene transfection of mouse embryonic stem cells. *Cornea* **2007**, *26*, 1220–1227.

44. Ahmad, S.; Stewart, S.R.; Yung, S.; Kolli, S.; Armstrong, L.; Stojkovic, M.; Figueiredo, F.; Lako, M. Differentiation of human embryonic stem cells into corneal epithelial-like cells by *in vitro* replication of the corneal epithelial stem cell niche. *Stem Cells* **2007**, *25*, 1145–1155.

45. Hanson, C.; Hardarson, T.; Ellerstrom, C.; Nordberg, M.; Caisander, G.; Rao, M.; Hyllner, J.; Stenevi, U. Transplantation of human embryonic stem cells onto a partially wounded human cornea *in vitro*. *Acta Ophthalmol.* **2013**, *91*, 127–130.

46. Gao, N.; Wang, Z.; Huang, B.; Ge, J.; Lu, R.; Zhang, R.; Fan, Z.; Lu, L.; Peng, Z.; Cui, G. Putative epidermal stem cell convert into corneal epithelium-like cell under corneal tissue *in vitro*. *Sci. China C Life Sci.* **2007**, *50*, 101–110.

47. Yang, X.; Qu, L.; Wang, X.; Zhao, M.; Li, W.; Hua, J.; Shi, M.; Moldovan, N.; Wang, H.; Dou, Z. Plasticity of epidermal adult stem cells derived from adult goat ear skin. *Mol. Reprod. Dev.* **2007**, *74*, 386–396.

48. Yang, X.; Moldovan, N.I.; Zhao, Q.; Mi, S.; Zhou, Z.; Chen, D.; Gao, Z.; Tong, D.; Dou, Z. Reconstruction of damaged cornea by autologous transplantation of epidermal adult stem cells. *Mol. Vis.* **2008**, *14*, 1064–1070.

49. Ma, Y.; Xu, Y.; Xiao, Z.; Yang, W.; Zhang, C.; Song, E.; Du, Y.; Li, L. Reconstruction of chemically burned rat corneal surface by bone marrow-derived human mesenchymal stem cells. *Stem Cells* **2006**, *24*, 315–321.

50. Jiang, T.S.; Cai, L.; Ji, W.Y.; Hui, Y.N.; Wang, Y.S.; Hu, D.; Zhu, J. Reconstruction of the corneal epithelium with induced marrow mesenchymal stem cells in rats. *Mol. Vis.* **2010**, *16*, 1304–1316.

51. Gu, S.; Xing, C.; Han, J.; Tso, M.O.; Hong, J. Differentiation of rabbit bone marrow mesenchymal stem cells into corneal epithelial cells *in vivo* and *ex vivo*. *Mol. Vis.* **2009**, *15*, 99–107.

52. Omoto, M.; Miyashita, H.; Shimmura, S.; Higa, K.; Kawakita, T.; Yoshida, S.; McGrogan, M.; Shimazaki, J.; Tsubota, K. The use of human mesenchymal stem cell-derived feeder cells for the cultivation of transplantable epithelial sheets. *Invest. Ophthalmol. Vis. Sci.* **2009**, *50*, 2109–2115.

53. Hu, N.; Zhang, Y.Y.; Gu, H.W.; Guan, H.J. Effects of bone marrow mesenchymal stem cells on cell proliferation and growth factor expression of limbal epithelial cells *in vitro*. *Ophthalmic Res.* **2012**, *48*, 82–88.

54. Martínez-Conesa, E.M.; Espel, E.; Reina, M.; Casaroli-Marano, R.P. Characterization of ocular surface epithelial and progenitor cell markers in human adipose stromal cells derived from lipoaspirates. *Invest. Ophthalmol. Vis. Sci.* **2012**, *53*, 513–520.

55. Nieto-Miguel, T.; Galindo, S.; Reinoso, R.; Corell, A.; Martino, M.; Pérez-Simón, J.A.; Calonge, M. *In vitro* simulation of corneal epithelium microenvironment induces a corneal epithelial-like cell phenotype from human adipose tissue mesenchymal stem cells. *Curr. Eye Res.* **2013**, *38*, 933–944.

56. Ho, J.H.; Ma, W.H.; Tseng, T.C.; Chen, Y.F.; Chen, M.H.; Lee, O.K. Isolation and characterization of multi-potent stem cells from human orbital fat tissues. *Tissue Eng. Part A* **2011**, *17*, 255–266.

57. Lin, K.J.; Loi, M.X.; Lien, G.S.; Cheng, C.F.; Pao, H.Y.; Chang, Y.C.; Ji, A.T.; Ho, J.H. Topical administration of orbital fat-derived stem cells promotes corneal tissue regeneration. *Stem Cell Res. Ther.* **2013**, *4*, doi:10.1186/scrt223.

58. Chen, S.Y.; Mahabole, M.; Horesh, E.; Wester, S.; Goldberg, J.L.; Tseng, S.C. Isolation and Characterization of Mesenchymal Progenitor Cells from Human Orbital Adipose Tissue. *Invest Ophthalmol. Vis. Sci.* **2014**, *55*, 4842–4852.

59. Monteiro, B.G.; Serafim, R.C.; Melo, G.B.; Silva, M.C.; Lizier, N.F.; Maranduba, C.M.; Smith, R.L.; Kerkis, A.; Cerruti, H.; Gomes, J.A.; *et al.* Human immature dental pulp stem cells share key characteristic features with limbal stem cells. *Cell Prolif.* **2009**, *42*, 587–594.

60. Gomes, J.A.; Geraldes Monteiro, B.; Melo, G.B.; Smith, R.L.; Cavenaghi Pereira da Silva, M.; Lizier, N.F.; Kerkis, A.; Cerruti, H.; Kerkis, I. Corneal reconstruction with tissue-engineered cell sheets composed of human immature dental pulp stem cells. *Invest. Ophthalmol. Vis. Sci.* **2010**, *51*, 1408–1414.

61. Blazejewska, E.A.; Schlotzer-Schrehardt, U.; Zenkel, M.; Bachmann, B.; Chankiewitz, E.; Jacobi, C.; Kruse, F.E. Corneal limbal microenvironment can induce transdifferentiation of hair follicle stem cells into corneal epithelial-like cells. *Stem Cells* **2009**, *27*, 642–652.

62. Meyer-Blazejewska, E.A.; Call, M.K.; Yamanaka, O.; Liu, H.; Schlotzer-Schrehardt, U.; Kruse, F.E.; Kao, W.W. From hair to cornea: Toward the therapeutic use of hair follicle-derived stem cells in the treatment of limbal stem cell deficiency. *Stem Cells* **2011**, *29*, 57–66.

63. Reza, H.M.; Ng, B.Y.; Phan, T.T.; Tan, D.T.; Beuerman, R.W.; Ang, L.P. Characterization of a novel umbilical cord lining cell with CD227 positivity and unique pattern of P63 expression and function. *Stem Cell Rev.* **2011**, *7*, 624–638.

64. Reza, H.M.; Ng, B.Y.; Gimeno, F.L.; Phan, T.T.; Ang, L.P. Umbilical cord lining stem cells as a novel and promising source for ocular surface regeneration. *Stem Cell Rev.* **2011**, *7*, 935–947.

65. Kanayama, S.; Nishida, K.; Yamato, M.; Hayashi, R.; Sugiyama, H.; Soma, T.; Maeda, N.; Okano, T.; Tano, Y. Analysis of angiogenesis induced by cultured corneal and oral mucosal epithelial cell sheets *in vitro*. *Exp. Eye Res.* **2007**, *85*, 772–781.

66. Kanayama, S.; Nishida, K.; Yamato, M.; Hayashi, R.; Maeda, N.; Okano, T.; Tano, Y. Analysis of soluble vascular endothelial growth factor receptor-1 secreted from cultured corneal and oral mucosal epithelial cell sheets *in vitro*. *Br. J. Ophthalmol.* **2009**, *93*, 263–267.

67. ClinicalTrials.gov, a service of US National Institute of Health. Available online: https://clinicaltrials.gov/ (accessed 30 December 2014).

68. Takahashi, K.; Yamanaka, S. Induction of pluripotent stem cells from mouse embryonic and adult fibroblast cultures by defined factors. *Cell* **2006**, *126*, 663–676.

69. Yu, J.; Vodyanik, M.A.; Smuga-Otto, K.; Antosiewicz-Bourget, J.; Frane, J.L.; Tian, S.; Nie, J.; Jonsdottir, G.A.; Ruotti, V.; Stewart, R.; *et al.* Induced pluripotent stem cell lines derived from human somatic cells. *Science* **2007**, *318*, 1917–1920.

70. Yamanaka, S. Induced pluripotent stem cells: Past, present, and future. *Cell Stem Cell* **2012**, *10*, 678–684.

71. Kelaini, S.; Cochrane, A.; Margariti, A. Direct reprogramming of adult cells: Avoiding the pluripotent state. *Stem Cells Cloning* **2014**, *15*, 19–29.

72. Pietronave, S.; Prat, M. Advances and applications of induced pluripotent stem cells. *Can. J. Physiol. Pharmacol.* **2012**, *90*, 317–325.

73. Yang, K.; Jiang, Z.; Wang, D.; Lian, X.; Yang, T. Corneal epithelial-like transdifferentiation of hair follicle stem cells is mediated by pax6 and beta-catenin/Lef-1. *Cell Biol. Int.* **2009**, *33*, 861–866.

74. Saichanma, S.; Bunyaratvej, A.; Sila-Asna, M. *In vitro* transdifferentiation of corneal epithelial-like cells from human skin-derived precursor cells. *Int. J. Ophthalmol.* **2012**, *5*, 158–163.

75. Casaroli-Marano, R.P.; Zarbin, M.A. Cell-based therapy for retinal degenerative disease. *Developments in Ophthalmology*; Karger: Basel, Switzerland, 2014; Volume 53.

76. Zhong, X.; Gutierrez, C.; Xue, T.; Hampton, C.; Vergara, M.N.; Cao, L.H.; Peters, A.; Park, T.S.; Zambidis, E.T.; Meyer, J.S. *et al.* Generation of three-dimensional retinal tissue with functional photoreceptors from human iPSCs. *Nat. Commun.* **2014**, *10*, doi:10.1038/ncomms5047.

77. Mekala, S.R.; Vauhini, V.; Nagarajan, U.; Maddileti, S.; Gaddipati, S.; Mariappan, I. Derivation, characterization and retinal differentiation of induced pluripotent stem cells. *J. Biosci.* **2013**, *38*, 123–134.

78. Notara, M.; Hernandez, D.; Mason, C.; Daniels, J.T. Characterization of the phenotype and functionality of corneal epithelial cells derived from mouse embryonic stem cells. *Regen. Med.* **2012**, *7*, 167–178.

79. Yu, D.; Chen, M.; Sun, X.; Ge, J. Differentiation of mouse induced pluripotent stem cells into corneal epithelial-like cells. *Cell Biol. Int.* **2013**, *37*, 87–94.

80. Hayashi, R.; Ishikawa, Y.; Ito, M.; Kageyama, T.; Takashiba, K.; Fujioka, T.; Tsujikawa, M.; Miyoshi, H.; Yamato, M.; Nakamura, Y.; *et al.* Generation of corneal epithelial cells from induced pluripotent stem cells derived from human dermal fibroblast and corneal limbal epithelium. *PLoS One* **2012**, *7*, e45435.

81. Sareen, D.; Saghizadeh, M.; Ornelas, L.; Winkler, M.A.; Narwani, K.; Sahabian, A.; Funari, V.A.; Tang, J.; Spurka, L.; Punj, V.; *et al.* Differentiation of Human Limbal-Derived Induced Pluripotent Stem Cells Into Limbal-Like Epithelium. *Stem Cells Transl. Med.* **2014**, *3*, 1002–1012.

82. Mikhailova, A.; Ilmarinen, T.; Uusitalo, H.; Skottman, H. Small-molecule induction promotes corneal epithelial cell differentiation from human induced pluripotent stem cells. *Stem Cell Rep.* **2014**, *6*, 219–231.

83. Zhu, J.; Zhang, K.; Sun, Y.; Gao, X.; Li, Y.; Chen, Z.; Wu, X. Reconstruction of functional ocular surface by acellular porcine cornea matrix scaffold and limbal stem cells derived from human embryonic stem cells. *Tissue Eng. Part A* **2013**, *19*, 2412–2425.

84. Taylor, C.J.; Peacock, S.; Chaudhry, A.N.; Bradley, J.A.; Bolton, E.M. Generating an iPSC bank for HLA-matched tissue transplantation based on known donor and recipient HLA types. *Cell Stem Cell* **2012**, *11*, 147–152.

85. Alexandrova, E.M.; Petrenko, O.; Nemajerova, A.; Romano, R.A.; Sinha, S.; Moll, U.M. ΔNp63 regulates select routes of reprogramming via multiple mechanisms. *Cell Death Differ.* **2013**, *20*, 1698–1708.

86. Ng, W.L.; Chen, G.; Wang, M.; Wang, H.; Story, M.; Shay, J.W.; Zhang, X.; Wang, J.; Amin, A.R.; Hu, B.; *et al.* OCT4 as a target of miR-34a stimulates p63 but inhibits p53 to promote human cell transformation. *Cell Death Dis.* **2014**, *5*, doi:10.1038/cddis.2013.563.

87. Shalom-Feuerstein, R.; Serror, L.; Aberdam, E.; Müller, F.J.; van Bokhoven, H.; Wiman, K.G.; Zhou, H.; Aberdam, D.; Petit, I. Impaired epithelial differentiation of induced pluripotent stem cells from ectodermal dysplasia-related patients is rescued by the small compound APR-246/PRIMA-1MET. *Proc. Natl. Acad. Sci. USA* **2013**, *110*, 2152–2156.

88. Shalom-Feuerstein, R.; Serror, L.; de La Forest Divonne, S.; Petit, I.; Aberdam, E.; Camargo, L.; Damour, O.; Vigouroux, C.; Solomon, A.; Gaggioli, C.; *et al.* Pluripotent stem cell model reveals essential roles for miR-450b-5p and miR-184 in embryonic corneal lineage specification. *Stem Cell* **2012**, *30*, 898–909.

89. Li, X.; Pei, D.; Zheng, H. Transitions between epithelial and mesenchymal states during cell fate conversions. *Protein Cell* **2014**, *5*, 580–591.

90. Grocott, T.; Johnson, S.; Bailey, A.P.; Streit, A. Neural crest cells organize the eye via TGF-β and canonical Wnt signalling. *Nat. Commun.* **2011**, *2*, doi:10.1038/ncomms1269.

91. Chan, A.A.; Hertsenberg, A.J.; Funderburgh, M.L.; Mann, M.M.; Du, Y.; Davoli, K.A.; Mich-Basso, J.D.; Yang, L.; Funderburgh, J.L. Differentiation of human embryonic stem cells into cells with corneal keratocyte phenotype. *PLoS One* **2013**, *8*, e56831.

92. Chien, Y.; Liao, Y.W.; Liu, D.M.; Lin, H.L.; Chen, S.J.; Chen, H.L.; Peng, C.H.; Liang, C.M.; Mou, C.Y.; Chiou, S.H. Corneal repair by human corneal keratocyte-reprogrammed iPSCs and amphiphatic carboxymethyl-hexanoyl chitosan hydrogel. *Biomaterials* **2012**, *33*, 8003–8016.

93. Fukuta, M.; Nakai, Y.; Kirino, K.; Nakagawa, M.; Sekiguchi, K.; Nagata, S.; Matsumoto, Y.; Yamamoto, T.; Umeda, K.; Heike, T.; *et al.* Derivation of Mesenchymal Stromal Cells from Pluripotent Stem Cells through a Neural Crest Lineage using Small Molecule Compounds with Defined Media. *PLoS One* **2014**, *9*, e112291.

94. Gore, A.; Li, Z.; Fung, H.; Young, J.E.; Agarwal, S.; Antosiewicz-Bourget, J.; Canto, I.; Giorgetti, A.; Israel, M.A.; Kiskinis, E.; *et al.* Somatic coding mutations in human induced pluripotent stem cells. *Nature* **2011**, *471*, 63–67.

Chapter 4:
Spinal Cord Injury

The Potential for iPS-Derived Stem Cells as a Therapeutic Strategy for Spinal Cord Injury: Opportunities and Challenges

Mohamad Khazaei, Ahad M. Siddiqui and Michael G. Fehlings

Abstract: Spinal cord injury (SCI) is a devastating trauma causing long-lasting disability. Although advances have occurred in the last decade in the medical, surgical and rehabilitative treatments of SCI, the therapeutic approaches are still not ideal. The use of cell transplantation as a therapeutic strategy for the treatment of SCI is promising, particularly since it can target cell replacement, neuroprotection and regeneration. Cell therapies for treating SCI are limited due to several translational roadblocks, including ethical and practical concerns regarding cell sources. The use of iPSCs has been particularly attractive, since they avoid the ethical and moral concerns that surround other stem cells. Furthermore, various cell types with potential for application in the treatment of SCI can be created from autologous sources using iPSCs. For applications in SCI, the iPSCs can be differentiated into neural precursor cells, neurons, oligodendrocytes, astrocytes, neural crest cells and mesenchymal stromal cells that can act by replacing lost cells or providing environmental support. Some methods, such as direct reprogramming, are being investigated to reduce tumorigenicity and improve reprogramming efficiencies, which have been some of the issues surrounding the use of iPSCs clinically to date. Recently, iPSCs have entered clinical trials for use in age-related macular degeneration, further supporting their promise for translation in other conditions, including SCI.

Reprinted from *J. Clin. Med.* Cite as: Mohamad Khazaei, Ahad M. Siddiqui and Michael G. Fehlings. The Potential for iPS-Derived Stem Cells as a Therapeutic Strategy for Spinal Cord Injury: Opportunities and Challenges. *J. Clin. Med.* **2015**, *4*, 37–65.

1. Current Outlook on the Pathophysiology and Treatment of Spinal Cord Injury

1.1. Epidemiology of Spinal Cord Injury

Dislocation or fracture of the spine in the neck or back as a result of vehicle accidents, falls, sports accidents, work accidents or other causes commonly results in spinal cord injury (SCI). The seriousness of the damage varies depending on the severity of the injury and the level of injury. Over half of SCIs occur at the cervical level of the spinal cord [1]. The global prevalence of SCI varies between 250 and 906 per million of the population depending on global region [1–3]. There have been many advances in the medical, surgical and rehabilitative treatment of SCI in the last few decades; however, these treatments result in limited functional recovery after injury.

1.2. Pathophysiology of SCI

The mechanical crushing, stretching or rupture of the spinal cord at the time of injury leads to axonal damage, quick necrotic death and loss of neurons and glia, which are collectively referred to as the primary injury [4–6]. Axon damage and disruption of the cell membrane that occurs during the primary injury results in a cascade of molecular and signaling pathways that initiate a series of secondary injuries to the spinal cord. Formation of free radicals and oxidative stress as a consequence of secondary injuries result in more neuronal and glial death, mainly due to apoptosis [7]. Disintegration of myelin and demyelination are another consequence of secondary injury in the spinal cord. The mechanical insult to the spinal cord also results in the disruption of the blood spinal cord barrier (BSCB). This increases the permeability of the BSCB, allowing the infiltration of immune cells from the blood and increasing inflammation, which augment secondary injury [8]. The activation of astrocytes results in reactive gliosis and subsequent formation of the glial scar which acts as a physical and chemical barrier that inhibits axon regeneration. Progressive loss of neurons and glial cells results in the formation of a cystic cavity in the spinal cord [5,9,10].

1.3. Approaches and Progresses towards the Treatment of SCI

The current treatment options for SCI are mainly focused on stabilizing the spine, preventing the progress of secondary injuries and controlling inflammation. Fractured vertebrae and bone fragments that compress the spinal cord may need to be surgically removed by spinal decompression surgery [11]. Corticosteroid drugs (like methylprednisolone) may be used within 8 h of the injury, although their application is controversial. Methylprednisolone appears to work by modulating inflammation near the site of injury and reducing damage to nerve cells [12]. After the initial treatment and stabilization of patients with an SCI, much of the current treatment approaches are geared toward rehabilitation. However, there are many promising advancements in research towards protecting surviving neural cells from further damage, stimulating axonal regeneration and replacing damaged nerve or glial cells. Several medications that can increase neuronal survival and reduce inflammation are in clinical trials, including corticosteroids, minocycline, erythropoietin and gangliosides [12]. Riluzole is a drug with neuroprotective effects that has been investigated by our laboratory as a part of an international, multicenter effort sponsored by AOSpine and the North American Clinical Trial Network [13]. Therapeutic interventions to promote axonal regeneration have also entered clinical trials. In a phase I/IIa clinical trial, in which our laboratory was also involved, the RhoA inhibitor C3 transferase (Cethrin) was tested on patients with SCI. The observed motor recovery in this open-label trial suggests that inactivation of RhoA may increase neurological recovery after complete SCI [14,15].

1.4. Cell Therapy: Promise and Progress

Stem cell transplantation is a promising therapeutic strategy for the treatment of SCI that works through several different mechanisms [16,17]. Preclinical studies have shown encouraging beneficial effects of cell therapies in animal models of SCI. Cell therapies have been shown to have their therapeutic effect through many mechanisms that target different events occurring during the primary and secondary phases of SCI. One of these mechanisms is the replacement of cells that are lost or damaged during the injury, through differentiation or transdifferentiation into mature neurons and through myelination of oligodendrocytes. Some transplanted cells render their therapeutic effect by providing neurotrophic factors that are crucial in order to enhance neuronal regeneration and survival. Some other cell types are beneficial to SCI through downregulation of inhibitory molecules, immunomodulation, modulation of the environment and extracellular matrix or by providing scaffold support for the regeneration of axons [16–18].

Several differentiated, multipotent or pluripotent cell types have been investigated so far for the treatment of SCI. Some of these cells have entered clinical trials. One such study is a phase I/II trial using human neural progenitor cells (NPCs) sponsored by Stem Cells Inc. (Newark, CA, United States of America). Our centre (Toronto Western Hospital) is involved in this trial, in collaboration with other centers at the University of Calgary and the University of Zurich. The first patient in this trial was treated in Toronto in February, 2014. Despite these advances, stem cell therapy for SCI is limited by the availability of the ideal cell source, the control and safety of the transplantation and the ethical and logistical challenges surrounding the use of stem cells.

Here, we briefly describe some of the most important cell types that have been investigated so far for the treatment of SCI. For a more thorough review on the application of these cells, refer to the recent review from our laboratory on this topic [17].

1.4.1. Neural Progenitor Cells

Neural progenitor cells (NPCs) have attracted great interest as a potential source for replacing damaged or lost neurons and glia in SCI [16]. Our laboratory and others have shown that transplantation of rodent and human NPCs into the spinal cord improves neural repair and regeneration, as well as functional recovery following traumatic SCI in rodents. This occurs via cell replacement and plasticity, remyelination and nutrient secretion, increasing axonal regeneration and immunomodulatory effects [19–24]. Although adult NPCs, derived from the CNS, are attractive for use after SCI due to their neural commitment and lack of tumorigenicity [20,22,24], the derivation of adult or embryonic NPCs for autologous transplantation is not feasible. This is due to the fact that these cells are collected from the brains of aborted fetuses or post-mortem patients, which possibly excludes their application in the clinical treatment of SCI. Furthermore, concerns regarding donor cell rejection have been problematic in SCI, in which activated inflammatory responses can present an intrinsically hostile environment to any allogeneic grafts.

1.4.2. Mesenchymal Stromal Cells

Mesenchymal stromal cells (MSCs) are multipotent cells that originate from the mesodermal germ layer. Several labs have studied the effect of MSCs for the treatment of SCI. These studies demonstrate that MSCs exert their beneficial effect mostly by providing immunomodulation, trophic support, environmental modification and by providing physical scaffolding for elongating axons [25–28], resulting in improvement of locomotor function [29–33]. Due to poor engraftment and limited differentiation under *in vivo* conditions, MSCs do not have the potential to be used for cell replacement therapy for SCI, and their therapeutic effect is limited to providing trophic support. An additional limitation is the potential of MSCs to differentiate into unwanted mesenchymal lineages.

1.4.3. Schwann Cells

Schwann cells (SCs) are one of the first cell types to have been used for the treatment of SCI. In the past two decades, many studies have demonstrated positive results and potential for SC transplantation as a therapy for SCI. They may do this by sustaining regeneration and through remyelination of damaged CNS axons, as well as by secreting several neurotrophic factors (such as NGF, BDNF and CNTF) [34] that aid the survival and intrinsic regeneration ability of damaged neurons. SCs have also been investigated in a clinical trial for the treatment of SCI [35]. In this trial, SCs were transplanted into the spinal cord one year after injury. This study demonstrated no adverse effects from SC transplantation, and one patient showed improvements in motor and sensory functions combined with extensive rehabilitation [35].

1.4.4. Olfactory Ensheathing Glia

Olfactory ensheathing glia (OEG) are a type of myelinating cell derived from the olfactory mucosa. Like SCs, OEGs have also been transplanted as myelinating cells for the treatment of SCI in numerous studies in animal models of SCI. OEGs have been shown to facilitate remyelination and tissue scaffolding and can stimulate the regeneration of lesioned axons [36,37]. OEGs have also entered into clinical trials for the treatment of SCI. In one trial, no complications were reported one year after transplantation of OEG, but no functional recovery on the ASIA (American Spinal Injury Association) scale was found [38,39].

1.4.5. Embryonic Stem Cell-Derived Cells

The isolation and propagation of the various cells types discussed above is difficult, and it is often a tedious and lengthy process to produce sufficient cells for treatment of SCI. The optimal time point for the application of cell therapy for SCI patients is 2–4 weeks after the injury [22,40], and it is important to have a sufficient amount of cells at this time window ready for transplantation. Embryonic stem cells (ESCs) are pluripotent cells derived from the inner cell mass of blastocysts with the ability to replicate indefinitely and the potential to differentiate into the cell types discussed above and, thus, may be useful as an accessible source for providing these cells for SCI treatment. Several studies have shown the beneficial effects of cells derived from ESCs in functional recovery in animal models of SCI [41–46]. Although providing a sufficient quantity of multipotent cells and differentiated ESCs is more feasible and requires less time, there are ethical issues concerning the destruction of human embryos or fertilized oocytes to obtain such stem cells. This has been a major impediment to developing clinically useful stem cell sources and to using them in clinical applications. Furthermore, there is the possibility of tumorigenesis due to incomplete differentiation.

2. Induced Pluripotent Stem Cells

The discovery of induced pluripotent stem cells (iPSCs) by Takahashi and Yamanaka in 2006 [47] opened novel opportunities in providing pluripotent stem cells for the treatment of patients with SCI and other injuries/diseases. They showed that stem cells with properties similar to ESCs could be generated from mouse fibroblasts by simultaneously introducing four factors: Oct4, Sox2, Klf2 and c-Myc [47]. In 2007, they reported that a similar approach was applicable for human fibroblasts to generate human iPSCs [48]. At the same time, James Thomson's group also reported the generation of human iPSCs using a different combination of factors including: Oct4, Sox2, Nanog and Lin28 [49]. Since iPSCs can be derived directly from adult tissues, they can be made in a patient-specific manner that circumvents ethical and moral concerns while allowing for autologous transplantation.

2.1. Methods of Generating iPSCs

It is very important to have a safe and reliable method for the generation of iPSCs for clinical purposes. To reprogram the somatic cells into a pluripotent state, reprogramming factors should be introduced to the cells. Different combinations of reprogramming factors can be used with different efficiency and outcomes [50,51], which may be critical for clinical applications. Reprogramming methods that do not use the oncogene, c-Myc, are desirable to reduce the risk of tumor formation, but methods that exclude c-Myc are associated with significantly lower reprogramming efficiency [52]. Recently, the Yamanaka group has shown that the transcription factor, Glis1, can be used as a substitute for c-Myc for the induction of pluripotency [53].

The suitability of iPSCs for use in the clinic is also dependent on the method by which the reprogramming factors are delivered to the cell. Traditionally, lentiviruses have been used to deliver the reprogramming factors, but random integration of the lentivirus DNA into the host genome raises concerns about the risk of tumorigenicity and the safety of this method. Other viruses, like adenovirus [54] and Sendai virus (SeV) [55], have also been used as less risky options. Adenovirus is considered to be safer than lentivirus, because it does not incorporate any of its own genes into the targeted host and, thus, avoids the potential for insertional mutagenesis [54]. SeV has higher efficiency in infecting a wide spectrum of host cell species and tissues compared to adenoviruses. Furthermore, SeV vectors replicate in the form of negative-sense single-stranded RNA in the cytoplasm of infected cells, which do not go through a DNA phase nor integrate into the host genome [55].

Various studies have recently described the induction of pluripotency without the use of viruses, but instead by using recombinant proteins [56], mRNAs [57], microRNAs [58], episomal vectors [59] and even removable transposons [60]. The piggyBac transposons have been shown to be able to deliver the reprogramming factors without leaving any footprint mutations in the host cell genome. The piggyBac system involves the re-excision of exogenous genes, which eliminates issues, such as insertional mutagenesis [61].

Another exciting approach that has been investigated recently is the use of small molecules and chemical compounds that can mimic the effects of transcription factors. The histone deacetylase

(HDAC) inhibitor, valproic acid, has been shown to be able to mimic the signaling that is caused by the transcription factor, c-Myc, and can be used instead of c-Myc for reprogramming [62]. A similar type of compensatory mechanism has been proposed to mimic the effects of Sox2 by inhibition of histone methyl transferase (HMT) with BIX-01294 in combination with the activation of calcium channels in the plasma membrane [63]. More recently, Deng *et al.* (2013) showed that iPSCs could be created without any genetic modification. They used a cocktail of seven small-molecule compounds, including DZNep (3-deazaneplanocin A), to induce mouse somatic cells into stem cells, which they called CiPS (chemically induced pluripotent stem) cells, with an efficiency of 0.2%, comparable to those using standard iPSC production techniques [64].

2.2. Cell Sources for Generating iPSCs

Along with choosing the right reprogramming factors and delivery method for the generation of iPSCs, it is also important to use a source of cells that will generate the desirable cell types for transplantation into the spinal cord. Several different types of cells have been used to produce iPSCs, including fibroblasts, neural progenitor cells, keratinocytes, melanocytes, CD34$^+$ cells, hepatocytes, cord blood cells and adipose stem cells (Figure 1).

iPSCs can even be derived from terminally-differentiated post-mitotic neurons. The cell types that are reprogrammed to become iPSCs can influence the differentiation capacity of the resultant iPSCs, due to epigenetic memory and genetic variations of their original cell line (Figure 2) [65–69]. The ideal iPSC source for the treatment of SCI should reprogram efficiently, be able to be isolated in large quantities in a reasonable period of time and, more importantly, should be able to differentiate into the desired multipotent/differentiated cell types that are required for the treatment of SCI. The efficiency of cell reprogramming varies among different cell types. For example, human keratinocytes from skin biopsies can be reprogrammed to pluripotency at a much higher frequency and more quickly than fibroblasts [70]. On the other hand, the iPSCs derived from keratinocytes have an increased tendency to differentiate into NPCs than do iPSCs from CD34$^+$ blood cells [66]. More research is needed to determine the best starting somatic cell for iPSC generation that allows for reproducible differentiation into NPCs and other multipotent cell types for transplantation into SCI.

2.2.1. Skin Fibroblasts

Skin fibroblasts are one of the most used cell types for reprogramming. Adult human fibroblasts can be easily isolated and maintained in culture [71,72], which makes them ideal for autologous transplantation in SCI patients. However, it takes a long time to reprogram these cells into iPSCs. Three to four weeks are required for expanding fibroblasts taken from human skin biopsy [73]. It takes another three to four weeks for iPSC colonies to appear [73]. Even after two months of culturing, the reprogramming efficiency of adult human fibroblasts from the skin is only 0.01% when the four Yamanaka factors are used and can be even lower if three or less of the factors are used [62]. Yamanaka postulated that since fibroblasts are terminally-differentiated cells, they require greater energy to reprogram than cells that are less differentiated [74]. However, recent studies have shown that it is possible to enhance the efficiency of iPSC generation by up to 100-fold, by using different combinations of reprogramming factors [51].

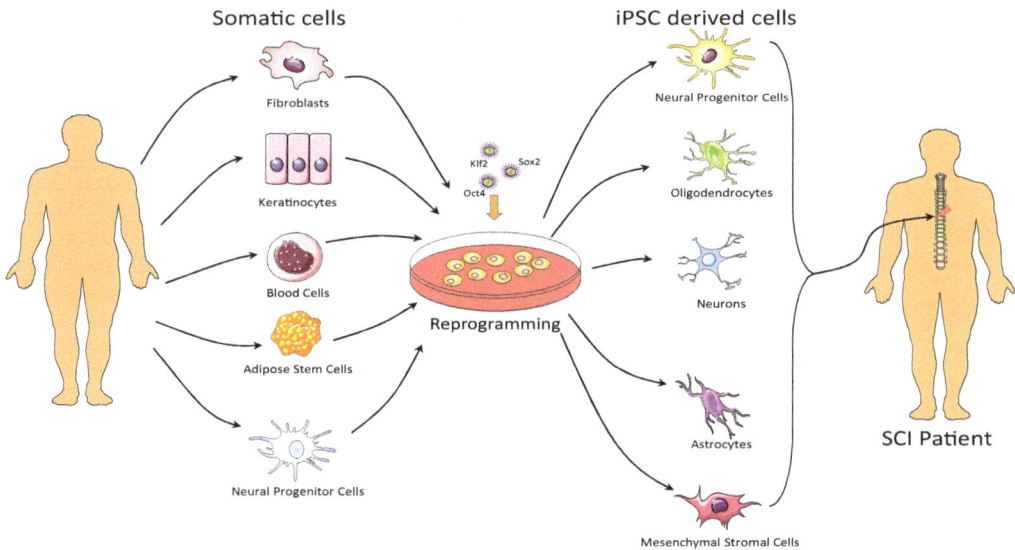

Figure 1. Several different types of cells have been used to produce iPSCs, including fibroblasts, neural progenitor cells, keratinocytes, melanocytes, CD34[+] cells, cord blood cells and adipose stem cells. The next step, after generating iPSCs, towards the treatment of spinal cord injury (SCI) is to differentiate the iPSCs to the appropriate multipotent or differentiated cell type that can be used for the treatment of SCI. To date, several different cell types have been successfully derived from iPSCs and have been transplanted into SCI animal models, including neuronal progenitor cells, neurons, oligodendrocytes, astrocytes, neural crest cells and mesenchymal stromal cells.

2.2.2. Keratinocytes

There has been some interest in using keratinocytes for reprogramming, because they can be easily obtained from the human foreskin with minimal invasiveness [75]. This presents the opportunity to use keratinocyte-derived iPSCs for autologous transplantation in patients with SCI. Keratinocytes take longer to expand than fibroblasts, but can be reprogrammed more quickly (10 days) and have a higher reprogramming efficiency [76]. The higher reprogramming efficiency may be due to the higher levels of endogenous Klf4 and C-Myc [76], meaning that these cells require less energy to reach pluripotency. Although it is thought that cells isolated from younger sources are better suited for reprogramming, Linta *et al.* were able to achieve a reprogramming efficiency of 2.8% using adult keratinocytes transfected with the Yamanaka factors using lentiviruses [77].

This demonstrates the importance of considering the appropriate age and reprogramming conditions, as well as the cell type when determining the ideal method for developing iPSCs.

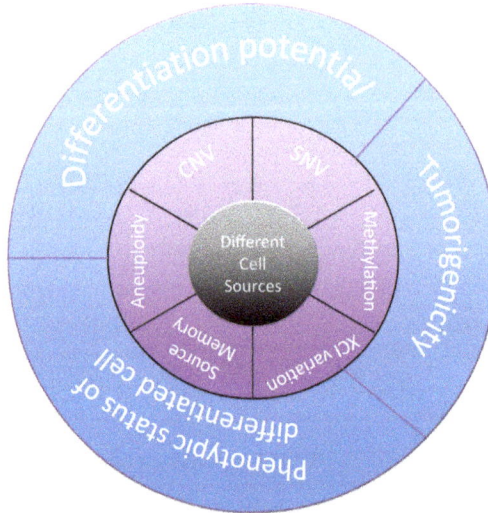

Figure 2. The epigenetic and genetic variations among different cell sources used for reprogramming can affect the properties of the iPSC and its differentiation to the target cell type. The characteristics of the different cell sources are at the core of defining how easily hiPSCs (human induced pluripotent stem cells) can be produced and their characteristics. Variations in aneuploidy, subchromosomal copy number variations (CNV), single-nucleotide variations (SNV), methylation, X chromosome inactivation (XCI) and source memory in the different cell sources can affect the differentiation potential, tumorigenicity and phenotypic status of hiPSCs. Aneuploidy is an abnormality in chromosome number. It is estimated that 13% of hiPSC cultures have karyotype abnormalities, commonly trisomy 12 [68]. CNVs are alterations in the DNA that lead to an abnormal number of a segment of the chromosome. They can occur around pluripotency genes, such as NANOG on chromosome 12 [67]. There can be as many as a dozen SNVs in a hiPSC line that may be inherited from their somatic cell source [69]. XCI is a process where one of the X chromosomes in the cell isolated from a female source is inactivated, so that it does not receive a double dose of the gene product. Reprogramming of certain cells may be more prone to XCI variations than others. Different lines of hiPSCs may have different methylation states, as shown by the fact that blood-derived iPSCs have an enhanced ability to become blood cells. This type of source memory is important to consider, since iPSCs can dedifferentiate after reprogramming to the source cell type [78].

2.2.3. Melanocytes

Like fibroblasts, melanocytes can also be isolated from skin biopsies. Melanocytes contain high levels of endogenous Sox2, so they can be reprogrammed using just the other three factors [79]. In addition, melanocytes take only 10 days to reprogram and have been shown to have a reprogramming efficiency of 0.19% [79]. All of this suggests that melanocytes may be a better option for use as sources for iPSCs than fibroblasts for autologous transplantation.

2.2.4. CD34+ Cells

CD34+ cells isolated from human umbilical cord blood and peripheral blood have been used to generate iPSCs [80]. The collection of CD34+ cells from the peripheral blood of SCI patients is not thought to be ideal, since it has to be collected from patients undergoing granulocyte colony stimulating factor (G-CSF) mobilization [80]. G-CSF use is associated with increased risk of complications and side effects [81], which might not be well tolerated by SCI patients. CD34+ cells have a low reprogramming efficiency of 0.01%–0.02% with the Yamanaka factors [80]. The reprogramming efficiency is even lower for CD34+ cells isolated from umbilical cord blood [82].

2.2.5. Cord Blood Cells

Umbilical cord blood may be a better source of iPSCs, since the method of isolation is less invasive, and they can be cryopreserved for more than five years and still be used to generate iPSCs [83]. Another benefit of cord blood is that many cord blood banks exist worldwide. CD133+ cells from umbilical cord blood can be reprogrammed to iPSCs using just Oct4 and Sox2 with a reprogramming efficiency of 0.45% [83]. Endothelial cells can also be isolated from cord blood and reprogrammed to iPSCs [84]. Cell isolated from the umbilical cord have primitive characteristics that make them ideal for reprogramming, since they may be epigenetically closer to iPSCs than other differentiated cells [85]. However, iPSCs derived from the umbilical cord cannot be considered as sources of autologous transplantation for SCI patients, unless the patient had already deposited his/her umbilical cord in cord blood banks after birth.

2.2.6. Adipose Stem Cells

Adipose stem cells are multipotent cells that are collected by lipoaspiration [86]. As many as 100 million cells can be isolated from a 300-mL sample and can be expanded for reprogramming in approximately 48 h [87]. Using the Yamanaka factors, adipose stem cells can be reprogrammed in 10 to 15 days at a reprogramming efficiency of 0.2% [87]. Adipose stem cells express high levels of Klf4, and their multipotent nature would theoretically make them require fewer epigenetic changes to reach pluripotency [88].

2.2.7. Neural Progenitor Cells

Multipotent cells, such as neural progenitor cells (NPCs), require fewer factors to be reprogrammed. Human fetal NPCs can be reprogrammed in seven to eight weeks using only

Oct4 [89]. However, the reprogramming efficiency is very low, at 0.004%. NPCs are not an ideal source for generating iPSCs for use in the treatment of SCI, because they are not readily available and there are ethical issues associated with their use.

3. Using iPSC-Derived Cells for Treatment of SCI

The next step towards the treatment of SCI after generating iPSCs is to differentiate the iPSCs into the appropriate multipotent or differentiated cell type that can be used for the treatment of SCI (Figure 1). Due to the high risk of teratoma formation, the differentiation process should be "definitively" completed, and the cell population should be devoid of pluripotent cells. The direct injection of iPSCs into the injured spinal cord can be problematic. In an un-published study, Hodgetts *et al.* transplanted undifferentiated hiPSCs into the spinal cord in a thoracic level 7 (T7) contusion model of SCI in nude rats at seven days post injury [90]. They did not observe any significant improvement in motor function by five weeks after SCI with this method, despite subtle differences in some neuronal marker expressions at the lesion site [90].

To date, several different cell types have been successfully derived from iPSCs and have been transplanted into animal models of SCI. These studies have provided a proof of principle that iPSCs can be successfully differentiated *in vitro* to yield desirable progeny. They can be safely transplanted into models of SCI and survive, integrate and differentiate into desired phenotypes, as well as promoting functional recovery with an outcome comparable to the counterpart ESC therapy. iPSC-derived cells can be useful in the treatment of SCI through cell replacement and restoration of lost myelin and through trophic support, which results in the induction of neuroprotection and a reduction in cell loss. They may also be a source of increased regeneration and neuroplasticity. Cytokines and chemokines, which are secreted by iPSC-derived cells, can also have immunomodulatory effects. iPSC-derived cells can help remodel the physical structure of the tissue following injury to make it a less inhibitory and more permissive substrate for neural regeneration. The influence of iPSC-derived cells on astrogliosis at the early stages of injury can halt the expansion of the cystic cavity. The different potential cellular and molecular mechanisms through which iPSC-derived cells can exert their therapeutic effects in SCI are illustrated in Figure 3.

3.1. iPSC-Derived NPCs

One of the most promising cell types that has been studied so far for the treatment of SCI are NPCs. However, as discussed in the previous section, the availability of adult NPCs for SCI patients is limited, if even available at all. NPCs can also be derived from ESCs. However, the logistical and ethical issues surrounding the use of ESCs are quite significant. iPSCs present an alternative and potentially clinically attractive approach for the derivation of NPCs.

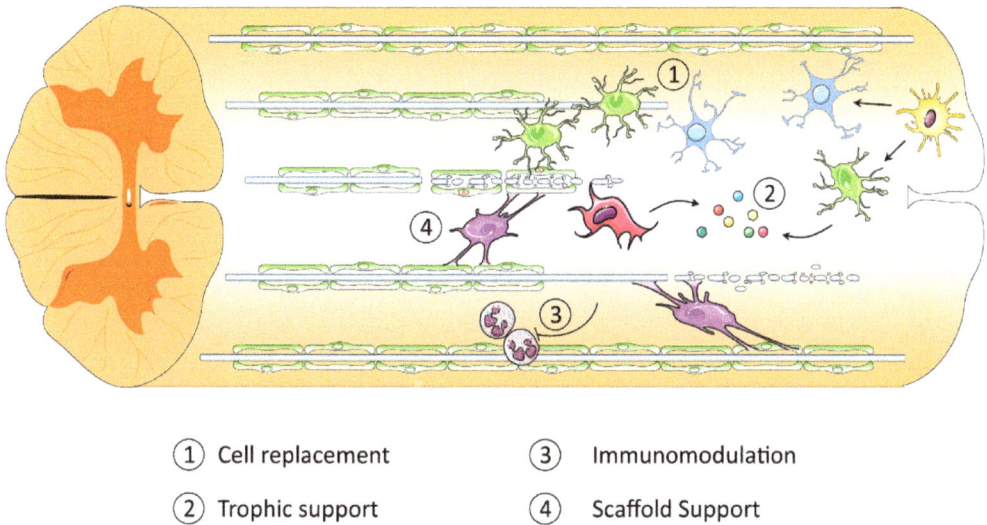

① Cell replacement   ③ Immunomodulation

② Trophic support   ④ Scaffold Support

Figure 3. iPSC-derived cells exert their therapeutic effects for the treatment of SCI through different mechanisms. Some transplanted cells, like iPSC-derived neural progenitor cells (NPCs), can replace lost or damaged cells through differentiation or transdifferentiation into mature neurons and oligodendrocytes ①. iPSC-derived neurons and oligodendrocytes can also potentially replace lost or damaged cells. iPSC-derived cells, such as mesenchymal stromal cells (MSCs), NPCs astrocytes and oligodendrocytes, provide neurotrophic factors (like GDNF, NGF, BDNF and CNTF), which are crucial to enhancing neuronal regeneration and survival ②. iPSC-derived MSCs can also be beneficial to SCI by downregulating inhibitory molecules and immunomodulation ③. iPSC-derived astrocytes and oligodendrocytes can potentially modulate the environment and provide a scaffold support for the regeneration of axons ④.

Several protocols have been developed to differentiate iPSCs into neural precursors and specific neuronal and glial lineages. In our lab, definitive neural progenitor cells were recently generated from piggy-Bac transposon iPSCs, and by inducing the NOTCH signaling pathway, we enhanced NPC generation with reduced expression of pluripotency and nonectodermal markers [61]. We have shown that this method is safe and effective [61]. Other studies using iPSC-NPCs in rodent and primate models of SCI have indicated that transplanted cells differentiate into neurons and glia *in vivo*, enhance remyelination and axon regeneration, supporte the survival of endogenous neurons and promote locomotor recovery and sensory responses [91–93]. These pre-clinical studies led to the launch of a collaborative team by Okano and Yamanaka laboratories, who are currently planning a clinical trial for hiPSC-derived NPC transplantation for SCI patients in the sub-acute phase. This study will use clinical-grade integration-free human iPSC lines that will be generated by Kyoto University's Center for iPS Cell Research and Application (CiRA).

The Okano group has done several pioneering studies examining the transplantation of iPSC-derived NPCs for the treatment of SCI [92,94,95]. They tested different iPSC lines derived from mouse embryonic fibroblasts (MEF) or mouse tail tip fibroblasts (TTF). The iPSCs were differentiated into NPCs, and the tumorigenicity of each NPC line was pre-evaluated by transplantation into the brains of immunocompromised mice. They proposed that each iPSC line has to be pre-evaluated to assess teratoma formation after cell transplantation in animal models due to the differences among iPSC lines in differentiation capacity and teratoma formation. In this study, around 9.5×10^5 cells were transplanted into the spinal cord in a T10 contusion mouse model of SCI at nine days after injury, the time window when most of the inflammatory responses are reduced. The survival rate of transplanted cells was around 20%, and they differentiated into 30% neurons, 50% astrocytes and 15% oligodendrocytes. In the transplantation group, motor function was restored for a long period of time without tumors developing. This study showed that the functional recovery after transplantation of iPSC-derived neurospheres is attributable to three possible mechanisms: (1) remyelination by mouse iPSC-derived oligodendrocytes; (2) axonal regrowth; and (3) trophic support. Those transplanted cells that differentiated into immature astrocytes may play a role in the guidance of regenerating axons [95]. The Okano group next proceeded to test the efficiency of iPSCs derived from human fibroblasts [94]. hiPSC-derived NPCs were transplanted into the spinal cord of NOD-SCID (non-obese diabetic-server combine immunodeficiency) mice with a T10 contusion injury. Transplanted cells survived, migrated and differentiated toward all neural cell fates (50% neurons, astrocytes and oligodendrocytes) and contributed to restoring motor function. These neurons could integrate into the host tissue and functioned as interneurons. They formed synapses with the host neurons and contributed to the reconstruction of neural circuits. This preclinical study serves to validate hiPSCs as a source of neural cells and represents an important step towards clinical practice [94]. In their next step towards the clinical application of hiPSC-NPCs in the treatment of SCI, they used a primate model of SCI [92]. This primate study demonstrated that hiPSC-NPCs can promote long-term functional recovery without tumorigenicity [92]. Similarly, Fujimoto *et al.* (2012) have shown that the transplantation of hiPSC-derived NPCs into a T9 contusion model of SCI in NOD-SCID mice could result in functional recovery [91]. NPCs were derived from iPSCs in a monolayer procedure, and around 10×10^5 cells were transplanted into the lesion epicenter at seven days post-SCI. Grafted cells showed a survival rate of 20% and differentiated into 75% neurons, 20% astrocytes and 1% oligodendrocytes. Differentiated neurons were able to form synapses with endogenous neurons [91].

In a highly clinically-relevant study of chronic cervical SCI, Nutt *et al.* (2013) used a human iPSC line derived from human fetal lung fibroblasts for the generation of NPCs. This study transplanted 2×10^5 cells into a C4 contusion rat model of SCI at the chronic time point of four weeks after injury. By four weeks after transplant, hiPSC-NPCs were mainly differentiated to astrocytes (30%) and neurons (15%), but no oligodendrocyte marker was detected. However by eight weeks after transplantation, transplanted cells with an oligodendrocyte marker (17%) were detected, though none could convincingly form myelin. Despite thorough integration and differentiation into both neurons and glia, assessment of behavioral recovery indicated that transplantation of hiPSC-NPCs did not confer any significant improvement in functional recovery. This study suggests that the best time for cell transplantation for the treatment of SCI is likely to be in the acute phases [93]. In concordance, Romanyuk *et al.*, 2014, transplanted hiPSC-NPCs into the spinal cord one week after a balloon-induced compression SCI at T8–T9. The animals were subjected to triple drug immunosuppression. Cell transplantation resulted in increased axonal regrowth, reduced lesion cavity size and improved hindlimb functional recovery, which may be due to trophic support from the cell transplant to the spared axons [96].

In a recent study by the Tuszynski group, human iPSCs derived from the dermal fibroblasts of an 89-year-old man were differentiated into NPCs [97]. These hiPSC-NPCs were used for transplantation into the spinal cord two weeks after C5 hemisection SCI in immunodeficient rats. Grafted hiPSC-NPCs showed a high survival rate three months post-transplantation and were distributed through most of the lesion. The majority of grafted hiPSC-NPCs (71%) were differentiated into neurons, and around 18% of grafted cells differentiated into astrocytes, but no oligodendrocytes were detected amongst transplanted cells. The differentiated neurons could extend their axons directly out of the lesion site and into the host spinal cord. Interestingly, these axons extended over very long distances in the host spinal cord, continuing to extend into the brain and even reaching the olfactory bulb. However, graft-derived human axons were not detectably myelinated by rat host oligodendrocytes. The synaptic structures were also formed between graft-derived human axons and host dendrites. Furthermore, host axons were shown to be capable of growing into grafted hiPSC-derived NPCs [97].

3.2. iPSC-Derived Oligodendrocyte Progenitor Cells

Results from our laboratory and others show that functional recovery after NPC transplantation may be chiefly attributed to remyelination of host axons by myelinating oligodendrocyte progenitors differentiated from NPCs [22,23,98–101]. Therefore, a more direct approach of transplanting oligodendrocyte progenitor cells (OPCs) straight into the spinal cord may be warranted. Several protocols have been established to generate OPCs from iPSCs [102,103], including one protocol from our group, though none of these iPSC-derived OPCs have been used in models of SCI yet. However, there has been extensive research on the application of ESC-derived OPCs for the treatment of SCI, and the application of iPSC-derived OPCs is reinforced by this. The ESC-derived OPC experiments showed that their transplantation resulted in remyelination of spared axons [24,104], improved behavioral and electrophysiological outcomes [105], restoration of forelimb motor function, improved forelimb stride length, reduced cavitation and resulted in better white and gray matter sparing [24,104]. These exciting results led to FDA approval for the world's first phase I clinical trial by Geron Corporation for the transplantation of hESC-derived OPCs into individuals with thoracic (T3–T11) SCI on January 23, 2009. hESC-OPCs were administered into the lesion site within 14 days of injury with a low dose of two million cells. The follow-up studies on the five patients have shown no serious side effects after cell transplantation. In four of the five patients, MRI scans showed that the injury site shrank and that the cells may have had some positive effects in reducing the deterioration of spinal cord tissue. However in November, 2011, Geron announced that it had ended its SCI stem cell research program for financial reasons [106,107]. In 2013, Asterias Biotherapeutics, Inc. purchased Geron's hESC-OPCs and recently obtained FDA approval for a dose escalation study of patients with spinal cord injury with high level (cervical) injuries [108].

3.3. iPSC Derived Motor Neurons

Stem cell-derived motor neurons (MNs) are increasingly utilized as cellular replacement strategies for the treatment of SCI. Motor neurons (MNs) and motor neuron progenitors (MNPs) have been successfully generated from iPSCs [109]. There are several protocols established for the generation of MNs from iPSCs. In one protocol, the exogenous expression of MN-specific factors, neurogenin 2 (NGN2), islet-1 (ISL-1) and LIM/homeobox protein 3 (LHX3), in hiPSCs derived from human fibroblasts resulted in the generation of motor neurons. There are also some other successful protocols for the generation of MNPs and MNs from iPSCs involving the sequential use of reprogramming factors, such as bFGF, activin, retinoic acid (RA) and Sonic hedgehog (SHH), in addition to growth factors, such as GDNF, BDNF and CNTF [110,111]. Although the efficiency of iPSC-derived MNs has not been tested yet for the treatment of SCI, previous data from ESC-derived MNs suggest that the application of iPSC-derived MNs may be promising. Transplantation of ESC-derived MNPs into the spinal cord of an adult rat after SCI resulted in enhanced sprouting of endogenous axons [44,45], and MNPs were shown to be able to mature into MNs and resulted in the improvement of functional recovery when transplanted *in vivo* [112].

3.4. iPSC-Derived Neural Crest Cells

Neural crest cells originate from cells at the border between the neuroectoderm and the surface ectoderm. They are a transient population of cells that give rise to neurons and the glial cells of the peripheral nervous system. They can be differentiated *in vitro* into Schwann cells (SC) by neuregulin-1 [113], which are capable of myelinating sensory axons *in vitro* [114], and can potentially be used for transplantation into SCI. Neural crest stem cells (NCSCs) are capable of integrating into spinal cord tissue and differentiating into neurons and myelinating oligodendrocytes [115,116]. However, human neural crest cells are difficult to obtain, because of their transient nature and the limited availability of human fetal cells [114]. There are several protocols established to derive NCSCs from iPSCs [117,118]. These iPSC-derived NCSCs can also be differentiated into Schwann cells [117,118]. hiPSC-derived NCSCs have been used *in vivo* for neural tissue engineering in athymic rat models of peripheral nerve injury. They were shown to differentiate into Schwann cells and participate in the myelination of regenerating axons [119]. The first description of iPSC-NCSC survival and integration into the spinal cord was demonstrated in a lamb spina bifida model [120], findings that support the potential application of iPSC-derived NCSCs for the treatment of SCI.

3.5. iPSC Derived Astrocytes

Although reactive astrocytes proliferate, form a glial scar, and secrete inhibitory agents, such as chondroitin sulfate proteoglycan, there are reports showing that the transplantation of purified astrocytes promotes axonal regeneration and functional recovery in a rat model of SCI [121]. The compaction of the lesion center and seclusion of inflammatory cells by migrating reactive astrocytes seem to underlie this beneficial effect [122,123]. Astrocytes can be derived from iPSCs [124–126]. In one study, astrocytes derived from iPSCs were transplanted three and seven days after T9–10 level SCI in rats. The transplanted cells survived in the spinal cords eight weeks after transplantation, but they did not result in significant locomotor recovery. However, astrocyte transplantation increased the sensitivity to mechanical stimulus and thermal hyperalgesia [125].

3.6. iPSC-Derived MSCs

MSCs are a promising cell source for the treatment of SCI. Although easy access to MSCs is recognized as a great advantage, extended *in vitro* culture reduces the differentiation potential of MSCs, limiting their therapeutic efficacy. Bone marrow-derived MSCs, have a limited capacity to proliferate, quickly lose differentiation potential and reduce protective factors during *ex vivo* expansion before possible therapeutic use [127]. MSCs derived from iPSCs have the potential to be expanded indefinitely without senescence [128]. To overcome the limitations of MSCs, iPSC-derived MSCs have been considered as a promising alternative for cell therapy.

MSCs have been successfully generated from iPSCs [127,129], and interestingly, they have been shown to have greater regenerative potential compared to MSCs derived from bone marrow [127]. This may be attributable to superior survival and engraftment after transplantation, because of higher telomerase activity and less senescence as compared to bone marrow-derived MSCs [127]. Future studies should examine the efficiency of iPSC-derived MSCs on different clinically relevant SCI models and compare them to umbilical cord-derived or bone marrow-derived MSCs.

4. Future Approaches and Prospects

4.1. Using Directly Reprogrammed Cells for the Treatment of SCI

The process of deriving iPSC lines and subsequently inducing differentiation is very time consuming and inefficient (0.01%–1% cell yield). In addition, the use of pluripotent-derived cells might lead to the development of tumors if not properly controlled. The transdifferentiation of one mature somatic cell into another mature somatic cell without undergoing an intermediate pluripotent state or progenitor cell type has become possible in recent years. It is now possible to directly convert fully differentiated mature cells into a variety of other cell types, while bypassing an intermediate pluripotent state. Bypassing the intermediate pluripotent state reduces the time required for generating a specific cell type and, more importantly, reduces the risk of teratoma formation. It is postulated that the future direction of cell therapy will shift from iPSCs to directly reprogrammed cells. Different cell types with potential application for the treatment of SCI have been generated recently using direct reprogramming methods [130].

4.1.1. iNPC

Several studies have recently demonstrated the direct induction of neural progenitor cells (NPCs) from human and mouse fibroblasts using a range of pluripotent and neural transcription factors. Kim *et al.* (2012) have shown that fibroblasts can be directly reprogrammed into NPCs (iNPCs) by using a combination of Yamanaka factors and growth factors in culture media [130]. These iNPCs could not be maintained for more than three to five passages and lacked the potential to differentiate into oligodendrocytes. Later on, the Wernig lab overcame this problem and were able to generate self-renewing tripotent NPCs that could be differentiated not only into neurons and astrocytes, but also into oligodendrocytes [131]. In their method, they used Sox2, FoxG1 and Brn2 reprogramming factors. Removing Brn2 from this combination gave rise to the formation of bipotent iNPCs that could only differentiate into astrocytes and neurons [131]. Several other combinations of factors that can directly reprogram mouse or human fibroblast into iNPCs have subsequently been discovered [132–134]. Interestingly, all of these combinations had SOX2 in common. However, recently, Mitchel *et al.* (2014) showed that tripotent iNPCs can be generated from human fibroblast using only one reprogramming factor, Oct4 [135].

4.1.2. iOPC

As discussed earlier, myelination by transplanted cells has a great impact on functional recovery after SCI. Myelination is mainly accomplished by oligodendrocyte progenitor cells (OPCs) [136]. However, sources of OPCs are largely restricted, and they have limited expansion capacity. Recently, Najm *et al.* (2013) have succeeded in the direct generation of OPCs (iOPCs) from mice fibroblasts by using eight reprogramming factors (Olig1, Olig2, Nkx2.2, Nkx6.2, Sox10, ST18, Myrf and Myt1), collectively referred to as 8TF (eight transcription factors). These iOPCs were capable of generating compact myelin in hypomyelinated shiverer mice [137]. More recently, the Wernig group was able to generate iOPCs from rodent fibroblasts just by using the three factors, Sox10, Olig2 and Zfp536. These iOPCs had the ability to differentiate into oligodendrocytes *in vitro* and to myelinate host axons after transplantation into the demyelinated shiverer mouse brain [138].

4.1.3. iN

Transplantation of neurons and motor neurons has also shown promise as a cellular therapy in animal models of SCI. Several studies have demonstrated that combinations of neural transcription factors and/or microRNAs can directly convert both mouse and human fibroblasts into neuronal cells, including dopaminergic and motor neurons [139–141]. The Wernig group has recently shown that the three factors, Ascl1, Brn2 and Myt1l, are sufficient to rapidly and efficiently convert mouse embryonic and human postnatal fibroblasts into functional neurons [140,141]. In another attempt, microRNA (miR-124) and two transcription factors (Myt1l and Brn2) [142] or just Ascl1 [143] were shown to be sufficient to directly reprogram postnatal and adult human primary dermal fibroblasts into hiN (human-induced neurons). Functionally induced motor neurons (iMNs) can be generated from mouse or human fibroblasts by using seven to eight factors (Ascl1, Brn2, Myt1l, Lhx3, Hb9, Isl1, Ngn2 and NeuroD1) [144]. iMNs displayed the electrophysiological characteristics of MNs, and they formed functional synapses with muscle fibers in culture. They were also capable of extending axons into the periphery when transplanted into the developing chick spinal cord [144].

4.2. World's First iPSC Clinical Trial

The start of the first ever clinical trial using human iPSCs at the RIKEN (Rikagaku Kenkyūjo) Center for Developmental Biology in Japan has raised a lot of hope for the treatment of human injury and disease, including SCI. This trial is using retinal pigment epithelium (RPE) cells derived from hiPSCs to treat age-related macular degeneration (AMD).

The Takahashi group at the RIKEN Center for Developmental Biology in Japan began a clinical pilot study to determine the safety and feasibility of using autologous hiPSC-derived RPE cell sheets in the treatment of wet AMD. The first patient was implanted with a 1.3 by 3.0-mm hiPSC-derived RPE sheet on September 12, 2014, in a 2-h procedure [145]. No initial complications from the surgery have been reported, and the patient will be followed up monthly for the first 24 weeks, bi-monthly for the next 28 weeks and then yearly for the next three years. Stem cell scientists around the world will be following this trial with interest.

5. Conclusions

There have been considerable advances in cell therapies for the treatment of SCI, some of which have entered clinical trials. iPSCs provide a cell source that has characteristics of embryonic stem cells, but are associated with fewer ethical and moral issues. In addition, they can be sourced from autologous sources, which may decrease the risk of immune rejection. However, there are some concerns about the use of iPSCs clinically, since many of the induction methods can increase the risk of tumors and have reprogramming efficiencies that would be too low for clinical use. In some cases, the issue of tumorigenicity may be due to partial reprogramming of the iPSCs, which may result in differentiated iPSCs reverting back to a pluripotent state [146]. Another limitation of using iPSCs clinically is that the histocompatibility of the cells may increase the risk of immune rejection. MHC I molecules make iPSCs a target of direct or indirect allorecognition [147]. Therefore, there is a need to develop histocompatible iPSC lines or to rely on patient-specific iPSCs, which adds to the time required before the treatment of the patient can begin. Lastly, there is a need to optimize the growth and expansion of iPSCs for clinical use. There is a common reliance on mouse fibroblast feeder cells to support the growth of iPSCs and the use of animal products either in the culture media or matrices used to grow the cells. This increases the risk of graft rejection [148]. One solution to this has been the use of TeSR™ media (STEMCELL Technologies, BC, Canada), which is free of animal products and does not require feeder cells to support the growth of iPSCs [149]. We also need to be able to culture the cells for use in patients at appropriate numbers, which 2D culturing systems cannot support. Microcarrier systems can be used to culture the cells in bioreactors. However, the appropriate coating, size and materials used in the microcarrier systems need to be optimized to support the growth of iPSCs, since these factors have been shown to affect cell yields of hESCs [150]. There are many methods under investigation to address these issues, including non-viral induction and direct reprogramming. With continued investigation into these methods and the start of a clinical trial using iPSCs to treat AMD, the translation to clinical use for SCI is on the horizon.

Author Contributions

Mohamad Khazaei and Ahad M. Siddiqui co-wrote the paper with greater contribution from Mohamad Khazaei. Michael G. Fehlings was the principal supervising author of this paper, providing editing and content advice and giving approval for the final version.

Conflicts of Interest

The authors declare no conflict of interest.

References

1. Sekhon, L.H.; Fehlings, M.G. Epidemiology, demographics, and pathophysiology of acute spinal cord injury. *Spine* **2001**, *26* (Suppl. S24), 2–12.
2. Fehlings, M.G.; Tator, C.H. An evidence-based review of decompressive surgery in acute spinal cord injury: Rationale, indications, and timing based on experimental and clinical studies. *J. Neurosurg.* **1999**, *91*, 1–11.
3. Fehlings, M.; Singh, A.; Tetreault, L.; Kalsi-Ryan, S.; Nouri, A. Global prevalence and incidence of traumatic spinal cord injury. *Clin. Epidemiol.* **2014**, *2014*, 309–331.
4. Baptiste, D.C.; Fehlings, M.G. Pharmacological approaches to repair the injured spinal cord. *J. Neurotrauma* **2006**, *23*, 318–334.
5. Rowland, J.W.; Hawryluk, G.W.J.; Kwon, B.; Fehlings, M.G. Current status of acute spinal cord injury pathophysiology and emerging therapies: Promise on the horizon. *Neurosurg. Focus* **2008**, *25*, doi:10.3171/FOC.2008.25.11.E2.
6. Tator, C.H.; Duncan, E.G.; Edmonds, V.E.; Lapczak, L.I.; Andrews, D.F. Changes in epidemiology of acute spinal cord injury from 1947 to 1981. *Surg. Neurol.* **1993**, *40*, 207–215.
7. Austin, J.W.; Fehlings, M.G. Molecular mechanisms of Fas-mediated cell death in oligodendrocytes. *J. Neurotrauma* **2008**, *25*, 411–426.
8. Tzekou, A.; Fehlings, M.G. Treatment of spinal cord injury with intravenous immunoglobulin G: Preliminary evidence and future perspectives. *J. Clin. Immunol.* **2014**, *34* (Suppl. S1), 132–138.
9. Fehlings, M.G.; Sekhon, L.H.; Tator, C. The role and timing of decompression in acute spinal cord injury: What do we know? What should we do? *Spine* **2001**, *26* (Suppl. S24), 101–110.
10. Tator, C.H.; Fehlings, M.G. Review of the secondary injury theory of acute spinal cord trauma with emphasis on vascular mechanisms. *J. Neurosurg.* **1991**, *75*, 15–26.
11. Wilson, J.R.; Fehlings, M.G. Emerging approaches to the surgical management of acute traumatic spinal cord injury. *Neurotherapeutics* **2011**, *8*, 187–194.
12. Fehlings, M.G.; Baptiste, D.C. Current status of clinical trials for acute spinal cord. *Injury* **2005**, *36* (Suppl. S2), 113–122.
13. Wu, Y.; Satkunendrarajah, K.; Fehlings, M.G. Riluzole improves outcome following ischemia-reperfusion injury to the spinal cord by preventing delayed paraplegia. *Neuroscience* **2014**, *265*, 302–312.

14. Fehlings, M.G.; Theodore, N.; Harrop, J.; Maurais, G.; Kuntz, C.; Shaffrey, C.I.; Kwon, B.K.; Chapman, J.; Yee, A.; Tighe, A.; *et al.* A phase I/IIa clinical trial of a recombinant RHO protein antagonist in acute spinal cord injury. *J. Neurotrauma* **2011**, *28*, 787–796.

15. McKerracher, L.; Anderson, K.D. Analysis of Recruitment and Outcomes in the Phase I/IIa Cethrin Clinical Trial for Acute Spinal Cord Injury. *J. Neurotrauma* **2013**, *30*, 1795–1804.

16. Tetzlaff, W.; Okon, E.B.; Karimi-Abdolrezaee, S.; Hill, C.E.; Sparling, J.S.; Plemel, J.R.; Plunet, W.T.; Tsai, E.C.; Baptiste, D.; Smithson, L.J.; *et al.* A systematic review of cellular transplantation therapies for spinal cord injury. *J. Neurotrauma* **2011**, *28*, 1611–1682.

17. Vawda, R.; Wilcox, J.; Fehlings, M. Current stem cell treatments for spinal cord injury. *Indian J. Orthop.* **2012**, *46*, 10–18.

18. Tobias, C.A.; Shumsky, J.S.; Shibata, M.; Tuszynski, M.H.; Fischer, I.; Tessler, A.; Murray, M. Delayed grafting of BDNF and NT-3 producing fibroblasts into the injured spinal cord stimulates sprouting, partially rescues axotomized red nucleus neurons from loss and atrophy, and provides limited regeneration. *Exp. Neurol.* **2003**, *184*, 97–113.

19. Alexanian, A.R.; Svendsen, C.N.; Crowe, M.J.; Kurpad, S.N. Transplantation of human glial-restricted neural precursors into injured spinal cord promotes functional and sensory recovery without causing allodynia. *Cytotherapy* **2011**, *13*, 61–68.

20. Cummings, B.J.; Uchida, N.; Tamaki, S.J.; Salazar, D.L.; Hooshmand, M.; Summers, R.; Gage, F.H.; Anderson, A.J. Human neural stem cells differentiate and promote locomotor recovery in spinal cord-injured mice. *Proc. Natl. Acad. Sci. USA* **2005**, *102*, 14069–14074.

21. Emgård, M.; Holmberg, L.; Samuelsson, E.-B.; Bahr, B.A.; Falci, S.; Seiger, A.; Sundström, E. Human neural precursor cells continue to proliferate and exhibit low cell death after transplantation to the injured rat spinal cord. *Brain Res.* **2009**, *1278*, 15–26.

22. Karimi-Abdolrezaee, S.; Eftekharpour, E.; Wang, J.; Morshead, C.M.; Fehlings, M.G. Delayed transplantation of adult neural precursor cells promotes remyelination and functional neurological recovery after spinal cord injury. *J. Neurosci. Off. J. Soc. Neurosci.* **2006**, *26*, 3377–3389.

23. Karimi-Abdolrezaee, S.; Eftekharpour, E.; Wang, J.; Schut, D.; Fehlings, M.G. Synergistic effects of transplanted adult neural stem/progenitor cells, chondroitinase, and growth factors promote functional repair and plasticity of the chronically injured spinal cord. *J. Neurosci. Off. J. Soc. Neurosci.* **2010**, *30*, 1657–1676.

24. Keirstead, H.S.; Nistor, G.; Bernal, G.; Totoiu, M.; Cloutier, F.; Sharp, K.; Steward, O. Human embryonic stem cell-derived oligodendrocyte progenitor cell transplants remyelinat and restore locomotion after spinal cord injury. *J. Neurosci. Off. J. Soc. Neurosci.* **2005**, *25*, 4694–4705.

25. Carrade, D.D.; Affolter, V.K.; Outerbridge, C.A.; Watson, J.L.; Galuppo, L.D.; Buerchler, S.; Kumar, V.; Walker, N.J.; Borjesson, D.L. Intradermal injections of equine allogeneic umbilical cord-derived mesenchymal stem cells are well tolerated and do not elicit immediate or delayed hypersensitivity reactions. *Cytotherapy* **2011**, *13*, 1180–1192.

26. Hofstetter, C.P.; Schwarz, E.J.; Hess, D.; Widenfalk, J.; el Manira, A.; Prockop, D.J.; Olson, L. Marrow stromal cells form guiding strands in the injured spinal cord and promote recovery. *Proc. Natl. Acad. Sci. USA* **2002**, *99*, 2199–2204.

27. Malgieri, A.; Kantzari, E.; Patrizi, M.P.; Gambardella, S. Bone marrow and umbilical cord blood human mesenchymal stem cells: State of the art. *Int. J. Clin. Exp. Med.* **2010**, *3*, 248–269.

28. Mothe, A.J.; Bozkurt, G.; Catapano, J.; Zabojova, J.; Wang, X.; Keating, A.; Tator, C.H. Intrathecal transplantation of stem cells by lumbar puncture for thoracic spinal cord injury in the rat. *Spinal Cord* **2011**, *49*, 967–973.

29. Boido, M.; Garbossa, D.; Fontanella, M.; Ducati, A.; Vercelli, A. Mesenchymal stem cell transplantation reduces glial cyst and improves functional outcome after spinal cord compression. *World Neurosurg.* **2014**, *81*, 183–190.

30. Karaoz, E.; Kabatas, S.; Duruksu, G.; Okcu, A.; Subasi, C.; Ay, B.; Musluman, M.; Civelek, E. Reduction of lesion in injured rat spinal cord and partial functional recovery of motility after bone marrow derived mesenchymal stem cell transplantation. *Turk. Neurosurg.* **2012**, *22*, 207–217.

31. Park, W.B.; Kim, S.Y.; Lee, S.H.; Kim, H.-W.; Park, J.-S.; Hyun, J.K. The effect of mesenchymal stem cell transplantation on the recovery of bladder and hindlimb function after spinal cord contusion in rats. *BMC Neurosci.* **2010**, *11*, doi:10.1186/1471-2202-11-119.

32. Urdzíková, L.; Jendelová, P.; Glogarová, K.; Burian, M.; Hájek, M.; Syková, E. Transplantation of bone marrow stem cells as well as mobilization by granulocyte-colony stimulating factor promotes recovery after spinal cord injury in rats. *J. Neurotrauma* **2006**, *23*, 1379–1391.

33. Urdzíková, L.M.; Růžička, J.; LaBagnara, M.; Kárová, K.; Kubinová, S.; Jiráková, K.; Murali, R.; Syková, E.; Jhanwar-Uniyal, M.; Jendelová, P. Human mesenchymal stem cells modulate inflammatory cytokines after spinal cord injury in rat. *Int. J. Mol. Sci.* **2014**, *15*, 11275–11293.

34. Park, H.-W.; Lim, M.-J.; Jung, H.; Lee, S.-P.; Paik, K.-S.; Chang, M.-S. Human mesenchymal stem cell-derived Schwann cell-like cells exhibit neurotrophic effects, via distinct growth factor production, in a model of spinal cord injury. *Glia* **2010**, *58*, 1118–1132.

35. Saberi, H.; Moshayedi, P.; Aghayan, H.-R.; Arjmand, B.; Hosseini, S.-K.; Emami-Razavi, S.-H.; Rahimi-Movaghar, V.; Raza, M.; Firouzi, M. Treatment of chronic thoracic spinal cord injury patients with autologous Schwann cell transplantation: An interim report on safety considerations and possible outcomes. *Neurosci. Lett.* **2008**, *443*, 46–50.

36. Dlouhy, B.J.; Awe, O.; Rao, R.C.; Kirby, P.A.; Hitchon, P.W. Autograft-derived spinal cord mass following olfactory mucosal cell transplantation in a spinal cord injury patient. *J. Neurosurg. Spine* **2014**, *21*, 618–622.

37. Gingras, M.; Beaulieu, M.-M.; Gagnon, V.; Durham, H.D.; Berthod, F. *In vitro* study of axonal migration and myelination of motor neurons in a three-dimensional tissue-engineered model. *Glia* **2008**, *56*, 354–364.

38. Féron, F.; Perry, C.; Cochrane, J.; Licina, P.; Nowitzke, A.; Urquhart, S.; Geraghty, T.; Mackay-Sim, A. Autologous olfactory ensheathing cell transplantation in human spinal cord injury. *Brain J. Neurol.* **2005**, *128*, 2951–2960.

39. Mackay-Sim, A.; Féron, F.; Cochrane, J.; Bassingthwaighte, L.; Bayliss, C.; Davies, W.; Fronek, P.; Gray, C.; Kerr, G.; Licina, P.; *et al.* Autologous olfactory ensheathing cell transplantation in human paraplegia: A 3-year clinical trial. *Brain J. Neurol.* **2008**, *131*, 2376–2386.

40. Ogawa, Y.; Sawamoto, K.; Miyata, T.; Miyao, S.; Watanabe, M.; Nakamura, M.; Bregman, B.S.; Koike, M.; Uchiyama, Y.; Toyama, Y.; *et al.* Transplantation of *in vitro*-expanded fetal neural progenitor cells results in neurogenesis and functional recovery after spinal cord contusion injury in adult rats. *J. Neurosci. Res.* **2002**, *69*, 925–933.

41. Hatami, M.; Mehrjardi, N.Z.; Kiani, S.; Hemmesi, K.; Azizi, H.; Shahverdi, A.; Baharvand, H. Human embryonic stem cell-derived neural precursor transplants in collagen scaffolds promote recovery in injured rat spinal cord. *Cytotherapy* **2009**, *11*, 618–630.

42. Johnson, P.J.; Tatara, A.; McCreedy, D.A.; Shiu, A.; Sakiyama-Elbert, S.E. Tissue-engineered fibrin scaffolds containing neural progenitors enhance functional recovery in a subacute model of SCI. *Soft Matter* **2010**, *6*, 5127–5137.

43. Lukovic, D.; Valdés-Sanchez, L.; Sanchez-Vera, I.; Moreno-Manzano, V.; Stojkovic, M.; Bhattacharya, S.S.; Erceg, S. Brief Report: Astrogliosis Promotes Functional Recovery of Completely Transected Spinal Cord Following Transplantation of hESC-Derived Oligodendrocyte and Motoneuron Progenitors: Reactive Astrocytes in Spinal Cord Injury. *Stem Cells* **2014**, *32*, 594–599.

44. Nógrádi, A.; Pajer, K.; Márton, G. The role of embryonic motoneuron transplants to restore the lost motor function of the injured spinal cord. *Ann. Anat.* **2011**, *193*, 362–370.

45. Rossi, S.L.; Nistor, G.; Wyatt, T.; Yin, H.Z.; Poole, A.J.; Weiss, J.H.; Gardener, M.J.; Dijkstra, S.; Fischer, D.F.; Keirstead, H.S. Histological and functional benefit following transplantation of motor neuron progenitors to the injured rat spinal cord. *PLoS One* **2010**, *5*, e11852.

46. Salewski, R.P.; Mitchell, R.A.; Shen, C.; Fehlings, M.G. Transplantation of Neural Stem Cells Clonally Derived from Embryonic Stem Cells Promotes Recovery of the Injured Mouse Spinal Cord. *Stem Cells Dev.* **2014**, doi:10.1089/scd.2014.0096.

47. Takahashi, K.; Yamanaka, S. Induction of Pluripotent Stem Cells from Mouse Embryonic and Adult Fibroblast Cultures by Defined Factors. *Cell* **2006**, *126*, 663–676.

48. Takahashi, K.; Tanabe, K.; Ohnuki, M.; Narita, M.; Ichisaka, T.; Tomoda, K.; Yamanaka, S. Induction of pluripotent stem cells from adult human fibroblasts by defined factors. *Cell* **2007**, *131*, 861–872.

49. Yu, J.; Vodyanik, M.A.; Smuga-Otto, K.; Antosiewicz-Bourget, J.; Frane, J.L.; Tian, S.; Nie, J.; Jonsdottir, G.A.; Ruotti, V.; Stewart, R.; *et al.* Induced pluripotent stem cell lines derived from human somatic cells. *Science* **2007**, *318*, 1917–1920.

234

50. Meng, X.; Neises, A.; Su, R.-J.; Payne, K.J.; Ritter, L.; Gridley, D.S.; Wang, J.; Sheng, M.; William Lau, K.-H.; Baylink, D.J.; *et al.* Efficient Reprogramming of Human Cord Blood CD34⁺ Cells into Induced Pluripotent Stem Cells with OCT4 and SOX2 Alone. *Mol. Ther.* **2012**, *20*, 408–416.

51. Zhao, Y.; Yin, X.; Qin, H.; Zhu, F.; Liu, H.; Yang, W.; Zhang, Q.; Xiang, C.; Hou, P.; Song, Z.; *et al.* Two supporting factors greatly improve the efficiency of human iPSC generation. *Cell Stem Cell* **2008**, *3*, 475–479.

52. Nakagawa, M.; Koyanagi, M.; Tanabe, K.; Takahashi, K.; Ichisaka, T.; Aoi, T.; Okita, K.; Mochiduki, Y.; Takizawa, N.; Yamanaka, S. Generation of induced pluripotent stem cells without Myc from mouse and human fibroblasts. *Nat. Biotechnol.* **2008**, *26*, 101–106.

53. Maekawa, M.; Yamaguchi, K.; Nakamura, T.; Shibukawa, R.; Kodanaka, I.; Ichisaka, T.; Kawamura, Y.; Mochizuki, H.; Goshima, N.; Yamanaka, S. Direct reprogramming of somatic cells is promoted by maternal transcription factor GLIS1. *Nature* **2011**, *474*, 225–229.

54. Zhou, W.; Freed, C.R. Adenoviral gene delivery can reprogram human fibroblasts to induced pluripotent stem cells. *Stem Cells* **2009**, *27*, 2667–2674.

55. Ban, H.; Nishishita, N.; Fusaki, N.; Tabata, T.; Saeki, K.; Shikamura, M.; Takada, N.; Inoue, M.; Hasegawa, M.; Kawamata, S.; *et al.* Efficient generation of transgene-free human induced pluripotent stem cells (iPSCs) by temperature-sensitive Sendai virus vectors. *Proc. Natl. Acad. Sci. USA* **2011**, *108*, 14234–14239.

56. Kim, D.; Kim, C.-H.; Moon, J.-I.; Chung, Y.-G.; Chang, M.-Y.; Han, B.-S.; Ko, S.; Yang, E.; Cha, K.Y.; Lanza, R.; *et al.* Generation of Human Induced Pluripotent Stem Cells by Direct Delivery of Reprogramming Proteins. *Cell Stem Cell* **2009**, *4*, 472–476.

57. Warren, L.; Manos, P.D.; Ahfeldt, T.; Loh, Y.-H.; Li, H.; Lau, F.; Ebina, W.; Mandal, P.K.; Smith, Z.D.; Meissner, A.; *et al.* Highly Efficient Reprogramming to Pluripotency and Directed Differentiation of Human Cells with Synthetic Modified mRNA. *Cell Stem Cell* **2010**, *7*, 618–630.

58. Subramanyam, D.; Lamouille, S.; Judson, R.L.; Liu, J.Y.; Bucay, N.; Derynck, R.; Blelloch, R. Multiple targets of miR-302 and miR-372 promote reprogramming of human fibroblasts to induced pluripotent stem cells. *Nat. Biotechnol.* **2011**, *29*, 443–448.

59. Yu, J.; Hu, K.; Smuga-Otto, K.; Tian, S.; Stewart, R.; Slukvin, I.I.; Thomson, J.A. Human Induced Pluripotent Stem Cells Free of Vector and Transgene Sequences. *Science* **2009**, *324*, 797–801.

60. Woltjen, K.; Michael, I.P.; Mohseni, P.; Desai, R.; Mileikovsky, M.; Hämäläinen, R.; Cowling, R.; Wang, W.; Liu, P.; Gertsenstein, M.; *et al. PiggyBac* transposition reprograms fibroblasts to induced pluripotent stem cells. *Nature* **2009**, *458*, 766–770.

61. Salewski, R.P.; Buttigieg, J.; Mitchell, R.A.; van der Kooy, D.; Nagy, A.; Fehlings, M.G. The generation of definitive neural stem cells from PiggyBac transposon-induced pluripotent stem cells can be enhanced by induction of the NOTCH signaling pathway. *Stem Cells Dev.* **2013**, *22*, 383–396.

62. Huangfu, D.; Maehr, R.; Guo, W.; Eijkelenboom, A.; Snitow, M.; Chen, A.E.; Melton, D.A. Induction of pluripotent stem cells by defined factors is greatly improved by small-molecule compounds. *Nat. Biotechnol.* **2008**, *26*, 795–797.

63. Shi, Y.; Desponts, C.; Do, J.T.; Hahm, H.S.; Schöler, H.R.; Ding, S. Induction of pluripotent stem cells from mouse embryonic fibroblasts by Oct4 and Klf4 with small-molecule compounds. *Cell Stem Cell* **2008**, *3*, 568–574.

64. Hou, P.; Li, Y.; Zhang, X.; Liu, C.; Guan, J.; Li, H.; Zhao, T.; Ye, J.; Yang, W.; Liu, K.; *et al.* Pluripotent Stem Cells Induced from Mouse Somatic Cells by Small-Molecule Compounds. *Science* **2013**, *341*, 651–654.

65. Kim, K.; Doi, A.; Wen, B.; Ng, K.; Zhao, R.; Cahan, P.; Kim, J.; Aryee, M.J.; Ji, H.; Ehrlich, L.I.R.; *et al.* Epigenetic memory in induced pluripotent stem cells. *Nature* **2010**, *467*, 285–290.

66. Kim, K.; Zhao, R.; Doi, A.; Ng, K.; Unternaehrer, J.; Cahan, P.; Hongguang, H.; Loh, Y.-H.; Aryee, M.J.; Lensch, M.W.; *et al.* Donor cell type can influence the epigenome and differentiation potential of human induced pluripotent stem cells. *Nat. Biotechnol.* **2011**, *29*, 1117–1119.

67. Laurent, L.C.; Ulitsky, I.; Slavin, I.; Tran, H.; Schork, A.; Morey, R.; Lynch, C.; Harness, J.V.; Lee, S.; Barrero, M.J.; *et al.* Dynamic changes in the copy number of pluripotency and cell proliferation genes in human ESCs and iPSCs during reprogramming and time in culture. *Cell Stem Cell* **2011**, *8*, 106–118.

68. Taapken, S.M.; Nisler, B.S.; Newton, M.A.; Sampsell-Barron, T.L.; Leonhard, K.A.; McIntire, E.M.; Montgomery, K.D. Karotypic abnormalities in human induced pluripotent stem cells and embryonic stem cells. *Nat. Biotechnol.* **2011**, *29*, 313–314.

69. Young, M.A.; Larson, D.E.; Sun, C.-W.; George, D.R.; Ding, L.; Miller, C.A.; Lin, L.; Pawlik, K.M.; Chen, K.; Fan, X.; *et al.* Background mutations in parental cells account for most of the genetic heterogeneity of induced pluripotent stem cells. *Cell Stem Cell* **2012**, *10*, 570–582.

70. Colman, A.; Dreesen, O. Pluripotent Stem Cells and Disease Modeling. *Cell Stem Cell* **2009**, *5*, 244–247.

71. Chen, J.; Lin, M.; Foxe, J.J.; Pedrosa, E.; Hrabovsky, A.; Carroll, R.; Zheng, D.; Lachman, H.M. Transcriptome comparison of human neurons generated using induced pluripotent stem cells derived from dental pulp and skin fibroblasts. *PLoS One* **2013**, *8*, e75682.

72. Maherali, N.; Ahfeldt, T.; Rigamonti, A.; Utikal, J.; Cowan, C.; Hochedlinger, K. A high-efficiency system for the generation and study of human induced pluripotent stem cells. *Cell Stem Cell* **2008**, *3*, 340–345.

73. Park, I.-H.; Lerou, P.H.; Zhao, R.; Huo, H.; Daley, G.Q. Generation of human-induced pluripotent stem cells. *Nat. Protoc.* **2008**, *3*, 1180–1186.

74. Yamanaka, S. Elite and stochastic models for induced pluripotent stem cell generation. *Nature* **2009**, *460*, 49–52.

75. Aasen, T.; Izpisúa Belmonte, J.C. Isolation and cultivation of human keratinocytes from skin or plucked hair for the generation of induced pluripotent stem cells. *Nat. Protoc.* **2010**, *5*, 371–382.

76. Aasen, T.; Raya, A.; Barrero, M.J.; Garreta, E.; Consiglio, A.; Gonzalez, F.; Vassena, R.; Bilić, J.; Pekarik, V.; Tiscornia, G.; *et al.* Efficient and rapid generation of induced pluripotent stem cells from human keratinocytes. *Nat. Biotechnol.* **2008**, *26*, 1276–1284.

77. Linta, L.; Stockmann, M.; Kleinhans, K.N.; Böckers, A.; Storch, A.; Zaehres, H.; Lin, Q.; Barbi, G.; Böckers, T.M.; Kleger, A.; *et al.* Rat embryonic fibroblasts improve reprogramming of human keratinocytes into induced pluripotent stem cells. *Stem Cells Dev.* **2012**, *21*, 965–976.

78. Hu, Q.; Friedrich, A.M.; Johnson, L.V.; Clegg, D.O. Memory in induced pluripotent stem cells: Reprogrammed human retinal-pigmented epithelial cells show tendency for spontaneous redifferentiation. *Stem Cells Dayt. Ohio* **2010**, *28*, 1981–1991.

79. Utikal, J.; Maherali, N.; Kulalert, W.; Hochedlinger, K. Sox2 is dispensable for the reprogramming of melanocytes and melanoma cells into induced pluripotent stem cells. *J. Cell Sci.* **2009**, *122*, 3502–3510.

80. Loh, Y.-H.; Agarwal, S.; Park, I.-H.; Urbach, A.; Huo, H.; Heffner, G.C.; Kim, K.; Miller, J.D.; Ng, K.; Daley, G.Q. Generation of induced pluripotent stem cells from human blood. *Blood* **2009**, *113*, 5476–5479.

81. Brockmann, F.; Kramer, M.; Bornhäuser, M.; Ehninger, G.; Hölig, K. Efficacy and side effects of granulocyte collection in healthy donors. *Transfus. Med. Hemother.* **2013**, *40*, 258–264.

82. Ramos-Mejía, V.; Montes, R.; Bueno, C.; Ayllón, V.; Real, P.J.; Rodríguez, R.; Menendez, P. Residual expression of the reprogramming factors prevents differentiation of iPSC generated from human fibroblasts and cord blood CD34$^+$ progenitors. *PLoS One* **2012**, *7*, e35824.

83. Giorgetti, A.; Montserrat, N.; Aasen, T.; Gonzalez, F.; Rodríguez-Pizà, I.; Vassena, R.; Raya, A.; Boué, S.; Barrero, M.J.; Corbella, B.A.; *et al.* Generation of induced pluripotent stem cells from human cord blood using OCT4 and SOX2. *Cell Stem Cell* **2009**, *5*, 353–357.

84. Haase, A.; Olmer, R.; Schwanke, K.; Wunderlich, S.; Merkert, S.; Hess, C.; Zweigerdt, R.; Gruh, I.; Meyer, J.; Wagner, S.; *et al.* Generation of induced pluripotent stem cells from human cord blood. *Cell Stem Cell* **2009**, *5*, 434–441.

85. Red-Horse, K.; Zhou, Y.; Genbacev, O.; Prakobphol, A.; Foulk, R.; McMaster, M.; Fisher, S.J. Trophoblast differentiation during embryo implantation and formation of the maternal-fetal interface. *J. Clin. Investig.* **2004**, *114*, 744–754.

86. Bunnell, B.A.; Flaat, M.; Gagliardi, C.; Patel, B.; Ripoll, C. Adipose-derived stem cells: Isolation, expansion and differentiation. *Methods San Diego Calif.* **2008**, *45*, 115–120.

87. Sun, N.; Panetta, N.J.; Gupta, D.M.; Wilson, K.D.; Lee, A.; Jia, F.; Hu, S.; Cherry, A.M.; Robbins, R.C.; Longaker, M.T.; *et al.* Feeder-free derivation of induced pluripotent stem cells from adult human adipose stem cells. *Proc. Natl. Acad. Sci. USA* **2009**, *106*, 15720–15725.

88. Qu, X.; Liu, T.; Song, K.; Li, X.; Ge, D. Induced pluripotent stem cells generated from human adipose-derived stem cells using a non-viral polycistronic plasmid in feeder-free conditions. *PLoS One* **2012**, *7*, e48161.

89. Kim, J.B.; Greber, B.; Araúzo-Bravo, M.J.; Meyer, J.; Park, K.I.; Zaehres, H.; Schöler, H.R. Direct reprogramming of human neural stem cells by OCT4. *Nature* **2009**, *461*, 649–653.

90. Kramer, A.S.; Harvey, A.R.; Plant, G.W.; Hodgetts, S.I. Systematic review of induced pluripotent stem cell technology as a potential clinical therapy for spinal cord injury. *Cell Transplant.* **2013**, *22*, 571–617.

91. Fujimoto, Y.; Abematsu, M.; Falk, A.; Tsujimura, K.; Sanosaka, T.; Juliandi, B.; Semi, K.; Namihira, M.; Komiya, S.; Smith, A.; *et al.* Treatment of a mouse model of spinal cord injury by transplantation of human induced pluripotent stem cell-derived long-term self-renewing neuroepithelial-like stem cells. *Stem Cells Dayt. Ohio* **2012**, *30*, 1163–1173.

92. Kobayashi, Y.; Okada, Y.; Itakura, G.; Iwai, H.; Nishimura, S.; Yasuda, A.; Nori, S.; Hikishima, K.; Konomi, T.; Fujiyoshi, K.; *et al.* Pre-Evaluated Safe Human iPSC-Derived Neural Stem Cells Promote Functional Recovery after Spinal Cord Injury in Common Marmoset without Tumorigenicity. *PLoS One* **2012**, *7*, e52787.

93. Nutt, S.E.; Chang, E.-A.; Suhr, S.T.; Schlosser, L.O.; Mondello, S.E.; Moritz, C.T.; Cibelli, J.B.; Horner, P.J. Caudalized human iPSC-derived neural progenitor cells produce neurons and glia but fail to restore function in an early chronic spinal cord injury model. *Exp. Neurol.* **2013**, *248*, 491–503.

94. Nori, S.; Okada, Y.; Yasuda, A.; Tsuji, O.; Takahashi, Y.; Kobayashi, Y.; Fujiyoshi, K.; Koike, M.; Uchiyama, Y.; Ikeda, E.; *et al.* Grafted human-induced pluripotent stem-cell—Derived neurospheres promote motor functional recovery after spinal cord injury in mice. *Proc. Natl. Acad. Sci. USA* **2011**, *108*, 16825–16830.

95. Tsuji, O.; Miura, K.; Okada, Y.; Fujiyoshi, K.; Mukaino, M.; Nagoshi, N.; Kitamura, K.; Kumagai, G.; Nishino, M.; Tomisato, S.; *et al.* Therapeutic potential of appropriately evaluated safe-induced pluripotent stem cells for spinal cord injury. *Proc. Natl. Acad. Sci. USA* **2010**, *107*, 12704–12709.

96. Romanyuk, N.; Amemori, T.; Turnovcova, K.; Prochazka, P.; Onteniente, B.; Sykova, E.; Jendelová, P. Beneficial effect of human induced pluripotent stem cell-derived neural precursors in spinal cord injury repair. *Cell Transplant.* **2014**, doi:10.3727/096368914X684042.

97. Lu, P.; Woodruff, G.; Wang, Y.; Graham, L.; Hunt, M.; Wu, D.; Boehle, E.; Ahmad, R.; Poplawski, G.; Brock, J.; *et al.* Long-Distance Axonal Growth from Human Induced Pluripotent Stem Cells after Spinal Cord Injury. *Neuron* **2014**, *83*, 789–796.

98. Hawryluk, G.W.J.; Mothe, A.J.; Chamankhah, M.; Wang, J.; Tator, C.; Fehlings, M.G. *In vitro* characterization of trophic factor expression in neural precursor cells. *Stem Cells Dev.* **2012**, *21*, 432–447.

99. Hawryluk, G.W.J.; Spano, S.; Chew, D.; Wang, S.; Erwin, M.; Chamankhah, M.; Forgione, N.; Fehlings, M.G. An Examination of the Mechanisms by Which Neural Precursors Augment Recovery Following Spinal Cord Injury: A Key Role for Remyelination. *Cell Transplant.* **2014**, *23*, 365–380.

100. Karimi-Abdolrezaee, S.; Schut, D.; Wang, J.; Fehlings, M.G. Chondroitinase and growth factors enhance activation and oligodendrocyte differentiation of endogenous neural precursor cells after spinal cord injury. *PLoS One* **2012**, *7*, e37589.

101. Yasuda, A.; Tsuji, O.; Shibata, S.; Nori, S.; Takano, M.; Kobayashi, Y.; Takahashi, Y.; Fujiyoshi, K.; Hara, C.M.; Miyawaki, A.; *et al.* Significance of remyelination by neural stem/progenitor cells transplanted into the injured spinal cord. *Stem Cells Dayt. Ohio* **2011**, *29*, 1983–1994.

102. Douvaras, P.; Wang, J.; Zimmer, M.; Hanchuk, S.; O'Bara, M.A.; Sadiq, S.; Sim, F.J.; Goldman, J.; Fossati, V. Efficient Generation of Myelinating Oligodendrocytes from Primary Progressive Multiple Sclerosis Patients by induced Pluripotent Stem Cells. *Stem Cell Rep.* **2014**, *3*, 250–259.

103. Wang, S.; Bates, J.; Li, X.; Schanz, S.; Chandler-Militello, D.; Levine, C.; Maherali, N.; Studer, L.; Hochedlinger, K.; Windrem, M.; *et al.* Human iPSC-Derived Oligodendrocyte Progenitor Cells Can Myelinate and Rescue a Mouse Model of Congenital Hypomyelination. *Cell Stem Cell* **2013**, *12*, 252–264.

104. Sharp, J.; Frame, J.; Siegenthaler, M.; Nistor, G.; Keirstead, H.S. Human embryonic stem cell-derived oligodendrocyte progenitor cell transplants improve recovery after cervical spinal cord injury. *Stem Cells Dayt. Ohio* **2010**, *28*, 152–163.

105. Kerr, C.L.; Letzen, B.S.; Hill, C.M.; Agrawal, G.; Thakor, N.V.; Sterneckert, J.L.; Gearhart, J.D.; All, A.H. Efficient differentiation of human embryonic stem cells into oligodendrocyte progenitors for application in a rat contusion model of spinal cord injury. *Int. J. Neurosci.* **2010**, *120*, 305–313.

106. Bretzner, F.; Gilbert, F.; Baylis, F.; Brownstone, R.M. Target Populations for First-In-Human Embryonic Stem Cell Research in Spinal Cord Injury. *Cell Stem Cell* **2011**, *8*, 468–475.

107. Wilcox, J.T.; Cadotte, D.; Fehlings, M.G. Spinal cord clinical trials and the role for bioengineering. *Neurosci. Lett.* **2012**, *519*, 93–102.

108. Treatment for Spinal Cord Injury to Start Clinical Trial Funded by California's Stem Cell Agency. Available online: http://www.cirm.ca.gov/about-cirm/newsroom/press-releases/08262014/treatment-spinal-cord-injury-start-clinical-trial-funded (accessed on 24 November 2014).

109. Sareen, D.; O'Rourke, J.G.; Meera, P.; Muhammad, A.K.M.G.; Grant, S.; Simpkinson, M.; Bell, S.; Carmona, S.; Ornelas, L.; Sahabian, A.; *et al.* Targeting RNA Foci in iPSC-Derived Motor Neurons from ALS Patients with a C9ORF72 Repeat Expansion. *Sci. Transl. Med.* **2013**, *5*, doi:10.1126/scitranslmed.3007529.

110. Jha, B.S.; Rao, M.; Malik, N. Motor Neuron Differentiation from Pluripotent Stem Cells and Other Intermediate Proliferative Precursors that can be Discriminated by Lineage Specific Reporters. *Stem Cell Rev.* **2014**, doi:10.1007/s12015-014-9541-0.

111. Karumbayaram, S.; Novitch, B.G.; Patterson, M.; Umbach, J.A.; Richter, L.; Lindgren, A.; Conway, A.E.; Clark, A.T.; Goldman, S.A.; Plath, K.; *et al.* Directed differentiation of human-induced pluripotent stem cells generates active motor neurons. *Stem Cells Dayt. Ohio* **2009**, *27*, 806–811.

112. Erceg, S.; Ronaghi, M.; Oria, M.; Roselló, M.G.; Aragó, M.A.P.; Lopez, M.G.; Radojevic, I.; Moreno-Manzano, V.; Rodríguez-Jiménez, F.-J.; Bhattacharya, S.S.; *et al.* Transplanted oligodendrocytes and motoneuron progenitors generated from human embryonic stem cells promote locomotor recovery after spinal cord transection. *Stem Cells Dayt. Ohio* **2010**, *28*, 1541–1549.

113. Sieber-Blum, M.; Grim, M.; Hu, Y.F.; Szeder, V. Pluripotent neural crest stem cells in the adult hair follicle. *Dev. Dyn.* **2004**, *231*, 258–269.

114. Liu, Q.; Spusta, S.C.; Mi, R.; Lassiter, R.N.T.; Stark, M.R.; Höke, A.; Rao, M.S.; Zeng, X. Human neural crest stem cells derived from human ESCs and induced pluripotent stem cells: Induction, maintenance, and differentiation into functional Schwann cells. *Stem Cells Transl. Med.* **2012**, *1*, 266–278.

115. Sieber-Blum, M.; Schnell, L.; Grim, M.; Hu, Y.F.; Schneider, R.; Schwab, M.E. Characterization of epidermal neural crest stem cell (EPI-NCSC) grafts in the lesioned spinal cord. *Mol. Cell. Neurosci.* **2006**, *32*, 67–81.

116. Trolle, C.; Konig, N.; Abrahamsson, N.; Vasylovska, S.; Kozlova, E.N. Boundary cap neural crest stem cells homotopically implanted to the injured dorsal root transitional zone give rise to different types of neurons and glia in adult rodents. *BMC Neurosci.* **2014**, *15*, doi:10.1186/1471-2202-15-60.

117. Kreitzer, F.R.; Salomonis, N.; Sheehan, A.; Huang, M.; Park, J.S.; Spindler, M.J.; Lizarraga, P.; Weiss, W.A.; So, P.-L.; Conklin, B.R. A robust method to derive functional neural crest cells from human pluripotent stem cells. *Am. J. Stem Cells* **2013**, *2*, 119–131.

118. Lee, G.; Chambers, S.M.; Tomishima, M.J.; Studer, L. Derivation of neural crest cells from human pluripotent stem cells. *Nat. Protoc.* **2010**, *5*, 688–701.

119. Wang, A.; Tang, Z.; Park, I.-H.; Zhu, Y.; Patel, S.; Daley, G.Q.; Song, L. Induced Pluripotent Stem Cells for Neural Tissue Engineering. *Biomaterials* **2011**, *32*, 5023–5032.

120. Saadai, P.; Wang, A.; Nout, Y.S.; Downing, T.L.; Lofberg, K.; Beattie, M.S.; Bresnahan, J.C.; Li, S.; Farmer, D.L. Human induced pluripotent stem cell-derived neural crest stem cells integrate into the injured spinal cord in the fetal lamb model of myelomeningocele. *J. Pediatr. Surg.* **2013**, *48*, 158–163.

121. Davies, J.E.; Huang, C.; Proschel, C.; Noble, M.; Mayer-Proschel, M.; Davies, S.J.A. Astrocytes derived from glial-restricted precursors promote spinal cord repair. *J. Biol.* **2006**, *5*, doi:10.1186/jbiol35.

122. Faulkner, J.R.; Herrmann, J.E.; Woo, M.J.; Tansey, K.E.; Doan, N.B.; Sofroniew, M.V. Reactive astrocytes protect tissue and preserve function after spinal cord injury. *J. Neurosci.* **2004**, *24*, 2143–2155.

123. Renault-Mihara, F.; Okada, S.; Shibata, S.; Nakamura, M.; Toyama, Y.; Okano, H. Spinal cord injury: Emerging beneficial role of reactive astrocytes' migration. *Int. J. Biochem. Cell Biol.* **2008**, *40*, 1649–1653.

124. Emdad, L.; D'Souza, S.L.; Kothari, H.P.; Qadeer, Z.A.; Germano, I.M. Efficient Differentiation of Human Embryonic and Induced Pluripotent Stem Cells into Functional Astrocytes. *Stem Cells Dev.* **2011**, *21*, 404–410.

125. Hayashi, K.; Hashimoto, M.; Koda, M.; Naito, A.T.; Murata, A.; Okawa, A.; Takahashi, K.; Yamazaki, M. Increase of sensitivity to mechanical stimulus after transplantation of murine induced pluripotent stem cell-derived astrocytes in a rat spinal cord injury model. *J. Neurosurg. Spine* **2011**, *15*, 582–593.

126. Juopperi, T.A.; Kim, W.R.; Chiang, C.-H.; Yu, H.; Margolis, R.L.; Ross, C.A.; Ming, G.; Song, H. Astrocytes generated from patient induced pluripotent stem cells recapitulate features of Huntington's disease patient cells. *Mol. Brain* **2012**, *5*, doi:10.1186/1756-6606-5-17.

127. Lian, Q.; Zhang, Y.; Zhang, J.; Zhang, H.K.; Wu, X.; Zhang, Y.; Lam, F.F.-Y.; Kang, S.; Xia, J.C.; Lai, W.-H.; *et al.* Functional mesenchymal stem cells derived from human induced pluripotent stem cells attenuate limb ischemia in mice. *Circulation* **2010**, *121*, 1113–1123.

128. Jung, Y.; Bauer, G.; Nolta, J.A. Concise review: Induced pluripotent stem cell-derived mesenchymal stem cells: Progress toward safe clinical products. *Stem Cells* **2012**, *30*, 42–47.

129. Himeno, T.; Kamiya, H.; Naruse, K.; Cheng, Z.; Ito, S.; Kondo, M.; Okawa, T.; Fujiya, A.; Kato, J.; Suzuki, H.; *et al.* Mesenchymal stem cell-like cells derived from mouse induced pluripotent stem cells ameliorate diabetic polyneuropathy in mice. *BioMed. Res. Int.* **2013**, *2013*, doi:10.1155/2013/259187.

130. Kim, J.; Efe, J.A.; Zhu, S.; Talantova, M.; Yuan, X.; Wang, S.; Lipton, S.A.; Zhang, K.; Ding, S. Direct reprogramming of mouse fibroblasts to neural progenitors. *Proc. Natl. Acad. Sci. USA* **2011**, *108*, 7838–7843.

131. Lujan, E.; Chanda, S.; Ahlenius, H.; Südhof, T.C.; Wernig, M. Direct conversion of mouse fibroblasts to self-renewing, tripotent neural precursor cells. *Proc. Natl. Acad. Sci. USA* **2012**, *109*, 2527–2532.

132. Han, D.W.; Tapia, N.; Hermann, A.; Hemmer, K.; Höing, S.; Araúzo-Bravo, M.J.; Zaehres, H.; Wu, G.; Frank, S.; Moritz, S.; *et al.* Direct reprogramming of fibroblasts into neural stem cells by defined factors. *Cell Stem Cell* **2012**, *10*, 465–472.

133. Ring, K.L.; Tong, L.M.; Balestra, M.E.; Javier, R.; Andrews-Zwilling, Y.; Li, G.; Walker, D.; Zhang, W.R.; Kreitzer, A.C.; Huang, Y. Direct reprogramming of mouse and human fibroblasts into multipotent neural stem cells with a single factor. *Cell Stem Cell* **2012**, *11*, 100–109.

134. Zou, Q.; Yan, Q.; Zhong, J.; Wang, K.; Sun, H.; Yi, X.; Lai, L. Direct conversion of human fibroblasts into neuronal restricted progenitors. *J. Biol. Chem.* **2014**, *289*, 5250–5260.

135. Mitchell, R.R.; Szabo, E.; Benoit, Y.D.; Case, D.T.; Mechael, R.; Alamilla, J.; Lee, J.H.; Fiebig-Comyn, A.; Gillespie, D.C.; Bhatia, M. Activation of Neural Cell Fate Programs toward Direct Conversion of Adult Human Fibroblasts into Tri-Potent Neural Progenitors Using OCT-4. *Stem Cells Dev.* **2014**, *23*, 1937–1946.

136. Franklin, R.J.M.; Ffrench-Constant, C. Remyelination in the CNS: From biology to therapy. *Nat. Rev. Neurosci.* **2008**, *9*, 839–855.

137. Najm, F.J.; Lager, A.M.; Zaremba, A.; Wyatt, K.; Caprariello, A.V.; Factor, D.C.; Karl, R.T.; Maeda, T.; Miller, R.H.; Tesar, P.J. Transcription factor-mediated reprogramming of fibroblasts to expandable, myelinogenic oligodendrocyte progenitor cells. *Nat. Biotechnol.* **2013**, *31*, 426–433.

138. Yang, N.; Zuchero, J.B.; Ahlenius, H.; Marro, S.; Ng, Y.H.; Vierbuchen, T.; Hawkins, J.S.; Geissler, R.; Barres, B.A.; Wernig, M. Generation of oligodendroglial cells by direct lineage conversion. *Nat. Biotechnol.* **2013**, *31*, 434–439.

139. Caiazzo, M.; Dell'Anno, M.T.; Dvoretskova, E.; Lazarevic, D.; Taverna, S.; Leo, D.; Sotnikova, T.D.; Menegon, A.; Roncaglia, P.; Colciago, G.; *et al.* Direct generation of functional dopaminergic neurons from mouse and human fibroblasts. *Nature* **2011**, *476*, 224–227.

140. Pang, Z.P.; Yang, N.; Vierbuchen, T.; Ostermeier, A.; Fuentes, D.R.; Yang, T.Q.; Citri, A.; Sebastiano, V.; Marro, S.; Südhof, T.C.; *et al.* Induction of human neuronal cells by defined transcription factors. *Nature* **2011**, *476*, 220–223.

141. Vierbuchen, T.; Ostermeier, A.; Pang, Z.P.; Kokubu, Y.; Südhof, T.C.; Wernig, M. Direct conversion of fibroblasts to functional neurons by defined factors. *Nature* **2010**, *463*, 1035–1041.

142. Ambasudhan, R.; Talantova, M.; Coleman, R.; Yuan, X.; Zhu, S.; Lipton, S.A.; Ding, S. Direct Reprogramming of Adult Human Fibroblasts to Functional Neurons under Defined Conditions. *Cell Stem Cell* **2011**, *9*, 113–118.

143. Chanda, S.; Ang, C.E.; Davila, J.; Pak, C.; Mall, M.; Lee, Q.Y.; Ahlenius, H.; Jung, S.W.; Südhof, T.C.; Wernig, M. Generation of Induced Neuronal Cells by the Single Reprogramming Factor ASCL1. *Stem Cell Rep.* **2014**, *3*, 282–296.

144. Son, E.Y.; Ichida, J.K.; Wainger, B.J.; Toma, J.S.; Rafuse, V.F.; Woolf, C.J.; Eggan, K. Conversion of mouse and human fibroblasts into functional spinal motor neurons. *Cell Stem Cell* **2011**, *9*, 205–218.

145. Cyranoski, D. Japanese woman is first recipient of next-generation stem cells. Available online: http://www.nature.com/news/japanese-woman-is-first-recipient-of-next-generation-stem-cells1.15915 (acessed on 15 September 2014).

146. Chen, J.; Liu, H.; Liu, J.; Qi, J.; Wei, B.; Yang, J.; Liang, H.; Chen, Y.; Chen, J.; Wu, Y.; *et al.* H3K9 methylation is a barrier during somatic cell reprogramming into iPSCs. *Nat. Genet.* **2013**, *45*, 34–42.

147. Scaron, T.; Frenzel, L.P.; Hescheler, J. Immunological Barriers to Embryonic Stem Cell-Derived Therapies. *Cells Tissues Organs* **2008**, *188*, 78–90.

148. Ludwig, T.E.; Levenstein, M.E.; Jones, J.M.; Berggren, W.T.; Mitchen, E.R.; Frane, J.L.; Crandall, L.J.; Daigh, C.A.; Conard, K.R.; Piekarczyk, M.S.; *et al.* Derivation of human embryonic stem cells in defined conditions. *Nat. Biotechnol.* **2006**, *24*, 185–187.

149. Chen, A.K.-L.; Reuveny, S.; Oh, S.K.W. Application of human mesenchymal and pluripotent stem cell microcarrier cultures in cellular therapy: Achievements and future direction. *Biotechnol. Adv.* **2013**, *31*, 1032–1046.

150. Chen, A.K.-L.; Chen, X.; Choo, A.B.H.; Reuveny, S.; Oh, S.K.W. Critical microcarrier properties affecting the expansion of undifferentiated human embryonic stem cells. *Stem Cell Res.* **2011**, *7*, 97–111.

The State of Play with iPSCs and Spinal Cord Injury Models

Stuart I. Hodgetts, Michael Edel and Alan R. Harvey

Abstract: The application of induced pluripotent stem cell (iPSC) technologies in cell based strategies, for the repair of the central nervous system (with particular focus on the spinal cord), is moving towards the potential use of clinical grade donor cells. The ability of iPSCs to generate donor neuronal, glial and astrocytic phenotypes for transplantation is highlighted here, and we review recent research using iPSCs in attempts to treat spinal cord injury in various animal models. Also discussed are issues relating to the production of clinical grade iPSCs, recent advances in transdifferentiation protocols for iPSC-derived donor cell populations, concerns about tumourogenicity, and whether iPSC technologies offer any advantages over previous donor cell candidates or tissues already in use as therapeutic tools in experimental spinal cord injury studies.

Reprinted from *J. Clin. Med.* Cite as: Stuart I. Hodgetts, Michael Edel and Alan R. Harvey. The State of Play with iPSCs and Spinal Cord Injury Models. *J. Clin. Med.* **2015**, *4*, 193–203.

1. Introduction

Spinal cord injury (SCI) is characterised by damage to sensory and motor function, the extent of any functional loss dependent on the location, extent (severity) and type of injury (contusion *vs.* transection, incomplete *vs.* complete). Sensorimotor loss that results from a primary mechanical injury is a result of many interacting pathological factors, including: axonal damage, loss of neurons, activation of astrocytes and microglia, degeneration of oligodendrocytes, and demyelination [1]. The extent of this initial damage is significantly increased by ensuing secondary cascades of ischaemia, anoxia, generation of damaging free-radicals, lipid peroxidation, excitotoxicity, and immune-mediated and inflammatory events (e.g., cytokines), which can stimulate further cell death and tissue loss. A region of spreading degeneration rostral and caudal to the injury site, together with inhibitor molecule production, eventually leads to cavitation as well as a glial scar rich in, among other things, various types of chondroitin sulphate proteoglycans (CSPG) that are extremely inhibitory to axonal regrowth. Strategies to induce repair and promote functional (locomotor) recovery generally aim to reduce the extent of secondary damage and demyelination, promote the re-myelination of damaged (but still viable) axons, induce axonal repair and/or regeneration, and perhaps stimulate an endogenous stem cell response. For decades, extensive research has been conducted into clinically relevant cell transplantation strategies to either promote regeneration or to replace damaged/missing cell populations using: fibroblasts, peripheral nerve grafts and Schwann cell bridges, olfactory ensheathing glia (OEG), embryonic stem cells (ESCs), oligodendroglial progenitor cells (OPCs), adult neural precursor cells (NPCs) and neural stem cells (NSCs), autologous macrophages and mesenchymal precursor cells (MPCs) isolated from bone marrow stroma (BMSCs) (for reviews see [2–5]). More recently, the possibility of developing strategies that use induced Pluripotent Stem Cell (iPSC) technology to generate donor cell populations has gathered momentum.

2. iPSCs as Neuronal and Glial Candidate Donor Populations

To date, iPSCs have been directed to generate neural crest cells [6,7], peripheral sensory neurons [8], neural stem cells and their neuronal progenitors including specific neuronal subtypes such as dopaminergic neurons [9–17] glutamatergic neurons [18–21], GABAergic neurons [18,19,22], motor neurons [23–26,27–29] (see also Faravelli *et al.* 2014 for review of methodologies of induction into motor neurons [30]), retinal neurons [31–34], as well as astrocytes [35–38] and oligodendrocyte lineages [37,39–43]. iPSCs and their derivatives have been tested in various *in vivo* animal models of neurological/neurodegenerative disorders including Parkinson's Disease [9–12,14,44], demyelination [37,39–43], retinal regeneration [32,33], stroke [45–48] and peripheral nerve regeneration [7] as well as others (see [49,50]). These studies provide proof-of-principle that iPSCs can be successfully differentiated *in vitro* to yield a desired progeny that, if necessary, can be effectively subjected to *ex vivo* gene therapy [51,52] and then transplanted with similar outcomes to other pluripotent ESC therapies [53–56].

3. iPSCs in Spinal Cord Injury

Despite a rapid increase in iPSC-based studies in recent years, currently there is only a small number of published preclinical studies describing the *in vivo* use of iPSCs in mouse [57–59], rat [36,50,57–62] or simian [37,60–62] models of SCI, or sub-dural parenchymal injections into non-injured rats [63].

Of these studies, rodent moderate contusion injuries were almost all made at the thoracic level (T9–T10) using the Infinite Horizon Impactor device (delivering 60–70 kDyne forces for mice and 200 kDyne force for rat). An exception was a study that used C4 contusions using the Ohio State Injury Device [61], and Lu *et al.* [60] recently used C5 lateral hemisections in rats. Simian contusions have to date been more severe (17 g 50 mm drop at C5 using the NYU impactor [37] or a 50 g 10 mm drop at T9 [62]). All published studies using contusive SCI (apart from [62]) have reported neuronal, glial and astrocytic marker expression within or near the lesion after transplantation, with two groups reporting differentiation of donor cells into at least one or all these various cell types [37,50,58–63]. These studies used iPSC donor cells that were pre-differentiated into either neurospheres (NS) [58,59], neural precursor cells (NPCs) [61,63], neural stem cells (NSCs) [60–62] astrocytes [36] or undifferentiated iPSCs [50]. Sareen *et al.* [63] found that NPCs derived from iPSCs showed variability in differentiation phenotype and survival characteristics following transplantation, but migrated and integrated within the uninjured cord. Superparamagnetic iron oxide labelled iPSC-derived NSCs were tracked non-invasively using magnetic resonance imaging (MRI) from the cell injection sites in monkeys that extended progressively to the lesion regions [62]. Transplanted iPSC-derived NPCs after early chronic cervical SCI were shown to form neurons, astrocytes and oligodendrocytes at 8 weeks post transplantation, however importantly failed to promote functional recovery in forelimb behavioural tasks.

Whilst murine SCI studies using iPSC-derived donor cells showed functional improvements, others have reported no significant differences in morphological or functional outcomes in another acute moderate contusion SCI model in rats [36,50,60]. Lu *et al.* [60] reported that 3 months after transplantation, surviving human iPSC-derived NSCs from an 86 year old donor male exhibited extraordinarily long distance axonal growth with the host rat spinal cord, with human axons growing rostral and caudal to the lesion site and forming synaptic structures with host neurons and dendrites. Such extensive growth of immature human cells within the rodent central nervous system (CNS) is similar to that obtained many years ago using grafts of human fetal tissue and neuroblasts (e.g., [64]). In the iPSC study, host axons grew into the donor grafts and also formed synaptic structures, again similar to previous work that used donor fetal material of some kind (e.g., [65]). Taken together the new iPSC work confirms that even in the injured adult CNS it is possible, in some cases, to overcome the inhibitory environment of the lesion and elicit substantial regenerative growth and circuit construction. The grafting technique used by Lu *et al.* 2014 [60] involved a cocktail of growth factors (including brain-derived neurotrophic factor, neurotrophin-3, platelet-derived growth factor-AA, insulin-like growth factor-1, epidermal growth factor, basic fibroblast growth factor, acidic fibroblast growth factor, glial cell line-derived neurotrophic factor, hepatocyte growth factor, and calpain inhibitor in a fibrin matrix) that previously was shown by the same group to promote robust engraftment of donor (non-iPSC derived) NSCs, extensive integration with host tissue, long-distance outgrowth of axons from grafts and extensive ingrowth of host axons into the graft after acute thoracic (T3) SCI [66].

Significant functional improvement was reported in the initial NSC study [66]; however more recently, Lu *et al.* (2014) in a C5 lateral hemisection study [60], reported no measurable improvement in forelimb function in host rats despite the use of the same growth cocktail, extensive axonal outgrowth and cellular integration. The authors suggest that the injury type itself, the rate of maturation of donor cells (so that insufficient numbers of mature neurons were present to support recovery), inadequate myelination, undesirable ectopic projections and/or insufficient expression of neurotransmitters could account for the discrepancy between the functional recovery observed between the two studies. Whilst the extent of hindlimb *versus* forelimb recovery may vary depending on the type and complexity of restored or adapted neural circuitry [60], it is also important to note that independent researchers that attempted to replicate this study (as part of the NIH "Facilities of Research Excellence-Spinal Cord Injury" project to support independent replication) revealed conflicting data relating to ingrowth of host axons into the grafts and behavioural outcomes [67]. Overall, these are very important and influential studies, but the extent to which reported differences also reflect, for example, variation in surgical procedures, the individual contributions of factors in the growth cocktail [68], or differences in the nature and response of the donor cell type after transplantation, needs to be established, and future work should yield valuable information in this regard.

The approach of using restricted or individual populations of donor cells in the hope of achieving regrowth or repair leading to morphological improvements and functional restoration has some limitations. The ability of a wide variety of adult somatic (e.g., Schwann cells, olfactory ensheathing glia) and precursor/progenitor (e.g., NPCs, NSCs, OPCs, MPCs) cells to undergo directed differentiation and perform functionally and phenotypically as required *in vitro* has not always been reproduced when cells are transplanted into the inhibitory environment of the injured spinal cord *in vivo*. Perhaps these well characterised donor cells that meet necessary research requirements in a wide variety of controlled settings other than the injured spinal cord, simply fail to "perform" in animal models *in vivo* because of the antagonistic, often inflammatory environment they find themselves in after transplantation [69]. Those donor cells that eventually survive the host immune response may be unable to successfully respond to the new and dynamic myriad of both inhibitory and growth promoting stimuli of the host's injured spinal cord that is known to occur in a temporal and spatial fashion after trauma. Simply, the "correct language" that equipped the donor cells with the ability to perform all of those functions observed under controlled conditions *in vitro*, is no longer able to be understood or followed *in vivo*. Perhaps by using combined populations of adult stem cell-derived oligodendrocyte, astrocyte and neuronal precursor cells in the same relative proportions as those found within the uninjured (normal) spinal cord, we may achieve a phenotypic state that will allow enhanced plasticity and optimal repair/regrowth.

It is crucial to ensure that appropriate cell controls are used in preclinical SCI studies to evaluate the extent of contribution of different cell phenotypes to the morphological and functional outcomes observed after treatment. This applies to any small populations of incompletely reprogrammed donor cells and/or incompletely pre-differentiated donor iPSCs. Whilst the studies mentioned may suggest that improved outcomes were observed in mouse but not necessarily in rat models of SCI, the disparity in overall results from these very limited number of studies suggest that iPSC-based therapy in SCI warrants more extensive and thorough testing. Ideally, research in this area should be conducted using clinically relevant injury regimes in at least mouse and rat models as outlined in the recommendations and guidelines developed by the International Campaign for Cures of Spinal Cord Injury Paralysis (ICCP) [70] (see also [71,72]). Experimental studies in larger species (e.g., cats and primates) with an ascending and descending tract configuration more similar to the human [73], and capable of more complex sensorimotor behaviors, should also be undertaken. In addition, it may be important to include more relevant control donor cell types, such as cells that have been freeze-thawed.

4. Conclusions

There is a clear need to develop a gold standard positive control for use of stem cells in animal models of SCI, to determine the validity and reliability for future clinical application. It is most likely that stem cell therapy alone will not work for SCI, but will require new efforts to combine stem cell therapy with other treatments perhaps, such as bio-scaffolds, immune response modifications, and the timing of the use of different treatments, although the consensus at present is "the earlier the better". The threat of tumorigenicity remains to be fully addressed. In SCI studies that used iPSC-derived donor cells, "unsafe" murine iPSC-derived donor cells, but not "safe" donor cells, produced teratomas [59], although another study did not report such teratoma formation [36]. Of those studies using human iPSC-derived donor cells, one study did not report on teratoma formation [57], whilst others reported no evidence of tumour formation [37,50,58,60–63]. For clinical applications, donor cells must be grown in animal cell-free and serum-free conditions and derivation of the first hESC line with these properties has been a major advance for clinical applications of stem cell therapy [74]. Despite their highly similar expression of genes related to pluripotency and development, there is evidence that iPSCs may occupy a distinct pluripotent "state" from ESCs [50,75], and therefore iPSCs may not have the same capacity as ESCs to generate the whole spectrum of region-specific neural progenitors and functional neuronal subtypes for SCI therapies (and other CNS disorders). Nevertheless, the approaching capacity to produce clinical grade iPSCs, together with advances in the efficiency of transdifferentiation protocols for iPSCs into the required phenotypes, marks a potential focus toward the use of iPSC-derived donor cell populations for cell based therapies. If hESC-derived OPCs can be used in SCI trials (Geron), this should surely herald the addition of the clinical grade iPSCs to the potential repertoire of donor cell candidates for SCI and other neurotrauma related therapies, as long as they are conducted in accordance with Good Clinical Practise (GCP) and the associated regulatory directives.

Author Contributions

All authors contributed intellectually to the contents of this commentary.

Conflicts of Interest

The authors declare no conflict of interest.

References

1. Hodgetts, S.; Plant, G.W.; Harvey, A. Spinal cord injury: Experimental animal models and relation to human therapy. In *The Spinal Cord: A Christopher and Dana Reeve Foundation Text and Atlas*; Watson, C., Paxinos, G., Kayalioglu, G., Heise, C., Eds.; Elsevier: London, UK, 2009; pp. 223–251.
2. Sahni, V.; Kessler, J.A. Stem cell therapies for spinal cord injury. *Nat. Rev. Neurol.* **2010**, *6*, 363–372.
3. Tetzlaff, W. *Essentials of Spinal Cord Injury: Basic Research to Clinical Practice*, 1st ed.; Fehlings, M.G., Vaccaro, A.R., Boakye, M., Eds.; Thieme: Leipzig, Germany, 2013; pp. 399–420.
4. Tetzlaff, W.; Okon, E.B.; Karimi-Abdolrezaee, S.; Hill, C.E.; Sparling, J.S.; Plemel, J.R.; Plunet, W.T.; Tsai, E.C.; Baptiste, D.; Smithson, L.J.; *et al.* A systematic review of cellular transplantation therapies for spinal cord injury. *J. Neurotrauma* **2011**, *28*, 1611–1682.
5. Volarevic, V.; Erceg, S.; Bhattacharya, S.S.; Stojkovic, P.; Horner, P.; Stojkovic, M. Stem cell-based therapy for spinal cord injury. *Cell Transplant.* **2013**, *22*, 1309–1323.
6. Lee, G.; Chambers, S.M.; Tomishima, M.J.; Studer, L. Derivation of neural crest cells from human pluripotent stem cells. *Nat. Protoc.* **2010**, *5*, 688–701.
7. Wang, A.; Tang, Z.; Park, I.H.; Zhu, Y.; Patel, S.; Daley, G.Q.; Li, S. Induced pluripotent stem cells for neural tissue engineering. *Biomaterials* **2011**, *32*, 5023–5032.
8. Kitazawa, A.; Shimizu, N. Differentiation of mouse induced pluripotent stem cells into neurons using conditioned medium of dorsal root ganglia. *N. Biotechnol.* **2011**, *28*, 326–333.

9. Wernig, M.; Zhao, J.P.; Pruszak, J.; Hedlund, E.; Fu, D.; Soldner, F.; Broccoli, V.; Constantine-Paton, M.; Isacson, O.; Jaenisch, R. Neurons derived from reprogrammed fibroblasts functionally integrate into the fetal brain and improve symptoms of rats with parkinson's disease. *Proc. Natl. Acad. Sci. USA* **2008**, *105*, 5856–5861.

10. Cai, J.; Yang, M.; Poremsky, E.; Kidd, S.; Schneider, J.S.; Iacovitti, L. Dopaminergic neurons derived from human induced pluripotent stem cells survive and integrate into 6-OHDA-lesioned rats. *Stem Cells Dev.* **2010**, *19*, 1017–1023.

11. Deleidi, M.; Hargus, G.; Hallett, P.; Osborn, T.; Isacson, O. Development of histocompatible primate-induced pluripotent stem cells for neural transplantation. *Stem Cells* **2011**, *29*, 1052–1063.

12. Rhee, Y.H.; Ko, J.Y.; Chang, M.Y.; Yi, S.H.; Kim, D.; Kim, C.H.; Shim, J.W.; Jo, A.Y.; Kim, B.W.; Lee, H.; *et al.* Protein-based human iPS cells efficiently generate functional dopamine neurons and can treat a rat model of parkinson disease. *J. Clin. Invest.* **2011**, *121*, 2326–2335.

13. Swistowski, A.; Peng, J.; Liu, Q.; Mali, P.; Rao, M.S.; Cheng, L.; Zeng, X. Efficient generation of functional dopaminergic neurons from human induced pluripotent stem cells under defined conditions. *Stem Cells* **2010**, *28*, 1893–1904.

14. Sanchez-Danes, A.; Consiglio, A.; Richaud, Y.; Rodriguez-Piza, I.; Dehay, B.; Edel, M.; Bove, J.; Memo, M.; Vila, M.; Raya, A.; *et al.* Efficient generation of A9 midbrain dopaminergic neurons by lentiviral delivery of LMX1A in human embryonic stem cells and induced pluripotent stem cells. *Hum. Gene Ther.* **2012**, *23*, 56–69.

15. Pfisterer, U.; Kirkeby, A.; Torper, O.; Wood, J.; Nelander, J.; Dufour, A.; Bjorklund, A.; Lindvall, O.; Jakobsson, J.; Parmar, M. Direct conversion of human fibroblasts to dopaminergic neurons. *Proc. Natl. Acad. Sci. USA* **2011**, *108*, 10343–10348.

16. Pfisterer, U.; Wood, J.; Nihlberg, K.; Hallgren, O.; Bjermer, L.; Westergren-Thorsson, G.; Lindvall, O.; Parmar, M. Efficient induction of functional neurons from adult human fibroblasts. *Cell Cycle* **2011**, *10*, 3311–3316.

17. Caiazzo, M.; Dell'Anno, M.T.; Dvoretskova, E.; Lazarevic, D.; Taverna, S.; Leo, D.; Sotnikova, T.D.; Menegon, A.; Roncaglia, P.; Colciago, G.; *et al.* Direct generation of functional dopaminergic neurons from mouse and human fibroblasts. *Nature* **2011**, *476*, 224–227.

18. Kim, J.E.; O'Sullivan, M.L.; Sanchez, C.A.; Hwang, M.; Israel, M.A.; Brennand, K.; Deerinck, T.J.; Goldstein, L.S.; Gage, F.H.; Ellisman, M.H.; *et al.* Investigating synapse formation and function using human pluripotent stem cell-derived neurons. *Proc. Natl. Acad. Sci. USA* **2011**, *108*, 3005–3010.

19. Marchetto, M.C.; Carromeu, C.; Acab, A.; Yu, D.; Yeo, G.W.; Mu, Y.; Chen, G.; Gage, F.H.; Muotri, A.R. A model for neural development and treatment of rett syndrome using human induced pluripotent stem cells. *Cell* **2010**, *143*, 527–539.

20. Pedrosa, E.; Sandler, V.; Shah, A.; Carroll, R.; Chang, C.; Rockowitz, S.; Guo, X.; Zheng, D.; Lachman, H.M. Development of patient-specific neurons in schizophrenia using induced pluripotent stem cells. *J. Neurogenet.* **2011**, *25*, 88–103.

21. Zeng, H.; Guo, M.; Martins-Taylor, K.; Wang, X.; Zhang, Z.; Park, J.W.; Zhan, S.; Kronenberg, M.S.; Lichtler, A.; Liu, H.X.; *et al.* Specification of region-specific neurons including forebrain glutamatergic neurons from human induced pluripotent stem cells. *PLoS One* **2010**, *5*, e11853.

22. Brennand, K.J.; Simone, A.; Jou, J.; Gelboin-Burkhart, C.; Tran, N.; Sangar, S.; Li, Y.; Mu, Y.; Chen, G.; Yu, D.; *et al.* Modelling schizophrenia using human induced pluripotent stem cells. *Nature* **2011**, *473*, 221–225.

23. Boulting, G.L.; Kiskinis, E.; Croft, G.F.; Amoroso, M.W.; Oakley, D.H.; Wainger, B.J.; Williams, D.J.; Kahler, D.J.; Yamaki, M.; Davidow, L.; *et al.* A functionally characterized test set of human induced pluripotent stem cells. *Nat. Biotechnol.* **2011**, *29*, 279–286.

24. Hester, M.E.; Murtha, M.J.; Song, S.; Rao, M.; Miranda, C.J.; Meyer, K.; Tian, J.; Boulting, G.; Schaffer, D.V.; Zhu, M.X.; *et al.* Rapid and efficient generation of functional motor neurons from human pluripotent stem cells using gene delivered transcription factor codes. *Mol. Ther.* **2011**, *19*, 1905–1912.

25. Hu, B.Y.; Weick, J.P.; Yu, J.; Ma, L.X.; Zhang, X.Q.; Thomson, J.A.; Zhang, S.C. Neural differentiation of human induced pluripotent stem cells follows developmental principles but with variable potency. *Proc. Natl. Acad. Sci. USA* **2010**, *107*, 4335–4340.

26. Karumbayaram, S.; Novitch, B.G.; Patterson, M.; Umbach, J.A.; Richter, L.; Lindgren, A.; Conway, A.E.; Clark, A.T.; Goldman, S.A.; Plath, K.; *et al.* Directed differentiation of human-induced pluripotent stem cells generates active motor neurons. *Stem Cells* **2009**, *27*, 806–811.

27. Amoroso, M.W.; Croft, G.F.; Williams, D.J.; O'Keeffe, S.; Carrasco, M.A.; Davis, A.R.; Roybon, L.; Oakley, D.H.; Maniatis, T.; Henderson, C.E.; *et al.* Accelerated high-yield generation of limb-innervating motor neurons from human stem cells. *J. Neurosci.* **2013**, *33*, 574–586.

28. Burkard, T.; Kaiser, C.A.; Brunner-La Rocca, H.; Osswald, S.; Pfisterer, M.E.; Jeger, R.V.; Investigators, B. Combined clopidogrel and proton pump inhibitor therapy is associated with higher cardiovascular event rates after percutaneous coronary intervention: A report from the basket trial. *J. Int. Med.* **2012**, *271*, 257–263.

29. Sareen, D.; O'Rourke, J.G.; Meera, P.; Muhammad, A.K.; Grant, S.; Simpkinson, M.; Bell, S.; Carmona, S.; Ornelas, L.; Sahabian, A.; *et al.* Targeting RNA foci in iPSC-derived motor neurons from ALS patients with a *C9ORF72* repeat expansion. *Sci. Transl. Med.* **2013**, *5*, doi:10.1126/scitranslmed.3007529.

30. Faravelli, I.; Bucchia, M.; Rinchetti, P.; Nizzardo, M.; Simone, C.; Frattini, E.; Corti, S. Motor neuron derivation from human embryonic and induced pluripotent stem cells: Experimental approaches and clinical perspectives. *Stem Cell Res. Ther.* **2014**, *5*, doi:10.1186/scrt476.

31. Hirami, Y.; Osakada, F.; Takahashi, K.; Okita, K.; Yamanaka, S.; Ikeda, H.; Yoshimura, N.; Takahashi, M. Generation of retinal cells from mouse and human induced pluripotent stem cells. *Neurosci. Lett.* **2009**, *458*, 126–131.

32. Parameswaran, S.; Balasubramanian, S.; Babai, N.; Qiu, F.; Eudy, J.D.; Thoreson, W.B.; Ahmad, I. Induced pluripotent stem cells generate both retinal ganglion cells and photoreceptors: Therapeutic implications in degenerative changes in glaucoma and age-related macular degeneration. *Stem Cells* **2010**, *28*, 695–703.

33. Tucker, B.A.; Park, I.H.; Qi, S.D.; Klassen, H.J.; Jiang, C.; Yao, J.; Redenti, S.; Daley, G.Q.; Young, M.J. Transplantation of adult mouse iPS cell-derived photoreceptor precursors restores retinal structure and function in degenerative mice. *PLoS One* **2011**, *6*, e18992.

34. Zhou, L.; Wang, W.; Liu, Y.; Fernandez de Castro, J.; Ezashi, T.; Telugu, B.P.; Roberts, R.M.; Kaplan, H.J.; Dean, D.C. Differentiation of induced pluripotent stem cells of swine into ROD photoreceptors and their integration into the retina. *Stem Cells* **2011**, *29*, 972–980.

35. Emdad, L.; D'Souza, S.L.; Kothari, H.P.; Qadeer, Z.A.; Germano, I.M. Efficient differentiation of human embryonic and induced pluripotent stem cells into functional astrocytes. *Stem Cells Dev.* **2012**, *21*, 404–410.

36. Hayashi, K.; Hashimoto, M.; Koda, M.; Naito, A.T.; Murata, A.; Okawa, A.; Takahashi, K.; Yamazaki, M. Increase of sensitivity to mechanical stimulus after transplantation of murine induced pluripotent stem cell-derived astrocytes in a rat spinal cord injury model. *J. Neurosurg. Spine* **2011**, *15*, 582–593.

37. Kobayashi, Y.; Okada, Y.; Itakura, G.; Iwai, H.; Nishimura, S.; Yasuda, A.; Nori, S.; Hikishima, K.; Konomi, T.; Fujiyoshi, K.; *et al.* Pre-evaluated safe human iPSC-derived neural stem cells promote functional recovery after spinal cord injury in common marmoset without tumorigenicity. *PLoS One* **2012**, *7*, e52787.

38. Krencik, R.; Weick, J.P.; Liu, Y.; Zhang, Z.J.; Zhang, S.C. Specification of transplantable astroglial subtypes from human pluripotent stem cells. *Nat. Biotechnol.* **2011**, *29*, 528–534.

39. Czepiel, M.; Balasubramaniyan, V.; Schaafsma, W.; Stancic, M.; Mikkers, H.; Huisman, C.; Boddeke, E.; Copray, S. Differentiation of induced pluripotent stem cells into functional oligodendrocytes. *Glia* **2011**, *59*, 882–892.

40. Ogawa, S.; Tokumoto, Y.; Miyake, J.; Nagamune, T. Induction of oligodendrocyte differentiation from adult human fibroblast-derived induced pluripotent stem cells. *In Vitro Cell Dev. Biol. Anim.* **2011**, *47*, 464–469.

41. Ogawa, S.; Tokumoto, Y.; Miyake, J.; Nagamune, T. Immunopanning selection of A2B5-positive cells increased the differentiation efficiency of induced pluripotent stem cells into oligodendrocytes. *Neurosci. Lett.* **2011**, *489*, 79–83.

42. Pouya, A.; Satarian, L.; Kiani, S.; Javan, M.; Baharvand, H. Human induced pluripotent stem cells differentiation into oligodendrocyte progenitors and transplantation in a rat model of optic chiasm demyelination. *PLoS One* **2011**, *6*, e27925.

43. Tokumoto, Y.; Ogawa, S.; Nagamune, T.; Miyake, J. Comparison of efficiency of terminal differentiation of oligodendrocytes from induced pluripotent stem cells *versus* embryonic stem cells *in vitro*. *J. Biosci. Bioeng.* **2010**, *109*, 622–628.

44. Hargus, G.; Cooper, O.; Deleidi, M.; Levy, A.; Lee, K.; Marlow, E.; Yow, A.; Soldner, F.; Hockemeyer, D.; Hallett, P.J.; *et al.* Differentiated parkinson patient-derived induced pluripotent stem cells grow in the adult rodent brain and reduce motor asymmetry in parkinsonian rats. *Proc. Natl. Acad. Sci. USA* **2010**, *107*, 15921–15926.

45. Chen, A.; Xu, X.M.; Kleitman, N.; Bunge, M.B. Methylprednisolone administration improves axonal regeneration into schwann cell grafts in transected adult rat thoracic spinal cord. *Exp. Neurol.* **1996**, *138*, 261–276.

46. Chen, S.J.; Chang, C.M.; Tsai, S.K.; Chang, Y.L.; Chou, S.J.; Huang, S.S.; Tai, L.K.; Chen, Y.C.; Ku, H.H.; Li, H.Y.; *et al.* Functional improvement of focal cerebral ischemia injury by subdural transplantation of induced pluripotent stem cells with fibrin glue. *Stem Cells Dev.* **2010**, *19*, 1757–1767.

47. Jiang, M.; Lv, L.; Ji, H.; Yang, X.; Zhu, W.; Cai, L.; Gu, X.; Chai, C.; Huang, S.; Sun, J.; *et al.* Induction of pluripotent stem cells transplantation therapy for ischemic stroke. *Mol. Cell. Biochem.* **2011**, *354*, 67–75.

48. Yamashita, T.; Kawai, H.; Tian, F.; Ohta, Y.; Abe, K. Tumorigenic development of induced pluripotent stem cells in ischemic mouse brain. *Cell Transplant.* **2011**, *20*, 883–891.

49. Saporta, M.A.; Grskovic, M.; Dimos, J.T. Induced pluripotent stem cells in the study of neurological diseases. *Stem Cell Res. Ther.* **2011**, *2*, 37.

50. Kramer, A.S.; Plant, G.W.; Harvey, A.R.; Hodgetts, S.I. Systematic review of induced pluripotent stem cell technology as a potential clinical therapy for spinal cord injury. *Cell Transplant.* **2012**, *22*, 571–617.

51. Hanna, J.; Wernig, M.; Markoulaki, S.; Sun, C.W.; Meissner, A.; Cassady, J.P.; Beard, C.; Brambrink, T.; Wu, L.C.; Townes, T.M.; *et al.* Treatment of sickle cell anemia mouse model with iPS cells generated from autologous skin. *Science* **2007**, *318*, 1920–1923.

52. Xu, D.; Alipio, Z.; Fink, L.M.; Adcock, D.M.; Yang, J.; Ward, D.C.; Ma, Y. Phenotypic correction of murine hemophilia a using an iPS cell-based therapy. *Proc. Natl. Acad. Sci. USA* **2009**, *106*, 808–813.

53. Chin, M.H.; Mason, M.J.; Xie, W.; Volinia, S.; Singer, M.; Peterson, C.; Ambartsumyan, G.; Aimiuwu, O.; Richter, L.; Zhang, J.; *et al.* Induced pluripotent stem cells and embryonic stem cells are distinguished by gene expression signatures. *Cell Stem Cell* **2009**, *5*, 111–123.

54. Chin, M.H.; Pellegrini, M.; Plath, K.; Lowry, W.E. Molecular analyses of human induced pluripotent stem cells and embryonic stem cells. *Cell Stem Cell* **2010**, *7*, 263–269.

55. Guenther, M.G.; Frampton, G.M.; Soldner, F.; Hockemeyer, D.; Mitalipova, M.; Jaenisch, R.; Young, R.A. Chromatin structure and gene expression programs of human embryonic and induced pluripotent stem cells. *Cell Stem Cell* **2010**, *7*, 249–257.

56. Newman, A.M.; Cooper, J.B. Lab-specific gene expression signatures in pluripotent stem cells. *Cell Stem Cell* **2010**, *7*, 258–262.

57. Fujimoto, Y.; Abematsu, M.; Falk, A.; Tsujimura, K.; Sanosaka, T.; Juliandi, B.; Semi, K.; Namihira, M.; Komiya, S.; Smith, A.; *et al.* Treatment of a mouse model of spinal cord injury by transplantation of human induced pluripotent stem cell-derived long-term self-renewing neuroepithelial-like stem cells. *Stem Cells* **2012**, *30*, 1163–1173.

58. Nori, S.; Okada, Y.; Yasuda, A.; Tsuji, O.; Takahashi, Y.; Kobayashi, Y.; Fujiyoshi, K.; Koike, M.; Uchiyama, Y.; Ikeda, E.; *et al.* Grafted human-induced pluripotent stem-cell-derived neurospheres promote motor functional recovery after spinal cord injury in mice. *Proc. Natl. Acad. Sci. USA* **2011**, *108*, 16825–16830.

59. Tsuji, O.; Miura, K.; Okada, Y.; Fujiyoshi, K.; Mukaino, M.; Nagoshi, N.; Kitamura, K.; Kumagai, G.; Nishino, M.; Tomisato, S.; *et al.* Therapeutic potential of appropriately evaluated safe-induced pluripotent stem cells for spinal cord injury. *Proc. Natl. Acad. Sci. USA* **2010**, *107*, 12704–12709.

60. Lu, P.; Woodruff, G.; Wang, Y.; Graham, L.; Hunt, M.; Wu, D.; Boehle, E.; Ahmad, R.; Poplawski, G.; Brock, J.; *et al.* Long-distance axonal growth from human induced pluripotent stem cells after spinal cord injury. *Neuron* **2014**, *83*, 789–796.

61. Nutt, S.E.; Chang, E.A.; Suhr, S.T.; Schlosser, L.O.; Mondello, S.E.; Moritz, C.T.; Cibelli, J.B.; Horner, P.J. Caudalized human iPSC-derived neural progenitor cells produce neurons and glia but fail to restore function in an early chronic spinal cord injury model. *Exp. Neurol.* **2013**, *248*, 491–503.

62. Tang, H.; Sha, H.; Sun, H.; Wu, X.; Xie, L.; Wang, P.; Xu, C.; Larsen, C.; Zhang, H.L.; Gong, Y.; *et al.* Tracking induced pluripotent stem cells-derived neural stem cells in the central nervous system of rats and monkeys. *Cell. Reprogram.* **2013**, *15*, 435–442.

63. Sareen, D.; Gowing, G.; Sahabian, A.; Staggenborg, K.; Paradis, R.; Avalos, P.; Latter, J.; Ornelas, L.; Garcia, L.; Svendsen, C.N. Human induced pluripotent stem cells are a novel source of neural progenitor cells (iNPCs) that migrate and integrate in the rodent spinal cord. *J. Comp. Neurol.* **2014**, *522*, 2707–2728.

64. Wictorin, K.; Brundin, P.; Gustavii, B.; Lindvall, O.; Bjorklund, A. Reformation of long axon pathways in adult rat central nervous system by human forebrain neuroblasts. *Nature* **1990**, *347*, 556–558.

65. Thompson, L.; Bjorklund, A. Survival, differentiation, and connectivity of ventral mesencephalic dopamine neurons following transplantation. *Prog. Brain Res.* **2012**, *200*, 61–95.

66. Lu, P.; Wang, Y.; Graham, L.; McHale, K.; Gao, M.; Wu, D.; Brock, J.; Blesch, A.; Rosenzweig, E.S.; Havton, L.A.; *et al.* Long-distance growth and connectivity of neural stem cells after severe spinal cord injury. *Cell* **2012**, *150*, 1264–1273.

67. Sharp, K.G.; Flanagan, L.A.; Yee, K.M.; Steward, O. A re-assessment of a combinatorial treatment involving schwann cell transplants and elevation of cyclic AMP on recovery of motor function following thoracic spinal cord injury in rats. *Exp. Neurol.* **2012**, *233*, 625–644.

68. Harvey, A.R.; Lovett, S.J.; Majda, B.T.; Yoon, J.H.; Wheeler, L.P.G.; Hodgetts, S.I. Neurotrophic factors for spinal cord repair: Wwhich, where, how and when to apply, and for what period of time? *Brain Res.* **2014**, in press.

69. Emsley, J.G.; Mitchell, B.D.; Kempermann, G.; Macklis, J.D. Adult neurogenesis and repair of the adult CNS with neural progenitors, precursors, and stem cells. *Prog. Neurobiol.* **2005**, *75*, 321–341.

70. Fawcett, J.W.; Curt, A.; Steeves, J.D.; Coleman, W.P.; Tuszynski, M.H.; Lammertse, D.; Bartlett, P.F.; Blight, A.R.; Dietz, V.; Ditunno, J.; *et al.* Guidelines for the conduct of clinical trials for spinal cord injury as developed by the iccp panel: Spontaneous recovery after spinal cord injury and statistical power needed for therapeutic clinical trials. *Spinal Cord* **2007**, *45*, 190–205.

71. Lemmon, V.P.; Abeyruwan, S.; Visser, U.; Bixby, J.L. Facilitating transparency in spinal cord injury studies using data standards and ontologies. *Neural Regen. Res.* **2014**, *9*, 6–7.

72. Lemmon, V.P.; Ferguson, A.R.; Popovich, P.G.; Xu, X.M.; Snow, D.M.; Igarashi, M.; Beattie, C.E.; Bixby, J.L. Minimum information about a spinal cord injury experiment: A proposed reporting standard for spinal cord injury experiments. *J. Neurotrauma* **2014**, *31*, 1354–1361.

73. Watson, C.R.R.; Harvey, A.R. Projections from the brain to the spinal cord. In *The Spinal Cord: A Christopher and Dana Reeve Foundation Text and Atlas*; Watson, C., Paxinos, G., Kayalioglu, G., Heise, C., Eds.; Elsevier: London, UK, 2009; pp. 182–193.

74. Klimanskaya, I.; Chung, Y.; Meisner, L.; Johnson, J.; West, M.D.; Lanza, R. Human embryonic stem cells derived without feeder cells. *Lancet* **2005**, *365*, 1636–1641.

75. Lister, R.; Mukamel, E.A.; Nery, J.R.; Urich, M.; Puddifoot, C.A.; Johnson, N.D.; Lucero, J.; Huang, Y.; Dwork, A.J.; Schultz, M.D.; *et al.* Global epigenomic reconfiguration during mammalian brain development. *Science* **2013**, *341*, doi:10.1126/science.1237905.

Chapter 5:
Liver

Potential and Challenges of Induced Pluripotent Stem Cells in Liver Diseases Treatment

Yue Yu, Xuehao Wang and Scott L. Nyberg

Abstract: Tens of millions of patients are affected by liver disease worldwide. Many of these patients can benefit from cell therapy involving living metabolically active cells, either by treatment of their liver disease, or by prevention of their disease phenotype. Cell therapies, including hepatocyte transplantation and bioartificial liver (BAL) devices, have been proposed as therapeutic alternatives to the shortage of transplantable livers. Both BAL and hepatocyte transplantation are cellular therapies that avoid use of a whole liver. Hepatocytes are also widely used in drug screening and liver disease modelling. However, the demand for human hepatocytes, heavily outweighs their availability by conventional means. Induced pluripotent stem cells (iPSCs) technology brings together the potential benefits of embryonic stem cells (ESCs) (*i.e.*, self-renewal, pluripotency) and addresses the major ethical and scientific concerns of ESCs: embryo destruction and immune-incompatibility. It has been shown that hepatocyte-like cells (HLCs) can be generated from iPSCs. Furthermore, human iPSCs (hiPSCs) can provide an unlimited source of human hepatocytes and hold great promise for applications in regenerative medicine, drug screening and liver diseases modelling. Despite steady progress, there are still several major obstacles that need to be overcome before iPSCs will reach the bedside. This review will focus on the current state of efforts to derive hiPSCs for potential use in modelling and treatment of liver disease.

Reprinted from *J. Clin. Med.* Cite as: Yu, Y.; Wang, X.; Nyberg, S.L. Potential and Challenges of Induced Pluripotent Stem Cells in Liver Diseases Treatment. *J. Clin. Med.* **2014**, *6*, 3727–3733.

1. Introduction

Tens of millions of patients are affected by liver disease worldwide. Liver transplantation, the ultimate cell therapy, is presently the only proven treatment for many medically refractory liver diseases including end-stage liver disease and many inherited liver diseases. However, there is a profound shortage of transplantable donor livers. Regenerative medicine, which focuses on innovative approaches to repairing and replacing cells, tissues and organs, is undergoing significant revolution do to the unprecedented world-wide demand for organs. Many of the liver disease patients can benefit from cell therapy involving metabolically active cells. Cell therapies, including hepatocyte transplantation and bioartificial liver (BAL) devices, have been proposed as therapeutic alternatives to the shortage of transplantable livers. BAL is an extracorporeal supportive therapy developed to bridge patients with liver failure to liver transplantation or to recovery of the native liver. Hepatocyte transplantation is best suited for patients with metabolic liver disease for which smaller number of cells (<10% of liver mass) may be curative. Both BAL and hepatocyte transplantation are cellular therapies that avoid use of a whole liver. Hepatocytes are also widely used in drug screening and liver disease modelling. However, conventional methods of obtaining hepatocytes cannot meet clinical demand because of the shortage of donor livers from which high quality hepatocytes can be isolated. Furthermore, hepatocytes are not easily maintained in culture over extended periods of time. Moreover, hepatocyte propagation is minimal *in vitro*, even in the presence of growth factors such as hepatocyte growth factor [1]. Hepatocytes are also difficult to cryopreserve and highly susceptible to freeze-thaw damage [2]. The demand for human hepatocytes, therefore, heavily outweighs their availability.

The recent discovery that human induced pluripotent stem cells (hiPSCs) can be derived from human somatic cells through forced expression of defined transcription factors such as OCT4 (O), SOX2 (S), KLF4 (K), and c-MYC (M) (so called OSKM cocktail) or O, S, NANOG (N) and LIN28 (L) (so called OSNL), has renewed hopes for regenerative medicine and *in vitro* disease modelling, as these cells are easily accessible. iPSC technology brings together the potential benefits of embryonic stem cells (ESCs) (*i.e.*, self-renewal, pluripotency) and addresses major ethical and scientific concerns of ESCs: (1) iPSCs bypass the ethical concerns of embryo destruction since they are produced from somatic cells *in vitro* without embryonic tissues or oocytes; (2) the immune-compatibility issues since they are generated from patient-specific cell types. The field of iPSCs has undergone tremendous growth, and differentiated cell types produced from a patient's iPSCs have demonstrated many potential therapeutic applications, including their use in tissue replacement and gene therapy. It was shown that HLCs could be generated from iPSCs. Our previous study [3] and others' reports [4] of the potential benefits of HLCs generated from hiPSCs have described their secretion of human albumin, alpha-1-antitrypsin (A1AT), and hepatocyte nuclear factor 4-alpha (HNF4α), synthesis of urea, and expression of cytochrome P450 (CYP) enzymes *in vitro*. Therefore, in theory, hiPSCs could provide an unlimited source of human hepatocytes and hold great promise for applications in regenerative medicine, drug screening and liver diseases modelling. More recently, investigators have reported that HLCs differentiated from hiPSCs of patients with the inherited metabolic conditions may be used to model inherited liver diseases [5]. Transplantation of HLCs derived from hiPSCs may provide alternatives to liver transplantation for the treatment of acute liver failure (ALF), liver cirrhosis, viral hepatitis, and the correction of inherited metabolic liver disorders. This review will focus on the current state of efforts to derive hiPSCs for potential use in modelling and treatment of liver disease.

2. Hepatic Differentiation of iPSCs *in Vitro*

We will first address the hepatic differentiation of iPSCs. The term HLCs refers to cells produced *in vitro* that possess some of the properties of mature hepatocytes. Song *et al.* [6] first demonstrated that hiPSCs can be induced to HLCs directly by the administration of various growth factors in a time dependent manner. The sequence of differentiation follows the normal sequence of human liver development, and includes: Stage 1-endoderm induction, Stage 2-hepatic specification, Stage 3-hepatoblast expansion and Stage 4-hepatic maturation. Subsequent reports have focused on optimizing this method by adding modifications and improvements to the differentiation protocols. In addition to growth factors, a variety of factors have been used to enhance the differentiation of hiPSCs towards the hepatic lineage. For example, small molecules (*i.e.*, dimethyl sulfoxide (DMSO), dexamethasone) have been shown to extend the hepatic differentiation of iPSCs. The characteristics of pluripotent stem cell derived HLCs produced from various differentiation protocols have been critically reviewed [7]. Zhang *et al.* induced efficient generation of highly differentiated HLCs from mouse iPSCs by a combination of cytokines and sodium butyrate [8]. To promote hepatic maturation, Takayama utilized transduction of the hepatocyte HNF4α gene, which is known as a master regulator of liver-specific gene expression. Over expression of HNF4α in hepatoblasts derived from iPSCs led to up-regulation of markers of epithelial and mature hepatic development, such as CYP enzymes. HNF4α also promoted hepatic maturation by activating the mesenchymal-to-epithelial transition. The Takayama method is also a valuable tool for the efficient generation of functional hepatocytes derived from human ESCs and iPSCs, and these HLCs have been used for predicting drug toxicity [9]. A limitation of these four-stage protocols is that they are time consuming, usually requiring more than 20 days. In contrast, Chen [10] reported rapid generation of HLCs from hiPSCs by an efficient three-step protocol. Using Chen's system, the differentiation of hiPSCs into functional HLCs requires only 12 days. Chen's method is different from the typical protocols as they apply HGF in the first stage (endoderm induction), rather than during the hepatocyte maturation stage. It is expected that future research will facilitate the differentiated of iPSCs to fully mature functional hepatocyte.

3. Applications of iPSCs in Liver Diseases

The applications of iPSCs in liver diseases will be outlined in the Table 1.

3.1. Regenerative Medicine

iPSCs-Derived HLCs from normal individuals can be used in the establishment of cell banks for applications in regenerative medicine. Results from various studies have demonstrated the therapeutic potential of iPSCs-derived HLCs in liver diseases. Examples of the therapeutic potential of iPSC-derived HLC's in rodent models include *vivo* transplantation of HLCs to reverse lethal fulminant hepatic failure [10], both the functional and proliferative potential of HLCs for enhanced liver regeneration [11], reduced liver fibrosis [12], and stabilization of chronic liver disease [13]. Disease models have utilized immunodeficient mice and immunosuppression to demonstrate a therapeutic benefit of human HLC's. For human application, generating hiPSC-derived HLCs from selected adults and construction of libraries of cell lines with known genotypes, providing patients with a close HLA/MHC match, may minimize the need for immunosuppression to achieve cell engraftment. hiPSCs also introduce the possibility of patient-derived HLCs which will be discussed later.

Table 1. Applications of iPSCs in liver diseases.

Applications	Diseases	iPSCs from Donor	References
Regenerative Medicine	fulminant hepatic failure	mouse normal iPSCs	[10]
	liver regeneration	mouse normal iPSCs	[11]
	liver fibrosis	mouse normal iPSCs	[12]
	chronic liver disease	mouse normal iPSCs	[13]
BAL	liver failure	human normal iPSCs	[14]
Gene Therapy	A1AT deficiency	A1AT deficiency patient iPSCs	[15]
	WD	WD patient	[16]
Liver Diseases Model	HBV, HCV	human normal iPSCs	[17]
	HCV	human normal iPSCs	[18,19]
	A1AT deficiency GSD, FH, Crigler-Najjar syndrome, hereditary tyrosinemia	patients iPSCs	[5,20]
Drug Discovery and Hepatoxicity Screening	Normal liver	patients iPSCs or human normal iPSCs	[5,21–25]

3.2. BAL

The incidence of ALF is approximately 2500 cases per year in the United States and is much higher worldwide [26]. The shortage of liver donor for transplantation leads to approximately 40% of listed patients per year not receiving a liver transplant with a significant number of these patients either dying or becoming too sick to transplant. BAL is an extracorporeal supportive therapy developed to bridge patients with liver failure to liver transplantation or to recovery of the native liver. The BAL system removes toxins by filtration or adsorption (artificial liver) while performing biotransformation and synthetic functions of biochemically active hepatocytes. A major question in the clinical application of liver support devices is how to supply them with adequate numbers of functional hepatocytes to improve patient survival. Fortunately, cells in the BAL are separated from the patient's circulation by a semi-permeable membrane to prevent allogenic rejection, thus patient-specific hepatocytes are not needed.

To date, the various cell types that have been used in BAL devices have included primary human hepatocytes, primary porcine hepatocytes, immortalized human cell lines, fetal liver cells, and stem cell-derived cells. Primary human hepatocytes are not available in sufficient amounts needed for clinical usage of BAL, exceeding 200 grams per treatment. Furthermore, primary hepatocytes are limited by the short duration that they retain functionality and viability *in vitro*. Porcine hepatocytes are limited by immunogenic reactions resulting from the xenogenicity of porcine hepatocyte products and the possibility of xenozoonotic retroviral infection of patients with porcine endogenous retrovirus (PERV). However, the BAL membrane mitigates these concerns (the risk has never been quantified since no cases exist). Also of concern, immortalized cell lines lack essential functions, particularly the loss of urea cycle activity and lack of CYP enzyme expression [27]. Transfection methods to enable overexpression of CYP enzymes in these cells have been adopted, but this approach is limited by the expression of one CYP isoform per cell line and therefore does not fully recapitulate the metabolic capacity of a fully functional hepatocyte [28]. Alternatively, human ESCs and iPSCs differentiated HLCs show great promise as cell sources for BAL devices. Patient specific iPSCs-HLCs transplantation can provide effective treatment to liver diseases. Of concern in acute situations, such as ALF, time to make, mature, and expand the patient's somatic cells into iPSCs and then HLCs may be prohibitive for treatment of ALF, either as a cell transplant or BAL therapy. The cell banks of normal individual-derived iPSCs with close HLA/MHC match to the ALF patient and then rapid differentiation into HLCs for use in BAL and temporary treatment of ALF deserves further investigation.

The Fox group has reported an implantable BAL device containing HLCs derived from ESCs in a murine model of liver failure [29]. They differentiated mouse ESCs into HLCs by coculture with a combination of human liver nonparenchymal cell lines and cytokines. Functional hepatocytes were isolated using albumin promoter-based cell sorting. The coculture differentiation strategy induced a 50% increase in the number of ESCs becoming albumin positive, and resulted in 68.7% of the entire cell population differentiating toward a hepatocyte phenotype. This may be due to the heterotopic interactions between hepatocytes and hepatic nonparenchymal cells in liver development. Treatment of 90% hepatectomized mice with a subcutaneously implanted BAL seeded with ESCs-derived HLCs improved liver function and prolonged survival. Iwamuro [14] tested a BAL system whose cell source was HLC's derived from mouse iPSCs. These cells were injected into a hollow fiber module with a 0.2-µm pore size. The murine HLC's adhered to the hollow fiber surface and produced albumin and urea for 7 days. Although further investigation and improvement of the device and the differentiation process are required, the authors concluded that the combination of a 0.2-µm pore membrane and iPSC-derived HLCs showed promise as an improved BAL system. This paper provides the basic concept and preliminary data for BAL as an individualized treatment system employing the patient's own cells. Despite the paucity of reports addressing functionality of HLCs derived from hiPSCs in BAL systems, we believe hiPSCs-HLCs are a promising resource for BAL therapy.

3.3. Gene Therapy in Hereditary Liver Disease

The liver is affected by many types of diseases, including inherited metabolic disorders. A major indication for hepatocyte transplantation is inherited metabolic liver diseases in children. The liver is a vital organ that represents a promising target for cell therapy, because of its ability to functionally integrate transplanted hepatocytes. Hepatocyte transplantation has been performed as a treatment for inherited liver diseases, either for bridging to whole organ transplantation or for long-term correction of the underlying metabolic deficiency [30]. However, as mentioned earlier, the both shortage of donor organs from which to isolate high quality primary hepatocytes and the possibility of allogeneic rejection hamper the advance of hepatocyte transplantation. Patient-specific cell therapy is an ideal option to prevent cell rejection. However, isolation of autologous hepatocytes requires a lobectomy (resection of at least 20% of the liver), a procedure with risk in patients. Fortunately, development of iPSCs from patient somatic tissues and then differentiation into HLCs may provide patient specific hepatocyte source for treatment for inherited liver diseases. In the case of monogenic inherited metabolic liver diseases, in which all the cells from the body initially carry the disease-causing mutation in their genomic DNA, a gene correction approach is required to generate disease-free autologous cells. Thus, a combination of *ex vivo* gene therapy and cell transplantation has been considered [31,32].

iPSC-based gene/cell therapies have been applied in several animal models of liver-based metabolic disorders, with encouraging results. Yusa performed targeted gene correction of A1AT deficiency in iPSCs [15]. Mutation in A1AT gene is most commonly associated with Pizz-associated liver disease leading to cirrhosis. These investigators used the combined method of zinc finger nucleases (ZFNs) and piggyBac (PB) technology in hiPSCs to achieve biallelic correction of the culprit point mutation (Glu342Lys) in the A1AT gene. Genetic correction of hiPSCs restored the structure and function of HLC's *in vitro* and subsequently corrected A1AT *in vivo*. Transplantation of these iPSC-derived HLCs into immunodeficient mice was able to produce albumin and provide functional A1AT protein. This approach is significantly more efficient than other gene-targeting technology currently available, and does not require homologous recombination that leaves residual sequences in the targeted genome, and which leads to unintended consequences. These studies provide the first proof of principle that combining genetic correction in hiPSCs will generate clinically relevant cells for autologous cell-based therapies.

Wilson's disease (WD) is an autosomal recessive inborn error of copper metabolism. Mutations in the ATP7B gene (located in chromosome 13) are responsible for WD with a prevalence of 1 in 30,000–100,000 [33]. Zhang *et al.* [16] described the generation of iPSCs from a Chinese patient with WD bearing the R778L "Chinese hotspot" mutation in the ATP7B gene. These iPSCs were pluripotent and could be readily differentiated into HLCs that displayed abnormal cytoplasmic localization of mutated ATP7B and defective copper transport. This phenomenon is susceptible to correction using a chaperone drug. Gene correction was performed in HLCs using a self-inactivating lentiviral vector that expresses codon optimized-ATP7B. The newly produced HLCs reversed the functional defect *in vitro*. Hence, their work describes an attractive model for studying the pathogenesis of WD that is valuable for screening compounds or gene therapy approaches aimed to correct the abnormality. This approach may be used for other diagnosis and correction of diseases susceptible to gene therapy. Genetically corrected, characterized lines of patient-specific iPSCs can be obtained in 4–5 months [34].

3.4. iPSCs in Liver Diseases Model

Liver tissue from patients is difficult to obtain and only reveals the disease aftermath, so several genetic disorders have been modeled in rodents and large animals [7]. Although these models of human inherited metabolic disease are invaluable, they provide a limited representation of human pathophysiology [35]. Animal models, especially those in rodents, do not always faithfully mimic human diseases, and most are imperfect [7]. Therefore, new advances in experimental techniques are needed to develop new models of human liver disease, especially large animal models that may be of greater clinical relevance [36]. Transplantation of hiPSCs into immunodeficient pigs with formation of humanized xenografts offers great potential [37].

3.4.1. iPSCs from Normal Individuals

Disease modelling and drug screening are two immediate applications of the reprogramming technology and the resulting iPSCs differentiated cells. hiPSCs offer the ability to produce host-specific differentiated cells and thus have the potential to transform the study of infectious disease. HLCs derived from hiPSCs are particularly important for patients with liver diseases who cannot undergo surgical biopsy for the isolation of hepatocytes for transplantation. Disease modelling using iPSCs has been achieved for a variety of genetic diseases [38].

Research on HBV or HCV has been hampered by difficulty in culturing human primary hepatocytes, which tend to dedifferentiate and lose hepatic function after a limited time *in vitro*. Thus, alternative models have been used. *In vitro* models using animal hepatocytes, human HCC cell lines, or *in vivo* transgenic mouse models have contributed to understanding the pathogenesis of HBV and HCV [17]. However, host tropism of HBV or HCV is limited to human and chimpanzee. HBV and HCV infection has never been fully understood because there are few conventional models for hepatotropic virus infection. hiPSCs-derived HLCs from normal individuals would be useful for modelling susceptibility to infectious diseases. These hybrid cells provide an opportunity to elucidate the genetic basis of the mechanisms underlying cell susceptibility or resistance to viruses. In particular, HLCs derived from iPSCs of normal subjects are an appropriate target for studying the interactions between the host and virus with hepatic tropism.

HCV is a prototypic pathogen for which host genetic factors have been implicated in modulating disease natural history and treatment response but whose functions remain poorly understood because of the lack of robust experimental systems. Yoshida [18] group investigated the entry and genomic replication of HCV in iPSCs-derived HLCs by using HCV pseudotype virus (HCVpv) and HCV subgenomic replicons, respectively. They showed that iPSCs-derived HLCs, but not iPSCs, were susceptible to infection with HCVpv. The iPSCs-derived HLCs expressed HCV receptors. HCV RNA genome replication occurred in the iPSCs-derived HLCs. Anti-CD81 antibody, an inhibitor of HCV entry, and interferon, an inhibitor of HCV genomic replication, dose-dependently attenuated HCVpv entry and HCV subgenomic replication in iPSCs-derived HLCs, respectively. These findings suggest that iPSCs-derived HLCs are suitable *in vitro* models of hepatocytes for the study of HCV infection. Schwartz reported that hiPSC-derived HLCs support the entire life cycle of HCV [19], including inflammatory responses to infection, enabling studies of how host genetics impact viral pathogenesis. Such models will advance our understanding of host-pathogen interactions and help realize the potential of personalized medicine.

3.4.2. iPSCs from Patients

Monogenic metabolic disorders of the liver are an ideal platform to explore the complexity of gene–environment interactions and the role of genetic variation in the onset and progression of liver disease. The use of human hepatocyte cultures may circumvent the problems of animal models of human diseases in some sense. Many traditional cell-based models have been used to study pathogenesis and to screen for candidate drugs. However, none has used symptom-relevant human cell types since these cells are difficult to obtain, and under monolayer culture conditions hepatocytes lose their liver specific functions within a few days. Disease-relevant cell types could accurately reflect disease pathogenesis *in vitro*. iPSCs generated from patients who have monogenic inherited liver diseases and HLCs derived from iPSCs can be used as instruments to study the pathogenesis, disease mechanism(s) and possible cures for inherited liver disorders.

Current animal models of WD, including the toxic milk mouse, ATP7B2/2 mouse and Long-Evans Cinnamon rat, have provided very useful representation concerning its pathogenesis. However, physiological differences in phenotype between species limit the conclusions. As mentioned earlier, Zhang reported establishment of an *in vitro* disease model using iPSCs from WD patients [16].

Recently, several liver-specific disease iPSCs, such as familial hypercholesterolemia (FH), glycogen storage diseases (GSD), Crigler-Najjar syndrome, A1AT deficiency and FH have been launched [5,20]. These cells can be used as suitable specific models to study the pathogenesis, mechanism(s) and possible treatment for inherited liver disorders.

Rashid *et al.* demonstrate the possibility of modeling groups of diseases whose phenotypes are a consequence of complex protein dysregulation within adult cells. They derived iPSCs from the skin fibroblasts of patients with A1AT deficiency, GSD type 1a, FH, Crigler-Najjar syndrome type 1 and hereditary tyrosinemia. These iPSCs were then differentiated into HLCs, and characterized with special attention to the phenotypic properties specific to the corresponding diseases [5]. Rashid *et al.*'s results demonstrated that hiPSCs-derived HLCs can be generated from multiple patients of varied genetic and disease backgrounds. Their system has proved to be an efficient methodology for screening of early-stage safety and therapeutic effect of liver-targeted compounds of potential relevance to the pharmaceutical industry.

Ghodsizadeh [20] derived iPSCs from liver-specific patients with tyrosinemia, GSD, progressive familial hereditary cholestasis, and two siblings with Crigler-Najjar syndrome. The hepatic lineage-directed differentiation of the iPSCs showed that the HLCs expressed hepatocyte-specific markers. Functionality of these cells was confirmed by glycogen storage and lipid storage activity, secretion of albumin, alpha-fetoprotein, and urea, CYP metabolic activity, as well as LDL and indocyanine green uptake. The large array of iPSCs lines produced in these studies will permit more in-depth characterization of disease phenotypes. The patient-derived HLCs from iPSCs can also be used as suitable specific models to study the pathogenesis, mechanism(s) and possible treatment for inherited liver disorders.

3.5. In Drug Discovery and Hepatoxicity Screening

An added benefit of iPSCs is that they can be used for drug screening. Adverse drug reactions continue to pose a major problem to the clinician, the pharmaceutical industry and the regulatory authorities. Amongst the different types of adverse drug reactions, drug-induced liver injury (DILI) is the most prominent cause of patient morbidity and mortality. Thus, a multitude of new drugs need to be efficiently screened every year to assess their potential for toxicity. A major challenge for drug discovery is to develop appropriate preclinical models. Human primary hepatocytes have become a major liver model for hepatotoxicity tests. Unfortunately, as mentioned above, there is also a shortage of primary hepatocytes, and it is difficult to culture the hepatocytes *in vivo* without losing their depth and breadth of specialized functions, and their limited availability, inter-donor differences, variable viability following isolation and rapid dedifferentiation of the hepatocyte phenotype in culture, particularly in the loss of CYP enzyme expression, impede their use. The pluripotent nature and the indefinite proliferative potential of ESCs are two major detractions of using ESCs in safety research in the fields of pharmacology and toxicology. However, directed differentiation of human ESCs to mature hepatocyte phenotypes *in vitro* could provide a readily available source of hepatocytes for early stage safety testing. Today, approximately 70% of the top 20 pharmaceutical companies utilize stem cells in their research and among these, 64% use human ESCs or their derivatives. Human ESCs and their derivatives do not encompass all the variances within a population or between ethnicities. Alternatively, ideal cells for drug screening could be obtained from iPSCs-derived HLCs. Since cells from patients with many different metabolism phenotypes must be tested to establish safety, hiPSCs-derived HLCs from this wide range of patients are expected to improve the drug discovery process [5,21] and may lead to personalized drug administration. Specifically, iPSC-hepatocytes generated from individuals with different CYP polymorphisms would be of great value for study of drug metabolism and toxicity prediction of new drugs [7]. Moreover, iPSCs offer the opportunity to generate liver cells at different stages of maturation, as well as the potential to give rise to all the composite cells of the adult liver, which may provide extra advantages and substantially expand the scope of traditional studies in drug metabolism and toxicology [22]. Choi *et al.* used patient-specific iPSCs, screened the clinical-ready drug library (the JHDL), and identified and validated several hits for novel treatment of A1AT deficiency. With emerging new tools and technologies for gene manipulation, such as transcription activator-like effector nucleases (TALENs) and clustered regularly interspaced short palindromic repeats (CRISPRs), the feasibility of iPSC-based large-scale drug screening and highly efficient gene correction are anticipated. Integration of patient-specific iPSC-based screening in early stages of drug development will help to more accurately predict drug effects in humans, thereby significantly shortening the timeline and reducing the costs associated with clinical trials and high failure rates [23]. In view of the potential of hiPSCs in providing an alternative model for safety pharmacology and toxicology applications, many pharmaceutical and biotechnology companies in recent years have invested or have developed joint collaborations with academia, to develop *in vitro* systems based on hiPSCs [24]. Moreover, the potential to make genetically corrected hiPSCs from a diverse number of diseases and genetic subtypes also allows for the development of reliable models for studying the development and progression of genetic diseases *in vitro* [23,25]. For example, disease-causing gene mutation and/or correction of hiPSCs offer ideal controls for comparative studies of pharmaceutical agents *in vitro*.

4. Challenges of iPSCs Application

4.1. Large Expansion System of iPSCs

A major technical hurdle that must be overcome before iPSCs can be implemented clinically is scalability, referring to the reproducible production of cells and their differentiated progeny on a large scale. All of the iPSCs lines established thus far have been generated and expanded under static tissue culture protocols, which are time-consuming and suffer from batch-to-batch variability.

Additionally, monolayer culture provides limited numbers of iPSCs, only sufficient for research. Therefore, large scale systems for rapid expansion and maintenance of iPSC's and their differentiated progeny are required for further research as well as future clinical applications.

Shafa reported expansion and long-term maintenance of iPSCs in a stirred suspension bioreactor (SSB) [39]. Their study showed that murine iPSCs can be maintained and expanded in SSB without loss of pluripotency over a long-term period. Kehoe also reported scalable SSB culture of hiPSCs [40]. They demonstrated SSB cultured iPSCs as aggregates, and the iPSCs aggregates retained the ability to express pluripotency markers, as well as the potential for multi-lineage differentiation *in vitro* and *in vivo*. Chen described the use of microcarriers (MCs) in suspension culture bioreactors for iPSCs cultivation [41]. Such a 3-dimensional culture system represents an efficient process for the large-scale expansion and maintenance of iPSCs, which is an important first step in their clinical application.

4.2. Immaturity of the HLCs Derived from iPSCs

Prior to clinical application, HLCs derived from iPSCs must be compared to primary liver-derived cells and shown to have similar morphology and functional properties such as nutrient processing, detoxification, plasma protein synthesis, and engraftment after transplantation into a suitable animal model. While a wealth of studies highlight the promise of iPSC-derived HLCs for transplantation therapies, several obstacles remain. So far, neither ESCs nor iPSCs can differentiate to fully mature hepatocytes *in vitro*. Researchers have then termed such populations of cells derived from iPSCs or ESCs as hepatocyte-like cells or "HLCs". HLCs indicates that only some of the properties of mature hepatocytes are present. In general, HLCs demonstrate lower rates of albumin production, incomplete urea cycle activity, lower CYP activity, immature mitochondria and lower oxygen consumption than primary hepatocytes [3]. HLCs also show persistent expression and high levels of AFP production, suggesting that HLCs exhibit an inability to turn off early stage gene(s) as the mechanism of persistent immature phenotype [42]. Moreover, despite recent advances, the efficiency of human ESCs and iPSCs directed-differentiation into HLCs is highly variable and cell line-dependent. Since the undifferentiated iPSCs have the potential to form teratoma, research must be actively pursued to gain more information in order to clearly delineate the differentiation pathways of iPSC into specific cell types to ensure similar function and physiology.

To address the issue of maturation of HLCs from iPSCs, Ogawa [43] used a method of modified growth factor and a 32-day 3D differentiation to show that the combination of 3D cell aggregation and cAMP signaling enhanced the maturation of hiPSCs-derived hepatoblasts to a hepatocyte-like population. The resulting cells displayed expression profiles and metabolic enzyme levels comparable to those of primary human hepatocytes. Importantly, they also demonstrated that generation of the hepatoblast population capable of responding to cAMP is dependent on appropriate activin/nodal signaling in the definitive endoderm at early stages of differentiation. Together, these findings provide new insights into the pathways that regulate maturation of iPSCs-derived HLCs. In doing so, they provide a simple and reproducible approach for generating metabolically functional hepatocytes.

Shan [44] used a screening approach involving two different classes of small molecules to identify factors that induce the proliferation of mature primary human hepatocytes or induce the maturation of HLCs from hiPSCs. The first class induced functional proliferation of primary human hepatocytes *in vitro*. The second class enhanced hepatocyte functions and promoted the differentiation of iPSCs-derived HLCs toward a more mature phenotype than what was previously obtainable. Gene expression profiles showed that HLCs treated with small molecules more closely resembled mature hepatocytes. Marked increases in the amount of albumin and CYP3A were seen with treated cells *vs.* untreated cells. Of particular interest, AFP was largely absent in treated cells. The identification of these small molecules may have an impact on several areas of research, including maturation of other iPSCs-derived cell types, expansion of other "terminally" differentiated cell types, and the translational potential of these cell types.

Zhang *et al.* [8] directly compared the hepatic-differentiation capacity of mouse iPSCs with three different induction approaches: conditions via embryonic body formation plus cytokines, conditions by combination of DMSO, and sodium butyrate, and chemically defined N2B27 medium, serum free monolayer conditions. In the mid-term induction stage, the investigators added sodium butyrate, a short-chain fatty acid and a histone deacetylase inhibitor. Sodium butyrate has been reported to induce growth arrest, differentiation, and apoptosis of cancer cells in chemically defined, serum free medium. Among these three induction conditions, more homogenous populations can be promoted under serum free conditions. Although efficient hepatic differentiation was achieved by these modifications, the present protocols are far from perfect. Further optimization is needed for clinical application of iPSCs-derived HLCs. Efforts are underway to define an ideal hepatic induction strategy for future individualized hepatocyte transplantation.

The induction of HLCs from iPSCs is a complicated process that will eventually be replaced by less complex technology. Huang *et al.* demonstrated the direct induction of functional HLCs (named as iHep cells) from mouse tail-tip fibroblasts. Direct induction was accomplished by single step transduction of Gata4, Hnf1a and Foxa3, and inactivation of p19^{Arf}. iHep cells show typical epithelial morphology, express hepatic genes, and perform hepatocyte functions. Notably, iHep cells showed an expression profile and hepatic function very similar to mature hepatocytes. Donor iHep cells repopulate the livers of FAH-deficient mice and rescued almost half of recipients from death by restoring liver functions. More importantly, iHep cells did not form tumors in immunodeficient mice. Their study provides a novel strategy to generate functional HLCs for the purpose of liver regenerative medicine [45].

4.3. Strategies to Purify the HCLs Differentiated from iPSCs

Under current situations, transplantation of differentiated iPSCs into patients is risky as the residual undifferentiated iPSCs may retain the possibility of tumor formation. Therefore, the safety of clinical cell transplantation using differentiated hiPSC derivatives is contingent on novel methods to remove the undifferentiated iPSCs [46]. To date, strategies for purifying a given cell population have used either a cell surface protein specific for the target cell population, such as a cell surface marker specific to hepatic progenitors, or lentivectors expressing a reporter gene under the control of a specific promoter [47]. For example, to purify HLCs from a heterogeneic population, elegant experiments by Basma *et al.* [48] generated human HLCs through embryoid bodies. These cell aggregates were purified using fluorescence-activated cell sorting for the asialoglycoprotein receptor. Purified epithelial cell adhesion molecule EpCAM-positive cells from fetal and postnatal livers have also been used to generate mature hepatocytes [49]. The EpCAM marker is also expressed in the visceral endoderm and in several progenitor cell populations and cancers, and is associated with undifferentiated hESCs [50,51]. Therefore, to date, purification of progenitors and mature cells generated from either ESCs or iPSCs remains challenging with use of conventional methods. More studies need to be carried out to develop better purification methods before iPSC can be used clinically.

Yang *et al.* [52] reported the use of lentivectors encoding green fluorescent protein (GFP) driven by the liver-specific apoliprotein A-II (APOA-II) promoter to purify human hepatic progenitors. The investigators first differentiated a human ESC line into hepatic progenitors using a chemically defined protocol. Subsequently, cells were transduced with GFP and sorted at day 16 of differentiation to obtain a cell population enriched in hepatic progenitor cells. After sorting, more than 99% of these APOA-II-GFP-positive cells expressed hepatoblast markers such as AFP and cytokeratin 19. When cultured for an additional 16 days, the sorted hepatoblasts underwent differentiation into more mature cells and exhibited hepatocyte properties such as albumin secretion. Moreover, they were devoid of viral DNA integration. Their strategy produces a novel tool that could be used not only for cell therapy but also for *in vitro* applications such as drug screening. The present strategy should also be suitable for the purification of a broad range of cell types derived from either iPSCs or adult stem cells.

4.4. Low Efficiency of Engraftment

Functionality of human cells differentiated *in vitro* is currently best tested by transplantation into immunodeficient rodent models. However, low efficiency of engraftment and proliferation of transplanted cells into the host parenchyma is a limitation that must be considered. Alternatively, a selective growth advantage of donor cells over endogenous cells may address this limitation. For example, in some models, the survival and/or proliferation of native hepatocytes is impaired by a genetic or inherited inability to regenerate, as in fumarylacetoacetate hydrolase (FAH)-deficient mice and urokinase (Alb-uPA) transgenic mice [53,54]. These two murine models have been crossed with immunodeficient mice with a different genetic background [1]. Even with a suitable animal model, human HLCs generated from pluripotent or multipotent stem cells currently repopulate transplanted livers less efficiently than primary human hepatocytes [55]. These results suggest that fully mature donor HLCs may achieve higher engraftment efficiency.

4.5. EP Cell Lines from iPSCs

Besides the high variability and efficiency of differentiation, the pluripotent nature of ESCs and iPSCs results in production of cells types from different germ layers in most differentiation protocols. Thus, it is difficult to produce pure monolineage cultures of a desired cell type from iPSCs [56]. An effective method to direct iPSCs differentiation is to use an established definitive germ layer stem cell line, such as a definitive endoderm (DE) progenitor line. The spectrum of differentiation of definitive germ layer stem cells is relatively narrow. Thus, the efficiency of directional differentiation from definitive germ layer stem cells to a specific cell type can be increased. On the other hand, definitive germ layer stem cells have broader differentiation potential than tissue stem cells, which is economical. Furthermore, definitive germ layer stem cell lines are less tumorigenic than ESCs and iPSCs. Endoderm stem cells can differentiate to the liver, pancreas, intestines, stomach, lung and other organs cells, but not teratomas. Therefore, endoderm stem cells have potential in clinical application.

As noted earlier, differentiation from iPSCs toward hepatic lineage cells mimics *in vivo* step-wise developmental processes. Therefore, hiPSCs-derived hepatic progenitor-like cells (HPCs) might exist at an appropriate time point during similar *in vitro* differentiation steps. Yanagida reported that after differentiating with defined cytokines, HPCs from hiPSCs can be highly purified using cell surface markers CD13 and CD133. Further investigation revealed that hiPSCs-derived HPCs exhibit a long-term proliferative potential and maintain bipotent differentiation toward hepatocytic cells and cholangiocytic cells [57]. Their human HPCs derived from iPSCs may be useful for the analysis of human hepatic cell development. In addition, mature hepatocytes lose proliferative ability after cryopreservation. In contrast, hiPSCs-derived HPCs have a highly proliferate ability even after cryopreservation. Thus, the *in vitro* expansion system of HPCs may contribute to regenerative therapies of liver diseases using functional human hepatic progenitor cells and hepatocytes.

Recently, Cheng *et al.* [58] generated self-renewing DE progenitor lines from both human ESCs and iPSCs. These cells, termed endodermal progenitor (EP) cell lines, displayed a proliferative capacity similar to ESCs, yet lacked teratoma-forming ability. In addition, EP cell lines generated endodermal tissues representing liver, pancreas, and intestine, both *in vitro* and *in vivo*. EP cell lines provide a powerful reagent to study gut tissues from a common multipotent endodermal progenitor and to optimize monolineage differentiation. Moreover, creation of EP cells from ESCs/iPSCs may represent a strategy to optimize the production of pure, non-tumorigenic cells for tissue replacement therapies.

4.6. Large Expansion System of HLCs and Engineering Liver with iPSCs

Large scale production of HLCs is needed for their clinical application. As mentioned earlier, generation of HLCs from iPSCs is very time consuming under monolayer culture conditions. Vosough [59] reported their generation of functional HLCs from hiPSCs in a scalable suspension culture with rapamycin for "priming" and activin A for induction. After transplantation of these HLCs into the spleens of mice with acute liver injury, an increased rate of survival was observed. Improved survival correlated with cell engraftment in the liver and hepatic function (*i.e.*, albumin secretion after implantation). This novel enrichment strategy provides a new platform for generating HLCs, and it may open new windows in the clinical and pharmaceutical application of these cells.

It has been shown that the efficient function of multiple cell types, including hepatocytes and islet hormone-producing cells, is dependent on matrix-producing cells and endothelial cells that provide a 3D support structure and sufficient vascularization [60–62]. Thus, the liver extracellular matrix presents an ideal scaffold for stem-cell differentiation into hepatocytes [63,64]. It is known that local environmental factors induce hepatocyte homing, differentiation, and proliferation, and studies indicate that stem cells may differentiate toward mature hepatocytes following transfer into an injured liver. Therefore, the decellularized liver matrix has significant potential as the scaffold for hepatocyte maturation. This process may be further promoted by the sequential delivery of factors involved in the initiation and maturation of stem cells to liver cells [48], allowing temporal and spatial control over differentiation. Hannan [65] described a 25-day protocol to direct the differentiation of human pluripotent stem cells into a near homogenous population of HLCs. They demonstrated that day 25 of this protocol represents the earliest time point at which cells can be used to model basic hepatic metabolic function. However, cells differentiated at day 35 systematically displayed the highest level of albumin secretion and CYP activity, suggesting that the later date was optimal for functional analyses and toxicology screening. This delayed approach enables the generation of a larger quantities of hESCs/hiPSCs for differentiation into hepatocyte-like cells and their clinical applications.

4.7. In Vivo Differentiation of iPSCs

Because even a small number of undifferentiated cells can result in teratoma formation, a goal of iPSCs differentiation is to avoid production of undifferentiated cells. To date, no iPSCs-derived differentiation protocol has succeeded in yielding high purity HLCs that fulfill both functional engraftment and response to proliferative stimuli in the diseased liver. Alternative strategies are needed to obtain mature hepatocytes. To exclude compensation by hepatocytes not derived from iPSCs, Espejel et al. transferred wild-type mouse iPSCs into the embryos of FAH-deficient mice to generate chimeric mice. These mice demonstrated the ability of iPSCs to develop into hepatocytes in vivo. Furthermore, recipient FAH-deficient mice were protected from developing hepatic failure [11]. Zhao also produced mice using iPSCs and tetraploid complementation [66], which can provide the liver organ for engineering liver. The tumor formation potential of these cells has not been completely eliminated.

Takebe and his team grew bioengineered liver tissue from hiPSCs by reprogramming human skin cells to an embryo-like state. The researchers first placed the iPSCs on growth plates in a custom medium. After nine days, the mature cells were characterized by biochemical markers as hepatocytes. Umbilical endothelial cells and mesenchymal cells were then added to the culture system to induce formation of blood vessels and stroma, respectively. Two days later, 3D tissues of 5 mm width were observed, which the researchers described as a "liver bud" at an early stage of liver development [67]. The liver-buds were transplanted and examined histologically at multiple time points. Of the cells from the hiPSC-derived liver buds, 32.9% are albumin positive. These buds quickly attached to nearby blood vessels and grew rigorously after transplantation. The vascular networks of liver buds were similar in density and morphology to those of adult livers after transplantation.

Chan reported that they directly transplanted iPSCs into CCl4-induced liver injured mice [68]. They found that mice with transplants of iPSCs performed better than mice with transplants of iPSCs-derived HLCs. Performance was assessed by levels of serum alanine aminotransferase, aspartate aminotransferase, and liver necrosis. The protective effects of iPSCs were associated with increased chemokine inducible protein 10 (IP-10), a potential regulatory factor for amelioration of liver injury *in vivo*.

Other possibilities for large scale expansion and maturation of HLCs include a genetically engineered large animal model [36] to serve as an *in vivo* hepatocyte incubator [69]. Prior studies have established immunodeficient FAH−/− mice for this purpose [55]. Exposure to damaged liver tissue stimulates liver cell regeneration and can enhance homing and differentiation of stem cells to a hepatocyte phenotype. The future success of *ex vivo* cell therapies depends on novel techniques to provide an abundant, high quality supply of functionally normal hepatocytes.

5. Conclusions

iPSCs present exciting possibilities for the study and treatment of liver diseases. Areas of study and treatment include *in vitro* modeling, *in vivo* modeling of diseases, drug development, tissue engineering, and development of BAL devices. iPSCs also provide novel opportunities for autologous cell therapies and cell transplantation without risk of immune rejection. However, there are still several obstacles that need to be overcome before iPSCs reach the bedside. These include: (i) improved efficiency of iPSCs generation without viral integration; (ii) avoidance of animal feeders to culture hiPSCs; (iii) novel differentiation protocols for more efficient and economical production of mature cell types whose functionality are comparable to their *in vivo* counterparts; (iv) rapid differentiation protocols for emergent usage; and (v) enrichment of desired (mature) cells and removal of undesired (undifferentiated) cell types that have the potential for tumor formation *in vivo*. A recent report [70] that undifferentiated iPSCs elicit T-cell-dependent immune responses in syngeneic mice will require further investigation. This report suggests that host immune responses may be important for the removal of undifferentiated cells due to their abnormal expression of antigens following genetic manipulation.

A thorough preclinical assessment of iPSCs in suitable large-animal models is prudent to ensure that the proposed treatment with iPSC-derived cells is both safe and effective before testing in humans. It has reported recently that transplantation of undifferentiated iPSCs demonstrated T-cell-dependent immune response in recipient syngeneic mice due to the abnormal expression of antigens following genetic manipulation [70]. Therefore, critical aspects need to be further addressed, including the long-term safety, tolerability, and efficacy of the iPSC-based treatments. It is paramount to conduct well-designed clinical trials to fully establish the safety profile of such therapies and to define the target patient groups with efficacy assessed by standardized protocols. Despite their limitations, iPSC-derived hepatocytes remain a promising population for liver cell therapies. Moreover, engineered donor grafts derived from iPSCs, including re-cellularized biomatrix [71] and liver buds produced from iPSCs [67], may someday provide organs for liver transplantation. These results highlight the enormous therapeutic potential for treating organ failure.

Acknowledgments

This work was supported by grant(s) from the Wallace H. Coulter Foundation (SLN), National Natural Science Foundation of China (81070361 to Yue Yu), Jiangsu Province's Outstanding

Medical Academic key program (RC2011067 to Yue Yu), Natural Science Foundation of Jiangsu Provincial Department of Education (10KJB320006), and Jiangsu Province "Six adults just" high peak (12-WS-026 to Yue Yu).

Author Contributions

Yue Yu drafted the manuscript. Xuehao Wang helped to draft the manuscript. Scott Nyberg participated in the design of the study and critically revised the manuscript. All authors read and approved the final manuscript.

Abbreviations

A1AT, alpha-1-antitrypsin; ALF, acute liver failure; APOA-II, apoliprotein A-II; BAL, bioartificial liver; CYP, cytochrome P450; DMSO, dimethyl sulfoxide; DE, definitive endoderm; EP, endodermal progenitor; ESCs, embryonic stem cells; FAH, fumarylacetoacetate hydrolase; hiPSCs, human iPSCs; HNF4α, hepatic nuclear factor 4-alpha; HPCs, hepatic progenitor-like cells; iPSCs, induced pluripotent stem cells; HLC, hepatocyte-like cells; WD, Wilson's disease.

Conflicts of Interest

The authors declare that they have no conflict of interest.

References

1. Dianat, N.; Steichen, C.; Vallier, L.; Weber, A.; Dubart-Kupperschmitt, A. Human pluripotent stem cells for modelling human liver diseases and cell therapy. *Curr. Gene Ther.* **2013**, *13*, 120–132.
2. Terry, C.; Dhawan, A.; Mitry, R.R.; Lehec, S.C.; Hughes, R.D. Optimization of the cryopreservation and thawing protocol for human hepatocytes for use in cell transplantation. *Liver Transpl.* **2010**, *16*, 229–237.
3. Yu, Y.; Hongling, L.; Ikeda, Y.; Amiot, B.; Rinaldo, P.; Duncan, S.; Nyberg, S. Hepatocyte-like cells differentiated from human induced pluripotent stem cells: Relevance to cellular therapies. *Stem Cell Res.* **2012**, *9*, 196–207.
4. Si-Tayeb, K.; Noto, F.K.; Nagaoka, M.; Li, J.; Battle, M.A.; Duris, C.; North, P.E.; Dalton, S.; Duncan, S.A. Highly efficient generation of human hepatocyte-like cells from induced pluripotent stem cells. *Hepatology* **2010**, *51*, 297–305.
5. Rashid, S.T.; Corbineau, S.; Hannan, N.; Marciniak, S.J.; Miranda, E.; Alexander, G.; Huang-Doran, I.; Griffin, J.; Ahrlund-Richter, L.; Skepper, J.; *et al.* Modeling inherited metabolic disorders of the liver using human induced pluripotent stem cells. *J. Clin. Investig.* **2010**, *120*, 3127–3136.
6. Song, Z.; Cai, J.; Liu, Y.; Zhao, D.; Yong, J.; Duo, S.; Song, X.; Guo, Y.; Zhao, Y.; Qin, H.; *et al.* Efficient generation of hepatocyte-like cells from human induced pluripotent stem cells. *Cell Res.* **2009**, *19*, 1233–1242.

7. Asgari, S.; Pournasr, B.; Salekdeh, G.H.; Ghodsizadeh, A.; Ott, M.; Baharvand, H. Induced pluripotent stem cells: A new era for hepatology. *J. Hepatol.* **2010**, *53*, 738–751.

8. Zhang, Q.; Yang, Y.; Zhang, J.; Wang, G.Y.; Liu, W.; Qiu, D.B.; Hei, Z.Q.; Ying, Q.L.; Chen, G.H. Efficient derivation of functional hepatocytes from mouse induced pluripotent stem cells by a combination of cytokines and sodium butyrate. *Chin. Med. J.* **2011**, *124*, 3786–3793.

9. Takayama, K.; Inamura, M.; Kawabata, K.; Katayama, K.; Higuchi, M.; Tashiro, K.; Nonaka, A.; Sakurai, F.; Hayakawa, T.; Furue, M.K.; *et al.* Efficient generation of functional hepatocytes from human embryonic stem cells and induced pluripotent stem cells by HNF4α transduction. *Mol. Ther.* **2012**, *20*, 127–137.

10. Chen, Y.F.; Tseng, C.Y.; Wang, H.W.; Kuo, H.C.; Yang, V.W.; Lee, O.K. Rapid generation of mature hepatocyte-like cells from human induced pluripotent stem cells by an efficient three-step protocol. *Hepatology* **2011**, *55*, 1193–1203.

11. Espejel, S.; Roll, G.R.; McLaughlin, K.J.; Lee, A.Y.; Zhang, J.Y.; Laird, D.J.; Okita, K.; Yamanaka, S.; Willenbring, H. Induced pluripotent stem cell-derived hepatocytes have the functional and proliferative capabilities needed for liver regeneration in mice. *J. Clin. Investig.* **2010**, *120*, 3120–3126.

12. Asgari, S.; Moslem, M.; Bagheri-Lankarani, K.; Pournasr, B.; Miryounesi, M.; Baharvand, H. Differentiation and Transplantation of Human Induced Pluripotent Stem Cell-derived Hepatocyte-like Cells. *Stem Cell Rev.* **2013**, *9*, 493–504.

13. Choi, S.M.; Kim, Y.; Liu, H.; Chaudhari, P.; Ye, Z.; Jang, Y.Y. Liver engraftment potential of hepatic cells derived from patient-specific induced pluripotent stem cells. *Cell Cycle* **2011**, *10*, 2423–2427.

14. Iwamuro, M.; Shiraha, H.; Nakaji, S.; Furutani, M.; Kobayashi, N.; Takaki, A.; Yamamoto, K. A preliminary study for constructing a bioartificial liver device with induced pluripotent stem cell-derived hepatocytes. *Biomed. Eng. Online* **2012**, *11*, doi:10.1186/1475-925X-11-93.

15. Yusa, K.; Rashid, S.T.; Strick-Marchand, H.; Varela, I.; Liu, P.Q.; Paschon, D.E.; Miranda, E.; Ordonez, A.; Hannan, N.R.; Rouhani, F.J.; *et al.* Targeted gene correction of alpha1-antitrypsin deficiency in induced pluripotent stem cells. *Nature* **2011**, *478*, 391–394.

16. Zhang, S.; Chen, S.; Li, W.; Guo, X.; Zhao, P.; Xu, J.; Chen, Y.; Pan, Q.; Liu, X.; Zychlinski, D.; *et al.* Rescue of ATP7B function in hepatocyte-like cells from Wilson's disease induced pluripotent stem cells using gene therapy or the chaperone drug curcumin. *Hum. Mol. Genet.* **2011**, *20*, 3176–3187.

17. Zhou, X.L.; Sullivan, G.J.; Sun, P.; Park, I.H. Humanized murine model for HBV and HCV using human induced pluripotent stem cells. *Arch. Pharm. Res.* **2012**, *35*, 261–269.

18. Yoshida, T.; Takayama, K.; Kondoh, M.; Sakurai, F.; Tani, H.; Sakamoto, N.; Matsuura, Y.; Mizuguchi, H.; Yagi, K. Use of human hepatocyte-like cells derived from induced pluripotent stem cells as a model for hepatocytes in hepatitis C virus infection. *Biochem. Biophys. Res. Commun.* **2011**, *416*, 119–124.

19. Schwartz, R.E.; Trehan, K.; Andrus, L.; Sheahan, T.P.; Ploss, A.; Duncan, S.A.; Rice, C.M.; Bhatia, S.N. Modeling hepatitis C virus infection using human induced pluripotent stem cells. *Proc. Natl. Acad. Sci. USA* **2012**, *109*, 2544–2548.

20. Ghodsizadeh, A.; Taei, A.; Totonchi, M.; Seifinejad, A.; Gourabi, H.; Pournasr, B.; Aghdami, N.; Malekzadeh, R.; Almadani, N.; Salekdeh, G.H.; *et al.* Generation of liver disease-specific induced pluripotent stem cells along with efficient differentiation to functional hepatocyte-like cells. *Stem Cell Rev.* **2010**, *6*, 622–632.

21. Medine, C.N.; Lucendo-Villarin, B.; Storck, C.; Wang, F.; Szkolnicka, D.; Khan, F.; Pernagallo, S.; Black, J.R.; Marriage, H.M.; Ross, J.A.; *et al.* Developing high-fidelity hepatotoxicity models from pluripotent stem cells. *Stem Cells Transl. Med.* **2013**, *2*, 505–509.

22. Baxter, M.A.; Rowe, C.; Alder, J.; Harrison, S.; Hanley, K.P.; Park, B.K.; Kitteringham, N.R.; Goldring, C.E.; Hanley, N.A. Generating hepatic cell lineages from pluripotent stem cells for drug toxicity screening. *Stem Cell Res.* **2010**, *5*, 4–22.

23. Choi, S.M.; Kim, Y.; Shim, J.S.; Park, J.T.; Wang, R.H.; Leach, S.D.; Liu, J.O.; Deng, C.; Ye, Z.; Jang, Y.Y. Efficient drug screening and gene correction for treating liver disease using patient-specific stem cells. *Hepatology* **2013**, *57*, 2458–2468.

24. Prescott, C. The business of exploiting induced pluripotent stem cells. *Philos. Trans. R. Soc. Lond. B Biol. Sci.* **2011**, *366*, 2323–2328.

25. Zuba-Surma, E.K.; Wojakowski, W.; Madeja, Z.; Ratajczak, M.Z. Stem cells as a novel tool for drug screening and treatment of degenerative diseases. *Curr. Pharm. Des.* **2012**, *18*, 2644–2656.

26. Nyberg, S.L. Bridging the gap: Advances in artificial liver support. *Liver Transpl.* **2012**, *18*, doi:10.1002/lt.23506.

27. LeCluyse, E.L. Human hepatocyte culture systems for the *in vitro* evaluation of cytochrome P450 expression and regulation. *Eur. J. Pharm. Sci.* **2001**, *13*, 343–368.

28. Goldring, C.E.; Kitteringham, N.R.; Jenkins, R.; Lovatt, C.A.; Randle, L.E.; Abdullah, A.; Owen, A.; Liu, X.; Butler, P.J.; Williams, D.P.; *et al.* Development of a transactivator in hepatoma cells that allows expression of phase I, phase II, and chemical defense genes. *Am. J. Physiol. Cell Physiol.* **2006**, *290*, C104–C115.

29. Soto-Gutierrez, A.; Kobayashi, N.; Rivas-Carrillo, J.D.; Navarro-Alvarez, N.; Zhao, D.; Okitsu, T.; Noguchi, H.; Basma, H.; Tabata, Y.; Chen, Y.; *et al.* Reversal of mouse hepatic failure using an implanted liver-assist device containing ES cell-derived hepatocytes. *Nat. Biotechnol.* **2006**, *24*, 1412–1419.

30. Fox, I.J.; Chowdhury, J.R.; Kaufman, S.S.; Goertzen, T.C.; Chowdhury, N.R.; Warkentin, P.I.; Dorko, K.; Sauter, B.V.; Strom, S.C. Treatment of the Crigler-Najjar syndrome type I with hepatocyte transplantation. *N. Engl. J. Med.* **1998**, *338*, 1422–1426.

31. Simara, P.; Motl, J.A.; Kaufman, D.S. Pluripotent stem cells and gene therapy. *Transl. Res.* **2013**, *161*, 284–292.

32. Garate, Z.; Davis, B.R.; Quintana-Bustamante, O.; Segovia, J.C. New frontier in regenerative medicine: Site-specific gene correction in patient-specific induced pluripotent stem cells. *Hum. Gene Ther.* **2013**, *24*, 571–583.

33. Ala, A.; Walker, A.P.; Ashkan, K.; Dooley, J.S.; Schilsky, M.L. Wilson's disease. *Lancet* **2007**, *369*, 397–408.

34. Raya, A.; Rodriguez-Piza, I.; Navarro, S.; Richaud-Patin, Y.; Guenechea, G.; Sanchez-Danes, A.; Consiglio, A.; Bueren, J.; Belmonte, J.C.I. A protocol describing the genetic correction of somatic human cells and subsequent generation of iPS cells. *Nat. Protoc.* **2010**, *5*, 647–660.

35. Ordonez, M.P.; Goldstein, L.S. Using human-induced pluripotent stem cells to model monogenic metabolic disorders of the liver. *Semin. Liver Dis.* **2012**, *32*, 298–306.

36. Hickey, R.D.; Mao, S.A.; Glorioso, J.; Lillegard, J.B.; Fisher, J.E.; Amiot, B.; Rinaldo, P.; Harding, C.O.; Marler, R.; Finegold, M.J.; *et al.* Fumarylacetoacetate hydrolase deficient pigs are a novel large animal model of metabolic liver disease. *Stem Cell Res.* **2014**, *13*, 144–153.

37. Lee, K.; Kwon, D.N.; Ezashi, T.; Choi, Y.J.; Park, C.; Ericsson, A.C.; Brown, A.N.; Samuel, M.S.; Park, K.W.; Walters, E.M.; *et al.* Engraftment of human iPS cells and allogeneic porcine cells into pigs with inactivated RAG2 and accompanying severe combined immunodeficiency. *Proc. Natl. Acad. Sci. USA* **2014**, *111*, 7260–7265.

38. Park, I.H.; Arora, N.; Huo, H.; Maherali, N.; Ahfeldt, T.; Shimamura, A.; Lensch, M.W.; Cowan, C.; Hochedlinger, K.; Daley, G.Q. Disease-specific induced pluripotent stem cells. *Cell* **2008**, *134*, 877–886.

39. Shafa, M.; Sjonnesen, K.; Yamashita, A.; Liu, S.; Michalak, M.; Kallos, M.S.; Rancourt, D.E. Expansion and long-term maintenance of induced pluripotent stem cells in stirred suspension bioreactors. *J. Tissue Eng. Regen. Med.* **2012**, *6*, 462–472.

40. Kehoe, D.E.; Jing, D.; Lock, L.T.; Tzanakakis, E.S. Scalable stirred-suspension bioreactor culture of human pluripotent stem cells. *Tissue Eng. Part A* **2010**, *16*, 405–421.

41. Chen, A.K.; Reuveny, S.; Oh, S.K. Application of human mesenchymal and pluripotent stem cell microcarrier cultures in cellular therapy: Achievements and future direction. *Biotechnol. Adv.* **2013**, *31*, 1032–1046.

42. Yi, F.; Liu, G.H.; Belmonte, J.C.I. Human induced pluripotent stem cells derived hepatocytes: Rising promise for disease modeling, drug development and cell therapy. *Protein Cell* **2012**, *3*, 246–250.

43. Ogawa, S.; Surapisitchat, J.; Virtanen, C.; Ogawa, M.; Niapour, M.; Sugamori, K.S.; Wang, S.; Tamblyn, L.; Guillemette, C.; Hoffmann, E.; *et al.* Three-dimensional culture and cAMP signaling promote the maturation of human pluripotent stem cell-derived hepatocytes. *Development* **2013**, *140*, 3285–3296.

44. Shan, J.; Schwartz, R.E.; Ross, N.T.; Logan, D.J.; Thomas, D.; Duncan, S.A.; North, T.E.; Goessling, W.; Carpenter, A.E.; Bhatia, S.N. Identification of small molecules for human hepatocyte expansion and iPS differentiation. *Nat. Chem. Biol.* **2013**, *9*, 514–520.

45. Huang, P.; He, Z.; Ji, S.; Sun, H.; Xiang, D.; Liu, C.; Hu, Y.; Wang, X.; Hui, L. Induction of functional hepatocyte-like cells from mouse fibroblasts by defined factors. *Nature* **2011**, *475*, 386–389.

46. Hentze, H.; Soong, P.L.; Wang, S.T.; Phillips, B.W.; Putti, T.C.; Dunn, N.R. Teratoma formation by human embryonic stem cells: Evaluation of essential parameters for future safety studies. *Stem Cell Res.* **2009**, *2*, 198–210.

47. Hedlund, E.; Pruszak, J.; Ferree, A.; Vinuela, A.; Hong, S.; Isacson, O.; Kim, K.S. Selection of embryonic stem cell-derived enhanced green fluorescent protein-positive dopamine neurons using the tyrosine hydroxylase promoter is confounded by reporter gene expression in immature cell populations. *Stem Cells* **2007**, *25*, 1126–1135.

48. Basma, H.; Soto-Gutierrez, A.; Yannam, G.R.; Liu, L.; Ito, R.; Yamamoto, T.; Ellis, E.; Carson, S.D.; Sato, S.; Chen, Y.; *et al.* Differentiation and transplantation of human embryonic stem cell-derived hepatocytes. *Gastroenterology* **2009**, *136*, 990–999.

49. Schmelzer, E.; Zhang, L.; Bruce, A.; Wauthier, E.; Ludlow, J.; Yao, H.L.; Moss, N.; Melhem, A.; McClelland, R.; Turner, W.; *et al.* Human hepatic stem cells from fetal and postnatal donors. *J. Exp. Med.* **2007**, *204*, 1973–1987.

50. Lu, T.Y.; Lu, R.M.; Liao, M.Y.; Yu, J.; Chung, C.H.; Kao, C.F.; Wu, H.C. Epithelial cell adhesion molecule regulation is associated with the maintenance of the undifferentiated phenotype of human embryonic stem cells. *J. Biol. Chem.* **2010**, *285*, 8719–8732.

51. Yamashita, T.; Ji, J.; Budhu, A.; Forgues, M.; Yang, W.; Wang, H.Y.; Jia, H.; Ye, Q.; Qin, L.X.; Wauthier, E.; *et al.* EpCAM-positive hepatocellular carcinoma cells are tumor-initiating cells with stem/progenitor cell features. *Gastroenterology* **2009**, *136*, 1012–1024.

52. Yang, G.; Si-Tayeb, K.; Corbineau, S.; Vernet, R.; Gayon, R.; Dianat, N.; Martinet, C.; Clay, D.; Goulinet-Mainot, S.; Tachdjian, G.; *et al.* Integration-deficient lentivectors: An effective strategy to purify and differentiate human embryonic stem cell-derived hepatic progenitors. *BMC Biol.* **2013**, *11*, 86.

53. Rhim, J.A.; Sandgren, E.P.; Palmiter, R.D.; Brinster, R.L. Complete reconstitution of mouse liver with xenogeneic hepatocytes. *Proc. Natl. Acad. Sci. USA* **1995**, *92*, 4942–4946.

54. Meuleman, P.; Libbrecht, L.; de Vos, R.; de Hemptinne, B.; Gevaert, K.; Vandekerckhove, J.; Roskams, T.; Leroux-Roels, G. Morphological and biochemical characterization of a human liver in a uPA-SCID mouse chimera. *Hepatology* **2005**, *41*, 847–856.

55. Azuma, H.; Paulk, N.; Ranade, A.; Dorrell, C.; Al-Dhalimy, M.; Ellis, E.; Strom, S.; Kay, M.A.; Finegold, M.; Grompe, M. Robust expansion of human hepatocytes in Fah-/-/Rag2-/-/Il2rg-/- mice. *Nat. Biotechnol.* **2007**, *25*, 903–910.

56. Murry, C.E.; Keller, G. Differentiation of embryonic stem cells to clinically relevant populations: Lessons from embryonic development. *Cell* **2008**, *132*, 661–680.

57. Yanagida, A.; Ito, K.; Chikada, H.; Nakauchi, H.; Kamiya, A. An *In Vitro* Expansion System for Generation of Human iPS Cell-Derived Hepatic Progenitor-Like Cells Exhibiting a Bipotent Differentiation Potential. *PLoS One* **2013**, *8*, e67541.

58. Cheng, X.; Ying, L.; Lu, L.; Galvao, A.M.; Mills, J.A.; Lin, H.C.; Kotton, D.N.; Shen, S.S.; Nostro, M.C.; Choi, J.K.; *et al.* Self-renewing endodermal progenitor lines generated from human pluripotent stem cells. *Cell Stem Cell* **2012**, *10*, 371–384.

59. Vosough, M.; Omidinia, E.; Kadivar, M.; Shokrgozar, M.A.; Pournasr, B.; Aghdami, N.; Baharvand, H. Generation of functional hepatocyte-like cells from human pluripotent stem cells in a scalable suspension culture. *Stem Cells Dev.* **2013**, *22*, 2693–2705.

60. Matsumoto, K.; Yoshitomi, H.; Rossant, J.; Zaret, K.S. Liver organogenesis promoted by endothelial cells prior to vascular function. *Science* **2001**, *294*, 559–563.

61. Konstantinova, I.; Lammert, E. Microvascular development: Learning from pancreatic islets. *Bioessays* **2004**, *26*, 1069–1075.

62. Hammar, E.; Parnaud, G.; Bosco, D.; Perriraz, N.; Maedler, K.; Donath, M.; Rouiller, D.G.; Halban, P.A. Extracellular matrix protects pancreatic beta-cells against apoptosis: Role of short- and long-term signaling pathways. *Diabetes* **2004**, *53*, 2034–2041.

63. Snykers, S.; de Kock, J.; Rogiers, V.; Vanhaecke, T. *In vitro* differentiation of embryonic and adult stem cells into hepatocytes: State of the art. *Stem Cells* **2009**, *27*, 577–605.

64. Flaim, C.J.; Chien, S.; Bhatia, S.N. An extracellular matrix microarray for probing cellular differentiation. *Nat. Methods* **2005**, *2*, 119–125.

65. Hannan, N.R.; Segeritz, C.P.; Touboul, T.; Vallier, L. Production of hepatocyte-like cells from human pluripotent stem cells. *Nat. Protoc.* **2013**, *8*, 430–437.

66. Zhao, X.Y.; Lv, Z.; Li, W.; Zeng, F.; Zhou, Q. Production of mice using iPS cells and tetraploid complementation. *Nat. Protoc.* **2010**, *5*, 963–971.

67. Takebe, T.; Sekine, K.; Enomura, M.; Koike, H.; Kimura, M.; Ogaeri, T.; Zhang, R.R.; Ueno, Y.; Zheng, Y.W.; Koike, N.; *et al.* Vascularized and functional human liver from an iPSC-derived organ bud transplant. *Nature* **2013**, *499*, 481–484.

68. Chan, C.C.; Cheng, L.Y.; Lu, J.; Huang, Y.H.; Chiou, S.H.; Tsai, P.H.; Huo, T.I.; Lin, H.C.; Lee, F.Y. The role of interferon-gamma inducible protein-10 in a mouse model of acute liver injury post induced pluripotent stem cells transplantation. *PLoS One* **2012**, *7*, e50577.

69. Hickey, R.D.; Lillegard, J.B.; Fisher, J.E.; McKenzie, T.J.; Hofherr, S.E.; Finegold, M.J.; Nyberg, S.L.; Grompe, M. Efficient production of Fah-null heterozygote pigs by chimeric adeno-associated virus-mediated gene knockout and somatic cell nuclear transfer. *Hepatology* **2011**, *54*, 1351–1359.

70. Zhao, T.; Zhang, Z.N.; Rong, Z.; Xu, Y. Immunogenicity of induced pluripotent stem cells. *Nature* **2011**, *474*, 212–215.

71. Uygun, B.E.; Yarmush, M.L.; Uygun, K. Application of whole-organ tissue engineering in hepatology. *Nat. Rev. Gastroenterol. Hepatol.* **2012**, *9*, 738–744.

Chapter 6:
Muscle

Myogenic Precursors from iPS Cells for Skeletal Muscle Cell Replacement Therapy

Isart Roca, Jordi Requena, Michael J. Edel and Ana Belén Alvarez-Palomo

Abstract: The use of adult myogenic stem cells as a cell therapy for skeletal muscle regeneration has been attempted for decades, with only moderate success. Myogenic progenitors (MP) made from induced pluripotent stem cells (iPSCs) are promising candidates for stem cell therapy to regenerate skeletal muscle since they allow allogenic transplantation, can be produced in large quantities, and, as compared to adult myoblasts, present more embryonic-like features and more proliferative capacity *in vitro*, which indicates a potential for more self-renewal and regenerative capacity *in vivo*. Different approaches have been described to make myogenic progenitors either by gene overexpression or by directed differentiation through culture conditions, and several myopathies have already been modeled using iPSC-MP. However, even though results in animal models have shown improvement from previous work with isolated adult myoblasts, major challenges regarding host response have to be addressed and clinically relevant transplantation protocols are lacking. Despite these challenges we are closer than we think to bringing iPSC-MP towards clinical use for treating human muscle disease and sporting injuries.

Reprinted from *J. Clin. Med.* Cite as: Roca, I.; Requena, J.; Edel, M.J.; Alvarez-Palomo, A.B. Myogenic Precursors from iPS Cells for Skeletal Muscle Cell Replacement Therapy. *J. Clin. Med.* **2015**, *4*, 243–259.

1. Introduction

Skeletal muscle is a dynamic organ in which an efficient regeneration process ensures repair after damage. The process of muscle regeneration creates new myofibers after necrosis resulting from injury or a degenerative process. The myonuclei of multinucleated myofibers are post mitotic, arrested in the G_0 phase of the cell cycle and unable to proliferate. A resident population of adult myogenic stem cells called "satellite cells" is the main player in the regeneration process. These cells reside in a quiescent state, located between the basal membrane and the plasmalemma of each myofiber. Upon signaling from the damaged myofibers, satellite cells become activated, undergo an asymmetric division to self-renew, and produce activated myoblasts that are able to proliferate, migrate to the site of injury, and fuse with the existing myofibers or to form new myotubes [1]. Besides satellite cells, other populations with stem cell properties have been described as capable of undergoing myogenesis and contribute to myofiber repair, such as mesangioblasts, bone marrow-derived stem cells, pericytes, or interstitial muscle-derived stem cells, though it appears that *in vivo* they contribute to a much smaller extent than satellite cells [2].

Repeated cycles of myofiber necrosis and regeneration in muscle dystrophies (MD), such as Duchenne muscular dystrophy (DMD) and some limb girdle dystrophies, result in exhaustion of satellite cell regenerative capacity in humans [3]. Similarly, neuromuscular diseases in which neuromuscular junctions are lost and muscles undergo subsequent atrophy, such as spinal muscle atrophy (SMA) and familiar amyotrophic lateral sclerosis (ALS), present deficiencies in the satellite cells compartment [4,5]. Moreover, the myofibers in both MDs and neuromuscular diseases present different abnormalities in their structure and functionality [6–8]. Other situations in which muscle regeneration is compromised are severe injury [9] and inflammatory myopathies [3]. Restoration of the satellite cell compartment with healthy cells would restore the regenerative capacity of the muscle and progressively substitute the defective myofibers. Therefore, in all of these conditions, myogenic cell replacement therapy provides a promising perspective for the treatment of degenerative myopathies.

2. Using Myoblasts as a Cell Therapy

Transplantation of donor myoblast or satellite cells isolated from healthy individuals has been tried extensively in the past with somewhat positive but insufficient results and scarce references to functional improvement [10]. In 1995, allogenic normal myoblasts were transferred into the biceps brachii arm muscles of DMD patients in order to restore the lack of dystrophin protein [11]. Although some fusion of donor nuclei into host myofibers was observed, there was no significant improvement in muscle function. Genetic correction has also been explored to allow for autologous transplantation of expanded myoblasts, but results again showed engraftment but a low contribution to host fibers [12]. Massive death of most of the transplanted cells within a few days after intramuscular delivery has been reported by several laboratories [13]. The reasons why the myoblasts die initially are not clear but probably relate to immune aspects, anoikis, and a hostile environment in the host damaged muscle. Moreover, using myoblasts as a donor source poses a limitation in the amount of original tissue for cell isolation from normal human muscle biopsies. It also limits the possibilities of *in vitro* expansion because myoblasts are limited to a few passages due to senescence and the decreased self-renewal capacity of the cells due to the expansion process [14]. Therefore, it is difficult to obtain a clinically relevant number of transplantable myoblasts from a donor source. The use of other adult stem cells, with high proliferative capacity, as an alternative source of myogenic cells has been investigated with disappointing or inconclusive results such as bone marrow-derived stem cells [15], pericytes [16], and mesangioblasts [17]. Further research is needed to establish the efficacy of cell therapy using these types of donor cells.

Clinical trials using myogenic cell therapy to treat muscular dystrophies started in the 1990s, showed some engraftment of the donor cells but no clear signals of disease recovery or symptom alleviation (see Table 1).

However, extensive preclinical and clinical work over the past few decades has helped to identify some relevant issues to address in order to improve cell therapy in muscular dystrophies. The main limitations of this therapy are transplanted cell engraftment and contribution to host myofibers, which seems to be highly dependent on survival—immunosuppression is thus required but other factors might be contributing as well—and migration out of the site of injection. The transplantation regime can also affect engraftment success [18].

Taking all this into account, the ideal donor cell for skeletal muscle regeneration should be easily accessible and able to expand extensively without losing myogenic and engraftment capacity, have a great survival and fusion rate with host myofibers (high myogenic capacity), and be highly motile to spread within the muscle. Moreover, it should contribute to the satellite cell compartment, enabling indefinite muscle regenerative capacity. Finally, the ideal myogenic donor cell should have low immunogenicity, and be able to be delivered systemically, since intramuscular injection does not seem a feasible approach given the large volume of muscle tissue to be treated.

However, extensive preclinical and clinical work over the past few decades has helped to identify some relevant issues to address in order to improve cell therapy in muscular dystrophies. The main limitations of this therapy are transplanted cell engraftment and contribution to host myofibers, which seems to be highly dependent on survival—immunosuppression is thus required but other factors might be contributing as well—and migration out of the site of injection. The transplantation regime can also affect engraftment success [18].

Taking all this into account, the ideal donor cell for skeletal muscle regeneration should be easily accessible and able to expand extensively without losing myogenic and engraftment capacity, have a great survival and fusion rate with host myofibers (high myogenic capacity), and be highly motile to spread within the muscle. Moreover, it should contribute to the satellite cell compartment, enabling indefinite muscle regenerative capacity. Finally, the ideal myogenic donor cell should have low immunogenicity, and be able to be delivered systemically, since intramuscular injection does not seem a feasible approach given the large volume of muscle tissue to be treated.

Table 1. Clinical trials using myogenic progenitors for the treatment of Duchenne's muscular dystrophy.

Year	N	Donor Cells	Injection	Immuno-Suppression	Results	Conclusions	Reference
1992	4	Allogeneic immunocompatible myoblasts	Intramuscular: tibialis anterior, biceps brachii, and/or extensor carpi radialis longus	No	Variable response. Hybrid myofibers and modest strength increase in 3 of the 4 patient. Slow decay over time.	No signs of immune rejection	[19]
1992	8	Allogeneic immunocompatible myoblasts	Intramuscular: tibialis anterior	Cyclosporin	PCR evidence of hybrid fibers after 1 moth for 3 patients (1 patient tested still positive after 6 months).	Younger patients with less fibrosis presented best outcomes	[20]
1993	5	Allogenic myoblasts	Intramuscular: biceps brachii, left tibialis anterior	No	0%–36% hybrid fibers after 1 month. Low dystrophin expression. Strong decrease in hybrid fibers at 6 months. No functional recovery.	Transplantation cannot be done without immuno-suppression	[21]
1993	8	Allogeneic myoblasts	Intramuscular: biceps brachii	Cyclosporin	Poor functional recovery and lack of donor-derived dystrophin.	Younger donor cells, regeneration induction and basal laminal fenestration could improve results	[22]
1993	1	Asymptomatic twin sibling myoblasts	Intramuscular: extensor carpi radialis, biceps	No	After 1 year, significant force gain (12%–31%) in wrist extension but not for elbow flexion. Small increase in dystrophin positive and type II fibers.	Small benefit may be due to a low level of spontaneous muscle regeneration	[23]

Table 1. *Cont.*

Year	N	Donor Cells	Injection	Immuno-Suppression	Results	Conclusions	Reference
1995	12	Allogeneic myoblasts	Intramuscular: biceps brachii Injection repeated monthly over 6 months	With and without Cyclosporin	There was no significant change in muscle strength. % of hybrid fiber varied between 10.3 (1 patient), 1 (3) and 0 (8).	Patient age did not correlate with outcome	[11]
1997	10	Allogeneic immune-compatible myoblasts	Intramuscular: tibialis anterior	Cyclosporin	Myoblast survival after 1 month in 3 patients and after 6 month in 1 patient. No recovery symptoms or clinically significant dystrophin expression.	-	[24]
2004	3	Allogeneic myoblasts	Intramuscular: tibialis anterior	Tacrolimus	Hybrid fibers observed in all 3 patients (9%, 6%, 8% and 11%)	-	[25]
2006	9	Allogeneic immuno-compatible myoblasts	Intramuscular Tibalis anterior. High density injections	Tacrolimus	At 4 weeks, 3.5%–26% hybrid fibers	Dystrophin expression restricted to injection site and mostly in short inter-injection distances	[26]
2007	1	Allogeneic myoblasts	Intramuscular Thenar eminence, biceps brachii and gastrocnemius High density injections	Tacrolimus	At 18 months, 34.5% hybrid myofibers in gastrocnemius but almost 0% in biceps brachii. Increased strength only observed in thumb.	-	[27]
On-going	-	Mesoan-gioblasts	Intra-arterial	Tacrolimus	Not yet	-	*

* EudraCT Number: 2011-000176-33; Sponsor Protocol Number: DMD03; Start Date *: 14 February 2011; Sponsor Name: FONDAZIONE CENTRO S; RAFFAELE DEL MONTE TABOR; Full Title: Cell Therapy of Duchenne Muscular Dystrophy by intra-arterial delivery of HLA-identical allogeneic mesoangioblasts.

3. Induced Pluripotent Stem Cells (iPSCs)-Derived Myogenic Progenitors (iPSC-MP)

Embryonic stem cells (ESC) are pluripotent stem cells derived from the inner cell mass of a blastocyst that are able to self-renew and to be differentiated in all tissues in the body. Induced PSCs share most of the features of ESCs but are derived from adult somatic cells, e.g., dermal fibroblasts, by the transient expression of a defined set of reprogramming factors [28]. The fact that iPSCs do not involve the destruction of embryos, with the consequent ethical issues, and allow for autologous production of the pluripotent cells has opened up an enormous range of possibilities for the regenerative cell therapy field. Since iPSCs have limitless replicative capacity *in vitro* and can differentiate into myoblast-like cells, they represent an attractive source of myogenic donors for muscle regeneration. Induced PSC-MP also represents a highly valuable tool for *in vitro* drug testing and disease modeling for muscular genetic conditions that were so far limited because of the difficulties of obtaining large quantities of tissue.

Initially, human ESCs (hESCs) proved to be difficult to differentiate into myogenic progenitors, probably due to the fact that paraxial mesoderm and subsequently the myogenic program are not well recapitulated during embryoid body (EB)—three-dimensional aggregates of pluripotent stem cells—formation [29]. The first protocols using different sequential culture conditions, including a mesenchymal differentiation step, were successful at producing myogenic progenitors capable of engrafting *in vivo* but these protocols were lengthy and inefficient [30]. It has been reported that the need for a mesodermal transition previous to a myogenic commitment is determined by the epigenetic landscape in human ESCs [31]. Higher efficiency and shorter protocols were designed by overexpression of myogenic transcription factors. Pax3 and Pax7 are paired box transcription factors that contribute to early striated muscle development and are expressed in the dermatomyotome of paraxial mesoderm. Darabi and colleagues showed that inducible expression of Pax3 using viral vectors at early EB formation overcame mesoderm patterning restrictions and yielded up to 50% myogenic cells within barely a week [29]. Albini *et al.* described how overexpression of MyoD1—a transcription factor that appears after Pax3 and Pax7 in muscle development and in activated satellite cells—alone could not induce myogenic commitment directly on hESCs, but concomitant overexpression of the chromatin remodeling complex component BAF60C overcame the mesodermal transition limitation [32]. In opposition to these results, Rao *et al.* describe hESC-derived myogenic progenitors by inducible lentiviral overexpression of MyoD1 directly on hESC cells, without a previous EB formation [33].

Other more efficient and genetic modification-free protocols have been described to obtain myogenic progenitors from hESCs, such as isolation of the PDGFRα$^+$ population from EB derived-paraxial mesoderm [34] or isolation of the SM/C-2.6$^+$—satellite cell-like—population from differentiating mouse ESC-derived EB cultured in high serum [35].

Since the appearance of iPSCs, extensive work has been done to obtain myogenic progenitors with a vision to their clinical application and disease modeling (Table 2). The first iPSC-MP came from mouse cells using a protocol similar to the one described above for ESC [35], based on spontaneous differentiation and sorting of SM/C2.6 positive cells [36]. Similarly, the group of Awaya reported a method of deriving mesenchymal cells with myogenic capacity from EB by a protocol based on selective enrichment though step-wise culture conditions [37]. The resulting cells showed long-term engraftment in immunocompromised mice pre-injured with cardiotoxin, and evidence of replenishing the satellite cell compartment. However, these protocols are long and not very efficient. Using an inducible lentiviral expression system, Darabi *et al.* produced satellite cell-like progenitors by overexpression of Pax7—a transcription factor required for somite myogenesis in the embryo and a marker for satellite cells in the adult—in EB from mice (miPSCs) and humans (hiPSCs) [38,39]. The resulting cells were able to engraft in a mouse model of muscular dystrophy and to produce regeneration and restore some muscle strength, and even showed evidence of donor-derived satellite cells—by expression of Pax7 and M-cadherin by the capacity of regeneration after a subsequent injury. They reported much better proliferative capacity of the myogenic progenitors *in vitro* and much better engraftment as compared to myoblasts. Lentiviral inducible overexpression of Pax3 in iPSCs from dystrophin-lacking mice, which were gene corrected with a truncated version of dystrophin (μ-utrophin), produced in a similar fashion myogenic progenitors that engrafted, differentiated, and repopulated the satellite cell compartment and exhibited neuromuscular synapses [40]. Goudenege and colleagues described a two-step protocol consisting of first culturing in a myogenic medium and then infecting with an adenovirus expressing MyoD1 that rendered myogenic progenitors able to engraft in the muscular dystrophy model mdx mice [41]. Also, using a self-contained, drug-inducible expression vector, based on the PiggyBac transposon for overexpression of MyoD1 and an efficient and quick conversion of undifferentiated iPSCs into myogenic progenitors with the ability to engraft in immunocompromised mice has been described [42]. A limitation on the use of MyoD1 for generating myogenic progenitors is the induction of cell cycle arrest when expressed too long at high levels; therefore, as an excellent proliferative capacity is needed to expand *in vitro* and survive *in vivo*, careful dosage and timing are necessary when using this transcription factor.

Though gene overexpression approaches are fast, efficient, and appropriate to generate myogenic precursors for disease modeling, the risk of undesired genetic recombination or reactivation makes them unsuitable for a future application in the clinic for regenerative cell therapy. Different ways to obtain transplantable myogenic progenitors that do not involve any genetic modification and are still efficient and fast have recently been described. Recently, several reports describe other protocols without gene overexpression that include high concentrations of bFGF and EGF on free floating spheres [32] and, faster and more efficient, the use of GSK3 inhibitors and bFGF [43,44] in one of the cases, producing myogenic progenitors that engrafted in immunocompromised mice that contributed to the satellite cell pool [43].

Table 2. Protocols for myogenic progenitor derivation from iPSC and *in vivo* testing.

Origin	Method	Myogenic Cells	Mice	Fiber Contribution	Satellite Cell	Ref.
miPSC	EB on high serum, culture on Matrigel+ SM/C2.6 Ab⁺ selection	Myoblast-like SM/C2.6⁺	- Irradiated mdx mice - Intramuscular - Cardiotoxin	- 58% fibers positive	Yes	[36]
hiPSC	EB + general differentiation +MyoD1 mRNA	Myoblast-like MyoD1⁺	No	-	-	[45]
miPSC	Inducible Pax7 expression on EB+ PDGFaR⁺FLK1⁻ selection	Myoblast-like PDGFaR⁺FLK1⁻	- Immuno-deficient - Intramuscular - Cardiotoxin	- 15%–20% fibers positive - Functional improvement	NA *	[38]
LGMD2 D hiPSC	Inducible lentiviral MyoD1 on iPSC-derived MAB-like	MyoD1 expressing mesangioblast- like	- Immuno-deficient - Intramuscular (1) - Intra-arterial (2)	- (1) 53% fibers positive - (2) Muscle colonization	NA	[46]
hiPSC	EB+ITS medium + myogenic medium	Myoblast-like MyoD1⁺, Pax7⁺, Myf 5⁺	- Irradiated immuno-deficient - Intramuscular - Cardiotoxin	- 10%–17% fibers positive	Yes	[37]
hiPSC	Inducible Pax7 expression on EB	Pax7⁺ myoblast-like	- Immuno-deficient control (1) - immuno-deficient mdx (2) - Intramuscular - Cardiotoxin (1)	(1) Yes (2) Yes (2) Functional improvement	Yes	[39]
DMD **-hiPSC	Mesenchyal-like lineage differentiation +adenoviral MyoD1 expression	Myoblast-like MyoD1⁺	- Mdx mice - Intramuscular - Cardiotoxin	Yes	NA	[41]

Table 2. *Cont.*

Origin	Method	Myogenic Cells	Mice	Fiber Contribution	Satellite Cell	Ref.
hiPSC	EB on Matrigel, GSK3 inh., forskolin, bFGF STEMdiff APEL medium	Myoblast-like MyoD1[+], Pax7[+], Myf 5[+], Gata2[+]	Immuno-deficient Intramuscular Cardiotoxin	Yes	Yes	[44]
hiPSC	ITS Medium+ GSK3 inh. + bFGF + AChR[+] sorting	Myoblast-like Pax3[+], Pax7[+]	No	-	-	[43]
hiPSC	Piggyback transposon inducible MyoD1	Myoblast-like MyoD1[+]	Immuno-deficient diabetic Intramuscular Cardiotoxin	Low numbers of positive fibers	NA	[32]
miPSC dKO	Inducible Pax3 expression on EB +PDGFαR[+]FLK1[−] selection +μUTR gene correction	Myoblast-like Pax3[+]	dKO dystrophin—utrophin mice Immunosuppr ession Intramuscular (1) Intra-arterial (1)	20% fibers positive (1). Muscle colonization (2) Functional recovery (1,2)	Yes	[40]
hiPSC BMD [&], SMA, ALS	Free floating spherical culture +FGF2, EGF	Myoblast-like	-	-	-	[42]

* NA = not assessed; ** Duchenne's Muscular Dystrophy; [&] Becker's Muscular Dystrophy; Ref.: Reference.

Another way of avoiding introducing exogenous DNA is the transfection of *in vitro*-synthesized mRNA to overexpress the required transcription factors for myogenic conversion. It was recently shown as a proof of principle that transfection of MyoD1 mRNA in hiPSCs produced myogenic cells with the ability to fully differentiate [45] *in vitro*.

Other cells with myogenic potential that are not myoblasts have been derived from iPSCs: the group of Tedesco has developed mesangioblast (pericyte progenitors)-like cells that have been tested in animal models [46].

4. Disease Modeling

The different approaches published so far to make myogenic progenitors from hiPSCs are good models of myogenesis *in vitro*, as the produced cells recapitulate the expression of markers observed *in vivo*. They are able to fuse to produce premature myofibers in the animal *in vitro* and in most cases they have been tested in animal models for engrafting and fusion with host fiber. Several reports describe the establishment of myogenic cell lines produced from iPSCs from patients with different types of muscular dystrophy. Human iPSC-MPs have been established using MyoD1 overexpression by a PiggyBac vector on hiPSCs: Miyoshi Myopathy, a distal myopathy caused by mutations in DYSFERLIN, patients' fibroblasts [42], and carnitine palmitoyltransferase II deficiency, is an inherited disorder that leads to rhabdomyolysis [47]. Duchenne muscular dystrophy, the most common type of MD, is due to a mutation in the dystrophin gene and has been modeled by adenoviral expression of MyoD1 [41] and by inducible lentiviral Pax3 overexpression [40]. The group of Hosoyama have also described the derivation of myogenic derivatives using their sphere-base culture system from hiPSCs from Becker's muscular dystrophy, spinal muscular atrophy, and amyotrophic lateral atrophy [42]. The created cell lines make great tools for drug screening and further research into the molecular mechanisms of the different myopathies, and can be obtained in large quantities with minimal patient invasion.

5. Future Challenges for Clinical Application

Myogenic progenitors made from iPSCs seem to be a promising candidate for stem cell therapy to regenerate skeletal muscle since they can be produced in large quantities and present more embryonic-like features, so are probably more motile and proliferative compared to adult myoblasts. However, even though results in animal models show an improvement from previous work with isolated myoblasts, in terms of fiber contribution and functional recovery [39,41], a clinically relevant transplantation protocol still needs to be designed.

5.1. In Vivo Survival, Engraftment and Migration

One of the major caveats of myoblast therapy was the massive death after transplantation. The inflammatory and immunological response to allogenic transplants probably played a role in the survival of the cells and also engraftment, migration, and differentiation [48]. However, myoblast death is seen before the onset of the immunological response and in the presence of immunosuppressors or for autologous transplantation, where there should be no immune response [21,23]. Also, anoikis and the toxic environment from the high oxidant stress that characterizes dystrophic muscles may play a role in the survival of cells. These challenges to survival will be encountered by hiPSCs-MP in the same ways as purified adult myoblasts. Regarding engraftment, all the published work on hiPSCs-MP in animal models shows *in vivo* engraftment and fusion with host cells, but greater extent is needed for a clinically relevant cell therapy protocol. Limited migration from the injection site, in part due to high mortality, but also to intrinsic capacity, is another major limitation that iPSC-derived cells must overcome to outperform myoblast therapy. Some authors describe iPSC-MP as resembling embryonic more than adult myoblasts [31]. The use of two markers expressed during embryogenesis by hypaxial migratory myogenic precursors, C-MET and CXCR4, has been proposed to isolate the most migratory fraction of hiPSC-MD [49]. Also, beta 1 integrin, expressed in satellite cells, is essential for engraftment [11] and can be another migratory phenotype selection marker.

5.2. Fibrosis

Another major limitation to regeneration is dense fibrotic tissue. TGF-β1 induces collagen I deposition from myogenic cells with subsequent fibrotic tissue formation. Fibrosis limits myoblast engraftment as well as motility and this prevents axons from arriving to myofibers. Unfortunately, there are no drugs on the market that can overcome fibrosis in MD patients. However, there is a report that bone marrow-derived stromal cell transplantation in the muscle of an ischemia model reduced fibrosis due to paracrine effects [50]. This inhibitory effect should be studied in hiPSCs-MP if they are to be a candidate for use in a clinical setting.

5.3. Creating the Perfect Niche

Tissue engineering can also be of great help for the survival of transplanted myogenic progenitors in the hostile environment of a damaged tissue. Creating a three-dimensional niche for the transplanted myogenic progenitors that resembles satellite cells' natural niche *in vivo* by using biomaterials (alginate, collagen, and hyaluran) will conserve the engrafted cells' homeostasis and allow asymmetric division and myogenic commitment [51]. The cells to be transplanted would be seeded in the 3D scaffold and a graft generated *in vitro*. To complete the niche, extracellular matrix components and signaling molecules to stimulate proliferation, migration, and angiogenesis should be included. Muscle flaps made with decellularized devices from large mammals and synthetic scaffolds complemented with an *in vitro*-produced extracellular matrix from cell cultures derived from the host provide suitable tools for translation to the clinic [52]. From the complex set of requirements for skeletal muscle tissue engineered implants to function and integrate *in vivo*, some issues have already been addressed, such as restoration of the muscular-tendon junction or vascularization, while others like reinnervation still need further work [49].

5.4. Genetic Correction vs. Immunocompatible Transplantation

When addressing genetic origin myopathies, the transplanted cells should contain the correct version of the gene. This can be achieved in two ways: by genetic correction of patient-derived cells or by allogenic transplantation of immunocompatible donor cells. One of the major features of iPSCs is the possibility of generating patient-derived tissues with minor invasion. Several groups have performed gene correction on patient iPSCs. iPSC-derived mesangioblasts, from a Limb-Girdle MD patient, in which the wild-type alpha-sarcoglycan gene had been restored by lentiviral delivery, engrafted, and fused with host fibers when transplanted in nude mice [46]. Lamin A/C (LMNA) has also been corrected in laminopathy patient-derived iPSCs using a helper-dependent adenoviral vector, which is safer than other viral vector approaches [53]. Duchenne MD iPSCs have also been corrected with μ-utrophin using a sleeping beauty transposon system [39]. In any case, gene therapy is still under development and a totally safe way of gene correction has still not been demonstrated.

Another approach is to transplant cells created from a healthy donor that are matched for the main antigens in the host immunological rejection, the HLA antigens. An HLA-typed bank of iPSCs could be created to provide a source of compatible donor cells for the individual patients. A relatively small number of donors can provide an acceptable match to a high percentage of the population [54]. This approach would also be more feasible as a therapeutic approach than the expensive and time-consuming generation of personalized iPSC-MP.

It is necessary to take into account that in the case of genetic diseases that lack the native protein, its expression from the grafted tissue will most likely induce a considerable immune response that needs to be carefully addressed.

5.5. Delivery Route

Moreover, the desirable myogenic progenitor should be able to cross the blood barrier to allow for systemic delivery. Treatment of local damage could be done by local intramuscular injections or bio-engineered grafts, but for a cell therapy for MD, SMA, and ALS, in which all muscles in the body are affected, a systemic delivery is necessary. Very few reports show successful engraftment after intra-arterial delivery [38,39,46]. The adequate dosage and regime of injections still needs further study.

5.6. Safety

For all the reported work in humans and animals models using muscle stem cells, neither adverse side effect has been described, nor colonization in other organs when systemically delivered [39]. Also, for iPSC-MP no teratoma formation has been detected [37,39]. However, the double reprogramming process—first to pluripotency and then to myogenic lineage—bring along the risk of chromosomal abnormalities and genetic instability [55]. Darabi *et al.* described how, from several clones tested for *in vivo* engraftment and fiber contribution, those that performed better were the ones with a normal karyotype [38]. In this sense, chromosomal, genetic, and epigenetic studies must be performed on the cells to be transplanted before taking them to the clinic application. Also, reprogramming and differentiation methods should not include exogenous DNA but use, for example, mRNA transfection; the use of the oncogene c-Myc should be avoided when reprogramming for clinical applications. Genes involved in epigenetic remodeling [56] and cell cycle regulation [57] have been proposed as alternatives to c-Myc in reprogramming. In this regard, variants of c-Myc with no oncogenic potential such as L-Myc or the W136E c-Myc mutant are also able to induce reprogramming to pluripotency with less tumorigenic potential [58].

5.7. Clinical Grade Protocols

Whatever the method of choice is for generating the myogenic progenitors, a clinical grade protocol must be designed for the cells to be used in patients. The generation process should not include any viral vector or exogenous DNA, should be free of animal products, and should use as far as possible defined media to increase reproducibility and comply with good manufacturing procedures. Such a protocol has not yet been described for either iPSC generation or the derivation of MP.

6. Conclusions

The use of hiPSCs as a source of myogenic progenitors for cell therapy for the treatment of muscle degenerative diseases overcomes several of the limitations encountered in adult myoblast therapy: (i) easy non-invasive source of donor cells; (ii) unlimited proliferative capacity *in vitro*, and (iii) better performance when tested in mouse models *in vivo*—possibly because of more embryonic-like features. In recent years, several protocols of derivation of myogenic progenitors from iPSCs have been described reaching very satisfactory efficiency in a short time. The use of transcription factors (Pax7, MyoD1) overexpression or GSK3β inhibitors has contributed greatly in this direction. However, a clinical grade protocol still needs to be described, including the definition of safety and genetic stability requirements for clinical applications. Also, isolation of the MP presenting the most promising features for successful regeneration *in vivo* could improve the performance of the cell therapy, such as selecting cells that are more migratory and proliferative or with the possibility of systemic delivery. Other limitations relating to the host—for example, the inflammatory and immune response and the appearance of fibrotic tissue—present a major hurdle to a cell therapy approach. More research with selective inhibitors or modulators of these processes is needed, and the use of bioengineering to create a 3D protective niche for the transplanted cells would contribute to the long-term success of a muscle stem cell therapy strategy.

Acknowledgments

Ana Belén Alvarez Palomo is supported by project grant BFU2011-26596 and FBG307900. Michael J. Edel is supported by the Program Ramon y Cajal (RYC-2010-06512) and project grant BFU2011-26596. We thank Miranda D. Grounds and Jovita Mezquita for critical readings of the manuscript.

Author Contributions

Isart Roca performed literature searches and bibliography compilations, contributed to prepare the tables, and to the writing of the manuscript. Jordi Requena contributed to literature searches and bibliography. Michael J. Edel contributed to draft, edit and revise the manuscript. Ana Belén Alvarez Palomo performed literature searches and bibliography compilations, drafted, formatted and wrote the manuscript, prepared the tables, and edited and revised the final manuscript.

Conflicts of Interest

The authors declare no conflict of interest.

References

1. Ciciliot, S.; Schiaffino, S. Regeneration of mammalian skeletal muscle. Basic mechanisms and clinical implications. *Curr. Pharm. Des.* **2010**, *16*, 906–914.
2. Ceafalan, L.C.; Popescu, B.O.; Hinescu, M.E. Cellular players in skeletal muscle regeneration. *BioMed Res. Int.* **2014**, *2014*, doi:10.1155/2014/957014.
3. Karpati, G.; Molnar, M.J. Muscle fiber regeneration in human skeletal muscle diseases. In *Skeletal Muscle Repair and Regeneration*; Schiaffino, S., Partridge, T., Eds.; Springer: New York, NY, USA, 2008; pp. 199–216.
4. Guettier-Sigrist, S.; Hugel, B.; Coupin, G.; Freyssinet, J.M.; Poindron, P.; Warter, J.M. Possible pathogenic role of muscle cell dysfunction in motor neuron death in spinal muscular atrophy. *Muscle Nerve* **2002**, *25*, 700–708.

5. Pradat, P.F.; Barani, A.; Wanschitz, J.; Dubourg, O.; Lombes, A.; Bigot, A.; Mouly, V.; Bruneteau, G.; Salachas, F.; Lenglet, T.; *et al.* Abnormalities of satellite cells function in amyotrophic lateral sclerosis. *Amyotroph. Lateral Scler.* **2011**, *12*, 264–271.

6. Rahimov, F.; Kunkel, L.M. The cell biology of disease: Cellular and molecular mechanisms underlying muscular dystrophy. *J. Cell Biol.* **2013**, *201*, 499–510.

7. Braun, S.; Croizat, B.; Lagrange, M.C.; Warter, J.M.; Poindron, P. Constitutive muscular abnormalities in culture in spinal muscular atrophy. *Lancet* **1995**, *345*, 694–695.

8. Dupuis, L.; Loeffler, J.P. Neuromuscular junction destruction during amyotrophic lateral sclerosis: Insights from transgenic models. *Curr. Opin. Pharmacol.* **2009**, *9*, 341–346.

9. Quintero, A.J.; Wright, V.J.; Fu, F.H.; Huard, J. Stem cells for the treatment of skeletal muscle injury. *Clin. Sports Med.* **2009**, *28*, 1–11.

10. Cerletti, M.; Jurga, S.; Witczak, C.A.; Hirshman, M.F.; Shadrach, J.L.; Goodyear, L.J.; Wagers, A.J. Highly efficient, functional engraftment of skeletal muscle stem cells in dystrophic muscles. *Cell* **2008**, *134*, 37–47.

11. Mendell, J.R.; Kissel, J.T.; Amato, A.A.; King, W.; Signore, L.; Prior, T.W.; Sahenk, Z.; Benson, S.; McAndrew, P.E.; Rice, R.; *et al.* Myoblast transfer in the treatment of Duchenne's muscular dystrophy. *N. Engl. J. Med.* **1995**, *333*, 832–838.

12. Quenneville, S.P.; Chapdelaine, P.; Rousseau, J.; Tremblay, J.P. Dystrophin expression in host muscle following transplantation of muscle precursor cells modified with the phiC31 integrase. *Gene Ther.* **2007**, *14*, 514–522.

13. Dubowitz, V. Therapeutic efforts in Duchenne muscular dystrophy; the need for a common language between basic scientists and clinicians. *Neuromuscul. Disord.* **2004**, *14*, 451–455.

14. Montarras, D.; Morgan, J.; Collins, C.; Relaix, F.; Zaffran, S.; Cumano, A.; Partridge, T.; Buckingham, M. Direct isolation of satellite cells for skeletal muscle regeneration. *Science* **2005**, *309*, 2064–2067.

15. White, J.D.; Grounds, M.D. Harnessing the therapeutic potential of myogenic stem cells. *Cytotechnology* **2003**, *41*, 153–164.

16. Dellavalle, A.; Sampaolesi, M.; Tonlorenzi, R.; Tagliafico, E.; Sacchetti, B.; Perani, L.; Innocenzi, A.; Galvez, B.G.; Messina, G.; Morosetti, R.; *et al.* Pericytes of human skeletal muscle are myogenic precursors distinct from satellite cells. *Nat. Cell Biol.* **2007**, *9*, 255–267.

17. Sampaolesi, M.; Blot, S.; D'Antona, G.; Granger, N.; Tonlorenzi, R.; Innocenzi, A.; Mognol, P.; Thibaud, J.L.; Galvez, B.G.; Barthelemy, I.; *et al.* Mesoangioblast stem cells ameliorate muscle function in dystrophic dogs. *Nature* **2006**, *444*, 574–579.

18. Skuk, D.; Goulet, M.; Tremblay, J.P. Intramuscular transplantation of myogenic cells in primates: Importance of needle size, cell number, and injection volume. *Cell Transplant.* **2014**, *23*, 13–25.

19. Huard, J.; Bouchard, J.P.; Roy, R.; Malouin, F.; Dansereau, G.; Labrecque, C.; Albert, N.; Richards, C.L.; Lemieux, B.; Tremblay, J.P. Human myoblast transplantation: Preliminary results of 4 cases. *Muscle Nerve* **1992**, *15*, 550–560.

20. Gussoni, E.; Pavlath, G.K.; Lanctot, A.M.; Sharma, K.R.; Miller, R.G.; Steinman, L.; Blau, H.M. Normal dystrophin transcripts detected in Duchenne muscular dystrophy patients after myoblast transplantation. *Nature* **1992**, *356*, 435–438.

21. Tremblay, J.P.; Malouin, F.; Roy, R.; Huard, J.; Bouchard, J.P.; Satoh, A.; Richards, C.L. Results of a triple blind clinical study of myoblast transplantations without immunosuppressive treatment in young boys with Duchenne muscular dystrophy. *Cell Transplant* **1993**, *2*, 99–112.

22. Karpati, G.; Ajdukovic, D.; Arnold, D.; Gledhill, R.B.; Guttmann, R.; Holland, P.; Koch, P.A.; Shoubridge, E.; Spence, D.; Vanasse, M.; *et al.* Myoblast transfer in Duchenne muscular dystrophy. *Ann. Neurol.* **1993**, *34*, 8–17.

23. Tremblay, J.P.; Bouchard, J.P.; Malouin, F.; Theau, D.; Cottrell, F.; Collin, H.; Rouche, A.; Gilgenkrantz, S.; Abbadi, N.; Tremblay, M.; *et al.* Myoblast transplantation between monozygotic twin girl carriers of Duchenne muscular dystrophy. *Neuromuscul. Disord.* **1993**, *3*, 583–592.

24. Miller, R.G.; Sharma, K.R.; Pavlath, G.K.; Gussoni, E.; Mynhier, M.; Lanctot, A.M.; Greco, C.M.; Steinman, L.; Blau, H.M. Myoblast implantation in Duchenne muscular dystrophy: The San Francisco study. *Muscle Nerve* **1997**, *20*, 469–478.

25. Skuk, D.; Roy, B.; Goulet, M.; Chapdelaine, P.; Bouchard, J.P.; Roy, R.; Dugre, F.J.; Lachance, J.G.; Deschenes, L.; Helene, S.; *et al.* Dystrophin expression in myofibers of Duchenne muscular dystrophy patients following intramuscular injections of normal myogenic cells. *Mol. Ther.* **2004**, *9*, 475–482.

26. Skuk, D.; Goulet, M.; Roy, B.; Chapdelaine, P.; Bouchard, J.P.; Roy, R.; Dugre, F.J.; Sylvain, M.; Lachance, J.G.; Deschenes, L.; *et al.* Dystrophin expression in muscles of duchenne muscular dystrophy patients after high-density injections of normal myogenic cells. *J. Neuropathol. Exp. Neurol.* **2006**, *65*, 371–386.

27. Skuk, D.; Goulet, M.; Roy, B.; Piette, V.; Cote, C.H.; Chapdelaine, P.; Hogrel, J.Y.; Paradis, M.; Bouchard, J.P.; Sylvain, M.; *et al.* First test of a "high-density injection" protocol for myogenic cell transplantation throughout large volumes of muscles in a Duchenne muscular dystrophy patient: Eighteen months follow-up. *Neuromuscul. Disord.* **2007**, *17*, 38–46.

28. Takahashi, K.; Yamanaka, S. Induction of pluripotent stem cells from mouse embryonic and adult fibroblast cultures by defined factors. *Cell* **2006**, *126*, 663–676.

29. Darabi, R.; Gehlbach, K.; Bachoo, R.M.; Kamath, S.; Osawa, M.; Kamm, K.E.; Kyba, M.; Perlingeiro, R.C. Functional skeletal muscle regeneration from differentiating embryonic stem cells. *Nat. Med.* **2008**, *14*, 134–143.

30. Barberi, T.; Bradbury, M.; Dincer, Z.; Panagiotakos, G.; Socci, N.D.; Studer, L. Derivation of engraftable skeletal myoblasts from human embryonic stem cells. *Nat. Med.* **2007**, *13*, 642–648.

31. Albini, S.; Coutinho, P.; Malecova, B.; Giordani, L.; Savchenko, A.; Forcales, S.V.; Puri, P.L. Epigenetic reprogramming of human embryonic stem cells into skeletal muscle cells and generation of contractile myospheres. *Cell Rep.* **2013**, *3*, 661–670.

32. Tanaka, A.; Woltjen, K.; Miyake, K.; Hotta, A.; Ikeya, M.; Yamamoto, T.; Nishino, T.; Shoji, E.; Sehara-Fujisawa, A.; Manabe, Y.; *et al.* Efficient and reproducible myogenic differentiation from human iPS cells: Prospects for modeling Miyoshi Myopathy *in vitro*. *PLoS One* **2013**, *8*, e61540.

33. Rao, L.; Tang, W.; Wei, Y.; Bao, L.; Chen, J.; Chen, H.; He, L.; Lu, P.; Ren, J.; Wu, L.; *et al.* Highly efficient derivation of skeletal myotubes from human embryonic stem cells. *Stem Cell Rev.* **2012**, *8*, 1109–1119.

34. Sakurai, H.; Okawa, Y.; Inami, Y.; Nishio, N.; Isobe, K. Paraxial mesodermal progenitors derived from mouse embryonic stem cells contribute to muscle regeneration via differentiation into muscle satellite cells. *Stem Cells* **2008**, *26*, 1865–1873.

35. Chang, H.; Yoshimoto, M.; Umeda, K.; Iwasa, T.; Mizuno, Y.; Fukada, S.; Yamamoto, H.; Motohashi, N.; Miyagoe-Suzuki, Y.; Takeda, S.; *et al.* Generation of transplantable, functional satellite-like cells from mouse embryonic stem cells. *Faseb. J.* **2009**, *23*, 1907–1919.

36. Mizuno, Y.; Chang, H.; Umeda, K.; Niwa, A.; Iwasa, T.; Awaya, T.; Fukada, S.; Yamamoto, H.; Yamanaka, S.; Nakahata, T.; *et al.* Generation of skeletal muscle stem/progenitor cells from murine induced pluripotent stem cells. *Faseb. J.* **2010**, *24*, 2245–2253.

37. Awaya, T.; Kato, T.; Mizuno, Y.; Chang, H.; Niwa, A.; Umeda, K.; Nakahata, T.; Heike, T. Selective development of myogenic mesenchymal cells from human embryonic and induced pluripotent stem cells. *PLoS One* **2012**, *7*, e51638.

38. Darabi, R.; Pan, W.; Bosnakovski, D.; Baik, J.; Kyba, M.; Perlingeiro, R.C. Functional myogenic engraftment from mouse iPS cells. *Stem Cell Rev.* **2011**, *7*, 948–957.

39. Darabi, R.; Arpke, R.W.; Irion, S.; Dimos, J.T.; Grskovic, M.; Kyba, M.; Perlingeiro, R.C. Human ES- and iPS-derived myogenic progenitors restore DYSTROPHIN and improve contractility upon transplantation in dystrophic mice. *Cell Stem Cell* **2012**, *10*, 610–619.

40. Filareto, A.; Parker, S.; Darabi, R.; Borges, L.; Iacovino, M.; Schaaf, T.; Chamberlain, J.S.; Ervasti, J.M.; McIvor, R.S.; Kyba, M.; *et al.* An *ex vivo* gene therapy approach to treat muscular dystrophy using inducible pluripotent stem cells. *Nat. Commun.* **2013**, *4*, 1549–1557.

41. Goudenege, S.; Lebel, C.; Huot, N.B.; Dufour, C.; Fujii, I.; Gekas, J.; Rousseau, J.; Tremblay, J.P. Myoblasts derived from normal hESCs and dystrophic hiPSCs efficiently fuse with existing muscle fibers following transplantation. *Mol. Ther.* **2012**, *20*, 2153–2167.

42. Hosoyama, T.; McGivern, J.V.; van Dyke, J.M.; Ebert, A.D.; Suzuki, M. Derivation of myogenic progenitors directly from human pluripotent stem cells using a sphere-based culture. *Stem Cells Transl. Med.* **2014**, *3*, 564–574.

43. Borchin, B.; Chen, J.; Barberi, T. Derivation and FACS-Mediated Purification of PAX3$^+$/PAX7$^+$ Skeletal Muscle Precursors from Human Pluripotent Stem Cells. *Stem Cell Rep.* **2013**, *1*, 620–631.

44. Xu, C.; Tabebordbar, M.; Iovino, S.; Ciarlo, C.; Liu, J.; Castilgioni, A.; Price, E.; Liu, M.; Barton, E.R.; Kahn, C.R.; *et al.* Azebrafish culture system defines factors that promote vertebrate myogenesis across species. *Cell* **2013**, *155*, 909–921.

45. Warren, L.; Manos, P.D.; Ahfeldt, T.; Loh, Y.H.; Li, H.; Lau, F.; Ebina, W.; Mandal, P.K.; Smith, Z.D.; Meissner, A.; *et al.* Highly efficient reprogramming to pluripotency and directed differentiation of human cells with synthetic modified mRNA. *Cell Stem Cell* **2010**, *7*, 618–630.

46. Tedesco, F.S.; Gerli, M.F.; Perani, L.; Benedetti, S.; Ungaro, F.; Cassano, M.; Antonini, S.; Tagliafico, E.; Artusi, V.; Longa, E.; *et al.* Transplantation of genetically corrected human iPSC-derived progenitors in mice with limb-girdle muscular dystrophy. *Sci. Transl. Med.* **2012**, *4*, doi:10.1126/scitranslmed.3003541.

47. Yasuno, T.; Osafune, K.; Sakurai, H.; Asaka, I.; Tanaka, A.; Yamaguchi, S.; Yamada, K.; Hitomi, H.; Arai, S.; Kurose, Y.; *et al.* Functional analysis of iPSC-derived myocytes from a patient with carnitine palmitoyltransferase II deficiency. *Biochem. Biophys. Res. Commun.* **2014**, *448*, 175–181.

48. Maffioletti, S.M.; Noviello, M.; English, K.; Tedesco, F.S. Stem cell transplantation for muscular dystrophy: The challenge of immune response. *BioMed Res. Int.* **2014**, *2014*, doi:10.1155/2014/964010.

49. Perniconi, B.; Coletti, D. Skeletal muscle tissue engineering: Best bet or black beast? *Frotiers Physiol.* **2014**, *5*, doi:10.3389/fphys.2014.00255.

50. Kinnaird, T.; Stabile, E.; Burnett, M.S.; Shou, M.; Lee, C.W.; Barr, S.; Fuchs, S.; Epstein, S.E. Local delivery of marrow-derived stromal cells augments collateral perfusion through paracrine mechanisms. *Circulation* **2004**, *109*, 1543–1549.

51. Rossi, C.A.; Pozzobon, M.; de Coppi, P. Advances in musculoskeletal tissue engineering: Moving towards therapy. *Organogenesis* **2010**, *6*, 167–172.

52. Citadella Vigodarzere, G.; Mantero, S. Skeletal muscle tissue engineering: Strategies for volumetric constructs. *Front. Physiol.* **2014**, *5*, doi:10.3389/fphys.2014.00362.

53. Liu, G.H.; Suzuki, K.; Qu, J.; Sancho-Martinez, I.; Yi, F.; Li, M.; Kumar, S.; Nivet, E.; Kim, J.; Soligalla, R.D.; *et al.* Targeted gene correction of laminopathy-associated LMNA mutations in patient-specific iPSCs. *Cell Stem Cell* **2011**, *8*, 688–694.

54. Taylor, C.J.; Peacock, B.; Chaudhry, A.N.; Bradley, J.A.; Bolton, D.M. Generating an iPSCs bank for HLA-matched tissue transplantation based on known donor and recipient HLA types. *Cell Stem Cell* **2012**, *11*, 147–152.

55. Gore, A.; Li, Z.; Fung, H.L.; Young, J.E.; Agarwal, S.; Antosiewicz-Bourget, J.; Canto, I.; Giorgetti, A.; Israel, M.A.; Kiskinis, E.; *et al.* Somatic coding mutations in human induced pluripotent stem cells. *Nature* **2011**, *471*, 63–67.

56. Onder, T.T.; Kara, N.; Cherry, A.; Sinha, A.U.; Zhu, C.; Bernt, K.M.; Cahan, P.; Marcarci, B.O.; Unternaehrer, J.; Gupta, P.B.; *et al.* Chromatin-modifying enzymes as modulators of reprogramming. *Nature* **2012**, *483*, 598–602.

57. McLenachan, S.; Menchon, C.; Raya, A.; Consiglio, A.; Edel, M.J. Cyclin A1 is essential for setting the pluripotent state and reducing tumorigenicity of induced pluripotent stem cells. *Stem Cells Dev.* **2012**, *21*, 2891–2899.

58. Nakagawa, M.; Takizawa, N.; Narita, M.; Ichisaka, T.; Yamanaka, S. Promotion of direct reprogramming by transformation-deficient Myc. *Proc. Natl. Acad. Sci. USA* **2010**, *107*, 14152–14157.

Chapter 7:
Bone

The Use of Patient-Specific Induced Pluripotent Stem Cells (iPSCs) to Identify Osteoclast Defects in Rare Genetic Bone Disorders

I-Ping Chen

Abstract: More than 500 rare genetic bone disorders have been described, but for many of them only limited treatment options are available. Challenges for studying these bone diseases come from a lack of suitable animal models and unavailability of skeletal tissues for studies. Effectors for skeletal abnormalities of bone disorders may be abnormal bone formation directed by osteoblasts or anomalous bone resorption by osteoclasts, or both. Patient-specific induced pluripotent stem cells (iPSCs) can be generated from somatic cells of various tissue sources and in theory can be differentiated into any desired cell type. However, successful differentiation of hiPSCs into functional bone cells is still a challenge. Our group focuses on the use of human iPSCs (hiPSCs) to identify osteoclast defects in craniometaphyseal dysplasia. In this review, we describe the impact of stem cell technology on research for better treatment of such disorders, the generation of hiPSCs from patients with rare genetic bone disorders and current protocols for differentiating hiPSCs into osteoclasts.

Reprinted from *J. Clin. Med.* Cite as: Chen, I.-P. The Use of Patient-Specific Induced Pluripotent Stem Cells (iPSCs) to Identify Osteoclast Defects in Rare Genetic Bone Disorders. *J. Clin. Med.* **2014**, *3*, 1490–1510.

1. Introduction

Studying rare genetic bone disorders is clinically highly relevant. Although individual diseases only affect a small percentage of the population (less than 200,000 people or about 1 in 1500 people in the United States), overall, a large number of people suffer from these skeletal disorders due to their frequency (almost 500 rare genetic bone disorders listed by NIH Office of Rare Disease Research). Many of these diseases become apparent early in life and are present throughout the patient's entire life. The diverse expressivities of clinical manifestations, from lethality of newborns to mild skeletal abnormalities, make the diagnosis of some of these disorders challenging. Moreover, most of these rare bone diseases are understudied due to the rarity of human specimens and unavailable animal models, and therefore treatment options are often limited or lacking. It is thus important to establish better models for studying such disorders.

Research focusing on genetic disorders of the skeleton is not only beneficial for future treatment of patients, but has significantly contributed to our knowledge on key concepts of bone biology. Rare genetic bone disorders have been linked to abnormal bone development and/or bone remodeling. Pathologically and embryologically these diseases can be subdivided into four major groups: (1) disorders affecting skeletal patterning; (2) disorders of condensation/differentiation of skeletal precursor structures; (3) disorders affecting growth and (4) disorders of bone homeostasis caused by perturbation of interaction between the bone forming osteoblasts and the bone resorbing osteoclasts [1]. Our group has been studying a rare genetic bone disorder, craniometaphyseal dysplasia (CMD) characterized by progressive thickening of craniofacial bones and widening of metaphyses in long bones, utilizing a knock-in mouse model [2]. We have identified defects of osteoblasts and osteoclasts in mice with a CMD mutation [3]. We currently study CMD in a human system using patient-specific induced pluripotent stem cells (hiPSCs) to identify osteoclast defects and we believe this strategy can be applied widely for studying other rare genetic disorders.

In this article, we review some of the rare genetic bone disorders with osteoclast defects, the generation of hiPSCs from patients with rare genetic bone disorders and the protocols for differentiating hiPSC into osteoclasts.

2. Rare Genetic Bone Disorders with Osteoclast Defects

Osteoclasts are cells responsible for resorbing bone and work in close concert with osteoblasts to model the skeleton during growth/development and to remodel the bone throughout life. Osteoclasts are derived from the monocyte/macrophage lineage of hematopoietic stem cells and are multinucleated giant cells expressing marker genes, such as tartrate-resistant acid phosphatase (Trap), Cathepsin K, calcitonin receptor, nuclear factor of activated T-cells, cytoplasmic 1 (Nfatc1). Development of osteoclasts (osteoclastogenesis) involves (1) the commitment of hematopoietic stem cells into osteoclast precursors; (2) the fusion of mononucleated osteoclast precursors into multinucleated osteoclast syncytia; (3) the differentiation/maturation to functional osteoclasts. During stage 1, transcription factors PU.1, MITF and c-FOS are important determinants of lineage specification [4–6]. In addition, M-CSF signaling is necessary for proliferation and survival of osteoclast progenitors as first became obvious by the osteopetrotic phenotype of mice lacking the *M-CSF* gene (op/op mice) [7]. Interaction of RANKL, a member of TNF family and strongly expressed by osteoblasts, with its receptor RANK on osteoclast progenitors is necessary for the fusion of osteoclast precursors. The activation of RANK/RANKL signaling initiates a cascade of gene expression, including the expression of chemokines such as Mcp-1 to attract RANK[+] mononuclear osteoclast precursors and molecules important for osteoclast fusion such as Atp6v0d2 and DC-Stamp [8,9]. The final step in differentiation to mature and functional osteoclasts involves the formation of a ruffled border and sealing zone. Lack of functional osteoclasts by disruption of these processes or failure of polarization and cytokine organization can lead to osteopetrosis [10].

Many rare genetic bone disorders are partially or primarily caused by osteoclast defects. Dysfunctional osteoclasts can result in too much bone while increased bone resorption can lead to decreased bone mass. Some diseases present a combination of osteosclerosis with osteolytic lesions. Studies on these disorders highlight the important roles of some specific proteins or signaling pathways during osteoclastogenesis.

2.1. Diseases of Decreased Osteoclast Resorption

Osteopetrosis: Three main forms of hereditary osteopetrosis are autosomal recessive osteopetrosis (ARO), intermediate autosomal recessive osteopetrosis (IARO) and adult dominant osteopetrosis (ADO), the most severe form being ARO. Mutations causing these diseases generally lead to lack of acid secretion in osteoclasts. ARO presents in infants with severe sclerosis of bone, an increased rate of fracture, extreme reduction of bone marrow space, hepatosplenomegaly, anemia, compression of cranial nerves and growth failure [11]. Infantile malignant osteopetrosis is generally lethal and can only be treated by early bone-marrow transplantation. IARO is a recessive form of osteopetrosis with renal tubular acidosis. The affected protein, carbonic anhydrase type II is highly abundant in osteoclasts, cerebral neurons and in renal intercalated cells. Clinical features of IARO patients include the milder form of osteopetrosis, mental retardation due to cerebral calcification and renal dysfunction [12]. Two distinct types of ADO are known [13]. ADO is characterized by a generalized diffuse osteosclerosis with the most pronounced thickening at the cranial vault in its type I form and the most pronounced abnormalities in vertebrae in type II (Albers Schonberg disease).

Pycnodysostosis: This is an autosomal recessive disorder and can be diagnosed during early infancy. The phenotype is milder than ARO with short stature, recurrent bone fracture, skull deformity and hypoplasia of facial bones, sinuses and clavicles. Long bones are hyperostotic with narrow medullary canals. The calvarium and base of the skull are sclerotic. The genetic defect for pycnodysostosis has been identified in Cathepsin K, a lysosomal cysteine protease required to degrade collagen in resorption lacunae of osteoclasts [14].

2.2. Diseases of Increased Osteoclast Resorption

Paget's disease of bone (PDB): PDB is a late onset bone disease starting at mid-life or later. Genetic predisposition together with environmental risks and other risk factors such as trauma or surgery contribute to its etiology. PDB affects single or multiple locations of the skeleton where focal bone resorption occurs and bone is replaced with soft, fibrous expansile tissue that result in characteristic enlarged and softened bone tissue. Clinical symptoms include bone pain, bone deformity, deafness, pathological fractures and osteoarthritis [15,16]. Although increased osteoclast activity is primarily the cause of PDB, excessive osteoblast activity reflected in elevated serum alkaline phosphatase has been reported [17], which could be a sign of increased bone turnover.

Juvenile PDB (JPDB): Different from Paget's disease of bone, JPDB usually occurs in infancy or early childhood, characterized by massive thickening of calvaria, widened diaphyses, and deformities of extremities and vertebrae [18]. Autosomal recessive mutations in *TNFRSF11B* result in a less efficient form of osteoprotegerin (OPG) with reduced affinity for RANKL or in a failure to express OPG protein. OPG is a decoy receptor for RANKL, thus regulating osteoclast formation. As a consequence, increased bone resorption coupled with increased bone formation, are seen in JPDB [19,20].

Familial expansile osteolysis (FEO): FEO is an autosomal dominant rare bone disorder characterized by osteolytic lesions in major bones of the appendicular skeleton during early adulthood. It can also result in deafness and premature tooth loss due to abnormalities in the middle ear and jaw [21,22]. Mutations identified in *TNFRSF11A* cause enhanced RANK-mediated nuclear factor-κB (NF-κB) signaling and increased bone remodeling [23].

Expansile skeletal hyperphosphatasia (ESH): ESH is characterized by expanding hyperostotic long bones, early onset deafness, premature tooth loss, episodic hypercalcemia and increased alkaline phosphatase activity; the skull and appendicular skeleton display hyperostosis and/or osteosclerosis [24].

Mutations responsible for these rare disorders affecting osteoclast activity are summarized in Table 1. Research of disorders mentioned above would be greatly enhanced if elaborate models for studying osteoclastogenesis and osteoclast function would be available. Induced pluripotent stem cells (iPSCs) could be one worthwhile avenue to study such disorders in humans. iPS cell approaches have been published for certain bone remodeling disorders described below.

Table 1. Mutations in rare genetic bone disorders with osteoclast defects.

Diseases with Decreased Bone Resorption				
Disease	**OMIM**	**Gene Affected**	**Protein Affected**	**Reference(s)**
ARO	259,700	*TCIRG1*	α3 Subunit of vacuolar proton pump H$^+$ ATPase	[1,25]
ARO	259,700	*CLCN7*	Chloride channel	[26]
ARO	259,700	*OSTM1*	GL	[27]
IARO	259,730	*CAII*	Carbonic anhydrase II	[12]
ADOI	166,600	*Lrp5*	Lrp5	[28]
ADOII	166,600	*CLCN7*	Chloride channel	[29]
Pycnodysostosis	265,800	*CTSK*	Cathepsin K	[14]
PDB	6,002,080	*SQSTM1*	P62	[30,31]
JPDB	239,000	*TNFRSF11B*	Osteoprotegerin (OPG)	[19]
FEO	174,810	*TNFRSF11A*	RANK	[23]
ESH	N/A	*TNFRSF11A*	RANK	[32]

ARO: autosomal recessive osteopetrosis; IARO: intermediate autosomal recessive osteopetrosis; ADOI: adult dominant osteopetrosis, type I; ADOII: adult dominant osteopetrosis type II; PDB: Paget's disease of bone; JPDB: Juvenile Paget's disease of bone; FEO: familial expansile osteolysis; ESH: expansile skeletal hyperphosphatasia; OMIM: Online Mendelian Inheritance in Man; GL: Grey lethal; N/A: not available.

3. Generation of hiPSCs from Rare Genetic Bone Disorders

hiPSCs, similar to human embryonic stem cells (hESCs), have the ability to self-renew indefinitely and in theory differentiate to any cell type when induced under appropriate conditions. The advances in hiPSCs technology opened new opportunities for medical research in disease modeling, drug screening, gene therapy and genome editing [33–35]. Generation of hiPSCs can, for example, be achieved by introduction of reprogramming factors, *OCT3/4*, *SOX2*, *KLF4* and *c-MYC* or *OCT3/4*, *SOX2*, *NANOG*, and *LIN28* [36–38]. Methods successfully delivering these reprogramming factors into somatic cells include transduction with retroviruses, lentiviruses, adenoviruses, piggyBac transposons, episomal vectors, RNA, or protein [37,39–44]. Many types of somatic cells have been reprogrammed into hiPSCs, including fibroblasts, keratinocytes, peripheral blood mononuclear cells, cord blood cells, T cells, dental pulp stem cells, dermal papilla cells from hair follicles and urinary cells [37,45–49]. Patient-specific hiPSCs provide unique opportunities for researchers to dissect the pathogeneses and identify potential treatment strategies for the rare genetic bone disorders by providing a virtually unlimited source of cells carrying the disease-causing mutations. hiPSCs can be differentiated into functional cells of interest in the skeletal system, including osteoclasts. hiPSC disease modeling has been established for several non-skeletal disorders including type I and type II diabetes, muscular dystrophy, amyotrophic lateral sclerosis, Parkinson's disease, glioblastoma, familial platelet disorder with predisposition to acute myeloid leukemia (FPD) [36,50–55]. There have been only few attempts to establish hiPSCs from patients with rare genetic bone disorders (see also Table 2).

Table 2. iPSCs generated from patients with rare genetic bone disorders.

Disease	Source of Somatic Cells	Method	Reprogramming Factors	Patient Numbers	Reference
OI	MSC derived from bone fragments	(1) lentivirus	(1) *OCT4, SOX2, LIN28* or *NANOG*	6	[56]
		(2) floxed, polycystronic foamy virus	(2) *OCT4, SOX2, KLF4* and *c-MYC*		
CMD	5–7 mL peripheral blood	Sendai virus	*OCT3/4, SOX2, KLF4* and *c-MYC*	8	[57]
FOP	Dermal fibroblasts	(1) retrovirus	(1) *OCT4, SOX2, KLF4* and *c-MYC*	5	[58]
		(2) episomal vectors	(2) *SOX2, KLF4, OCT4, L-MYC, LIN28, p53*		
MFS	Dermal fibroblasts	retrovirus	*OCT4, SOX2, KLF4* and *c-MYC*	2	[59]

OI: osteogenesis imperfecta; CMD: craniometaphyseal dysplasia; FOP: Fibrodysplasia ossificans progressiva; MFS: Marfan syndrome; MSC: mesenchymal stem cells.

Osteogenesis Imperfecta (OI): OI, also known as brittle bone disease, is characterized by brittle bones that are prone to fracture and are caused by mutations in the *COL1A1* or *COL1A2* genes in the majority of cases. Misfolded collagen overwhelms the protein degradation machinery of cells and leads to abnormal bone matrix deposition by osteoblasts. 8 Types of OI have been identified. There is currently no cure for OI and treatment focuses on the prevention of fractures and the maintenance of mobility [60]. Deyle *et al.* established mesenchymal cell cultures from discarded bone fragments of OI patients undergoing surgery and further inactivated mutant collagen genes by adeno-associated virus (AAV)-mediated gene targeting, thus preventing the expression of misfolded collagen protein. OI and gene-targeted OI mesenchymal cells have been reprogrammed to hiPSCs [56].

Craniometaphyseal dysplasia (CMD): CMD is characterized by progressive hyperostosis of craniofacial bones and widened metaphyses of long bones. Patients often suffer from blindness, deafness, facial paralysis and severe headache due to hyperostosis and compression of the brain and nerves. Mutations for the autosomal dominant form of CMD have been identified in of progressive ankylosis (*ANKH*) gene and for a recessive form in Connexin 43 (*Cx43*) [61–63]. Our group identified dysfunctional osteoclasts in knock-in (KI) mice carrying a Phe377del mutation and in human osteoclast cultures [2,3]. The increased bone mass phenotype in CMD mice ($Ank^{KI/KI}$ mice) can partially be rescued by bone marrow transplantation. We have established a simple and efficient method to generate integration-free hiPSCs from peripheral blood of CMD patients and healthy controls using the Sendai virus, a cytoplasmic RNA viral vector [57], that can easily be removed from cells after reprogramming to iPSCs.

Fibrodysplasia ossificans progressiva (FOP): FOP is a rare genetic disorder caused by hyperactive mutations in the bone morphogenetic protein (BMP) type I receptor ACVR1 [64]. It is characterized by progressive ossification of soft tissues. The mechanism of heterotopic ossification is endochondral bone formation which involves pre-cartilaginous, fibro-proliferative and mineralization stages. Matsumoto *et al.* generated hiPSCs from skin fibroblasts of FOP patients and controls and showed increased *in vitro* chondrogenic differentiation and mineralization in FOP hiPSCs compared to wild type hiPSCs [58].

Marfan syndrome (MFS): MFS is a life-threatening, autosomal dominant disease with mutations identified in *FIBRILLIN-1* (*FBN1*) [65]. It is a disorder of fibrous connective tissue involving three systems: skeletal, cardiovascular and ocular. Skeletal features include long limbs and digits, deformities of vertebrae (scoliosis, thoracic lordosis) and anterior chest, increased height, and mild to moderate joint laxity. Quarto *et al.* generated hiPSCs from MFS patients and studied the pathogenic skeletogenesis *in vitro* [59]. They show that MFS-hiPSC faithfully represent the impaired osteogenic differentiation as a consequence of activation of TGF-β signaling and revealed a crosstalk between BMP and TGF-β signaling in MFS [66].

4. Differentiating hiPSCs into Osteoclasts

4.1. Differentiating Mouse Embryonic Stem Cells (mESCs) into Osteoclasts

Several studies have reported the generation of osteoclasts from mESC lines by culturing mESCs directly on a culture plate or by co-culturing mESCs with mouse bone marrow-derived stromal cells (ST2) or with the newborn calvaria-derived stromal cell line (OP9) from mice deficient in macrophage colony-stimulating factor (M-CSF) or through EB formation (for details see Table 3). Information gained from these mouse ESCs/iPSCs studies provided the fundamentals for establishing methods to generate osteoclasts from human ESCs and iPSCs.

Table 3. Protocols for differentiating mESCs/iPSCs to osteoclasts.

Methods	Mouse ESC Lines	Factors Added in OC Medium	Results	Reference	Lessons Learned
mESCs on 24-well plates	D3, J1	hM-CSF, hRANKL, A.A, VitD₃, Dexa	TRAP+ cells (day 14)	[67]	A.A. increased total cell recovery and OC precursors through increasing Flk-1-positive cells when added during the initial 4 days.
Co-culture 1-step, 2-step, 3-step	D3	hM-CSF (for OP9 coculture) VitD₃, Dexa	TRAP+ cells (day 11–16)	[68]	ST2 supported osteoclastogenesis more efficiently than OP9. C-fms signaling is required for OC development from mESCs.
Co-culture 1-step, 2-step, 3-step	CCE, D3, J1, CJ7	hM-CSF (for CFU assay) VitD₃, Dexa	TRAP+ cells (day 11–16)	[69]	SCL is indispensable for osteoclastogenesis. GATA-2 is required for osteoclastogenesis at early but not terminal differentiation stage.
Co-culture 1-step	D3	VitD₃, Dexa, hRANKL, hM-CSF (for some exp.)	TRAP+ cells c-Kit, c-fms, β2-integrin, CD31 expression (day 3–17)	[70]	Temporal expression of markers: c-Kit → β2-integrin → c-fms, TRAP. Exogenous hM-CSF and hRANKL promote osteoclastogenesis. Continuous hM-CSF can reduce number of TRAP+ cells.
Co-culture 1-step, 2-step, 3-step	D3, CCE	VitD₃, Dexa	TRAP+ cells	[71]	Blocking VEGFR-mediated signaling is inhibitory to OC development.
EB	mESCs	mM-CSF, mRANKL	TRAP+ (≥3 nuclei) (day 13)	[72]	Efficiency of OC generation: 3-step coculture > EB method > 1-step coculture.
EB, monolayer culture	J1, miPSCs (38c2, 20D17)	M-CSF, RANKL	TRAP+ (≥3 nuclei) (day 19)	[73]	A new *in vitro* culture method to differentiate mES/iPSCs into osteoclasts.

A.A: 50 μg/mL ascorbic acid; VitD₃: 10⁻⁸ M 1α,25-dihydroxyvitamin D₃; Dexa: 10⁻⁷ M dexamethasone; 1-step: mESCs are cocultured with ST2 cells for 10 days; 2-step: mESCs are cocultured with OP9 cells for 5 days and transferred onto ST2 cells for 6 days; 3-step: mESCs are cocultured with OP9 cells for 5 days, transferred to new OP9 for further 5 days, transferred onto ST2 cells for 6 more days; OC: osteoclasts; Exp.: experiments.

4.2. Commitment of Human ESCs/hiPSCs into Hematopoietic Lineages/OC Precursors

Consistent and adequate hematopoietic differentiation of hiPSCs is a prerequisite step for differentiating hiPSCs into osteoclasts. Hematopoiesis during embryogenesis starts with the formation of the primitive streak, mesoderm differentiation and hematopoietic specification. *In vitro* studies have shown that hiPSCs can be differentiated into different hematopoietic lineages through similar processes. Inducing hematopoiesis from human embryonic stem cells (hESCs) or hiPSCs has been reported by several extensive studies using three systems: (1) differentiation by coculturing hESC/hiPSCs with stromal cells; (2) differentiation through formation of embryoid bodies (EB), which can be differentiated into the three germ layers including mesoderm; (3) differentiation by monolayer culture of hESCs/hiPSCs on extracellular matrix protein coated-plates, such as collagen IV. We summarize culture conditions of these protocols in Table 4.

There are advantages and disadvantages inherent to these protocols. Differentiation efficiency of co-culture methods relies largely on optimized cell densities of hESCs/hiPSCs and the mouse stromal cell lines. It can be challenging to have both cell culture systems ready for co-culture at the same time. On the other hand, co-culture method requires less hematopoietic cytokines and is therefore relatively inexpensive compared to protocols involving EB and monolayer cultures. Concentrations of cytokines used are critical in those cultures. Stimulatory or inhibitory effects of cytokines towards hematopoiesis can be observed depending on the concentrations used. It is difficult to directly compare the lengths of cell culture time or hematopoietic differentiation efficiencies among the approaches described in Table 4. Variability of culture conditions used for the experiments among these protocols is discussed below.

4.3. Marker Genes for Mesodermal Formation and Hematopoietic Differentiation

Marker genes for mesodermal and hematopoietic lineages have been used to determine the efficiency of hematopoietic differentiation protocols during *in vitro* differentiation. Temporal expression patterns of certain marker genes are reliable indicators of mesoderm and hematopoietic differentiation from undifferentiated hESCs or hiPSCs. Early mesoderm formation is indicated by the expression of marker genes such as *Brachyury* (*T*), *Mix paired-like homeobox* (*Mixl1*), *Goosecoid homeobox* (*GSC*), and silencing of the pluripotency genes [74,75]. While kinase insert domain receptor (a type III receptor tyrosine kinase, *KDR*), also known as endothelial growth factor receptor 2 (*VEGFR-2*) or fetal liver kinase 1 (*Flk1*), is already detected in hESC/hiPSCs, its expression increases during the transition from mesoderm to hematopoietic lineage [76]. In addition, transcription factors stem cell leukemia (*Scl/Tal-1*), runt-related transcription factor 1 (*Runx1*), globin transcription factor 1 (*GATA-1*) and *GATA-2* play important roles in hematopoietic commitment during embryogenesis [77–79]. Combinations of surface marker expression are used to detect the hematopoietic stem cells (HSC) or the maturation of HSCs into specific hematopoietic cells. CD34, CD31 and VE-cadherin are expressed in early hematopoietic cells and vascular associated tissues [76]. CD45 is a pan-leukocyte marker [80]. Lin$^-$CD34$^+$CD43$^+$CD45$^+$ cells represent a population of enriched myeloid progenitors [81].

Table 4. Protocols for hematopoietic differentiation from hiPSCs.

Methods	hES/iPSCs & Medium	Differentiation medium	Results	Reference	Protocol Time Line
Monolayer	KhES-1, KhES-3, 201B7, 253G4 mTeSR1, Stemline II	Stemline II + ITS	T + Mixl1+ cells (d4) KDR+ CD34$^+$CD45 cells (d6) 36% CD235a$^-$; 53% CD45$^-$ (d30)	[82]	day 0 ⟶ 4 ⟶ 6 Bmp4 (40) VEGF (40) Bmp4 (20); VEGF (40); SCF (50); TPO (10); IL3 (50) SCF (50) Flt-3 (50); G-CSF (50); FP6 (50); EPO (5 U/ml))
Monolayer (Collagen IV)	WA01 hiPSCs Matrigel/mTeSR1	IMDM, BIT, MTG, NEAA, l-glu	95% CD43$^-$, 53% CD34$^-$, 59% CD41a$^+$, 60% CD235a$^+$, 35% CD45$^-$ (d14)	[83]	day -1 ⟶ 0 ⟶ 6 ⟶ 10-14 mTeSR1 Bmp4(50); VEGF(50); Heparin (5U/ml); TPO (25); SCF bFGF (50) (25); Flt-3 (25); IL-3 (10); IL-6 (10)
EB monolayer (gelatin)	hiPSCs MEF/hESC medium	EB^1 medium/ monocyte differentiation medium	90% CD14$^+$ (d15 of attached, flatten EBs on gelatin plates)	[84]	day 0 ⟶ 4 ⟶ 8 EB medium M-CSF (50); IL-3 (25) M-CSF (100); IL-3 (25)
EB	WA01, H9 Matrigel/condition medium	Knockout DMEM, FBS, NEAA, L-glu, ME	9 3% CD45$^+$ (d15)	[85]	day 0 ⟶ 1 ⟶ 15 EB Bmp4 (50); SCF (300); Flt-3 (300); IL-3 (10); IL-6 (10); G-CSF (50)
EB	WA01, ES02 MEF/hESC medium	StemPro-34 + MTG + l-glu + A.A.	Mesoderm induction and hemangioblast development (d1-8), increased *T* (d3), CD34, SCL (d5), CD117$^-$CD31$^-$ (d8)	[76]	day 0 ⟶ 1 ⟶ 4 ⟶ 7-8 Bmp4 (10) Bmp4 (10); Bmp4 (10); bFGF (5); bFGF (5) VEGF (10)

Table 4. *Cont.*

Methods	hES/iPSCs & Medium	Differentiation Medium	Results	Reference	Protocol Time Line
EB	hFib2-iPS5 MEF/hESC medium	EB² medium	29% CD34⁺, 27% CD45⁺, 16% CD34⁺CD45⁺ (d17)	[86]	day 0 1 ... 17; SCF (300); Flt-3 (300); IL-3 (10); IL-6 (10); G-CSF (50); Bmp4 (50)
EB	WA01, ES02, MSC-iPS1 matrigel/ hESC medium	StemPro34 + MTG + L-glu + A.A.	15%–59% CD45⁺ (d14); 38%–72% CD45⁺ (d22)	[87]	day 0 1 4 8 18-22; Bmp4 (10) Bmp4 (10) VEGF (10); bFGF(1); IL-6(10); VEGF (10);EPO (4 U/ml); bFGF (5) IL3 (40); IL-11 (5), SCF (100) TPO (50); IL-6 (10);IL3 (40); IL-11 (5), SCF (100)
EB	hiPSCs Matrigel/hESC medium	StemPro-34, L-glu, A.A., transferrin, MTG	Myeloid, erythroid, megakaryocytic cells released into the medium (d14)	[88]	day 0 2 4 8; Bmp4 (25); Bmp4 (25); VEGF (50); SCF (50); TPO (50); VEGF(50) SCF (50); TPO (50); TPO (50); Flt-3 (50); IL-3 (10); IL-11 (5); Flt-3 (50);bFGF (20) bFGF (20) EPO (2U/ml); IGF-1 (25)
Co-culture (S17/C166)	H1, H1.1, H9 2 MEF/hESC medium	DMEM, FBS, L-glu, ME, NEAA	1%–2% CD34 CD38 (d17)	[89]	day 0 ... 17; hES-S17 or C166; DMEM+ 20%FBS
Co-culture (AM-20, UG26, IL08, AGM, FL)	H1, H9, hES-NCL1 MEF/hESC medium	Knockout DMEM, FCS, ME, L-glu, NEAA, antibiotics	16% CD34⁺, 5%CD45⁺, 8% CD31⁺, 6% CD34⁺CD31⁻ (d18)	[90]	day 0 ... 17; hES-AM20 or UG26, IL08, primary AGM or FL; DMEM+ 20%FBS
Co-culture (OP9)	WA01, WA09, iPS-1, iPSCs (SK46)-M-4-10 MEF/hESC medium	α-MEM, FBS, MTG	9.8% CD43⁺, 14% CD45⁻ (d9); 94% CD43⁺, 78% CD45 (d11); 98% CD43⁺, 97% CD45⁻ (d17)	[81]	day 0 9 11-17; hiPSCs-OP9 Expansion of OC differentiation; lin CD34⁺CD45⁺ cells GM-CSF (50); VitD (200nM); GM-CSF (200) RANKL (25)

hESC medium: DMEM/F12, 15% KnockOut SR replacer, 2 mM L-glutamine. 0.1 mM β-mercaptoethanol, bFGF. FP6: complex of IL-6 and IL-6 receptor; A.A.: ascorbic acid (50 μg/mL); MTG: 4 × 10⁻⁴ M monothioglycerol; L-glu: 2 mM glutamine; EB¹ medium: DMEM-F12, 20% Knockout Serum Replacement, 0.1 mM nonessential amino acids (NEAA), 0.1 mM β-mercaptoethanol (ME), 1 mM L-glutamine; EB² medium: Knockout Dulbecco modified Eagle medium, 20% fetal calf serum, 0.1 mM nonessential amino acids (NEAA), 0.1 mM β-mercaptoethanol (ME), 1 mM L-glutamine, 50 μg/mL ascorbic acid, 201 μg/mL human holo-transferrin; S17: murine bone marrow cell line; C166: murine yolk sac endothelial cell lineAM20, UG26, EL08: stromal cell lines, AGM or FL: primary stromal cells from aorta-gonad-mesonephros (AGM) or fetal liver (FL); BIT: bovin serum albumin, human recombinant insulin, human transferrin; cytokine concentration (ng/mL).

4.4. Factors and Cytokines to Promote Hematopoiesis

Defined factors/cytokines can be added to support hematopoietic cell proliferation or differentiation under controlled conditions. BMP4 alone can induce primitive streak and early hematopoietic gene expression, including *Mixl1*, *Brachyury*, *Goosecoid*, *KDR*, *Runx1* and *Gata2* while BMP4 together with VEGF can increase expression of *Scl* and *CD34* [91]. The addition of FGF2 during hematopoietic differentiation of hESCs increases total cell number by improving cell proliferation but not cell survival [91]. A mixture of cytokines including stem cell factor (SCF), fms-like tyrosine kinase receptor-3 ligand (Flt-3), interleukin-3 (IL-3), interleukin-6 (IL-6) and granulocyte colony-stimulating factor (G-CSF) and thrombopoietin (TPO) is commonly used in hematopoietic differentiation protocols for hESCs. These cytokines have been shown to play important roles in maintenance of human hematopoietic cells [92,93]. Addition of SCF in the presence of BMP4, VEGF and FGF can significantly increase the yields of hematopoietic progenitors and mature cells *in vitro* [91]. When added to IL-3 and GM-CSF, SCF has profound effects on *in vitro* proliferation of primitive hematopoietic progenitors [94].

4.5. Variability among Hematopoietic Differentiation Protocols

Some studies showed variable efficiencies for deriving hematopoietic cell populations from hESCs/hiPSCs. Many factors contribute to this variability including the somatic cell type used for hiPSC reprogramming; the method of deriving hiPSCs; incomplete removal of reprogramming transgenes in hiPSCs; the culture conditions for maintaining hiPSCs; the type of differentiating medium, growth factors and hematopoietic cytokines added in the differentiation protocol; the dosage of cytokines to promote hematopoiesis; the oxygen level of cultures (normal oxygen or hypoxia); and the size of EBs or the densities of stromal cell lines [95]. It has been suggested that epigenetic memory exists in hiPSCs and the differentiation phenotype may be influenced by their cells of origin [96]. Transgenes remaining in hiPSCs can have a negative impact on hiPSC differentiation [97]. Multiple concentrations of BMP4 (5, 10, 25, 50 ng/mL) were tested and showed no differences in promoting CD34$^+$CD45$^+$ populations [85] while Pick *et al.* showed BMP4 increases primitive streak and hematopoietic gene expressions in a dose-dependent manner [91]. It is therefore important to develop a method that eliminates as many variable factors as possible and that aims to obtain hematopoietic cells from hiPSCs by a reproducible and efficient protocol.

4.6. Differentiating hiPSCs-Derived Osteoclast Progenitors into Osteoclasts

Two publications describe the successful differentiation of hiPSCs to hematopoietic cell stage and further to mature OC progenitors and into functional osteoclasts. Choi *et al.* cultured a Lin$^-$CD34$^+$CD43$^+$Cd45$^+$ population in the presence of GM-CSF and vitamin D3 on poly (2-hydroxyethyl methacrylate)-coated plates for 2 days to expand osteoclast progenitors and then induced osteoclast maturation in cultures with α-MEM, 10% FBS, and MTG solution supplemented with GM-CSF (50 ng/mL), Vitamin D3 (200 nM) and RANKL (10 ng/mL) [81]. Grigoriadis *et al.* cultured myeloid precursors derived from hiPSCs in IMDM containing 10% FCS, M-CSF (10 ng/mL) and RANKL (10 ng/mL). Osteoclasts were defined as multinucleated cells (≥3 nuclei) by TRAP positive staining and the capability of resorbing bone/dentin chips. Expressions of OC marker genes such as Cathepsin K, calcitonin receptor, NFATc1 are increased in these functional OCs [87].

Studies summarized in Tables 3 and 4 demonstrate that osteoclasts can be generated from both, human and mouse ES/iPSCs. In general, differentiation of osteoclasts from hESCs/hiPSCs systems is more challenging than differentiation from mouse ESCs/iPSCs. Differentiation of hESCs/hiPSCs requires more hematopoietic cytokines, longer culture periods and generally results in less efficient osteoclast formation. However, the mechanisms behind differences between human and mouse osteoclastogenesis are still unclear.

4.7. Strategies of Using hiPSC-Osteoclasts to Study Rare Genetic Bone Diseases

hiPSC technology in general enables researchers to reprogram somatic cells into an ES-like state followed by differentiation into desired cell type. While human osteoclasts can be differentiated directly from peripheral blood, the big advantage of hiPSC technology is that osteoclasts can be generated without repeated sampling of patients. hiPSCs provide a virtually unlimited cell source to study molecular mechanisms of osteoclastogenesis with the potential to develop therapies, which is especially important when studying rare genetic bone diseases. Because of potential species-specific differences, studying abnormal osteoclastogenesis in the human system may be closer to clinical reality than using animal models.

A preferred strategy for studying defective osteoclastogenesis in rare genetic bone disorders using patient-specific hiPSCs is summarized in Figure 1. One challenge of hiPSC disease modeling *in vitro* is the lack of genetically matched controls. Using healthy subjects as controls may not be the best solution as individual hESCs and hiPSC lines differentiate to specific cell populations with variable efficiency because of biological variability [98]. Distinguishing mutation-relevant disease phenotypes from genetic/epigenetic variations becomes easier in isogenic hiPSCs, which only differ at disease-causing mutations. Correction or introduction of specific mutations into a cell can be achieved by genome editing using zinc-finger nucleases (ZFNs), transcription activator-like effector nucleases (TALENs) or the clustered regulatory interspaced short palindromic repeats/Cas9 system (CRISPR) [99–102]. Using step-wise OC differentiation protocols for differentiating hESCs or hiPSCs may allow researchers to identify which step of osteoclastogenesis is disrupted by a disease causing mutation. Analysis tools are available to study each step (lineage determination of precursors, precursor proliferation, fusion to multinucleated syncytia, maturation to functional osteoclasts) such as expression of marker genes, numbers of TRAP$^+$ mono/multinucleated cells, resorption efficiency, live-image migration assays and nuclear localization of NFATc1. Therapeutic strategies can be investigated once the pathologic mechanisms are understood.

Figure 1. Summary of generating osteoclasts from human iPSCs.

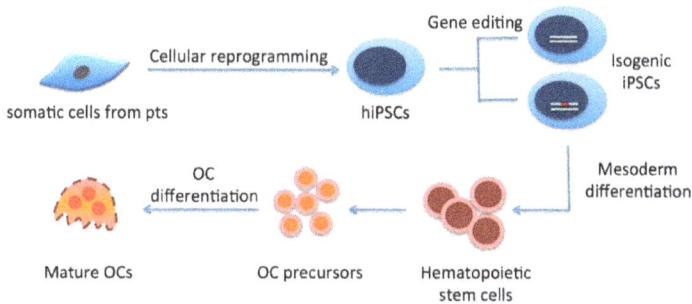

5. Conclusions

Osteoclast defects are involved in many rare genetic bone diseases as well as in some common bone diseases such as osteoporosis. Although human OC can be cultured from peripheral blood, being able to differentiate OCs from hiPSCs has at least two additional advantages: (1) eliminating the need to repeatedly obtain blood from study subjects; (2) serving as an *in vitro* model for studying hematopoiesis during embryogenesis. Lessons learned from embryology and differentiation studies are expected to improve protocols for consistent and efficient differentiation of hiPSCs into hematopoietic cells and further into osteoclasts. Similar concepts can be applied to differentiate hiPSCs to other bone cells such as osteoblasts. We believe this model will have great impact on a better understanding of bone diseases and to establish the bases for potential therapies.

Acknowledgments

This work is supported by National Institutes of Health funding (NIDCR, K99/R00 DE021442).

Conflicts of Interest

The author declares no conflict of interest.

References

1. Kornak, U.; Mundlos, S. Genetic disorders of the skeleton: A developmental approach. *Am. J. Hum. Genet.* **2003**, *73*, 447–474.
2. Chen, I.P.; Wang, C.J.; Strecker, S.; Koczon-Jaremko, B.; Boskey, A.; Reichenberger, E.J. Introduction of a Phe377del mutation in ANK creates a mouse model for craniometaphyseal dysplasia. *J. Bone Miner. Res.* **2009**, *24*, 1206–1215.
3. Chen, I.P.; Wang, L.; Jiang, X.; Aguila, H.L.; Reichenberger, E.J. A Phe377del mutation in ANK leads to impaired osteoblastogenesis and osteoclastogenesis in a mouse model for craniometaphyseal dysplasia (CMD). *Hum. Mol. Genet.* **2011**, *20*, 948–961.
4. Laslo, P.; Spooner, C.J.; Warmflash, A.; Lancki, D.W.; Lee, H.J.; Sciammas, R.; Gantner, B.N.; Dinner, A.R.; Singh, H. Multilineage transcriptional priming and determination of alternate hematopoietic cell fates. *Cell* **2006**, *126*, 755–766.
5. Kawaguchi, N.; Noda, M. Mitf is expressed in osteoclast progenitors *in vitro*. *Exp. Cell Res.* **2000**, *260*, 284–291.
6. Miyamoto, T.; Ohneda, O.; Arai, F.; Iwamoto, K.; Okada, S.; Takagi, K.; Anderson, D.M.; Suda, T. Bifurcation of osteoclasts and dendritic cells from common progenitors. *Blood* **2001**, *98*, 2544–2554.
7. Dai, X.M.; Ryan, G.R.; Hapel, A.J.; Dominguez, M.G.; Russell, R.G.; Kapp, S.; Sylvestre, V.; Stanley, E.R. Targeted disruption of the mouse colony-stimulating factor 1 receptor gene results in osteopetrosis, mononuclear phagocyte deficiency, increased primitive progenitor cell frequencies, and reproductive defects. *Blood* **2002**, *99*, 111–120.
8. Kim, M.S.; Day, C.J.; Morrison, N.A. MCP-1 is induced by receptor activator of nuclear factor-κb ligand, promotes human osteoclast fusion, and rescues granulocyte macrophage colony-stimulating factor suppression of osteoclast formation. *J. Biol. Chem.* **2005**, *280*, 16163–16169.
9. Lee, S.H.; Rho, J.; Jeong, D.; Sul, J.Y.; Kim, T.; Kim, N.; Kang, J.S.; Miyamoto, T.; Suda, T.; Lee, S.K.; *et al.* V-atpase V_0 subunit d_2-deficient mice exhibit impaired osteoclast fusion and increased bone formation. *Nat. Med.* **2006**, *12*, 1403–1409.
10. Faccio, R.; Teitelbaum, S.L.; Fujikawa, K.; Chappel, J.; Zallone, A.; Tybulewicz, V.L.; Ross, F.P.; Swat, W. Vav3 regulates osteoclast function and bone mass. *Nat. Med.* **2005**, *11*, 284–290.
11. Gerritsen, E.J.; Vossen, J.M.; van Loo, I.H.; Hermans, J.; Helfrich, M.H.; Griscelli, C.; Fischer, A. Autosomal recessive osteopetrosis: Variability of findings at diagnosis and during the natural course. *Pediatrics* **1994**, *93*, 247–253.
12. Sly, W.S.; Hewett-Emmett, D.; Whyte, M.P.; Yu, Y.S.; Tashian, R.E. Carbonic anhydrase II deficiency identified as the primary defect in the autosomal recessive syndrome of osteopetrosis with renal tubular acidosis and cerebral calcification. *Proc. Natl. Acad. Sci. USA* **1983**, *80*, 2752–2756.
13. Andersen, P.E., Jr.; Bollerslev, J. Heterogeneity of autosomal dominant osteopetrosis. *Radiology* **1987**, *164*, 223–225.

14. Gelb, B.D.; Shi, G.P.; Chapman, H.A.; Desnick, R.J. Pycnodysostosis, a lysosomal disease caused by cathepsin K deficiency. *Science* **1996**, *273*, 1236–1238.

15. Selby, P.L.; Davie, M.W.; Ralston, S.H.; Stone, M.D. Guidelines on the management of paget's disease of bone. *Bone* **2002**, *31*, 366–373.

16. Ralston, S.H.; Langston, A.L.; Reid, I.R. Pathogenesis and management of paget's disease of bone. *Lancet* **2008**, *372*, 155–163.

17. Tiegs, R.D. Paget's disease of bone: Indications for treatment and goals of therapy. *Clin. Ther.* **1997**, *19*, 1309–1329.

18. Golob, D.S.; McAlister, W.H.; Mills, B.G.; Fedde, K.N.; Reinus, W.R.; Teitelbaum, S.L.; Beeki, S.; Whyte, M.P. Juvenile paget disease: Life-long features of a mildly affected young woman. *J. Bone Miner. Res.* **1996**, *11*, 132–142.

19. Whyte, M.P.; Obrecht, S.E.; Finnegan, P.M.; Jones, J.L.; Podgornik, M.N.; McAlister, W.H.; Mumm, S. Osteoprotegerin deficiency and juvenile paget's disease. *N. Engl. J. Med.* **2002**, *347*, 175–184.

20. Cundy, T.; Hegde, M.; Naot, D.; Chong, B.; King, A.; Wallace, R.; Mulley, J.; Love, D.R.; Seidel, J.; Fawkner, M.; *et al.* A mutation in the gene *TNFRSF11B* encoding osteoprotegerin causes an idiopathic hyperphosphatasia phenotype. *Hum. Mol. Genet.* **2002**, *11*, 2119–2127.

21. Dickson, G.R.; Shirodria, P.V.; Kanis, J.A.; Beneton, M.N.; Carr, K.E.; Mollan, R.A. Familial expansile osteolysis: A morphological, histomorphometric and serological study. *Bone* **1991**, *12*, 331–338.

22. Takata, S.; Yasui, N.; Nakatsuka, K.; Ralston, S.H. Evolution of understanding of genetics of paget's disease of bone and related diseases. *J. Bone Miner. Res.* **2004**, *22*, 519–523.

23. Hughes, A.E.; Ralston, S.H.; Marken, J.; Bell, C.; MacPherson, H.; Wallace, R.G.; van Hul, W.; Whyte, M.P.; Nakatsuka, K.; Hovy, L.; *et al.* Mutations in *TNFRSF11A*, affecting the signal peptide of rank, cause familial expansile osteolysis. *Nat. Genet.* **2000**, *24*, 45–48.

24. Whyte, M.P.; Mills, B.G.; Reinus, W.R.; Podgornik, M.N.; Roodman, G.D.; Gannon, F.H.; Eddy, M.C.; McAlister, W.H. Expansile skeletal hyperphosphatasia: A new familial metabolic bone disease. *J. Bone Miner. Res.* **2000**, *15*, 2330–2344.

25. Frattini, A.; Orchard, P.J.; Sobacchi, C.; Giliani, S.; Abinun, M.; Mattsson, J.P.; Keeling, D.J.; Andersson, A.K.; Wallbrandt, P.; Zecca, L.; *et al.* Defects in TCIRG1 subunit of the vacuolar proton pump are responsible for a subset of human autosomal recessive osteopetrosis. *Nat. Genet.* **2000**, *25*, 343–346.

26. Frattini, A.; Pangrazio, A.; Susani, L.; Sobacchi, C.; Mirolo, M.; Abinun, M.; Andolina, M.; Flanagan, A.; Horwitz, E.M.; Mihci, E.; *et al.* Chloride channel *CICN7* mutations are responsible for severe recessive, dominant, and intermediate osteopetrosis. *J. Bone Miner. Res.* **2003**, *18*, 1740–1747.

27. Ramirez, A.; Faupel, J.; Goebel, I.; Stiller, A.; Beyer, S.; Stockle, C.; Hasan, C.; Bode, U.; Kornak, U.; Kubisch, C. Identification of a novel mutation in the coding region of the grey-lethal gene *OSTM1* in human malignant infantile osteopetrosis. *Hum. Mutat.* **2004**, *23*, 471–476.

28. Pangrazio, A.; Boudin, E.; Piters, E.; Damante, G.; Lo Iacono, N.; D'Elia, A.V.; Vezzoni, P.; van Hul, W.; Villa, A.; Sobacchi, C. Identification of the first deletion in the *LRP5* gene in a patient with autosomal dominant osteopetrosis type I. *Bone* **2011**, *49*, 568–571.

29. Cleiren, E.; Benichou, O.; van Hul, E.; Gram, J.; Bollerslev, J.; Singer, F.R.; Beaverson, K.; Aledo, A.; Whyte, M.P.; Yoneyama, T.; *et al.* Albers-schonberg disease (autosomal dominant osteopetrosis, type II) results from mutations in the *ClCN7* chloride channel gene. *Hum. Mol. Genet.* **2001**, *10*, 2861–2867.

30. Hocking, L.J.; Lucas, G.J.; Daroszewska, A.; Mangion, J.; Olavesen, M.; Cundy, T.; Nicholson, G.C.; Ward, L.; Bennett, S.T.; Wuyts, W.; *et al.* Domain-specific mutations in sequestosome 1 (SQSTM1) cause familial and sporadic Paget's disease. *Hum. Mol. Genet.* **2002**, *11*, 2735–2739.

31. Laurin, N.; Brown, J.P.; Morissette, J.; Raymond, V. Recurrent mutation of the gene encoding sequestosome 1 (SQSTM1/P62) in paget disease of bone. *Am. J. Hum. Genet.* **2002**, *70*, 1582–1588.

32. Whyte, M.P.; Hughes, A.E. Expansile skeletal hyperphosphatasia is caused by a 15-base pair tandem duplication in *TNFRSF11A* encoding RANK and is allelic to familial expansile osteolysis. *J. Bone Miner. Res.* **2002**, *17*, 26–29.

33. Cherry, A.B.; Daley, G.Q. Reprogrammed cells for disease modeling and regenerative medicine. *Ann. Rev. Med.* **2013**, *64*, 277–290.

34. Ding, Q.; Lee, Y.K.; Schaefer, E.A.; Peters, D.T.; Veres, A.; Kim, K.; Kuperwasser, N.; Motola, D.L.; Meissner, T.B.; Hendriks, W.T.; *et al.* A talen genome-editing system for generating human stem cell-based disease models. *Cell Stem Cell* **2013**, *12*, 238–251.

35. Emborg, M.E.; Liu, Y.; Xi, J.; Zhang, X.; Yin, Y.; Lu, J.; Joers, V.; Swanson, C.; Holden, J.E.; Zhang, S.C. Induced pluripotent stem cell-derived neural cells survive and mature in the nonhuman primate brain. *Cell Rep.* **2013**, *3*, 646–650.

36. Park, I.H.; Arora, N.; Huo, H.; Maherali, N.; Ahfeldt, T.; Shimamura, A.; Lensch, M.W.; Cowan, C.; Hochedlinger, K.; Daley, G.Q. Disease-specific induced pluripotent stem cells. *Cell* **2008**, *134*, 877–886.

37. Takahashi, K.; Tanabe, K.; Ohnuki, M.; Narita, M.; Ichisaka, T.; Tomoda, K.; Yamanaka, S. Induction of pluripotent stem cells from adult human fibroblasts by defined factors. *Cell* **2007**, *131*, 861–872.

38. Yu, J.; Vodyanik, M.A.; Smuga-Otto, K.; Antosiewicz-Bourget, J.; Frane, J.L.; Tian, S.; Nie, J.; Jonsdottir, G.A.; Ruotti, V.; Stewart, R.; *et al.* Induced pluripotent stem cell lines derived from human somatic cells. *Science* **2007**, *318*, 1917–1920.

39. Sommer, C.A.; Stadtfeld, M.; Murphy, G.J.; Hochedlinger, K.; Kotton, D.N.; Mostoslavsky, G. Induced pluripotent stem cell generation using a single lentiviral stem cell cassette. *Stem Cells* **2009**, *27*, 543–549.

40. Stadtfeld, M.; Nagaya, M.; Utikal, J.; Weir, G.; Hochedlinger, K. Induced pluripotent stem cells generated without viral integration. *Science* **2008**, *322*, 945–949.

41. Warren, L.; Manos, P.D.; Ahfeldt, T.; Loh, Y.H.; Li, H.; Lau, F.; Ebina, W.; Mandal, P.K.; Smith, Z.D.; Meissner, A.; *et al.* Highly efficient reprogramming to pluripotency and directed differentiation of human cells with synthetic modified mRNA. *Cell Stem Cell* **2010**, *7*, 618–630.

42. Woltjen, K.; Michael, I.P.; Mohseni, P.; Desai, R.; Mileikovsky, M.; Hamalainen, R.; Cowling, R.; Wang, W.; Liu, P.; Gertsenstein, M.; *et al.* Piggybac transposition reprograms fibroblasts to induced pluripotent stem cells. *Nature* **2009**, *458*, 766–770.

43. Yu, J.; Hu, K.; Smuga-Otto, K.; Tian, S.; Stewart, R.; Slukvin, I.I.; Thomson, J.A. Human induced pluripotent stem cells free of vector and transgene sequences. *Science* **2009**, *324*, 797–801.

44. Zhou, H.; Wu, S.; Joo, J.Y.; Zhu, S.; Han, D.W.; Lin, T.; Trauger, S.; Bien, G.; Yao, S.; Zhu, Y.; *et al.* Generation of induced pluripotent stem cells using recombinant proteins. *Cell Stem Cell* **2009**, *4*, 381–384.

45. Aasen, T.; Raya, A.; Barrero, M.J.; Garreta, E.; Consiglio, A.; Gonzalez, F.; Vassena, R.; Bilic, J.; Pekarik, V.; Tiscornia, G.; *et al.* Efficient and rapid generation of induced pluripotent stem cells from human keratinocytes. *Nat. Biotechnol.* **2008**, *26*, 1276–1284.

46. Giorgetti, A.; Montserrat, N.; Aasen, T.; Gonzalez, F.; Rodriguez-Piza, I.; Vassena, R.; Raya, A.; Boue, S.; Barrero, M.J.; Corbella, B.A.; *et al.* Generation of induced pluripotent stem cells from human cord blood using OCT4 and SOX2. *Cell Stem Cell* **2009**, *5*, 353–357.

47. Yan, X.; Qin, H.; Qu, C.; Tuan, R.S.; Shi, S.; Huang, G.T. IPS cells reprogrammed from human mesenchymal-like stem/progenitor cells of dental tissue origin. *Stem Cells Dev.* **2010**, *19*, 469–480.

48. Tsai, S.Y.; Bouwman, B.A.; Ang, Y.S.; Kim, S.J.; Lee, D.F.; Lemischka, I.R.; Rendl, M. Single transcription factor reprogramming of hair follicle dermal papilla cells to induced pluripotent stem cells. *Stem Cells* **2011**, *29*, 964–971.

49. Zhou, T.; Benda, C.; Dunzinger, S.; Huang, Y.; Ho, J.C.; Yang, J.; Wang, Y.; Zhang, Y.; Zhuang, Q.; Li, Y.; *et al.* Generation of human induced pluripotent stem cells from urine samples. *Nat. Protoc.* **2012**, *7*, 2080–2089.

50. Chen, C.; Wang, Y.; Goh, S.S.; Yang, J.; Lam, D.H.; Choudhury, Y.; Tay, F.C.; Du, S.; Tan, W.K.; Purwanti, Y.I.; *et al.* Inhibition of neuronal nitric oxide synthase activity promotes migration of human-induced pluripotent stem cell-derived neural stem cells toward cancer cells. *J. Neurochem.* **2013**, *126*, 318–330.

51. Dimos, J.T.; Rodolfa, K.T.; Niakan, K.K.; Weisenthal, L.M.; Mitsumoto, H.; Chung, W.; Croft, G.F.; Saphier, G.; Leibel, R.; Goland, R.; *et al.* Induced pluripotent stem cells generated from patients with als can be differentiated into motor neurons. *Science* **2008**, *321*, 1218–1221.

52. Kudva, Y.C.; Ohmine, S.; Greder, L.V.; Dutton, J.R.; Armstrong, A.; de Lamo, J.G.; Khan, Y.K.; Thatava, T.; Hasegawa, M.; Fusaki, N.; *et al.* Transgene-free disease-specific induced pluripotent stem cells from patients with type 1 and type 2 diabetes. *Stem Cells Trans. Med.* **2012**, *1*, 451–461.

53. Maehr, R.; Chen, S.; Snitow, M.; Ludwig, T.; Yagasaki, L.; Goland, R.; Leibel, R.L.; Melton, D.A. Generation of pluripotent stem cells from patients with type 1 diabetes. *Proc. Natl. Acad. Sci. USA* **2009**, *106*, 15768–15773.

54. Teo, A.K.; Windmueller, R.; Johansson, B.B.; Dirice, E.; Njolstad, P.R.; Tjora, E.; Raeder, H.; Kulkarni, R.N. Derivation of human induced pluripotent stem cells from patients with maturity onset diabetes of the young. *J. Biol. Chem.* **2013**, *288*, 5353–5356.

55. Connelly, J.P.; Kwon, E.M.; Gao, Y.; Trivedi, N.S.; Elkahloun, A.G.; Horwitz, M.S.; Cheng, L.; Liu, P.P. Targeted correction of RUNX1 mutation in FPD patient-specific induced pluripotent stem cells rescues megakaryopoietic defects. *Blood* **2014**, *124*, 1926–1930.

56. Deyle, D.R.; Khan, I.F.; Ren, G.; Wang, P.R.; Kho, J.; Schwarze, U.; Russell, D.W. Normal collagen and bone production by gene-targeted human osteogenesis imperfecta iPSCs. *Mol. Ther.* **2012**, *20*, 204–213.

57. Chen, I.P.; Fukuda, K.; Fusaki, N.; Iida, A.; Hasegawa, M.; Lichtler, A.; Reichenberger, E.J. Induced pluripotent stem cell reprogramming by integration-free sendai virus vectors from peripheral blood of patients with craniometaphyseal dysplasia. *Cell. Reprogram.* **2013**, *15*, 503–513.

58. Matsumoto, Y.; Hayashi, Y.; Schlieve, C.R.; Ikeya, M.; Kim, H.; Nguyen, T.D.; Sami, S.; Baba, S.; Barruet, E.; Nasu, A.; *et al.* Induced pluripotent stem cells from patients with human fibrodysplasia ossificans progressiva show increased mineralization and cartilage formation. *Orphanet J. Rare Dis.* **2013**, *8*, doi:10.1186/1750-1172-8-190.

59. Quarto, N.; Leonard, B.; Li, S.; Marchand, M.; Anderson, E.; Behr, B.; Francke, U.; Reijo-Pera, R.; Chiao, E.; Longaker, M.T. Skeletogenic phenotype of human marfan embryonic stem cells faithfully phenocopied by patient-specific induced-pluripotent stem cells. *Proc. Natl. Acad. Sci. USA* **2012**, *109*, 215–220.

60. Cole, W.G. Advances in osteogenesis imperfecta. *Clin. Orthop. Relat. Res.* **2002**, *401*, 6–16.

61. Reichenberger, E.; Tiziani, V.; Watanabe, S.; Park, L.; Ueki, Y.; Santanna, C.; Baur, S.T.; Shiang, R.; Grange, D.K.; Beighton, P.; *et al.* Autosomal dominant craniometaphyseal dysplasia is caused by mutations in the transmembrane protein ANK. *Am. J. Hum. Genet.* **2001**, *68*, 1321–1326.

62. Nurnberg, P.; Thiele, H.; Chandler, D.; Hohne, W.; Cunningham, M.L.; Ritter, H.; Leschik, G.; Uhlmann, K.; Mischung, C.; Harrop, K.; *et al.* Heterozygous mutations in ANKH, the human ortholog of the mouse progressive ankylosis gene, result in craniometaphyseal dysplasia. *Nat. Genet.* **2001**, *28*, 37–41.

63. Hu, Y.; Chen, I.P.; de Almeida, S.; Tiziani, V.; Do Amaral, C.M.; Gowrishankar, K.; Passos-Bueno, M.R.; Reichenberger, E.J. A novel autosomal recessive GJA1 missense mutation linked to craniometaphyseal dysplasia. *PLoS One* **2013**, *8*, e73576.

64. Shore, E.M.; Xu, M.; Feldman, G.J.; Fenstermacher, D.A.; Cho, T.J.; Choi, I.H.; Connor, J.M.; Delai, P.; Glaser, D.L.; LeMerrer, M.; *et al.* A recurrent mutation in the BMP type I receptor ACVR1 causes inherited and sporadic fibrodysplasia ossificans progressiva. *Nat. Genet.* **2006**, *38*, 525–527.

65. Pereira, L.; D'Alessio, M.; Ramirez, F.; Lynch, J.R.; Sykes, B.; Pangilinan, T.; Bonadio, J. Genomic organization of the sequence coding for fibrillin, the defective gene product in marfan syndrome. *Hum. mol. Genet.* **1993**, *2*, 961–968.

66. Quarto, N.; Li, S.; Renda, A.; Longaker, M.T. Exogenous activation of BMP-2 signaling overcomes TGFβ-mediated inhibition of osteogenesis in marfan embryonic stem cells and marfan patient-specific induced pluripotent stem cells. *Stem Cells* **2012**, *30*, 2709–2719.

67. Tsuneto, M.; Yamazaki, H.; Yoshino, M.; Yamada, T.; Hayashi, S. Ascorbic acid promotes osteoclastogenesis from embryonic stem cells. *Biochem. Biophys. Res. Commun.* **2005**, *335*, 1239–1246.

68. Yamane, T.; Kunisada, T.; Yamazaki, H.; Era, T.; Nakano, T.; Hayashi, S.I. Development of osteoclasts from embryonic stem cells through a pathway that is c-*fms* but not c-*kit* dependent. *Blood* **1997**, *90*, 3516–3523.

69. Yamane, T.; Kunisada, T.; Yamazaki, H.; Nakano, T.; Orkin, S.H.; Hayashi, S.I. Sequential requirements for SCL/tal-1, GATA-2, macrophage colony-stimulating factor, and osteoclast differentiation factor/osteoprotegerin ligand in osteoclast development. *Exp. Hematol.* **2000**, *28*, 833–840.

70. Hemmi, H.; Okuyama, H.; Yamane, T.; Nishikawa, S.; Nakano, T.; Yamazaki, H.; Kunisada, T.; Hayashi, S. Temporal and spatial localization of osteoclasts in colonies from embryonic stem cells. *Biochem. Biophys. Res. Commun.* **2001**, *280*, 526–534.

71. Okuyama, H.; Tsuneto, M.; Yamane, T.; Yamazaki, H.; Hayashi, S. Discrete types of osteoclast precursors can be generated from embryonic stem cells. *Stem Cells* **2003**, *21*, 670–680.

72. Goodman, M.L.; Chen, S.; Yang, F.C.; Chan, R.J. Novel method of murine embryonic stem cell-derived osteoclast development. *Stem Cells Dev.* **2009**, *18*, 195–200.

73. Nishikawa, K.; Iwamoto, Y.; Ishii, M. Development of an *in vitro* culture method for stepwise differentiation of mouse embryonic stem cells and induced pluripotent stem cells into mature osteoclasts. *J. Bone Miner. Metab.* **2014**, *32*, 331–336.

74. Herrmann, B.G. Expression pattern of the brachyury gene in whole-mount TWis/TWis mutant embryos. *Development* **1991**, *113*, 913–917.

75. Davis, R.P.; Ng, E.S.; Costa, M.; Mossman, A.K.; Sourris, K.; Elefanty, A.G.; Stanley, E.G. Targeting a GFP reporter gene to the *MIXL1* locus of human embryonic stem cells identifies human primitive streak-like cells and enables isolation of primitive hematopoietic precursors. *Blood* **2008**, *111*, 1876–1884.

76. Kennedy, M.; D'Souza, S.L.; Lynch-Kattman, M.; Schwantz, S.; Keller, G. Development of the hemangioblast defines the onset of hematopoiesis in human ES cell differentiation cultures. *Blood* **2007**, *109*, 2679–2687.

77. Porcher, C.; Swat, W.; Rockwell, K.; Fujiwara, Y.; Alt, F.W.; Orkin, S.H. The T cell leukemia oncoprotein SCL/tal-1 is essential for development of all hematopoietic lineages. *Cell* **1996**, *86*, 47–57.

78. Lacaud, G.; Gore, L.; Kennedy, M.; Kouskoff, V.; Kingsley, P.; Hogan, C.; Carlsson, L.; Speck, N.; Palis, J.; Keller, G. *Runx1* is essential for hematopoietic commitment at the hemangioblast stage of development *in vitro*. *Blood* **2002**, *100*, 458–466.

79. Orkin, S.H. Gata-binding transcription factors in hematopoietic cells. *Blood* **1992**, *80*, 575–581.

80. Woodford-Thomas, T.; Thomas, M.L. The leukocyte common antigen, CD45 and other protein tyrosine phosphatases in hematopoietic cells. *Semin. Cell Biol.* **1993**, *4*, 409–418.

81. Choi, K.D.; Vodyanik, M.A.; Slukvin, I.I. Generation of mature human myelomonocytic cells through expansion and differentiation of pluripotent stem cell-derived lin⁻CD34⁺CD43⁺CD45⁺ progenitors. *J. Clin. Invest.* **2009**, *119*, 2818–2829.

82. Niwa, A.; Heike, T.; Umeda, K.; Oshima, K.; Kato, I.; Sakai, H.; Suemori, H.; Nakahata, T.; Saito, M.K. A novel serum-free monolayer culture for orderly hematopoietic differentiation of human pluripotent cells via mesodermal progenitors. *PLoS One* **2011**, *6*, e22261.

83. Salvagiotto, G.; Burton, S.; Daigh, C.A.; Rajesh, D.; Slukvin, I.I.; Seay, N.J. A defined, feeder-free, serum-free system to generate *in vitro* hematopoietic progenitors and differentiated blood cells from hESCs and hiPSCs. *PLoS One* **2011**, *6*, e17829.

84. Panicker, L.M.; Miller, D.; Park, T.S.; Patel, B.; Azevedo, J.L.; Awad, O.; Masood, M.A.; Veenstra, T.D.; Goldin, E.; Stubblefield, B.K.; *et al.* Induced pluripotent stem cell model recapitulates pathologic hallmarks of gaucher disease. *Proc. Natl. Acad. Sci. USA* **2012**, *109*, 18054–18059.

85. Chadwick, K.; Wang, L.; Li, L.; Menendez, P.; Murdoch, B.; Rouleau, A.; Bhatia, M. Cytokines and BMP-4 promote hematopoietic differentiation of human embryonic stem cells. *Blood* **2003**, *102*, 906–915.

86. Lengerke, C.; Grauer, M.; Niebuhr, N.I.; Riedt, T.; Kanz, L.; Park, I.H.; Daley, G.Q. Hematopoietic development from human induced pluripotent stem cells. *Ann. NY Acad. Sci.* **2009**, *1176*, 219–227.

87. Grigoriadis, A.E.; Kennedy, M.; Bozec, A.; Brunton, F.; Stenbeck, G.; Park, I.H.; Wagner, E.F.; Keller, G.M. Directed differentiation of hematopoietic precursors and functional osteoclasts from human es and ips cells. *Blood* **2010**, *115*, 2769–2776.

88. Gandre-Babbe, S.; Paluru, P.; Aribeana, C.; Chou, S.T.; Bresolin, S.; Lu, L.; Sullivan, S.K.; Tasian, S.K.; Weng, J.; Favre, H.; *et al.* Patient-derived induced pluripotent stem cells recapitulate hematopoietic abnormalities of juvenile myelomonocytic leukemia. *Blood* **2013**, *121*, 4925–4929.

89. Kaufman, D.S.; Hanson, E.T.; Lewis, R.L.; Auerbach, R.; Thomson, J.A. Hematopoietic colony-forming cells derived from human embryonic stem cells. *Proc. Natl. Acad. Sci. USA* **2001**, *98*, 10716–10721.

90. Ledran, M.H.; Krassowska, A.; Armstrong, L.; Dimmick, I.; Renstrom, J.; Lang, R.; Yung, S.; Santibanez-Coref, M.; Dzierzak, E.; Stojkovic, M.; *et al.* Efficient hematopoietic differentiation of human embryonic stem cells on stromal cells derived from hematopoietic niches. *Cell Stem Cell* **2008**, *3*, 85–98.

91. Pick, M.; Azzola, L.; Mossman, A.; Stanley, E.G.; Elefanty, A.G. Differentiation of human embryonic stem cells in serum-free medium reveals distinct roles for bone morphogenetic protein 4, vascular endothelial growth factor, stem cell factor, and fibroblast growth factor 2 in hematopoiesis. *Stem Cells* **2007**, *25*, 2206–2214.

92. Bhatia, M.; Bonnet, D.; Kapp, U.; Wang, J.C.; Murdoch, B.; Dick, J.E. Quantitative analysis reveals expansion of human hematopoietic repopulating cells after short-term *ex vivo* culture. *J. Exp. Med.* **1997**, *186*, 619–624.

93. Zandstra, P.W.; Conneally, E.; Piret, J.M.; Eaves, C.J. Ontogeny-associated changes in the cytokine responses of primitive human haemopoietic cells. *Br. J. Haematol.* **1998**, *101*, 770–778.

94. Hoffman, R.; Tong, J.; Brandt, J.; Traycoff, C.; Bruno, E.; McGuire, B.W.; Gordon, M.S.; McNiece, I.; Srour, E.F. The *in vitro* and *in vivo* effects of stem cell factor on human hematopoiesis. *Stem Cells* **1993**, *11* (Suppl. 2), 76–82.

95. Kardel, M.D.; Eaves, C.J. Modeling human hematopoietic cell development from pluripotent stem cells. *Exp. Hematol.* **2012**, *40*, 601–611.

96. Bar-Nur, O.; Russ, H.A.; Efrat, S.; Benvenisty, N. Epigenetic memory and preferential lineage-specific differentiation in induced pluripotent stem cells derived from human pancreatic islet beta cells. *Cell Stem Cell* **2011**, *9*, 17–23.

97. Papapetrou, E.P.; Tomishima, M.J.; Chambers, S.M.; Mica, Y.; Reed, E.; Menon, J.; Tabar, V.; Mo, Q.; Studer, L.; Sadelain, M. Stoichiometric and temporal requirements of Oct4, Sox2, Klf4, and c-Myc expression for efficient human iPSC induction and differentiation. *Proc. Natl. Acad. Sci. USA* **2009**, *106*, 12759–12764.

98. Bock, C.; Kiskinis, E.; Verstappen, G.; Gu, H.; Boulting, G.; Smith, Z.D.; Ziller, M.; Croft, G.F.; Amoroso, M.W.; Oakley, D.H.; *et al.* Reference maps of human ES and iPS cell variation enable high-throughput characterization of pluripotent cell lines. *Cell* **2011**, *144*, 439–452.

99. Urnov, F.D.; Rebar, E.J.; Holmes, M.C.; Zhang, H.S.; Gregory, P.D. Genome editing with engineered zinc finger nucleases. *Nat. Rev. Genet.* **2010**, *11*, 636–646.

100. Wood, A.J.; Lo, T.W.; Zeitler, B.; Pickle, C.S.; Ralston, E.J.; Lee, A.H.; Amora, R.; Miller, J.C.; Leung, E.; Meng, X.; *et al.* Targeted genome editing across species using ZFNs and TALENs. *Science* **2011**, *333*, doi:10.1126/science.1207773.

101. Soldner, F.; Laganiere, J.; Cheng, A.W.; Hockemeyer, D.; Gao, Q.; Alagappan, R.; Khurana, V.; Golbe, L.I.; Myers, R.H.; Lindquist, S.; *et al.* Generation of isogenic pluripotent stem cells differing exclusively at two early onset parkinson point mutations. *Cell* **2011**, *146*, 318–331.

102. Cong, L.; Ran, F.A.; Cox, D.; Lin, S.; Barretto, R.; Habib, N.; Hsu, P.D.; Wu, X.; Jiang, W.; Marraffini, L.A.; *et al.* Multiplex genome engineering using CRISPR/Cas systems. *Science* **2013**, *339*, 819–823.

Chapter 8:
Germ Cells

Human iPS Cell-Derived Germ Cells: Current Status and Clinical Potential

Tetsuya Ishii

Abstract: Recently, fertile spermatozoa and oocytes were generated from mouse induced pluripotent (iPS) cells using a combined *in vitro* and *in vivo* induction system. With regard to germ cell induction from human iPS cells, progress has been made particularly in the male germline, demonstrating *in vitro* generation of haploid, round spermatids. Although iPS-derived germ cells are expected to be developed to yield a form of assisted reproductive technology (ART) that can address unmet reproductive needs, genetic and/or epigenetic instabilities abound in iPS cell generation and germ cell induction. In addition, there is still room to improve the induction protocol in the female germline. However, rapid advances in stem cell research are likely to make such obstacles surmountable, potentially translating induced germ cells into the clinical setting in the immediate future. This review examines the current status of the induction of germ cells from human iPS cells and discusses the clinical potential, as well as future directions.

Reprinted from *J. Clin. Med.* Cite as: Ishii, T. Human iPS Cell-Derived Germ Cells: Current Status and Clinical Potential. *J. Clin. Med.* **2014**, *3*, 1064–1083.

1. Introduction

There are various reasons to generate germ cells from human pluripotent stem cells in the laboratory. First, *in vitro* recapitulation of gametogenesis and early embryogenesis using such induced germ cells is expected to enhance our understanding of the basis of human reproduction because the inaccessibility to human eggs (oocytes) and embryos has hampered relevant research. Second, human germ cell induction research will establish a precious platform for modeling infertility and congenital anomalies that have been difficult to study using animals. Third, the *in vitro* induction of germ cells from autologous pluripotent stem cells should lead to a new form of assisted reproductive technology (ART) for infertile patients who wish to have genetically-related children.

Recent advances in stem cell research have made it conceivable that human sperm (spermatozoon) and oocytes will be induced from pluripotent stem cells in the near future. Notably, a Japanese group reported that mouse embryonic stem (ES) cells and induced pluripotent (iPS) cells could be differentiated into fertile spermatozoa and oocytes via primordial germ cell (PGC)—like cells, and demonstrated that viable offspring could be derived from pluripotent stem cells [1,2]. Although their protocols used gonadal tissues and an *in vivo* induction system, their work established an important step on the path to the *in vitro* recapitulation of gametogenesis. Significant progress has also been made in the differentiation from both human ES cells [3–8] and iPS cells [8–13] into human germ cells over the last decade. A recent report demonstrated that human iPS cells can be indirectly or directly differentiated into the male germline, including haploid, round spermatid-like cells [10,12,13]. Rapid advances in stem cell research would help to overcome the current technical issues and lead to the *in vitro* formation of bona fide human spermatozoa and oocytes.

If functional oocytes and spermatozoa can be differentiated from human iPS cells, the use of such cells for research will contribute to the molecular elucidation of gametogenesis, as well as the onset and progression of various diseases in obstetrics, gynecology, and neonatology/pediatrics. However, with regard to the reproductive use of such germ cells induced from autologous iPS cells, sufficient preclinical research will need to be performed to confirm the safety of the offspring. Remarkably, the overview of ART (Appendix) using induced germ cells appears to occur against the Weismann barrier, wherein hereditary information moves only from germ cells to somatic cells [14]. Such germ cells are likely to be subject to genetic and/or epigenetic instabilities during iPS cell generation and germ cell induction. Moreover, although assessing the biological function of induced germ cells involves the creation of embryos and subsequent culture for a short period, human embryo research is strictly regulated in most countries [15]. In this review article, the current status of germ cell induction from human iPS cells is examined and discussed in light of clinical potential and future directions.

2. Clinical Implications of Germ Cell Induction *in Vitro*

Two fundamental cell types constitute multicellular eukaryotes. Somatic cells proliferate by mitosis and form the tissues and organs comprising the body. Germ cells undergo meiosis as well as mitosis, resulting in the generation of gametes that can transfer half the genetic material to the next generation. The lineage of germ cells is referred to as the germline.

If germ cells can be efficiently induced from human iPS cells, the availability of such germ cells could contribute to various biomedical fields. First of all, the research use of human female germ cells and embryos is largely difficult owing to ethical reasons and the scarcity of oocytes and embryos for research. In contrast, patient-specific induced germ cells can model diseases that are derived from aberrant germ cells or that occur during embryogenesis. A wide variety of somatic cells which are differentiated from patient-specific iPS cells have already been used for disease-modeling to enhance the understanding of the pathogenesis of diseases [16]. Currently, the low efficiency of the differentiation of human iPS cells into germ cells has hampered the unveiling of the molecular pathogenesis of various diseases, including germ cell tumors [17], aneuploidy, sex chromosome abnormalities [11], and female and male infertilities.

If functional germ cells are induced from iPS cells, such germ cells are also expected to impact ART treatment (Figure 1). Although ART has helped many infertile patients to produce offspring, the current ART procedures are based on the premise that an infertile couple can produce fertile gametes in order to perform intrauterine insemination (IUI), *in vitro* fertilization (IVF), or intracytoplasmic sperm injection (ICSI) (Appendix). Otherwise, the couple must use donor gametes. This option has raised ethical issues and social confusion. ART using donor gametes results in the birth of genetically-unrelated children. Such children born of donor gametes frequently confront stigma that stems from being uninformed about their genetic parents or due to their lack of resemblance to their parents in shape and appearance [18]. In addition, some sperm donors have anonymously provided their gametes to a tremendous number of patients, creating social problems [19]. Such cases frequently occur because there are many prospective parents who have no viable gametes due to congenital anomalies, or because they have been rendered sterile by receiving chemotherapy and radiation therapy for cancer treatment [20–22], or because the females have undergone age-related oocyte senescence [23].

Recent progress in germ cell induction research is increasing the possibility of a new form of ART using germ cells induced from autologous iPS cells for patients with no viable gametes (Figure 1). If fertile spermatozoa can be induced from a male patient's iPS cells, performing IVF or ICSI will be possible using the generated spermatozoa. Similar approaches can be performed when fertile oocytes are generated from iPS cells. Even if no mature spermatozoa are obtained from the induction, *in vivo* spermatogenesis could be restored by transplanting spermatogonial stem cells (SSCs) derived from autologous iPS cells into the testis of a male patient [24–26]. In 1997, infusions of oocyte cytoplasm including mitochondria from donor oocytes was conducted in order to enhance the fertility of quality-compromised oocyte with mitochondrial defects [23], resulting in the birth of over 30 children [27]. However, the U.S. Food and Drug Administration concluded that further research was required for the use of this procedure in humans due to potential health risks to the progeny [28]. If this ooplasmic transfer procedure is sufficiently improved and induced female germ cells which genetically match the patient's oocytes can be obtained from iPS cells, such germ cells could be used as a resource for ooplasmic transfer. Following such ART procedures, the resulting embryos can be carefully examined for three to five days post-conception, and one or more viable embryo(s) can then be selected for embryo transfer. Thus, autologous iPS-derived germ cells are expected to meet the reproductive needs of infertile couples who have lost viable gametes for medical reasons or aging but wish to have genetically-related children.

Figure 1. The potential reproductive uses of iPS cell-based germ cells. Autologous iPS cells can be generated from somatic cells biopsied from infertile patients who have lost viable oocytes or spermatozoa. Subsequently, germ cells are induced from the iPS cells. The regenerated germ cells can be used for *in vitro* fertilization or intracytoplasmic sperm injection to create embryos for transfer. In cases of male infertility, spermatogonial stem cells (SSCs) could be transplanted into patients to restore spermatogenesis potential. In cases of female infertility, ooplasmic transfer to enhance the viability of quality-compromised oocytes is conceivable if female germ cells with a sufficient number of mitochondria can be induced from iPS cells.

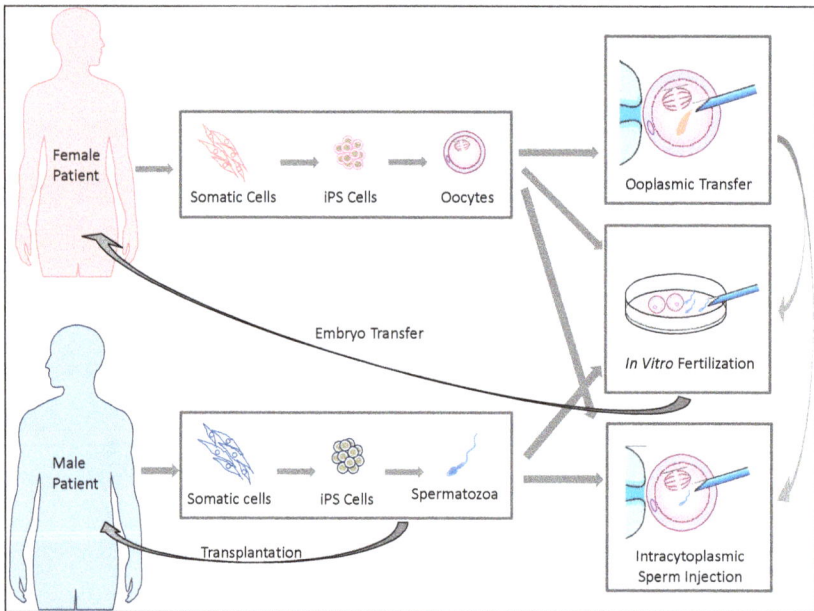

3. The Induction of Germ Cells from iPS Cells

Human iPS cells were initially generated from somatic cells by the ectopic expression of four transcription factor genes (OCT4, SOX2, KLF4, and c-MYC) in 2007 [29]. The current iPS cell generation methods vary in the choice of somatic origin, the set of reprogramming factors, and the transduction methodology [30]. The new pluripotent stem cells have become the starting material for germ cell induction, in which ES cells had been used (Table 1). Clinical applications of iPS-derived germ cells require scientific scrutiny in terms of meiosis, epigenetic programming, and the organization of the nucleus and mitochondria. Based on lessons learned from previous research on human ES cells [3–8] (Table 1), non-human primate ES cells [31], and mouse pluripotent stem cells [1,2,32–35], the current primary differentiation strategy involves differentiating human iPS cells into PGCs, and subsequently directing the PGCs to undergo meiosis, with some variations (Table 1). The PGC formation has been verified by the expression of marker genes or immunostaining for marker proteins including VASA (DDX4), cKIT, and SSEA1 (Figure 2). Confirming entrance into meiosis involves assessing the haploidy of differentiated cells as well as detecting meiosis-associated markers, such as acrosin, transition protein 1 (TP1), and protamine 1 (Prot1).

Table 1. Induction of germ cells from human pluripotent stem cells *in vitro* or *in vivo*.

Differentiation Method	Cell Lines Used			Differentiation Stage		Remarks	References
	iPS Cells	ES Cells	PGCs	Meiotic Cells	Haploid Cells		
EB formation	-	HSF-6(XX) HSF-1(XY) H9(XX)	-	-	-	Germ cell-like cells expressing VASA, SCP1, SCP3, BOULE, TEKT1, and GDF3 were observed.	Clark *et al.*, 2004 [3]
EB formation	-	NTU1(XX) NTU2(XX) NTU3(N.D.)	-	-	-	Germ cell-like cells expressing cKit, STELLA, VASA, and GDF9 were observed.	Chen *et al.*, 2006 [4]
Making colonies of fewer than 50 cells	-	HSF-6(XX) H9(XX)	Yes	-	-	Sertoli-like cells were simultaneously generated in this process.	Bucay *et al.*, 2008 [7]
Monolayer differentiation and FACS enrichment of SSEA1-positive cells	-	H9(XX) hES-NCL1(XX)	Yes	-	-	PGCs with removal of parental imprints and chromatin modification changes were generated.	Tilgner *et al.*, 2008 [6]
Differentiation on primary human fetal gonadal stromal cells, and isolation of a triple biomarker (cKIT, SSEA1, VASA)—positive cells	hIPS2(XY) hIPS1(XY)	HSF-6(XX) HSF-1(XY) H9(XX)	Yes	-	-	PGCs derived from human iPS cells did not initiate imprint erasure as efficiently.	Park *et al.*, 2009 [8]
Overexpression of DAZL, DAZ and BOULE following induction by BMPs	-	HSF-1(XY) HSF-6(XX) H1(XY) H9(XX)	Yes	Yes	Yes	DAZL functions in PGC formation, whereas DAZ and BOULE promote later stages of meiosis and development of haploid gametes.	Kee *et al.*, 2010 [5]
Overexpression of DAZ, DAZL, and BOULE following induction by BMPs	iPS(IMR90) (XX) iHUF4(XY)	H9(XX) HSF-1(XY)	Yes	Yes	Yes	Fetal-derived iPS cell line iPS (IMR90) and adult-derived iPS cell line iHUF4 were generated by lentiviral transfection with OCT3/4, SOX2, KLF4 and c-MYC.	Panula *et al.*, 2011 [10]

Table 1. *Cont.*

Differentiation Method	Cell Lines Used			Differentiation Stage		Remarks	References
	iPS Cells	ES Cells	PGCs	Meiotic Cells	Haploid Cells		
Overexpression of VASA and/or DAZL following differentiation on matrigel-coated plates	iPS(IMR90)(XX) iHUF4(XY)	iHUF3(XX) iHUF4(XY)	Yes	Yes	Yes	The same iPS cell lines described in Panula *et al.* were used.	Medrano *et al.*, 2011 [9]
Two step protocol: Culture in bFGF-depleted ES cell media; subsequently, RA added; Sorted cells are cultured with FRSK, rLIF, bFGF, and R115866	KiPS1(XY) KiPS2(XY) KiPS3(XY) KiPS4(XX) CBiPS1(XY) CBiPS2(XY) CBiPS3(XX) CBiPS4(XY) CBiPS5(XX)	HS306(XX) ES[6](XX)	-	Yes	Yes	iPS cells of different origin (keratinocytes and cord blood) were generated with a different number (2–4) of transcription factors.	Eguizabal *et al.*, 2011 [13]
Direct differentiation using mouse SSC culture conditions	H1(XY)	HFF1(XY)	-	Yes	Yes	iPS cells derived from male foreskin fibroblasts were used.	Easley *et al.*, 2012 [12]
1. Differentiation into PGCs with BMPs, RA, and hrLIF. 2. Induction of gonocytes by transplanting iPS cells directly into murine seminiferous tubules *in vivo*	iAZF1(XY) iAZF2(XY) iAZFΔbc(XY) iAZFΔc(XY) iAZFΔa(XY)	H1(XY)	Yes	-	-	iPS cells derived from dermal fibroblasts of males with intact Y chromosome (iAZF) and Y chromosome deletions (iAZFΔ) were used. Gonocytes expressing VASA, STELLA, UTF1, PLZF, and DAZ were induced.	Ramanthal *et al.*, 2014 [11]

PGCs: primordial germ cells; EB: embryoid body; BMPs: bone morphogenetic proteins; bFGF: basic fibroblast growth factor; FRSK: Forskolin; RA: retinoic acid; hrLIF: human recombinant leukemia inhibitory factor; SSC: spermatogonial stem cell.

326

Figure 2. Differentiation pathway from human iPS cells to germ cells. Human iPS cells are differentiated into primordial germ cells (PGCs), and further differentiated into meiotic cells. Indicated information regarding confirmed markers is derived from research reports regarding germ cell induction using human iPS cells. PGCs: primordial germ cells, SSCs: spermatogonial stem cells.

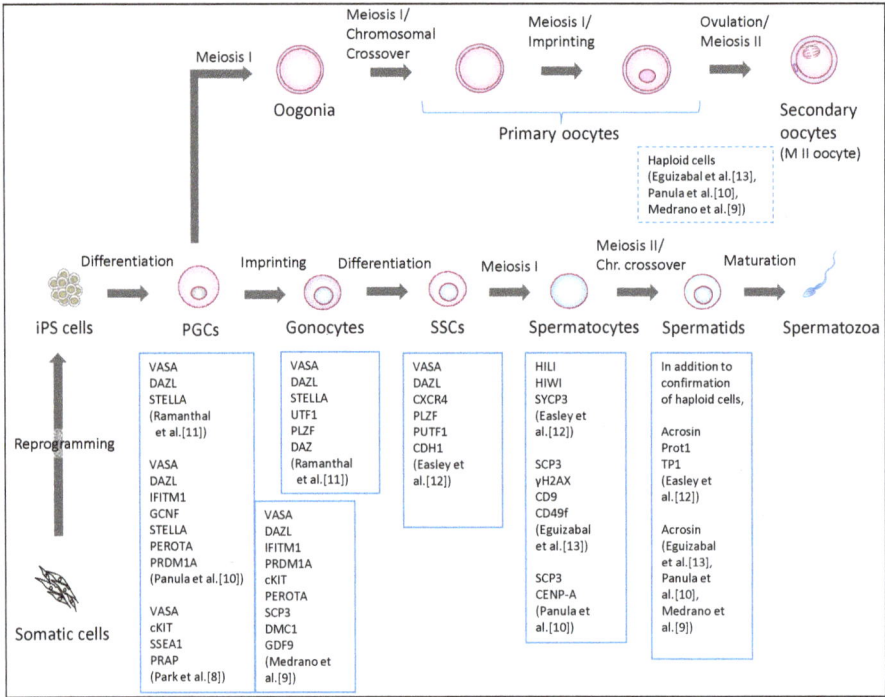

3.1. Induction of the Male Germline

The differentiation of human male iPS cells has so far produced PGCs [8–10], gonocytes [11], SSCs [12], spermatocytes [12,13], and haploid, round spermatid-like cells [10,12,13] (Figure 2, Table 1). As early as 2009, Park *et al.* [8] reported PGC induction from human iPS and ES cells. They used a triple biomarker (cKIT, SSEA1, VASA) assay to identify and isolate the PGCs, and demonstrated that culturing such human pluripotent stem cells on human fetal gonadal stromal cells, which were derived from a 10-week-old human fetus, significantly improved the efficiency of PGC formation. Moreover, the efficiency was comparable among various ES cell and iPS cell lines. Utilizing bisulfite sequencing, they showed that the PGCs initiate imprint erasure from differentially methylated imprinted regions (H19, PEG1, and SNRPN DMRs) by day seven of differentiation. However, PGCs derived from iPS cells did not initiate imprint erasure as efficiently, suggesting that further investigation is needed on the epigenetic status during germ cell induction from iPS cells.

In 2011, Panula *et al.* compared the potential of human iPS cells, derived from adult and fetal somatic cells to form primordial and meiotic germ cells [10]. As a consequence, approximately 5% of human iPS cells were found to have differentiated into PGCs with induction by bone morphogenetic proteins (BMPs). In addition, by overexpressing intrinsic regulator genes, including *DAZ*, *DAZL*, and *BOULE*, iPS cells formed meiotic cells with extensive synaptonemal complexes and post-meiotic haploid spermatid-like cells. These results show that human iPS cells generated from adult somatic cells can form germline cells other than PGCs. More recently, similar results using the overexpression of *VASA* and/or *DAZL* was reported, demonstrating that both human ES cells and iPS cells differentiated into PGCs, and the maturation and progression of these cells through meiosis was enhanced [9]. Again, post-meiotic male haploid cells were induced in 14 days following the overexpression of the two regulators. Moreover, the methylation pattern of the H19 locus, similar to that of normal germ cells, was observed following the expression of *VASA* alone. Therefore, such RNA-binding proteins appear to promote the meiotic progression of human iPS cell-derived germ cells *in vitro*.

In contrast to these studies, Eguizabal *et al.* demonstrated that without the overexpression of germline related factors, postmeiotic haploid cells were consistently obtained from human iPS cells of different origins (keratinocytes and cord blood), generated with a different number of transcription factors [13]. Their two-step differentiation protocol begins with iPS cell culture for three weeks with human ES cell media in the absence of bFGF. Subsequently, retinoic acid (RA) is added to the medium, and the culture continues for three more weeks. Then, the cells are sorted and reseeded onto culture plates in the presence of forskolin (FRSK), human recombinant leukemia inhibiting factor (rLIF), bFGF, and the CYP26 inhibitor, R115866, for at least two weeks. Consequently, the post-meiotic spermatid-like cells with acrosin-staining were identified. Moreover, Easley *et al.* also reported a similar direct differentiation approach without the overexpression of genes [12]. They adopted standardized mouse SSC culture conditions [36] and demonstrated that human ES cells and iPS cells differentiated directly into advanced male germ cell lineages, without genetic manipulation. They observed spermatogenesis *in vivo* by differentiating these pluripotent stem cells into UTF1-, PLZF-, and CDH1-positive spermatogonia-like cells; HIWI- and HILI positive spermatocyte-like cells; and haploid, round spermatid-like cells expressing acrosin, TP1, and Prot1. Such spermatids had uniparental genomic imprints similar to those of human sperm on two loci: H19 and IGF2. These results demonstrate that male iPS cells have the ability to differentiate directly into haploid, round spermatids *in vitro*.

Therefore, male germ cell induction from iPS cells has rapidly advanced since 2009. Although transplantation of autologous SSCs to restore spermatogenesis has already succeeded in infertile monkeys [37], clinical use of SSCs induced from iPS cells requires considerable caution. Notably, Amariglio *et al.* warned that transplantation of stem cells, not differentiated cells, in a patient could cause an adverse event [38]. They reported that a boy with ataxia telangiectasia treated with the intracerebellar and intrathecal injection of human fetal neural stem cells was diagnosed with a multifocal brain tumor four years after the first injection. One might consider using iPS cell-derived spermatids in the clinical setting. However, although oocytes have been fertilized with elongated spermatids [39,40], they were insufficiently fertilized with premature, round spermatids, resulting in poor embryonic development [41–43]. Successful fertilization of oocytes with more matured male germ cells *in vitro* needs to be examined in preclinical research.

Based on the recent mouse work by Hayashi *et al.* [1], primordial germ cell-like cells (PGCLCs) were generated from ES cells and iPS cells through epiblast-like cells (EpiLCs), a cellular state highly similar to pregastrulating epiblasts but distinct from epiblast stem cells (EpiSCs). To examine whether such PGCLCs undergo proper spermatogenesis, PGCLCs were transplanted into the seminiferous tubules neonatal mice lacking endogenous germ cells. As a result, fertile spermatozoa were produced in the thick tubules. The global transcription profiles, epigenetic reprogramming, such as imprinted genes (*Igf2r*, *Snrpn*, *H19*, and *Kcnq1ot1*), and cellular dynamics during PGCLC induction from EpiLCs resembled those associated with PGC specification from the epiblasts. Remarkably, they identified Integrin-b3 and SSEA1 as markers that could be used to isolate PGCLCs from differentiated cells. More recently, Ramathal *et al.* demonstrated that human iPS cells transplanted directly into mouse seminiferous tubules differentiated extensively to form germ cell-like cells with morphology indistinguishable from that of fetal germ cells, and these cells expressed PGC-specific proteins including VASA, DAZL, and STELLA [11].

These findings revealed the significance of differentiation pathway from iPS cells to germ cells and elaborated the need for culture conditions that mimic the stem cell niche in the testis to efficiently and effectively direct human iPS cells to form more advanced germ cells *in vitro*.

3.2. The Induction of Female Germline

In contrast to male germline induction, the differentiation of iPS cells or ES cells into female germ cells has been insufficiently studied (Table 1, Figure 2). Eguizabal *et al.* consistently observed between 1.0%–2.0% haploid cells per human female iPS cell line (derived from keratinocytes or cord blood) in their two-step differentiation protocol [13]. Their female iPS cells were differentiated into haploid cells following the detection of the SCP3 and H2AX proteins (indicators of meiotic competence). However, they observed that most of the iPS cell lines, including female cells, increased their methylation status of H19 (the maternally expressed, paternally imprinted gene), displaying a clear tendency toward paternal imprinting. Therefore, it appears that the germ cells induced from female iPS cells are certainly haploid, but are incomplete as mature female germ cells because oocytes only extrude the last polar body after fertilization. Panula *et al.* also reported a similar result regarding the differentiation of female iPS and ES cells into meiotic germ cells by the overexpression of the intrinsic regulators [10]. Moreover, Bucay *et al.* showed that germ cells differentiated from human ES cells *in vitro* express both male and female genetic programs regardless of their karyotype [7].

With regard to mouse systems, there have been attempts to induce female germ cells from ES cells since 2003 [44–48]. Although a follicle-like structure with oocyte-like cells was spontaneously observed, entrance into meiosis was not confirmed in those reports. Nicholas *et al.* clearly noted that mouse ES cell-derived oocyte maturation ultimately fails *in vitro* [48]. They transplanted ES cell-derived oocyte-like cells into an ovarian niche to direct their functional maturation and showed that the physiological niche of the ovary is required for their differentiation. Notably, Hayashi *et al.* showed that mouse female ES cells and iPS cells were differentiated into fertile oocytes via EpiLCs and PGCLCs [2], using a combined *in vitro* and *in vivo* system which led to the successful induction of fertile spermatozoa in 2011 [1]. When the PGCLCs were aggregated with female gonadal somatic cells as reconstituted ovaries, they underwent X-reactivation, imprint erasure, and cyst formation, and exhibited meiotic potential. After PGCLCs in the reconstituted ovaries were transplanted under the mouse ovarian bursa, such cells matured into germinal vesicle-stage oocytes, and contributed to fertile offspring after *in vitro* maturation and fertilization. Therefore, the differentiation of female iPS cells into germ cells largely depends on the use of an *in vivo* system.

The difficulty in female germ cell induction from pluripotent stem cells is more likely to reflect *in vivo* oogenesis. Human gametogenesis initiates around the 23–26th day post-conception [49]. The precursors of gametes, the PGCs, appear in the dorsal wall of the yolk sac near the developing allantois. The PGCs proliferate and migrate through the dorsal mesentery into the gonadal ridges. The PGCs are found in the gonads by the fourth week post-conception. Thereafter, female and male PGCs differentiate into oogonia (subsequently, oocytes) or gonocytes (subsequently, spermatozoa), respectively. The male germ cells undergo mitotic arrest until birth, whereas the female germ cells further enter meiotic arrest (Figure 2). Following birth, such germ cells are reactivated and resume meiosis, resulting in the beginning of the production of mature oocytes and spermatozoa after puberty. Therefore, human gametogenesis proceeds on a long-term basis with gender differences in meiotic progression.

In males, SSCs are maintained, and contribute to spermatogenesis by self-renewal *in vivo* for a long time. In addition, human SSCs can be maintained *in vitro* for a long term. Sadri-Ardekani *et al.* demonstrated that the human SSC numbers increased 53-fold within 19 days in testicular cell culture and increased 18,450-fold within 64 days in a germline stem cell subculture [50]. Conversely, it has generally been considered that most female germ cells enter meiosis I until birth, do not proliferate after birth, and that the number of the germ cells gradually declines until menopause (at approximately 40 years) [51]. The significant differences in the proceedings between spermatogenesis and oogenesis appear to impact the differentiation of human iPS cells into germ cells in the laboratory. However, there have been several unique reports regarding mammalian oogenesis. Some groups have reported the isolation of oogonial stem cell-like cells in mice and humans [52–55]. However, there are counterarguments about the existence of oogonial stem cells [56–58]. If the mitotically active oogonial cells can be isolated in a reproducible manner, the findings are expected to contribute to enhancing female germ cell induction as well as providing a mitochondrial resource for ooplasmic transfer.

4. Future Directions

In order to improve the induction efficiency and functional completeness of germ cell induction from human iPS cells, deeper insight into iPS cell generation and gametogenesis *in vivo* is vital. In addition, creating human embryos is likely to require the assessment of the developmental potential of induced germ cells. The conditions to permit the creation of human embryos for these functional assays should be discussed, because such experiments are frequently associated with ethical concerns or issues [15].

4.1. Genetic and Epigenetic Stability of Human iPS Cells

As mentioned in the Introduction, the ART using induced germ cells appears to be against the Weismann barrier. Induced germ cells are likely to be subject to genetic and/or epigenetic instabilities during iPS cell generation and germ cell induction. The genetic stability of iPS cells significantly impacts their research use, in addition to their safe medical use. Some cytogenetic analyses have suggested that human iPS cells and ES cells are likely to acquire trisomies in chromosome 12, and 17, indicating an underlying mechanism of growth advantage associated with culture adaptation [59–61]. Moreover, the tendency for large-scale chromosomal aberrations appears to have no dependence on the cell origin or iPS generation methods, although some of the chromosomal aberrations observed in PS cells were derived from the original somatic cells [59,60,62]. In addition, human iPS cell cultures are likely to undergo chromosomal changes at both early and late passages. A close examination of the genetic changes during culture indicated that the observed peak in occurrence of chromosomal aberrations is at around passage eight in iPS cells, while that in ES cells is at around passage 36 [59]. Moreover, smaller copy number variations (CNVs) in human iPS cell culture are present across chromosome 12, 17, and 20 [63]. Compared with human ES cells, iPS cells showed increased CNVs, and had more CNVs at low passages (18%) than at late passages (9%) [62,64]. Therefore, human iPS cells seem to be subject to genetic changes at earlier culture stage, mostly resulting from somatic cell reprogramming.

The genetic instabilities might occur not only in nuclear DNA, but also in mitochondrial DNA (mtDNA). The copy number of mtDNA, which encodes proteins required to produce ATP for motility of spermatozoon ranges from 2.8 to 226 copies of mtDNA [65]. In contrast, in oocytes, the mtDNA copy number ranges from 20,000 to 598,000 [66–69], significantly impacting the outcome of fertility in ART. Since proper ATP production by mitochondria is essential for accurate meiosis in oogenesis as well as normal embryonic development [66–69], the mtDNA integrity of human iPS cells needs to be addressed. Relative to the founder fibroblasts, a higher rate of heteroplasmic variation was observed in human iPS cells [70]. Although this phenomenon may imply an increased mutation load in the iPS cells, such iPS cell lines showed no significant metabolic differences. Van Haute *et al.* tested 16 human ES cell lines and showed that they carry a plethora of diverse mtDNA deletions [71]. The mtDNA mutations did not seem to correlate with the time in culture, and were detected in the early passage cells. Such deletions did not appear to impact the differentiation potential, and were still present in terminally differentiated cells. Conversely, Wahlestedt *et al.* reported a unique result using a mutator mouse model with an error-prone mtDNA polymerase [72]. They investigated the impact of an established mtDNA mutational load regarding the differentiation properties of mouse iPS cells. As a consequence, the mutator iPS cells displayed delayed proliferation kinetics and harbored extensive differentiation defects, although somatic cells with a heavy mtDNA mutation burden were amenable to reprogramming into iPS cells. These findings suggest the need for careful analyses of the nuclear DNA and mtDNA in human iPS cells prior to germ cell induction.

In addition, epigenetic aberrations in human iPS cells have been pointed out, indicating defects in DNA methylation, including regions subject to imprinting [73]. Interestingly, high-resolution DNA methylation profiles suggested that some iPS cell lines possess somatic memory [74,75]. Although iPS cell lines with such memory might readily differentiate into germ cells, careful assessment of the epigenetic status of human iPS cells is required to avoid a low efficiency differentiation or aberrant epigenetics in the resulting germ cells.

4.2. The Pluripotency State of Human iPS Cells

Human ES and iPS cells are more similar to mouse EpiSCs that were derived from epiblasts in postimplantation embryos than mouse naive, ground state ES cells [76,77]. The features of the ground state pluripotency include driving *Oct4* (also known as *Pou5f1*) transcription by its distal enhancer, globally reduced DNA methylation, prominent deposition of the repressive histone modification H3K27me3, and bivalent domain acquisition on lineage regulatory genes [78]. Moreover, human female ES and iPS cells frequently show a pronounced tendency for X chromosome inactivation. These lines of evidence suggest that human iPS cells represent a primed state of pluripotency that is distinct from the naive pluripotent ground state of mouse ES and iPS cells. Recently, some new methods to establish human iPS cells have been proposed [79–81]. These methods, which are based on 2i/LIF conditions (exogenous stimulation with leukemia inhibitory factor and small molecule inhibition of ERK1/ERK2 and GSK3β signaling) with additional components, demonstrated the establishment of human iPS cells in the naive ground state [79,81], or in the preimplantation epiblast state [80]. The use of human iPS cells generated by such methods are likely to facilitate the subsequent appropriate differentiation pathway to germ cells, as demonstrated by the two mouse experiments in which mouse pluripotent stem cells were differentiated into germ cells via EpiLCs [1,2].

4.3. Spatio-Temporal Factors in Gametogenesis

Currently, germ cell induction from human iPS cells is advancing primarily in the male germline. A better understanding of gametogenesis would facilitate the induction of female germ cells, as well as the terminal differentiation into spermatozoa. Following puberty, spermatogenesis occurs at the seminiferous tubules in the testis in which Sertoli cells co-exist with Leydig cells. In inducing male germ cells, co-culture with Sertoli cells that foster and differentiate spermatocytes *in vivo* has already been introduced to induce spermatogenesis *in vitro*. Park *et al.* improved PGC generation using a co-culture system with human fetal gonadal cells [8]. Moreover, Bucay *et al.* reported that PGC generation from human ES cells was accompanied by the development of Sertoli-like support cells [7]. Moreover, another article reported that testosterone, which the Leydig cells of the testes produce, was added to the culture medium in order to promote differentiation of mouse iPS cells into male germ cells *in vitro* [82]. More elaborate culture systems including Sertoli cells and Leydig cells may be effective to induce terminally differentiated male germ cells. However, fetal and adult populations of Leydig cells are distinct cells in terms of their physiology and function [83]. A recent report suggested that Sertoli cells support adult Leydig cell development in the prepubertal testis [84]. Regarding female germ cell development, oocytes are surrounded by a single layer of flattened ovarian follicular epithelial cells at meiotic arrest.

When stimulated at puberty, the oocyte enlarges, and the follicular cells continue to proliferate to form many layers surrounding the oocyte. These cells eventually become known as granulosa cells that secrete progesterone after ovulation. Qing *et al.* have used co-culture with ovarian granulosa cells in the induction of oocyte-like cells expressing oocyte-specific genes including Figalpha, GDF-9, and ZP1-3 from mouse ES cells [47]. Interestingly, when they were co-cultured with Chinese hamster ovary (CHO) cells or cultured in CHO cell-conditioned medium, these cells did not express all of these oocyte-specific markers during the germ cell induction. Moreover, Nicholas *et al.* differentiated mouse Oct4-GFP ES cells *in vitro*, isolated GFP positive germ cells by FACS and co-aggregated the cells with dissociated mouse newborn ovarian tissue [48]. Subsequently, they transplanted the co-aggregates under the kidney capsule of recipient mice. They observed ES cell-derived Oct4-GFP positive oocytes in the graft despite the efficiency being low. Furthermore, in a recent work [2], Hayashi *et al.* differentiated PGCLCs, which were induced from mouse ES and iPS cells into fertile oocytes, by using *in vitro* aggregation with female gonadal somatic cells and transplantation of germ cells under the mouse ovarian bursa. The spatio-temporal factors associated with human gametogenesis *in vivo* should be further considered to develop more elaborate culture or differentiation systems in order to increase the possibility of inducing more mature germ cells from human iPS cells.

4.4. Assessing the Developmental Potential of Induced Germ Cells

In order to confirm whether induced human germ cells possess the correct biological functions, creating embryos and culturing them for a short term is indispensable prior to considering the use for clinical applications. In doing so, a subsequent biological analysis would necessitate the establishment of ES cells from the embryos. Nonetheless, these experiments are likely to raise ethical concerns owing to the fact that such embryos are created and destroyed for research purposes, not for reproduction. In some countries, creating a human embryo and monitoring the development of human embryos until the 14th day post-conception or until the beginning of the formation of the primitive streak may be permitted with approval of an institutional review board (IRB) and/or national authorities [15]. However, such human embryo experiments require sufficient data to support their use based on animal experiments to confirm scientific or medical rationality. Since non-human primate (NHP) experiments are more scientifically comparable with the human conditions than experiments in lower animals such as rodents, the data obtained from NHP experiments are likely to be required by IRB or other bodies with regard to granting permission for human embryo research.

5. Conclusions

As discussed above, human germ cell induction has advanced primarily in the male germline, progressively reaching to a final differentiation stage. Meticulously selecting human iPS cell lines with higher pluripotency and genetic integrity is expected to improve the efficiency of the formation of PGCs and entrance into meiosis. Moreover, placing the differentiated cells in culture systems similar to the niche in human gonadal tissues will likely produce not only spermatozoa, but also female germ cells that are more similar to oocytes. Further considerations of the intrinsic regulators that could be overexpressed are also likely to advance meiotic progression, complete meiosis, and functionally mature these germ cells.

Rapid advances in stem cell research will likely enable human iPS cells to differentiate into elongated spermatids or *bona fide* spermatozoa within the next decade or less. Recently, perplexing ethical and social concerns associated with the careless use of induced germ cells have been raised [15]. The use of ART with induced germ cells might facilitate posthumous conception, the birth of many siblings in a region without their knowing their genetic relationships, and facilitating the birth of a "savior sibling" to provide HLA-matched transplantation therapy for a relative. The uncontrolled or unethical use of induced germ cells would make the current problems associated with ART more complicated. As human germ cell induction from human iPS cells proceeds, appropriate deployment of this stem cell technology in ART will become an urgent matter that will need to be addressed by both researchers and the general public, including prospective parents.

Acknowledgments

The author thanks Motoko Araki for supporting figure drawing. This work was supported by the Japan Society for the Promotion of Science (JSPS) KAKENHI Grant Number 26460586 (TI).

Appendix

Assisted Reproductive Technology (ART)

ART involves several types of medical procedures to achieve pregnancy. Types of ART include IUI, oocyte retrieval, IVF, and ICSI.

Intrauterine Insemination (IUI)

At the early stage of ART, IUI is performed by placing spermatozoa inside a woman's uterus in order to facilitate fertilization.

In Vitro Fertilization (IVF)

IVF begins with the induction of ovulation via hormonal stimulation, followed by oocyte retrieval. Subsequently, the retrieved oocytes are fertilized with spermatozoa in a petri dish. The resulting embryos are cultured for three to five days following fertilization, and one or more viable embryo is transferred to the uterus.

Intracytoplasmic Sperm Injection (ICSI)

In cases of male infertility, one spermatozoon is generally injected into an oocyte to facilitate fertilization under a microscope. The embryos are cultured and transferred as in IVF.

334

Ooplasmic Transfer [23,27,28]

In cases of female infertility, ooplasm, including mitochondria from fresh, mature or immature, or cryopreserved-thawed donor oocytes are directly injected into recipient oocytes via a modified ICSI technique to enhance the viability of the oocytes. Currently, there is a moratorium on this procedure in the U.S. and Canada due to the potential health risks to the progeny.

Conflicts of Interest

The author declares no conflict of interest.

References

1. Hayashi, K.; Ohta, H.; Kurimoto, K.; Aramaki, S.; Saitou, M. Reconstitution of the mouse germ cell specification pathway in culture by pluripotent stem cells. *Cell* **2011**, *146*, 519–532.
2. Hayashi, K.; Ogushi, S.; Kurimoto, K.; Shimamoto, S.; Ohta, H.; Saitou, M. Offspring from oocytes derived from *in vitro* primordial germ cell-like cells in mice. *Science* **2012**, *338*, 971–975.
3. Clark, A.T.; Bodnar, M.S.; Fox, M.; Rodriquez, R.T.; Abeyta, M.J.; Firpo, M.T.; Pera, R.A. Spontaneous differentiation of germ cells from human embryonic stem cells *in vitro*. *Hum. Mol. Genet.* **2004**, *13*, 727–739.
4. Chen, H.F.; Kuo, H.C.; Chien, C.L.; Shun, C.T.; Yao, Y.L.; Ip, P.L.; Chuang, C.Y.; Wang, C.C.; Yang, Y.S.; Ho, H.N. Derivation, characterization and differentiation of human embryonic stem cells: Comparing serum-containing *versus* serum-free media and evidence of germ cell differentiation. *Hum. Reprod.* **2007**, *22*, 567–577.
5. Kee, K.; Gonsalves, J.M.; Clark, A.T.; Pera, R.A. Bone morphogenetic proteins induce germ cell differentiation from human embryonic stem cells. *Stem Cells Dev.* **2006**, *15*, 831–837.
6. Tilgner, K.; Atkinson, S.P.; Golebiewska, A.; Stojkovic, M.; Lako, M.; Armstrong, L. Isolation of primordial germ cells from differentiating human embryonic stem cells. *Stem Cells* **2008**, *26*, 3075–3085.
7. Bucay, N.; Yebra, M.; Cirulli, V.; Afrikanova, I.; Kaido, T.; Hayek, A.; Montgomery, A.M. A novel approach for the derivation of putative primordial germ cells and sertoli cells from human embryonic stem cells. *Stem Cells* **2009**, *27*, 68–77.
8. Park, T.S.; Galic, Z.; Conway, A.E.; Lindgren, A.; van Handel, B.J.; Magnusson, M.; Richter, L.; Teitell, M.A.; Mikkola, H.K.; Lowry, W.E.; *et al.* Derivation of primordial germ cells from human embryonic and induced pluripotent stem cells is significantly improved by coculture with human fetal gonadal cells. *Stem Cells* **2009**, *27*, 783–795.
9. Medrano, J.V.; Ramathal, C.; Nguyen, H.N.; Simon, C.; Reijo Pera, R.A. Divergent RNA-binding proteins, DAZL and VASA, induce meiotic progression in human germ cells derived *in vitro*. *Stem Cells* **2012**, *30*, 441–451.
10. Panula, S.; Medrano, J.V.; Kee, K.; Bergström, R.; Nguyen, H.N.; Byers, B.; Wilson, K.D.; Wu, J.C.; Simon, C.; Hovatta, O.; *et al.* Human germ cell differentiation from fetal- and adult-derived induced pluripotent stem cells. *Hum. Mol. Genet.* **2011**, *20*, 752–762.

11. Ramathal, C.; Durruthy-Durruthy, J.; Sukhwani, M.; Arakaki, J.E.; Turek, P.J.; Orwig, K.E.; Reijo Pera, R.A. Fate of iPSCs Derived from Azoospermic and Fertile Men following Xenotransplantation to Murine Seminiferous Tubules. *Cell Rep.* **2014**, *7*, 1284–1297.

12. Easley, C.A., IV; Phillips, B.T.; McGuire, M.M.; Barringer, J.M.; Valli, H.; Hermann, B.P.; Simerly, C.R.; Rajkovic, A.; Miki, T.; Orwig, K.E.; *et al.* Direct Differentiation of Human Pluripotent Stem Cells into Haploid Spermatogenic Cells. *Cell Rep.* **2012**, *2*, 440–446.

13. Eguizabal, C.; Montserrat, N.; Vassena, R.; Barragan, M.; Garreta, E.; Garcia-Quevedo, L.; Vidal, F.; Giorgetti, A.; Veiga, A.; Izpisua Belmonte, J.C. Complete meiosis from human induced pluripotent stem cells. *Stem Cells* **2011**, *29*, 1186–1195.

14. Weismann, A.; Newton Parker, W.; Rönnfeldt, H. *Germ-Plasm, a Theory of Heredity*; Scribner's: New York, NY, USA, 1893.

15. Ishii, T.; Pera, R.A.; Greely, H.T. Ethical and legal issues arising in research on inducing human germ cells from pluripotent stem cells. *Cell Stem Cell* **2013**, *13*, 145–148.

16. Saha, K.; Jaenisch, R. Technical challenges in using human induced pluripotent stem cells to model disease. *Cell Stem Cell* **2009**, *5*, 584–595.

17. Lee, J.; Kanatsu-Shinohara, M.; Morimoto, H.; Kazuki, Y.; Takashima, S.; Oshimura, M.; Toyokuni, S.; Shinohara, T. Genetic reconstruction of mouse spermatogonial stem cell self-renewal *in vitro* by Ras-cyclin D2 activation. *Cell Stem Cell* **2009**, *5*, 76–86.

18. Becker, G.; Butler, A.; Nachtigall, R.D. Resemblance talk: A challenge for parents whose children were conceived with donor gametes in the US. *Soc. Sci. Med.* **2005**, *61*, 1300–1309.

19. De Melo-Martín, I. The ethics of anonymous gamete donation: is there a right to know one's genetic origins? *Hastings Cent Rep.* **2014**, *44*, 28–35.

20. Meistrich, M.L. Male gonadal toxicity. *Pediatr. Blood Cancer* **2009**, *53*, 261–266.

21. Howell, S.J.; Shalet, S.M. Spermatogenesis after cancer treatment: Damage and recovery. *J. Natl. Cancer Inst. Monogr.* **2005**, *34*, 12–17.

22. Smit, M.; van Casteren, N.J.; Wildhagen, M.F.; Romijn, J.C.; Dohle, G.R. Sperm DNA integrity in cancer patients before and after cytotoxic treatment. *Hum. Reprod.* **2010**, *25*, 1877–1883.

23. Bentov, Y.; Casper, R.F. The aging oocyte—Can mitochondrial function be improved? *Fertil. Steril.* **2013**, *99*, 18–22.

24. Nagano, M.; McCarrey, J.R.; Brinster, R.L. Primate spermatogonial stem cells colonize mouse testes. *Biol. Reprod.* **2001**, *64*, 1409–1416.

25. Nagano, M.; Patrizio, P.; Brinster, R.L. Long-term survival of human spermatogonial stem cells in mouse testes. *Fertil. Steril.* **2002**, *78*, 1225–1233.

26. Hermann, B.P.; Sukhwani, M.; Hansel, M.C.; Orwig, K.E. Spermatogonial stem cells in higher primates: Are there differences from those in rodents? *Reproduction* **2010**, *139*, 479–493.

27. Levy, R.; Elder, K.; Menezo, Y. Cytoplasmic transfer in oocytes: Biochemical aspects. *Hum. Reprod. Update* **2004**, *10*, 241–250.

28. Callaway, E. Reproductive medicine: The power of three. *Nature* **2014**, *509*, 414–417.

29. Takahashi, K.; Tanabe, K.; Ohnuki, M.; Narita, M.; Ichisaka, T.; Tomoda, K.; Yamanaka, S. Induction of pluripotent stem cells from adult human fibroblasts by defined factors. *Cell* **2007**, *131*, 861–872.

30. Li, J.; Song, W.; Pan, G.; Zhou, J. Advances in understanding the cell types and approaches used for generating induced pluripotent stem cells. *J. Hematol. Oncol.* **2014**, *7*, 50.

31. Teramura, T.; Takehara, T.; Kawata, N.; Fujinami, N.; Mitani, T.; Takenoshita, M.; Matsumoto, K.; Saeki, K.; Iritani, A.; Sagawa, N.; *et al.* Primate embryonic stem cells proceed to early gametogenesis *in vitro*. *Cloning Stem Cells* **2007**, *9*, 144–156.

32. Toyooka, Y.; Tsunekawa, N.; Akasu, R.; Noce, T. Embryonic stem cells can form germ cells *in vitro*. *Proc. Natl. Acad. Sci. USA* **2003**, *100*, 11457–11462.

33. Geijsen, N.; Horoschak, M.; Kim, K.; Gribnau, J.; Eggan, K.; Daley, G.Q. Derivation of embryonic germ cells and male gametes from embryonic stem cells. *Nature* **2004**, *427*, 148–154.

34. Nayernia, K.; Nolte, J.; Michelmann, H.W.; Lee, J.H.; Rathsack, K.; Drusenheimer, N.; Dev, A.; Wulf, G.; Ehrmann, I.E.; Elliott, D.J.; *et al. In vitro*—Differentiated embryonic stem cells give rise to male gametes that can generate offspring mice. *Dev. Cell* **2006**, *11*, 125–132.

35. Eguizabal, C.; Shovlin, T.C.; Durcova-Hills, G.; Surani, A.; McLaren, A. Generation of primordial germ cells from pluripotent stem cells. *Differentiation* **2009**, *78*, 116–123.

36. Kanatsu-Shinohara, M.; Ogonuki, N.; Inoue, K.; Miki, H.; Ogura, A.; Toyokuni, S.; Shinohara, T. Long-term proliferation in culture and germline transmission of mouse male germline stem cells. *Biol. Reprod.* **2003**, *69*, 612–616.

37. Hermann, B.P.; Sukhwani, M.; Winkler, F.; Pascarella, J.N.; Peters, K.A.; Sheng, Y.; Valli, H.; Rodriguez, M.; Ezzelarab, M.; Dargo, G.; *et al.* Spermatogonial stem cell transplantation into rhesus testes regenerates spermatogenesis producing functional sperm. *Cell Stem Cell* **2012**, *11*, 715–726.

38. Amariglio, N.; Hirshberg, A.; Scheithauer, B.W.; Cohen, Y.; Loewenthal, R.; Trakhtenbrot, L.; Paz, N.; Koren-Michowitz, M.; Waldman, D.; Leider-Trejo, L.; *et al.* Donor-derived brain tumor following neural stem cell transplantation in an ataxia telangiectasia patient. *PLoS Med.* **2009**, *6*, e1000029.

39. Antinori, S.; Versaci, C.; Dani, G.; Antinori, M.; Pozza, D.; Selman, H.A. Fertilization with human testicular spermatids: Four successful pregnancies. *Hum. Reprod.* **1997**, *12*, 286–291.

40. Sofikitis, N.V.; Yamamoto, Y.; Miyagawa, I.; Mekras, G.; Mio, Y.; Toda, T.; Antypas, S.; Kawamura, H.; Kanakas, N.; Antoniou, N.; *et al.* Ooplasmic injection of elongating spermatids for the treatment of non-obstructive azoospermia. *Hum. Reprod.* **1998**, *13*, 709–714.

41. Yamanaka, K.; Sofikitis, N.V.; Miyagawa, I.; Yamamoto, Y.; Toda, T.; Antypas, S.; Dimitriadis, D.; Takenaka, M.; Taniguchi, K.; Takahashi, K.; *et al.* Ooplasmic round spermatid nuclear injection procedures as an experimental treatment for nonobstructive azoospermia. *J. Assist. Reprod. Genet.* **1997**, *14*, 55–62.

42. Levran, D.; Nahum, H.; Farhi, J.; Weissman, A. Poor outcome with round spermatid injection in azoospermic patients with maturation arrest. *Fertil. Steril.* **2000**, *74*, 443–449.

43. Vicdan, K.; Isik, A.Z.; Delilbasi, L. Development of blastocyst-stage embryos after round spermatid injection in patients with complete spermiogenesis failure. *J. Assist. Reprod. Genet.* **2001**, *18*, 78–86.

44. Hübner, K.; Fuhrmann, G.; Christenson, L.K.; Kehler, J.; Reinbold, R.; de La Fuente, R.; Wood, J.; Strauss, J.F., III; Boiani, M.; Schöler, H.R. Derivation of oocytes from mouse embryonic stem cells. *Science* **2003**, *300*, 1251–1256.

45. Novak, I.; Lightfoot, D.A.; Wang, H.; Eriksson, A.; Mahdy, E.; Höög, C. Mouse embryonic stem cells form follicle-like ovarian structures but do not progress through meiosis. *Stem Cells* **2006**, *24*, 1931–1936.

46. Lacham-Kaplan, O.; Chy, H.; Trounson, A. Testicular cell conditioned medium supports differentiation of embryonic stem cells into ovarian structures containing oocytes. *Stem Cells* **2006**, *24*, 266–273.

47. Qing, T.; Shi, Y.; Qin, H.; Ye, X.; Wei, W.; Liu, H.; Ding, M.; Deng, H. Induction of oocyte-like cells from mouse embryonic stem cells by co-culture with ovarian granulosa cells. *Differentiation* **2007**, *75*, 902–911.

48. Nicholas, C.R.; Haston, K.M.; Grewall, A.K.; Longacre, T.A.; Reijo Pera, R.A. Transplantation directs oocyte maturation from embryonic stem cells and provides a therapeutic strategy for female infertility. *Hum. Mol. Genet.* **2009**, *18*, 4376–4389.

49. Felici, M.D. Origin, Migration, and Proliferation of Human Primordial Germ Cells. *Oogenesis*; Springer: London, UK, 2013.

50. Sadri-Ardekani, H.; Mizrak, S.C.; van Daalen, S.K.; Korver, C.M.; Roepers-Gajadien, H.L.; Koruji, M.; Hovingh, S.; de Reijke, T.M.; de la Rosette, J.J.; van der Veen, F.; *et al.* Propagation of human spermatogonial stem cells *in vitro*. *JAMA* **2009**, *302*, 2127–2134.

51. Zuckerman, S. The number of oocytes in the mature ovary. *Recent Prog. Horm. Res.* **1951**, *6*, 63–109.

52. Johnson, J.; Canning, J.; Kaneko, T.; Pru, J.K.; Tilly, J.L. Germline stem cells and follicular renewal in the postnatal mammalian ovary. *Nature* **2004**, *428*, 145–150.

53. Johnson, J.; Bagley, J.; Skaznik-Wikiel, M.; Lee, H.J.; Adams, G.B.; Niikura, Y.; Tschudy, K.S.; Tilly, J.C.; Cortes, M.L.; Forkert, R.; *et al.* Oocyte generation in adult mammalian ovaries by putative germ cells in bone marrow and peripheral blood. *Cell* **2005**, *122*, 303–315.

54. Zou, K.; Yuan, Z.; Yang, Z.; Luo, H.; Sun, K.; Zhou, L.; Xiang, J.; Shi, L.; Yu, Q.; Zhang, Y.; *et al.* Production of offspring from a germline stem cell line derived from neonatal ovaries. *Nat. Cell Biol.* **2009**, *11*, 631–636.

55. White, Y.A.; Woods, D.C.; Takai, Y.; Ishihara, O.; Seki, H.; Tilly, J.L. Oocyte formation by mitotically active germ cells purified from ovaries of reproductive-age women. *Nat. Med.* **2012**, *18*, 413–421.

56. Eggan, K.; Jurga, S.; Gosden, R.; Min, I.M.; Wagers, A.J. Ovulated oocytes in adult mice derive from non-circulating germ cells. *Nature* **2006**, *441*, 1109–1114.

57. Begum, S.; Papaioannou, V.E.; Gosden, R.G. The oocyte population is not renewed in transplanted or irradiated adult ovaries. *Hum. Reprod.* **2008**, *23*, 2326–2330.

58. Zhang, H.; Zheng, W.; Shen, Y.; Adhikari, D.; Ueno, H.; Liu, K. Experimental evidence showing that no mitotically active female germline progenitors exist in postnatal mouse ovaries. *Proc. Natl. Acad. Sci. USA* **2012**, *109*, 12580–12585.

59. Taapken, S.M.; Nisler, B.S.; Newton, M.A.; Sampsell-Barron, T.L.; Leonhard, K.A.; McIntire, E.M.; Montgomery, K.D. Karotypic abnormalities in human induced pluripotent stem cells and embryonic stem cells. *Nat. Biotechnol.* **2011**, *29*, 313–314.

60. Mayshar, Y.; Ben-David, U.; Lavon, N.; Biancotti, J.C.; Yakir, B.; Clark, A.T.; Plath, K.; Lowry, W.E.; Benvenisty, N. Identification and classification of chromosomal aberrations in human induced pluripotent stem cells. *Cell Stem Cell* **2010**, *7*, 521–531.

61. Amps, K.; Andrews, P.W.; Anyfantis, G.; Armstrong, L.; Avery, S.; Baharvand, H.; Baker, J.; Baker, D.; Munoz, M.B.; Beil, S.; *et al.* Screening ethnically diverse human embryonic stem cells identifies a chromosome 20 minimal amplicon conferring growth advantage. *Nat. Biotechnol.* **2011**, *29*, 1132–1144.

62. Martins-Taylor, K.; Nisler, B.S.; Taapken, S.M.; Compton, T.; Crandall, L.; Montgomery, K.D.; Lalande, M.; Xu, R.H. Recurrent copy number variations in human induced pluripotent stem cells. *Nat. Biotechnol.* **2011**, *29*, 488–491.

63. Laurent, L.C.; Ulitsky, I.; Slavin, I.; Tran, H.; Schork, A.; Morey, R.; Lynch, C.; Harness, J.V.; Lee, S.; Barrero, M.J.; *et al.* Dynamic changes in the copy number of pluripotency and cell proliferation genes in human ESCs and iPSCs during reprogramming and time in culture. *Cell Stem Cell* **2011**, *8*, 106–118.

64. Hussein, S.M.; Batada, N.N.; Vuoristo, S.; Ching, R.W.; Autio, R.; Närvä, E.; Ng, S.; Sourour, M.; Hämäläinen, R.; Olsson, C.; *et al.* Copy number variation and selection during reprogramming to pluripotency. *Nature* **2011**, *471*, 58–62.

65. Song, G.J.; Lewis, V. Mitochondrial DNA integrity and copy number in sperm from infertile men. *Fertil. Steril.* **2008**, *90*, 2238–2244.

66. Reynier, P.; May-Panloup, P.; Chrétien, M.F.; Morgan, C.J.; Jean, M.; Savagner, F.; Barrière, P.; Malthièry, Y. Mitochondrial DNA content affects the fertilizability of human oocytes. *Mol. Hum. Reprod.* **2001**, *7*, 425–429.

67. Barritt, J.A.; Kokot, M.; Cohen, J.; Steuerwald, N.; Brenner, C.A. Quantification of human ooplasmic mitochondria. *Reprod. Biomed. Online* **2002**, *4*, 243–247.

68. May-Panloup, P.; Chrétien, M.F.; Jacques, C.; Vasseur, C.; Malthièry, Y.; Reynier, P. Low oocyte mitochondrial DNA content in ovarian insufficiency. *Hum. Reprod.* **2005**, *20*, 593–597.

69. Steuerwald, N.; Barritt, J.A.; Adler, R.; Malter, H.; Schimmel, T.; Cohen, J.; Brenner, C.A. Quantification of mtDNA in single oocytes, polar bodies and subcellular components by real-time rapid cycle fluorescence monitored PCR. *Zygote* **2000**, *8*, 209–215.

70. Prigione, A.; Lichtner, B.; Kuhl, H.; Struys, E.A.; Wamelink, M.; Lehrach, H.; Ralser, M.; Timmermann, B.; Adjaye, J. Human induced pluripotent stem cells harbor homoplasmic and heteroplasmic mitochondrial DNA mutations while maintaining human embryonic stem cell-like metabolic reprogramming. *Stem Cells* **2011**, *29*, 1338–1348.

71. Van Haute, L.; Spits, C.; Geens, M.; Seneca, S.; Sermon, K. Human embryonic stem cells commonly display large mitochondrial DNA deletions. *Nat. Biotechnol.* **2013**, *31*, 20–23.

72. Wahlestedt, M.; Ameur, A.; Moraghebi, R.; Norddahl, G.L.; Sten, G.; Woods, N.B.; Bryder, D. Somatic cells with a heavy mitochondrial DNA mutational load render induced pluripotent stem cells with distinct differentiation defects. *Stem Cells* **2014**, *32*, 1173–1182.

73. Nazor, K.L.; Altun, G.; Lynch, C.; Tran, H.; Harness, J.V.; Slavin, I.; Garitaonandia, I.; Müller, F.J.; Wang, Y.C.; Boscolo, F.S.; *et al.* Recurrent variations in DNA methylation in human pluripotent stem cells and their differentiated derivatives. *Cell Stem Cell* **2012**, *10*, 620–634.

74. Lister, R.; Pelizzola, M.; Kida, Y.S.; Hawkins, R.D.; Nery, J.R.; Hon, G.; Antosiewicz-Bourget, J.; O'Malley, R.; Castanon, R.; Klugman, S.; *et al.* Hotspots of aberrant epigenomic reprogramming in human induced pluripotent stem cells. *Nature* **2011**, *471*, 68–73.

75. Ohi, Y.; Qin, H.; Hong, C.; Blouin, L.; Polo, J.M.; Guo, T.; Qi, Z.; Downey, S.L.; Manos, P.D.; Rossi, D.J.; *et al.* Incomplete DNA methylation underlies a transcriptional memory of somatic cells in human iPS cells. *Nat. Cell Biol.* **2011**, *13*, 541–549.

76. Tesar, P.J.; Chenoweth, J.G.; Brook, F.A.; Davies, T.J.; Evans, E.P.; Mack, D.L.; Gardner, R.L.; McKay, R.D. New cell lines from mouse epiblast share defining features with human embryonic stem cells. *Nature* **2007**, *448*, 196–199.

77. Brons, I.G.; Smithers, L.E.; Trotter, M.W.; Rugg-Gunn, P.; Sun, B.; Chuva de Sousa Lopes, S.M.; Howlett, S.K.; Clarkson, A.; Ahrlund-Richter, L.; Pedersen, R.A.; *et al.* Derivation of pluripotent epiblast stem cells from mammalian embryos. *Nature* **2007**, *448*, 191–195.

78. Marks, H.; Kalkan, T.; Menafra, R.; Denissov, S.; Jones, K.; Hofemeister, H.; Nichols, J.; Kranz, A.; Stewart, A.F.; Smith, A.; *et al.* The transcriptional and epigenomic foundations of ground state pluripotency. *Cell* **2012**, *149*, 590–604.

79. Gafni, O.; Weinberger, L.; Mansour, A.A.; Manor, Y.S.; Chomsky, E.; Ben-Yosef, D.; Kalma, Y.; Viukov, S.; Maza, I.; Zviran, A.; *et al.* Derivation of novel human ground state naive pluripotent stem cells. *Nature* **2013**, *504*, 282–286.

80. Chan, Y.S.; Göke, J.; Ng, J.H.; Lu, X.; Gonzales, K.A.; Tan, C.P.; Tng, W.Q.; Hong, Z.Z.; Lim, Y.S.; Ng, H.H. Induction of a human pluripotent state with distinct regulatory circuitry that resembles preimplantation epiblast. *Cell Stem Cell* **2013**, *13*, 663–675.

81. Theunissen, T.W.; Powell, B.E.; Wang, H.; Mitalipova, M.; Faddah, D.A.; Reddy, J.; Fan, Z.P.; Maetzel, D.; Ganz, K.; Shi, L.; *et al.* Systematic Identification of Culture Conditions for Induction and Maintenance of Naive Human Pluripotency. *Cell Stem Cell* **2014**, doi:10.1016/j.stem.2014.07.002.

82. Li, P.; Hu, H.; Yang, S.; Tian, R.; Zhang, Z.; Zhang, W.; Ma, M.; Zhu, Y.; Guo, X.; Huang, Y.; *et al.* Differentiation of induced pluripotent stem cells into male germ cells *in vitro* through embryoid body formation and retinoic acid or testosterone induction. *Biomed. Res. Int.* **2013**, *2013*, doi:10.1155/2013/608728.

83. Svechnikov, K.; Landreh, L.; Weisser, L.; Izzo, G.; Colón, E.; Svechnikova, I.; Söder, O. Origin, Development and Regulation of Human Leydig Cells. *Horm. Res. Paediatr.* **2010**, *73*, 93–101.

84. Rebourcet, D.; O'Shaughnessy, P.J.; Pitetti, J.L.; Monteiro, A.; O'Hara, L.; Milne, L.; Tsai, Y.T.; Cruickshanks, L.; Riethmacher, D.; Guillou, F.; *et al.* Sertoli cells control peritubular myoid cell fate and support adult Leydig cell development in the prepubertal testis. *Development* **2014**, *141*, 2139–2149.

Chapter9:
Genetic Disorders

Comparing ESC and iPSC—Based Models for Human Genetic Disorders

Tomer Halevy and Achia Urbach

Abstract: Traditionally, human disorders were studied using animal models or somatic cells taken from patients. Such studies enabled the analysis of the molecular mechanisms of numerous disorders, and led to the discovery of new treatments. Yet, these systems are limited or even irrelevant in modeling multiple genetic diseases. The isolation of human embryonic stem cells (ESCs) from diseased blastocysts, the derivation of induced pluripotent stem cells (iPSCs) from patients' somatic cells, and the new technologies for genome editing of pluripotent stem cells have opened a new window of opportunities in the field of disease modeling, and enabled studying diseases that couldn't be modeled in the past. Importantly, despite the high similarity between ESCs and iPSCs, there are several fundamental differences between these cells, which have important implications regarding disease modeling. In this review we compare ESC-based models to iPSC-based models, and highlight the advantages and disadvantages of each system. We further suggest a roadmap for how to choose the optimal strategy to model each specific disorder.

Reprinted from *J. Clin. Med.* Cite as: Halevy, T.; Urbach, A. Comparing ESC and iPSC—Based Models for Human Genetic Disorders. *J. Clin. Med.* **2014**, *3*, 1146–1162.

1. Introduction

Pluripotent stem cells have an unlimited self-renewal capacity and can differentiate into virtually any adult cell type [1] and even some extra-embryonic tissues [2,3]. These features make human pluripotent stem cells (hPSCs) a useful tool for disease modeling, which overcomes limitations observed in animal and adult human cellular models. While the use of animal models proved to be extremely valuable and successful in many cases [4], there are numerous diseases, such as Lesch-Nyhan syndrome [5], Turner syndrome [6] and Fragile X syndrome [7], that cannot be studied using animal models due to species-specific differences. The use of mature cells from patients can solve the species-specificity issue but this strategy is limited by the fact that it enables studying only a few types of cells at a specific developmental stage, and in many cases requires also transformation of the cells to enable their proliferation in culture. By contrast, due to their unique properties, hPSCs enable exploration of different types of cells, to study the effect of a specific mutation on differentiation or development and can proliferate *in vitro* without additional transformation. Indeed, since the generation of the first human embryonic stem cells (ESCs) based model (a model for Lesch-Nyhan syndrome by targeting of the *HPRT* gene in human ESCs) [5] dozens of disease models were generated by reprogramming of somatic cells from patients [1], by derivation of mutant ESCs from affected embryos diagnosed by *pre*-implantation genetic diagnosis (PGD) or by genetic manipulation of normal ESCs [8] (see Figure 1). While some models were used as a "proof of concept" to demonstrate that hPSCs can be derived from a wide range of disorders [9–11] or to show the feasibility of the mutant pluripotent cells to be used as a disease model [12], other models were further used to obtain novel mechanistic or physiological insights regarding the disorders. One example is a model for Amyotrophic Lateral Sclerosis (ALS) by Kiskinis *et al.* [13].

Figure 1. Human pluripotent stem cell-based models for genetic disorders can be generated by different techniques. Mutated human pluripotent stem cells can be derived by genetic manipulation of normal pluripotent stem cells, from affected embryos (identified by PGD), or from adult patients (by reprogramming of somatic cells).

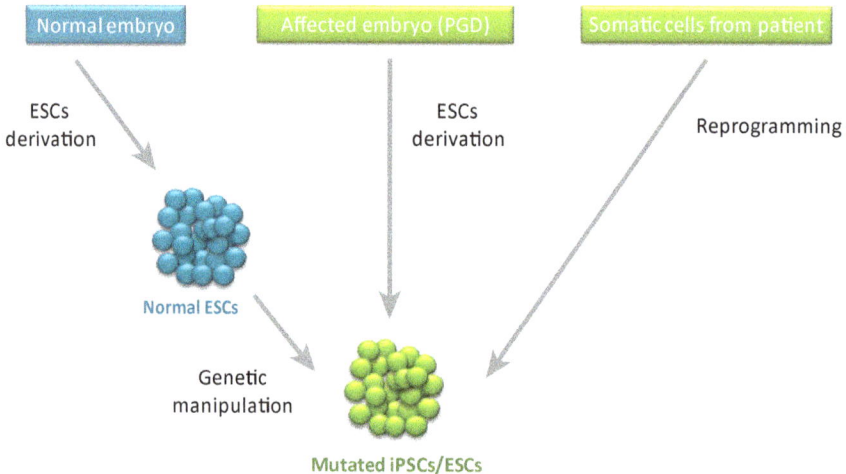

The general differences between ESCs and induced pluripotent stem cells (iPSCs) and the utilization of hPSCs for disease modeling has been discussed extensively in the literature [1,14–16]. In this review we will focus on the differences between ESC-based models and iPSC-based models, and discuss the effect of genome editing technologies on the field of disease modeling.

2. ESCs *vs.* iPSCs in Disease Modeling

Theoretically, a given disorder can be equally modeled by iPSCs and by ESCs, as both are pluripotent stem cells. However, several reasons have made iPSCs derived from patients the system of choice:

(1) The use of normal human ESCs to model a genetic disorder requires genetic manipulation to induce the specific mutation that one would like to study. The way to obtain a mutation that will be identical to the natural occurring mutation, seen in patients, is by genome editing. However, the efficiency of genome editing in human ESCs, before the establishment of gene targeting technologies as discussed below, was extremely low (especially in cases where a homozygous mutation was required) [17] and derivation of iPSCs that already contain the specific mutation obviates the needs for this inefficient process.

(2) While the above mentioned limitation can be overcome by derivation of mutant ESCs from affected embryos identified by Preimplantation Genetic Diagnosis (PGD), this procedure is limited to a small number of diseases in which PGD is normally preformed, and can be done only in labs that are associated with *in vitro* fertilization (IVF) units.

(3) By contrast to iPSCs from affected individuals, in the case of ESCs based models, the correlation between the genotype and the phenotype is not obvious, and the penetrance of the mutation might be low as a results of specific "protective" genetic background [18].

(4) Lastly, in some countries the use of human ESCs is limited or banned due to ethical and religious concerns regarding the use of human embryos for research purposes as was discussed by others [19,20].

Nevertheless, possible drawbacks in modeling genetic disorders by iPSCs suggest that some disorders or specific aspects within a given disease might be better modeled in ESCs than iPSCs. The generation of a faithful iPSC-based model might be disrupted due to the following reasons (see Figure 2): (1) Incomplete reprogramming as a result of "Epigenetic memory" of the original somatic cells [21–23]; (2) Mutations accumulated during the reprogramming process [24] and deleterious effects (such as chromosomal instability, [25]) of the reprogramming process on the genome integrity of iPSCs; (3) Genetic aberrations that significantly decrease the reprogramming efficiency [26]; (4) The absence of appropriate sources of somatic cells such as in the cases of genetic aberration and aneuploidies that lead to very early embryonic lethality [6].

To demonstrate the commonalities and differences between ESC- and iPSC-based models, we compared models for X-linked, autosomal recessive and autosomal dominant disorders in which disease-related phenotypes were observed in both models (Table 1). As expected, in some cases the ESC-based models and the iPSC-based models were similar (spinal muscular atrophy [27,28], Shwachman-Dimond syndrome [29], long QT syndrome [30], and some aspects of myotonic dystrophy [31,32]). However, in other cases the iPSCs were limited in their capacity to model the disorder or specific aspects within the disorders. To demonstrate some of these cases, and to discuss the principles behind them, we will focus on the following disorders: Turner syndrome, Fanconi Anemia, fragile X syndrome and Huntington's disease.

Figure 2. Limitations in the generation of iPSC-based disease models. The "X-axis" in this scheme depicts the specific stages during the formation of iPSC-based models that might be affected by the different factors that discussed in the main text.

Early lethality

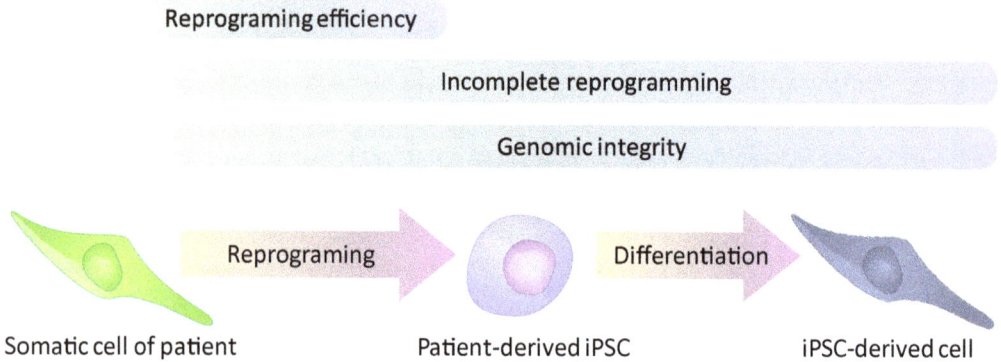

Reprograming efficiency

Incomplete reprogramming

Genomic integrity

Reprograming → Differentiation

Somatic cell of patient   Patient-derived iPSC   iPSC-derived cell

3. Turner Syndrome

X chromosome monosomy (XO) is one of the most common chromosomal abnormalities, as 3% of all pregnancies start with XO embryos [33]. Yet, approximately 99% of the XO embryos undergo miscarriage during the first trimester [33,34]. The 1% that survive to term are born with Turner syndrome which is characterized by several phenotypes; the most common among them are growth failure, gonadal dysgensis and webbed neck [34]. While Turner syndrome derived iPSCs can be used in order to study the phenotypes of the patient (pending the availability of the required differentiation protocols), they might be problematic in modeling the early lethality of XO embryos, as they represent the exceptional 1% of the cases that survived to term.

In agreement with this notion, gene expression analysis of XO ESCs (derived by screening for ESCs with normal karyotype that lost one of their X chromosomes) revealed a significant effect of X chromosome monosomy on the expression of placental genes and suggests that the reason for the early lethality is abnormal placental development [6]. By contrast, there was almost no effect of X chromosome monosomy on placental gene expression in iPSCs derived from Turner syndrome patients, and even from amniotes of a 20 weeks old embryo [35]. The results suggest that Turner syndrome iPSCs represent the rare cases in which the embryo survived despite the XO karyotype.

Table 1. Comparison between ESCs and iPSC models for human genetic disorders.

Disease		ESCs		iPSCs		ESCs vs. iPSCs
		Reference (ref #)	Method of Derivation of Mutate ESCs	Reference (ref #)	Reprogramming Method	
X-linked	Fragile X	Eiges 2007 [7]	PGD	Urbach 2009 [36]	Retroviruses	**ESCs > iPSCs** In iPSCs *FMR1* is already methylated and inactivated (due to an epigenetic memory), thus iPSCs can't be used to study the molecular mechanism related to *FMR1* gene silencing in Fragile X **ESCs < iPSCs** In iPSCs the *FMR1* gene is already inactivated, therefore iPSCs are a better system to study the effect of the gene silencing on neuronal development
	Rett syndrome	Li 2013 [37]	Gene targeting by TALEN	Cheung 2011 [38]	Retroviruses	**ESCs > iPSCs** Normal Female patients are heterogeneous in regard to the expression of *MECP2* (due to random X inactivation) but the iPSCs are homogeneous population of mutant cells (due to epigenetic memory of the inactivated X chromosome)
				Marchetto 2010 [39]	Retroviruses	**ESCs ~ iPSCs** iPSCs are heterogeneous population (Random X inactivation). Different phenotype has been examined in ESCs and iPSC's The discrepancy between the two iPSCs models illustrated the complexity of X inactivation in reprogramming
	Turner syndrome	Urbach 2011 [6]	Screen for XO colonies	Li 2012 [35]	Retroviruses and Lentiviruses	**ESCs > iPSCs** iPSCs represents the exceptional 1% of patients that survived to term and therefor can't be used in order to study the effect of X chromosome loss on early lethality

Table 1. *Cont.*

Disease		ESCs		iPSCs		ESCs vs. iPSCs
		Reference (ref #)	Method of Derivation of Mutate ESCs	Reference (ref #)	Reprogramming Method	
Autosomal recessive	Fanconi Anemia	Yung 2013 [25]; Tulpule 2010 [40]	Knockdown of FANCA and FANCD2	Yung 2013 [25]	Lentiviruses	**ESCs > iPSCs** Very low reprogramming efficiency. The mutated iPSCs have many chromosomal aberrations and didn't give rise to normal teratoma. Both ESCs and iPSCs showed hematopoietic phenotypes related to FA
		Liu 2014 [41]	Gene targeting by TALEN	Liu 2014 [41]	Episomal reprogramming	**ESCs ~ iPSCs** Very low reprogramming efficiency, however, iPSCs have normal karyotype and normal characterization of pluripotent cells. Both ESCs and iPSCs demonstrated FA related phenotypes
	Spinal muscular atrophy	Wang 2013 [27]	Knockdown of SMN	Ebert 2009 [28]	Lentiviruses	**ESCs ~ iPSCs** Different phenotypes has been examined in ESCs and iPSCs Both models demonstrated abnormal motor neuron phenotypes
	Shwachman-Diamond syndrome	Tulpule 2013 [29]	Knockdown of SBDS	Tulpule 2013 [29]	Retroviruses	**ESCs ~ iPSCs** Both models demonstrated SDS related phenotype
Autosomal dominant	Long QT	Bellin 2013 [30]	Gene targeting	Bellin 2013 [30]	Retroviruses	**ESCs ~ iPSCs** Both models demonstrated Long QT related phenotypes. ESCs derived cardiomyocytes were electrophysiologically less mature than those derived from the iPSCs. Could be explained due to inherent variability between specific iPSCs and ESCs lines

Table 1. *Cont.*

Disease		ESCs		iPSCs		ESCs vs. iPSCs
		Reference (ref #)	Method of Derivation of Mutate ESCs	Reference (ref #)	Reprogramming Method	
Autosomal dominant	Huntington's disease	Lu 2013 [42]	Over-expression of HTTexon1 with 23, 73 or 145 glutamine repeats in HESCs	HD iPSC Consortium 2012 [43]	Lentiviruses (OSKM + Nanog + Lin28)	**ESCs > iPSCs** (Based on Lu *et al.*) mHTT aggregated appeared only in ESCs based model
	Myotonic Dystrophy	Seriola 2011 [31]		Du 2013 [32]	Retroviruses	**ESCs ~ iPSCs** TNR becomes stable upon differentiation in ES and iPS. Down-regulation of MMR genes upon differentiation was observed only in ESCs

Representative examples of ESC and iPSC models for X linked, autosomal recessive and autosomal dominant disorders. As the primary intention of this review is to discuss the differences between the two model systems and to highlight cases in which the ESCs model is a better choice than the iPSCs model, only the characteristics or phenotypes that are relevance for the direct comparison between the two models were mentioned in the table. We refer the readers to the original papers to learn more details about each model. When several studies for a specific disorder were relevant for the comparison between the systems we cited all relevant studies.

4. Fanconi Anemia

Fanconi Anemia (FA) is an autosomal recessive disorder caused by a mutation in any of the 16 *FANC* genes and characterized by congenital abnormalities, cancer predisposition and progressive bone marrow failure [44]. Initial attempts to reprogram somatic cells from FA patients into iPSCs failed unless using fibroblasts that were first genetically corrected [45]. These results suggested that the FA pathway is essential for the reprogramming pathway (probably due to defective DNA repair and genomic instability of FA cells) and therefore that FA can't be easily modeled by iPSCs. However, further attempts to reprogram "uncorrected" somatic cells from FA patients under hypoxic conditions [26], and even under normoxic conditions [25], showed that iPSCs can be derived from FA somatic cells, albeit in a very low efficiency and revealed that "...somatic cells harboring mutations that render the FA pathway defective are resistant but not refractory to reprogramming" [26]. Nevertheless, significant chromosomal aberration in uncorrected FA-iPSCs [25], but not in FA-iPSCs derived from "corrected" somatic cells [26] or in human ESCs with stable knockdown of FANCC [25] suggests that the FA pathway is required to prevent DNA damage and chromosomal instabilities associated with the reprogramming process. The severe aneuploidy in the uncorrected FA-iPSCs but not in the ESC-based model for Fanconi anemia suggests that ESCs and not iPSCs should be used to study FA. Surprisingly though, it has been recently shown [41] that FA-iPSCs with a normal karyotype can be derived from FA somatic cells upon episomal reprogramming. Moreover, the FA-iPSCs were very similar to FA-ESCs that were generated by gene targeting of the *FANCA* gene using the TALEN mediated gene targeting [38]. The FA-iPSCs and the FA-ESCs were extensively studied and compared to isogenic control cells (the original ESCs and target corrected FA-iPSCs) and proved to be a very useful model for different aspects of Fanconi anemia. While the reasons for the differences in the chromosomal stability between the viruses mediated reprogramming and the integration-free episomal mediated reprogramming are still not clear, these results indicate that in some cases, the reprogramming method itself might have a dramatic effect on the quality of the iPSCs and thus, should be taken under consideration when choosing to generate a disease model by reprogramming of somatic cells from patients.

5. Fragile X Syndrome

Fragile X syndrome (FXS) is a trinucleotide repeat disorder and is the leading cause of inherited intellectual disability in males, affecting approximately one in every four thousand boys and one in eight thousand girls worldwide [46–49]. The mutation leading to the syndrome is a trinucleotide CGG expansion at the 5' untranslated region of the fragile X mental retardation 1 (*FMR1*) gene, which is accompanied by epigenetic changes, resulting in the silencing of the gene [49,50]. The product of the *FMR1* gene is the fragile X mental retardation protein (FMRP) which is most abundant in the brain and testis and plays a major role in synaptic plasticity [51].

In 2007 human ESCs from FXS affected embryos (FXS-ESCs) were derived for the first time through PGD and enabled the study of the development of the disease [7]. Interestingly, although carrying the full mutation, FXS-ESCs showed both *FMR1* mRNA expression and the presence of FMRP. This finding showed that the transcriptional silencing of *FMR1* is a developmentally regulated process. Moreover, the study indicated that *FMR1* is silenced in FXS embryos only during development and that the inactivation is initiated by chromatin modifications prior to DNA methylation [7]. Other studies on FXS-ESCs supported the finding that *FMR1* is expressed in full mutation embryos and is silenced only during differentiation and further demonstrated that *FMR1* plays an important role in early stages of neurogenesis and synaptic function [52,53]. Therefore, FX-ESCs are invaluable to study many aspects of FXS, first and foremost the epigenetic silencing mechanism. However, there are also limitations in the FX-ESCs model: FXS is represented by profound variability in patients, ranging from the varying length of the repeats, through the methylation levels, and to the neurological phenotype itself. The degree of intellectual impairment also varies between different individuals, as only about 30% of full mutation carriers display autistic behavior [54,55]. Additionally, some carriers of the full mutation allele do not display any of the syndrome's phenotypes [56,57]. As this variability is not inherited from the parents and is detected only after PGD analysis, the probability of acquiring numerous human embryonic stem cells displaying the entire spectrum of genetic and epigenetic differences is quite small and may take several years.

In contrast to the *FMR1* expression seen in FXS-ESCs, it seems that in FXS derived iPSCs (FXS-iPSCs), despite successful reprogramming of patients derived fibroblasts, the *FMR1* gene is resistant to the process and remains methylated and silent [36,58,59]. Thus, while the FXS model in human ESCs demonstrated the temporal silencing of *FMR1*, in FXS-iPSCs *FMR1* was already inactive in the undifferentiated state. This fundamental difference between FXS-ESCs and FXS-iPSCs controls the choice of model according to the question being asked. In order to better understand the different aspects of the initiating steps of the *FMR1* silencing such as CGG methylation and the epigenetic silencing, one should use the FXS-ESC model. On the other hand, if one wishes to model neural development, screen for new drugs or understand the CGG expansion mechanism it is preferential to use the FXS-iPSC model to understand the effects of lack of FMRP on developing neurons, as we do not fully understand at which time point during the differentiation process *FMR1* is silenced in ESCs *in vitro*. One example using FX-iPSCs to model Fragile X syndrome is a study aimed to evaluate the reactivation of *FMR1* in FXS-iPSCs and their neuronal derivatives through epigenetic modulation drugs. This study showed not only that reactivation is possible but also uncovered additional layers of epigenetic control on *FMR1* [60].

6. Huntington's Disease

Huntington's disease (HD) is an autosomal dominant neurological disorder caused by a trinucleotide repeat expansion and characterized by a late onset progressive neurodegeneration ending with death [61,62]. In HD, an expansion of a CAG repeat in the first exon of the Huntingtin (*HTT*) gene leads to a toxic gain of function activity of the mutant Huntingtin protein (mHTT), containing an increased number of polyglutamines at the *N* terminus [62]. These polyglutamine tails are then cleaved and accumulate as aggregates in the nuclei of neurons [63].

During the past few years, several groups have successfully created iPSC models for HD (HD-iPSCs) [11,43,64,65]. Some have further differentiated HD-iPSCs to neurons and showed increased caspase activity of neural precursors upon growth factor deprivation [64] or increased lysosomal activity in both HD-iPSCs and derived neurons [65]. The most comprehensive work done with the HD-iPSCs model system was performed by the HD-iPSC Consortium, in which several HD-iPSC lines were created and analyzed by a group of different labs [43]. In this work, HD-iPSCs were also differentiated into neural stem cells (NSCs) and neurons. HD-derived NSCs showed differential gene expression accompanied with changes at the protein level as well. Other changes observed were compromised energy metabolism, inability to fire action potential and increased cell death. Neurons also display increased death under different stress conditions most notably in lines containing longer repeats.

HD-iPSCs provide a useful model, however, it was never shown that they accumulate any insoluble aggregates, and thus cannot be used to study the formation and pathological contribution of this aggregates to the development of the disease. In order to study this aspect of the syndrome, normal ESCs were genetically engineered to express the polyglutamine repeats [42]. Neurons derived from these HD-ESCs matured over a period of several months and showed the polyglutamine aggregates. Similar to HD-iPSCs, HD-ESCs derived neurons exhibited progressive death under stress conditions. It was also shown using this model that reduction of mHTT by just 10% is sufficient to prevent toxicity and lowering the expression levels of *HTT* by up to 90% had no effect on neurons, opening the possibility to screen for new drugs to control the levels of mHTT. Thus, HD-ESCs may provide a stronger tool than HD-iPSCs in our understanding of the initiation and progression of the pathology of HD. However, work done on ESCs derived directly from an embryo with HD did not show the formation of polyglutamine aggregates [66]. Furthermore, HD embryos from PGD are not readily available, and due to the fact that HD is a late onset disease, we do not know the ultimate phenotype of these never developed embryos. In this case, more work should be done on both HD-ESCs and HD-iPSCs in an attempt to obtain more of the molecular phenotypes characteristic of the disease to create a better model system.

7. Disease Modeling by Gene Targeting of hPSCs

As mentioned above, hPSCs based models can be generated by the derivation of ESCs from affected embryos diagnosed by PGD or by genetic manipulation of normal hPSC cells. Down-regulation or over-expression of specific genes can be easily achieved by RNAi technologies (for down regulation) or by introduction of exogenous genes into the genome (for over-expression). While these methods proved to be very informative in some cases, they can't mimic the natural occurring mutation in the patients and therefore the relevance of the finding to the disease might be questionable in other cases. To overcome this problem, one has to induce a specific mutation that is identical to the mutation occurring in patients. However, until lately, genome editing in mammalian cells was an extremely inefficient process [17], and therefore it was challenging to generate homozygous mutations in human cells using the traditional methods for gene targeting. The development of new technologies for gene targeting, (reviewed in details in [17]) especially the TALEN technology and the Cas/CRISPER technology have dramatically increased the efficiency of gene targeting in mammalian cells and enabled to correct specific mutations or to obtained homozygous mutations in reasonable efficiency in human pluripotent stem cells.

These methods enable, for the first time, the comparison between isogenic cells that differ only in the specific mutation under investigation. This can be achieved by induction of a specific mutation in otherwise normal ESCs, by correction of a specific mutation in iPSCs or by combination of both methods [30,41] One possible drawback in these methods is the possible off-target effect that might result in additional unplanned genetic aberrations [17]. To overcome this possibility it is important to design the targeting sequence in a way that will decrease the off-target effects and to target different sequences of the same gene. Among these methods, the CRISPR technique will probably become the first choice for most labs due to the combination of accuracy, efficiency and accessibility.

8. "Guidelines" for Choosing the Optimal Model System for a Given Disease

The choice between modeling disorders with ESCs or iPSCs is dependent on several factors. We propose that the optimal model that probably overcomes most if not all the drawbacks mentioned above, is a model that combines both ESCs (that were genetically modified to carry a specific mutation) and iPSCs from patients (with an isogenic control of iPSCs from the same patient in which the mutation was corrected by genomic engineering). Such "combined methods" have been recently generated for long QT syndrome [30] and for Fanconi anemia [41]. However, as was discussed above, in some cases only one of the two methods is doable/informative. In Figure 3 we suggest general guidelines that should assist in choosing the right system for a given disorder. We generated this scheme based on the following assumptions:

Figure 3. Scheme depicting the steps in choosing the appropriate system for disease modeling. While in some cases there is only one possible option (either ESCs or iPSCs), in other cases both ESCs or iPSCs can be used and the decision between the two methods should be done after the consideration of the advantageous and disadvantageous of each one of the options (some of them are described in the scheme).

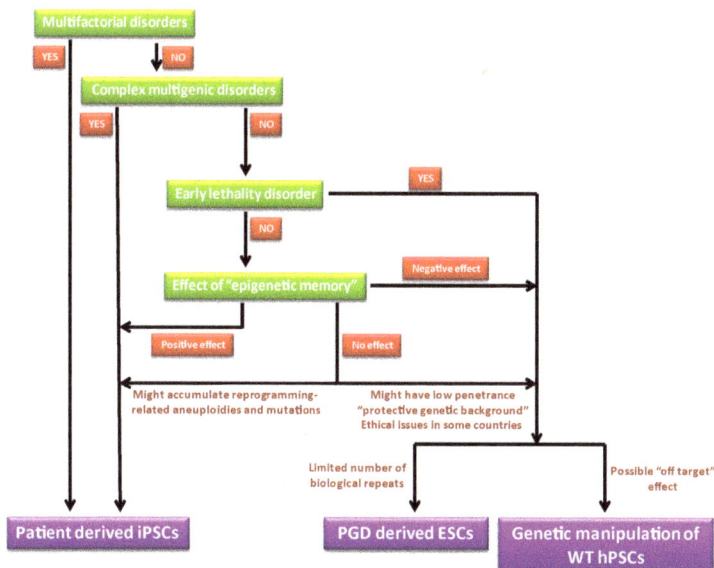

Multifactorial disorders in which there is a major contribution to factors other than genetic factors on the disease etiology can be modeled exclusively by iPSCs from patients that already manifested the disease and can't be modeled by ESCs. Similarly, iPSCs but not ESCs should be used to model multigenic disorders in which the genetic factor cannot be narrowed down into a single gene, (the discussion regarding the use of hPSCs to model these type of disorders is out of the scope of this review). Other than these two groups of disorders, "monogeneic" disorders can be modeled theoretically using both systems but under the following notions: (1) Genetic aberrations that lead to early lethality should not be modeled by iPSCs that derived from individuals that survived to term as they represent the exceptional cases (these rare cases however, can be used to study the effect of the genetic aberration on the phenotype of the exceptional embryos that survived to term and the genetic backgrounds that enable them to escape the early lethality); (2) Possible epigenetic memory in iPSCs has to be taken under consideration. While in general the epigenetic memory is considered to have a negative effect on iPSCs (as the pluripotent cells retain some of their previous identity of adult cells and therefore might not be equivalent to normal pluripotent cells), one can also utilize these phenomena in a positive manner. For example, in cases of hematopoietic disorders, iPSCs that were derived from blood cells might undergo hematopoietic differentiation in a greater efficiency than ESCs or iPSCs derived from other somatic cells [16]; (3) In cases in which no epigenetic effect is predicted, the best choice is to combine both model systems. When only one of the two systems will be used it is important to keep in mind the following limitations of each one of the methods: (a) The reprogramming process itself might results in accumulation of genetic aberrations that under some circumstances might affect the reliability of the model; (b) The penetrance of the mutation in the ESCs based model might not be completed (as a result of "protective" genetic background). By contrast, iPSCs are derived from patients that already manifested the phenotype and therefore one should not be concerned about "protective" genetic background; (c) In the case of PGD-based models the number of available samples (affected embryos) might be limited; (d) Gene targeting by the TALEN or CRISPER systems might lead to off-target effects.

9. Conclusions

Reprogramming of somatic cells from patients is a relatively easy procedure that doesn't involve the usage of human embryos, nor ethical issues, and results in the formation of iPSCs with the naturally occurring mutation. Therefore, since the first derivation of human iPSCs from normal donors [67–69] and from patients [11], this method was considered by many to be the optimal methodology for disease modeling by human pluripotent cells (due to scientific reasons as well as other reasons). Indeed, during the last several years numerous models for genetic disorders were generated by reprogramming of somatic cells from patients. Yet, in many cases the mutant cell lines were not further analyzed to study their relevance to the actual disorders. In this review we focused on iPSCs based models and ESCs based models that have been shown to have a phenotype related to the disease.

To demonstrate that iPSCs can't always replace ESCs in disease modeling, we focused on four models, each one emphasizes a specific aspect of the differences between ESC-based models and iPSC-based models. In addition to these specific examples, the reprogramming process itself might result in the generation of *de-novo* mutations [24] that might add "noise" to the system. On the other hand one general advantage of iPSC-based models compared to ESCs-based models is the fact that the patient chosen already manifested the phenotype associated with the mutation. This assures that there is no effect to the specific genetic background on the penetrance of the mutation. Based on the comparison between ESC-based models and iPSC-based models we suggested in Figure 3 a general guidelines to assist in choosing the appropriate model for a given disorder.

Lastly, the development of the "iPSCs technology" by Takahashi and Yamanaka some eight years ago [70], dramatically changed the entire field of pluripotent stem cells biology. While the most desirable application of this technology is probably for cell therapy, there is no doubt that currently the most common application of iPSCs is for disease modeling. In this review we highlighted some of the pros and cons of iPSCs compared to ESCs in regards to disease modeling and discussed the effect of advanced technologies for genome editing on the field. We believe that the field of disease modeling by hPSCs has reached a point wherein the challenge is not to derive pluripotent cells (ESCs or iPSCs) with a specific mutation but rather to better understand the pathophysiology of the disease and finding effective therapies.

Acknowledgments

The Authors would like to acknowledge Nissim Benvenisty for helpful discussions and critical comments on the manuscript.

Author Contributions

Tomer Halevy and Achia Urbach wrote the manuscript and designed the figures.

Conflicts of Interest

The authors declare no conflict of interest.

References

1. Robinton, D.A.; Daley, G.Q. The promise of induced pluripotent stem cells in research and therapy. *Nature* **2012**, *481*, 295–305.
2. Roberts, R.M.; Loh, K.M.; Amita, M.; Bernardo, A.S.; Adachi, K.; Alexenko, A.P.; Schust, D.J.; Schulz, L.C.; Telugu, B.P.V.L.; Ezashi, T.; *et al.* Differentiation of trophoblast cells from human embryonic stem cells: To be or not to be? *Reproduction* **2014**, *147*, doi:10.1530/REP-14-0080.
3. Xu, R.-H.; Chen, X.; Li, D.S.; Li, R.; Addicks, G.C.; Glennon, C.; Zwaka, T.P.; Thomson, J.A. BMP4 Initiates Human Embryonic Stem Cell Differentiation to Trophoblast. *Nat. Biotechnol.* **2002**, *20*, 1261–1264.
4. Vandamme, T.F. Use of rodents as models of human diseases. *J. Pharm. Bioallied Sci.* **2014**, *6*, 2–9.

5. Urbach, A.; Schuldiner, M.; Benvenisty, N. Modeling for Lesch-Nyhan disease by gene targeting in human embryonic stem cells. *Stem Cells* **2004**, *22*, 635–641.

6. Urbach, A.; Benvenisty, N. Studying early lethality of 45,XO (Turner's syndrome) embryos using human embryonic stem cells. *PLoS One* **2009**, *4*, doi:10.1371/journal.pone.0004175.

7. Eiges, R.; Urbach, A.; Malcov, M.; Frumkin, T.; Schwartz, T.; Amit, A.; Yaron, Y.; Eden, A.; Yanuka, O.; Benvenisty, N.; *et al.* Developmental study of fragile X syndrome using human embryonic stem cells derived from preimplantation genetically diagnosed embryos. *Cell Stem Cell* **2007**, *1*, 568–577.

8. Maury, Y.; Gauthier, M.; Peschanski, M.; Martinat, C. Human pluripotent stem cells for disease modelling and drug screening. *Bioessays* **2012**, *34*, 61–71.

9. Verlinsky, Y.; Strelchenko, N.; Kukharenko, V.; Rechitsky, S.; Verlinsky, O.; Galat, V.; Kuliev, A. Human embryonic stem cell lines with genetic disorders. *Reprod. Biomed. Online* **2005**, *10*, 105–110.

10. Mateizel, I.; Spits, C.; de Rycke, M.; Liebaers, I.; Sermon, K. Derivation, culture, and characterization of VUB hESC lines. *Vitr. Cell. Dev. Biol. Anim.* **2010**, *46*, 300–308.

11. Park, I.-H.; Arora, N.; Huo, H.; Maherali, N.; Ahfeldt, T.; Shimamura, A.; Lensch, M.W.; Cowan, C.; Hochedlinger, K.; Daley, G.Q. Disease-specific induced pluripotent stem cells. *Cell* **2008**, *134*, 877–886.

12. Dimos, J.T.; Rodolfa, K.T.; Niakan, K.K.; Weisenthal, L.M.; Mitsumoto, H.; Chung, W.; Croft, G.F.; Saphier, G.; Leibel, R.; Goland, R.; *et al.* Induced pluripotent stem cells generated from patients with ALS can be differentiated into motor neurons. *Science* **2008**, *321*, 1218–1221.

13. Kiskinis, E.; Sandoe, J.; Williams, L.; Boulting, G.; Moccia, R.; Wainger, B.; Han, S.; Peng, T.; Thams, S.; Mikkilineni, S.; *et al.* Pathways Disrupted in Human ALS Motor Neurons Identified through Genetic Correction of Mutant SOD1. *Cell Stem Cell* **2014**, *14*, 781–795.

14. Puri, M.C.; Nagy, A. Concise review: Embryonic stem cells *versus* induced pluripotent stem cells: The game is on. *Stem Cells* **2012**, *30*, 10–14.

15. Bilic, J.; Izpisua Belmonte, J.C. Concise review: Induced pluripotent stem cells *versus* embryonic stem cells: Close enough or yet too far apart? *Stem Cells* **2012**, *30*, 33–41.

16. Cherry, A.B.C.; Daley, G.Q. Reprogrammed cells for disease modeling and regenerative medicine. *Annu. Rev. Med.* **2013**, *64*, 277–290.

17. Kim, H.; Kim, J.-S. A guide to genome engineering with programmable nucleases. *Nat. Rev. Genet.* **2014**, *15*, 321–334.

18. Sandoe, J.; Eggan, K. Opportunities and challenges of pluripotent stem cell neurodegenerative disease models. *Nat. Neurosci.* **2013**, *16*, 780–789.

19. Robertson, J.A. Human embryonic stem cell research: Ethical and legal issues. *Nat. Rev. Genet.* **2001**, *2*, 74–78.

20. De Wert, G.; Mummery, C. Human embryonic stem cells: Research, ethics and policy. *Hum. Reprod.* **2003**, *18*, 672–682.

21. Kim, K.; Doi, A.; Wen, B.; Ng, K.; Zhao, R.; Cahan, P.; Kim, J.; Aryee, M.J.; Ji, H.; Ehrlich, L.I.; *et al.* Epigenetic memory in induced pluripotent stem cells. *Nature* **2010**, *467*, 285–290.

22. Bar-Nur, O.; Russ, H.A.; Efrat, S.; Benvenisty, N. Epigenetic memory and preferential lineage-specific differentiation in induced pluripotent stem cells derived from human pancreatic islet beta cells. *Cell Stem Cell* **2011**, *9*, 17–23.

23. Ma, H.; Morey, R.; O'Neil, R.C.; He, Y.; Daughtry, B.; Schultz, M.D.; Hariharan, M.; Nery, J.R.; Castanon, R.; Sabatini, K.; *et al.* Abnormalities in human pluripotent cells due to reprogramming mechanisms. *Nature* **2014**, *511*, 177–183.

24. Gore, A.; Li, Z.; Fung, H.-L.; Young, J.E.; Agarwal, S.; Antosiewicz-Bourget, J.; Canto, I.; Giorgetti, A.; Israel, M.A.; Kiskinis, E.; *et al.* Somatic coding mutations in human induced pluripotent stem cells. *Nature* **2011**, *471*, 63–67.

25. Yung, S.K.; Tilgner, K.; Ledran, M.H.; Habibollah, S.; Neganova, I.; Singhapol, C.; Saretzki, G.; Stojkovic, M.; Armstrong, L.; Przyborski, S.; *et al.* Brief report: Human pluripotent stem cell models of fanconi anemia deficiency reveal an important role for fanconi anemia proteins in cellular reprogramming and survival of hematopoietic progenitors. *Stem Cells* **2013**, *31*, 1022–1029.

26. Muller, L.U.W.; Milsom, M.D.; Harris, C.E.; Vyas, R.; Brumme, K.M.; Parmar, K.; Moreau, L.A.; Schambach, A.; Park, I.H.; London, W.B.; *et al.* Overcoming reprogramming resistance of Fanconi anemia cells. *Blood* **2012**, *119*, 5449–5457.

27. Wang, Z.-B.; Zhang, X.; Li, X.-J. Recapitulation of spinal motor neuron-specific disease phenotypes in a human cell model of spinal muscular atrophy. *Cell Res.* **2013**, *23*, 378–393.

28. Ebert, A.D.; Yu, J.; Rose, F.F.; Mattis, V.B.; Lorson, C.L.; Thomson, J.A.; Svendsen, C.N. Induced pluripotent stem cells from a spinal muscular atrophy patient. *Nature* **2009**, *457*, 277–280.

29. Tulpule, A.; Kelley, J.M.; Lensch, M.W.; McPherson, J.; Park, I.H.; Hartung, O.; Nakamura, T.; Schlaeger, T.M.; Shimamura, A.; Daley, G.Q. Pluripotent stem cell models of shwachman-diamond syndrome reveal a common mechanism for pancreatic and hematopoietic dysfunction. *Cell Stem Cell* **2013**, *12*, 727–736.

30. Bellin, M.; Casini, S.; Davis, R.P.; D'Aniello, C.; Haas, J.; Ward-van Oostwaard, D.; Tertoolen, L.G.J.; Jung, C.B.; Elliott, D.A.; Welling, A.; *et al.* Isogenic human pluripotent stem cell pairs reveal the role of a KCNH2 mutation in long-QT syndrome. *EMBO J.* **2013**, *32*, 3161–3175.

31. Seriola, A.; Spits, C.; Simard, J.P.; Hilven, P.; Haentjens, P.; Pearson, C.E.; Sermon, K. Huntington's and myotonic dystrophy hESCs: Down-regulated trinucleotide repeat instability and mismatch repair machinery expression bupon differentiation. *Hum. Mol. Genet.* **2011**, *20*, 176–185.

32. Du, J.; Campau, E.; Soragni, E.; Jespersen, C.; Gottesfeld, J.M. Length-dependent CTG.CAG triplet-repeat expansion in myotonic dystrophy patient-derived induced pluripotent stem cells. *Hum. Mol. Genet.* **2013**, *22*, 5276–5287.

33. Saenger, P. Turner's syndrome. *N. Engl. J. Med.* **1996**, *335*, 1749–1754.

34. Ranke, M.B.; Saenger, P. Turner's syndrome. *Lancet* **2001**, *358*, 309–314.

35. Li, W.; Wang, X.; Fan, W.; Zhao, P.; Chan, Y.C.; Chen, S.; Zhang, S.; Guo, X.; Zhang, Y.; Li, Y.; *et al.* Modeling abnormal early development with induced pluripotent stem cells from aneuploid syndromes. *Hum. Mol. Genet.* **2012**, *21*, 32–45.

36. Urbach, A.; Bar-Nur, O.; Daley, G.Q.; Benvenisty, N. Differential modeling of fragile X syndrome by human embryonic stem cells and induced pluripotent stem cells. *Cell Stem Cell* **2010**, *6*, 407–411.

37. Li, Y.; Wang, H.; Muffat, J.; Cheng, A.W.; Orlando, D.A.; Lovén, J.; Kwok, S.M.; Feldman, D.A.; Bateup, H.S.; Gao, Q.; *et al.* Global transcriptional and translational repression in human-embryonic-stem-cell-derived Rett syndrome neurons. *Cell Stem Cell* **2013**, *13*, 446–458.

38. Cheung, A.Y.L.; Horvath, L.M.; Grafodatskaya, D.; Pasceri, P.; Weksberg, R.; Hotta, A.; Carrel, L.; Ellis, J. Isolation of MECP2-null Rett Syndrome patient hiPS cells and isogenic controls through X-chromosome inactivation. *Hum. Mol. Genet.* **2011**, *20*, 2103–2115.

39. Marchetto, M.C.N.; Carromeu, C.; Acab, A.; Yu, D.; Yeo, G.W.; Mu, Y.; Chen, G.; Gage, F.H.; Muotri, A.R. A model for neural development and treatment of Rett syndrome using human induced pluripotent stem cells. *Cell* **2010**, *143*, 527–539.

40. Tulpule, A.; William Lensch, M.; Miller, J.D.; Austin, K.; D'Andrea, A.; Schlaeger, T.M.; Shimamura, A.; Daley, G.Q. Knockdown of Fanconi anemia genes in human embryonic stem cells reveals early developmental defects in the hematopoietic lineage. *Blood* **2010**, *115*, 3453–3462.

41. Liu, G.-H.; Suzuki, K.; Li, M.; Qu, J.; Montserrat, N.; Tarantino, C.; Gu, Y.; Yi, F.; Xu, X.; Zhang, W.; *et al.* Modelling Fanconi anemia pathogenesis and therapeutics using integration-free patient-derived iPSCs. *Nat. Commun.* **2014**, *5*, 4330.

42. Lu, B.; Palacino, J. A novel human embryonic stem cell-derived Huntington's disease neuronal model exhibits mutant huntingtin (mHTT) aggregates and soluble mHTT-dependent neurodegeneration. *FASEB J.* **2013**, *27*, 1820–1829.

43. HD iPSC Consortium. Induced pluripotent stem cells from patients with Huntington's disease show CAG-repeat-expansion-associated phenotypes. *Cell Stem Cell* **2012**, *11*, 264–278.

44. D'Andrea, A.D.; Grompe, M. Molecular biology of Fanconi anemia: Implications for diagnosis and therapy. *Blood* **1997**, *90*, 1725–1736.

45. Raya, A.; Rodríguez-Pizà, I.; Guenechea, G.; Vassena, R.; Navarro, S.; Barrero, M.J.; Consiglio, A.; Castellà, M.; Río, P.; Sleep, E.; *et al.* Disease-corrected haematopoietic progenitors from Fanconi anaemia induced pluripotent stem cells. *Nature* **2009**, *460*, 53–59.

46. Boyle, L.; Kaufmann, W.E. The behavioral phenotype of *FMR1* mutations. *Am. J. Med. Genet. Part C Semin. Med. Genet.* **2010**, *154C*, 469–476.

47. Penagarikano, O.; Mulle, J.G.; Warren, S.T. The pathophysiology of fragile X syndrome. *Annu. Rev. Genomics Hum. Genet.* **2007**, *8*, 109–129.

48. Wang, T.; Bray, S.M.; Warren, S.T. New perspectives on the biology of fragile X syndrome. *Curr. Opin. Genet. Dev.* **2012**, *22*, 256–263.

49. Callan, M.A.; Zarnescu, D.C. Heads-up: New roles for the fragile X mental retardation protein in neural stem and progenitor cells. *Genesis* **2011**, *49*, 424–440.

50. Santoro, M.R.; Bray, S.M.; Warren, S.T. Molecular mechanisms of fragile X syndrome: A twenty-year perspective. *Annu. Rev. Pathol.* **2012**, *7*, 219–245.

51. Devys, D.; Lutz, Y.; Rouyer, N.; Bellocq, J.P.; Mandel, J.L. The FMR-1 protein is cytoplasmic, most abundant in neurons and appears normal in carriers of a fragile X premutation. *Nat. Genet.* **1993**, *4*, 335–340.

52. Turetsky, T.; Aizenman, E.; Gil, Y.; Weinberg, N.; Shufaro, Y.; Revel, A.; Laufer, N.; Simon, A.; Abeliovich, D.; Reubinoff, B.E. Laser-assisted derivation of human embryonic stem cell lines from IVF embryos after preimplantation genetic diagnosis. *Hum. Reprod.* **2008**, *23*, 46–53.

53. Telias, M.; Segal, M.; Ben-Yosef, D. Neural differentiation of Fragile X human Embryonic Stem Cells reveals abnormal patterns of development despite successful neurogenesis. *Dev. Biol.* **2013**, *374*, 32–45.

54. Hatton, D.D.; Sideris, J.; Skinner, M.; Mankowski, J.; Bailey, D.B.; Roberts, J.; Mirrett, P. Autistic behavior in children with fragile X syndrome: Prevalence, stability, and the impact of FMRP. *Am. J. Med. Genet. Part A* **2006**, *140*, 1804–1813.

55. Kaufmann, W.E.; Cortell, R.; Kau, A.S.M.; Bukelis, I.; Tierney, E.; Gray, R.M.; Cox, C.; Capone, G.T.; Stanard, P. Autism spectrum disorder in fragile X syndrome: Communication, social interaction, and specific behaviors. *Am. J. Med. Genet. A* **2004**, *129A*, 225–234.

56. Pietrobono, R.; Tabolacci, E.; Zalfa, F.; Zito, I.; Terracciano, A.; Moscato, U.; Bagni, C.; Oostra, B.; Chiurazzi, P.; Neri, G. Molecular dissection of the events leading to inactivation of the *FMR1* gene. *Hum. Mol. Genet.* **2005**, *14*, 267–277.

57. Smeets, H.J.; Smits, A.P.; Verheij, C.E.; Theelen, J.P.; Willemsen, R.; van de Burgt, I.; Hoogeveen, A.T.; Oosterwijk, J.C.; Oostra, B.A. Normal phenotype in two brothers with a full *FMR1* mutation. *Hum. Mol. Genet.* **1995**, *4*, 2103–2108.

58. Sheridan, S.D.; Theriault, K.M.; Reis, S.A.; Zhou, F.; Madison, J.M.; Daheron, L.; Loring, J.F.; Haggarty, S.J. Epigenetic characterization of the *FMR1* gene and aberrant neurodevelopment in human induced pluripotent stem cell models of fragile X syndrome. *PLoS One* **2011**, *6*, e26203.

59. Alisch, R.S.; Wang, T.; Chopra, P.; Visootsak, J.; Conneely, K.N.; Warren, S.T. Genome-wide analysis validates aberrant methylation in fragile X syndrome is specific to the *FMR1* locus. *BMC Med. Genet.* **2013**, *14*, 18.

60. Bar-Nur, O.; Caspi, I.; Benvenisty, N. Molecular analysis of *FMR1* reactivation in fragile-X induced pluripotent stem cells and their neuronal derivatives. *J. Mol. Cell Biol.* **2012**, *4*, 180–183.

61. Martin, J.B.; Gusella, J.F. Huntington's disease. Pathogenesis and management. *N. Engl. J. Med.* **1986**, *315*, 1267–1276.

62. Huntington, T.; Macdonald, M.E.; Ambrose, C.M.; Duyao, M.P.; Myers, R.H.; Lin, C.; Srinidhi, L.; Barnes, G.; Taylor, S.A.; James, M.; Groat, N.; *et al.* A novel gene containing a trinucleotide repeat that is expanded and unstable on Huntington's disease chromosomes. The Huntington's Disease Collaborative Research Group. *Cell* **1993**, *72*, 971–983.

63. Landles, C.; Sathasivam, K.; Weiss, A.; Woodman, B.; Moffitt, H.; Finkbeiner, S.; Sun, B.; Gafni, J.; Ellerby, L.M.; Trottier, Y.; *et al.* Proteolysis of mutant huntingtin produces an exon 1 fragment that accumulates as an aggregated protein in neuronal nuclei in Huntington disease. *J. Biol. Chem.* **2010**, *285*, 8808–8823.

64. Zhang, N.; An, M.C.; Montoro, D.; Ellerby, L.M. Characterization of human Huntington's disease cell model from induced pluripotent stem cells. *PLoS Curr.* **2010**, *2*, 1–11.

65. Camnasio, S.; Carri, A.D.; Lombardo, A.; Grad, I.; Mariotti, C.; Castucci, A.; Rozell, B.; Riso, P.L.; Castiglioni, V.; Zuccato, C.; *et al.* The first reported generation of several induced pluripotent stem cell lines from homozygous and heterozygous Huntington's disease patients demonstrates mutation related enhanced lysosomal activity. *Neurobiol. Dis.* **2012**, *46*, 41–51.

66. Bradley, C.K.; Scott, H.A.; Chami, O.; Peura, T.T.; Dumevska, B.; Schmidt, U.; Stojanov, T. Derivation of Huntington's disease-affected human embryonic stem cell lines. *Stem Cells Dev.* **2011**, *20*, 495–502.

67. Takahashi, K.; Tanabe, K.; Ohnuki, M.; Narita, M.; Ichisaka, T.; Tomoda, K.; Yamanaka, S. Induction of Pluripotent Stem Cells from Adult Human Fibroblasts by Defined Factors. *Cell* **2007**, *131*, 861–872.

68. Park, I.-H.; Zhao, R.; West, J.A.; Yabuuchi, A.; Huo, H.; Ince, T.A.; Lerou, P.H.; Lensch, M.W.; Daley, G.Q. Reprogramming of human somatic cells to pluripotency with defined factors. *Nature* **2008**, *451*, 141–146.

69. Yu, J.Y.; Vodyanik, M.A.; Smuga-Otto, K.; Antosiewicz-Bourget, J.; Frane, J.L.; Tian, S.; Nie, J.; Jonsdottir, G.A.; Ruotti, V.; Stewart, R.; *et al.* Induced pluripotent stem cell lines derived from human somatic cells. *Science* **2007**, *318*, 1917–1920.

70. Takahashi, K.; Yamanaka, S. Induction of Pluripotent Stem Cells from Mouse Embryonic and Adult Fibroblast Cultures by Defined Factors. *Cell* **2006**, *126*, 663–676.

Design of a Tumorigenicity Test for Induced Pluripotent Stem Cell (iPSC)-Derived Cell Products

Shin Kawamata, Hoshimi Kanemura, Noriko Sakai, Masayo Takahashi and Masahiro J. Go

Abstract: Human Pluripotent Stem Cell (PSC)-derived cell therapy holds enormous promise because of the cells' "unlimited" proliferative capacity and the potential to differentiate into any type of cell. However, these features of PSC-derived cell products are associated with concerns regarding the generation of iatrogenic teratomas or tumors from residual immature or non-terminally differentiated cells in the final cell product. This concern has become a major hurdle to the introduction of this therapy into the clinic. Tumorigenicity testing is therefore a key preclinical safety test in PSC-derived cell therapy. Tumorigenicity testing becomes particularly important when autologous human induced Pluripotent Stem Cell (iPSC)-derived cell products with no immuno-barrier are considered for transplantation. There has been, however, no internationally recognized guideline for tumorigenicity testing of PSC-derived cell products for cell therapy. In this review, we outline the points to be considered in the design and execution of tumorigenicity tests, referring to the tests and laboratory work that we have conducted for an iPSC-derived retinal pigment epithelium (RPE) cell product prior to its clinical use.

Reprinted from *J. Clin. Med.* Cite as: Kawamata, S.; Kanemura, H.; Sakai, N.; Takahashi, M.; Go, M.J. Design of a Tumorigenicity Test for Induced Pluripotent Stem Cell (iPSC)-Derived Cell Products. *J. Clin. Med.* **2015**, *4*, 159–171.

1. Introduction

Several notable clinical trials using human Pluripotent Stem Cell (PSC)-derived cell products have been conducted recently. In the first, Geron used embryonic stem cell (ESC)-derived oligodendrocyte progenitor cells (GRNOPC1) for treatment of acute spinal cord injury [1]. Advanced Cell Technology initiated a study in which ESC-derived retinal pigment epithelium (RPE) was used for treatment of Stargardt's disease and dry type Age-related Macular Degeneration (AMD) [2]. More recently, a clinical study for wet type AMD using induced Pluripotent Stem Cell (iPSC)-derived RPE was started at Riken CDB [3–5].

While clinical applications are moving forward, there are concerns that transplantation of differentiated PSC might lead to the formation of tumors in the recipient. Thus, examination of this possible outcome of transplantation is critically important. Cell transplantation or infusion therapy is distinctly different from drug administration. One must consider that transplanted or infused cells can survive for long periods in the host and may form tumors at the site of transplantation or at distal sites. The extent of tumor formation can be influenced by the microenvironment at the transplantation site or the ultimate homing site of the host. Furthermore, once a tumor has formed, it may influence the physical condition of the host through secreted factor(s) [6].

The aforementioned aspects of cell therapy must be addressed with animal transplantation studies prior to clinical use. Tumorigenicity tests that can assess the tumor-forming potential of transplanted cells are particularly important in the case of PSC-based cell therapies. As PSC have "unlimited" proliferation potential as undifferentiated stem cells, they can generate teratomas if they remain in the final product. The chance of generating a teratoma will increase if the procedure uses an autologous iPSC-derived cell product that presents no immunologic barrier. PSC might accumulate chromosomal abnormalities by selecting cells with unusual proliferative advantages over a long culture period. Lund *et al.* reported that some 13% of ESC and iPSC maintained in research labs worldwide demonstrated some type of genetic abnormality [7]. For that reason, the timely assessment of the genetic stability of PSC is of major interest for both research labs and clinical PSC banks. In addition, it is important to assess the potential for differentiation resistance due to incomplete reprogramming or a differentiation bias due to epigenetic memory when iPSC-based therapy is considered. In this context, it is necessary to assess the tumor-forming potential of non-terminally differentiated cells as well.

Information regarding genetic stability, gene expression, differentiation marker expression, cell growth rate and how cells were generated must be collected and evaluated prior to commencement of tumorigenicity testing. Next, it is necessary to have a clear idea about the scope and objective of related safety parameters: toxicology tests, Proof of Concept (POC) tests, biodistribution tests and tumorigenicity tests that can be conducted concurrently.

Toxicology tests can be designed depending on the properties of testing reagents and the purpose of the tests. The Organisation for Economic Cooperation and Development (OECD) Guideline for the Testing of Chemicals [8] is an internationally recognized test guideline for toxicology testing. They should be conducted in a blinded fashion to minimize the bias of measurement and observation by operators. Short-term and long-term end points are to be defined. Toxicology tests should be conducted by using clinically relevant methods of administration so that they can provide insights into a safe range of therapeutic cell doses. Acute (early) and late phase end points should be established in this test.

POC tests often employ a genetically modified animal that offers a model of the disease in question (e.g., Tg, KI, KO or KD mice) or injured animals to address the potential benefit or efficacy of the investigational therapy and to define the range of the effective dose used in clinical application by escalating the doses. The administration route and the method should be as close as possible to the intended clinical use. Positive and negative events should be clearly defined. In such a POC study, indices such as physiological recovery of lost function or overall survival of transplanted cells that could underlie intended therapeutic use are examined. Measurement of indices should be conducted in a blinded fashion to minimize bias during data acquisition. The size of the test group should be large enough to permit meaningful statistical analysis.

Biodistribution tests should be conducted to address tumorigenic proliferation of transplanted cells at the ectopic site. *Alu* sequence PCR is commonly used to detect human cells in host tissues or organs. While this PCR test detects human cells over a 0.1% frequency in host tissue by DNA ratio [9], greater sensitivity is needed to detect small metastatic colonies. In PET technology, proliferative cell mass is labelled by taking in a metabolic probe such as ^{18}F FLT, providing a distribution of tumorigenic cell proliferation in the animal's body. However to trace the behavior of transplanted cells and their biodistribution over time requires labeling test cells by introducing marker genes by retrovirus or lentivirus that can emit a signal with a high S/N ratio. These approaches are currently under development.

2. Guidelines for Tumorigenicity Tests

Somatic cells with a normal chromosomal structure show limited proliferation potential. Tumorigenicity testing of mesenchymal stem cells may not reveal a serious problem [10]. However, in the case of PSC-derived cell products, the tumor-forming potential should be examined thoroughly because of the "unlimited" proliferation capacity of PSC and their genetic instability. However, there is no internationally recognized guideline for tumorigenicity testing of cells used for cell therapy. WHO TRS 878, "Recommendation for the evaluation of animal cell cultures as substrates for the manufacture of cell banks" [11,12] provides a guideline for animal cell substrates used for the production of biological medicinal products, but not for cells used for therapeutic transplantation into patients. Recently, FDA/CBER commented on the issues to be considered for cell-based products and associated challenges for preclinical animal study [13]. The report stated that when tumorigenicity testing of ESC-derived cellular products is undertaken, the tumorigenicity tests should be designed considering the nature of cell products to be transplanted and the anatomical location or microenvironment of the host animal. Tumorigenic test results from the administration of cells through nonclinical routes are not considered relevant as they would not assess the behavior of transplanted cells in the intended microenvironment to which the cells would be exposed. The study design should include groups of animals that have received undifferentiated ESCs, serial dilutions of undifferentiated ESCs combined with ESC-derived final products to infer the contamination of undifferentiated ESCs in the final product.

The aforementioned summarizes current discussions of tumorigenicity testing. However, we still need to answer a fundamental question: "How can we extrapolate animal tumorigenicity testing to humans?" The design of tumorigenicity tests should attempt to answer this question. For this, we must first estimate the risk that we will underestimate the incidence of tumor-forming events in humans by conducting an improper or non-informative animal study. So, how do we define such risk? For example, there is a risk that a study is unable to link unexpected tumor formation to genetic abnormalities of test cells presented before transplantation due to inadequate genetic information regarding test cells. In addition, there is a risk of obtaining "false" negative results by transplanting an insufficient dose, using an inadequate monitoring period, using an improper immunodeficient animal model that is insufficient to detect tumor, not transplanting into the right anatomical position, failure of transplantation itself or unexpected early death of transplanted cells in host tissue. We can address the risks by conducting quality control tests of test cells prior to transplantation and small scale pilot studies to determine the design of tumorigenicity tests. The following points should be considered in designing tumorigenicity tests.

1. The history of cell production (cultured in a research lab or Good Manufacturing Practice (GMP) grade cell processing facility).
2. Quality control records of test cells (e.g., phenotype, gene expression, sterility tests, genetic information, passage number and growth rate).

3. The type of immunodeficient animal model used and the route of administration (clinical route or subcutaneous route).

4. The method of transplantation (e.g., embedded with Matrigel or in sheets or in cell suspension).

5. Gender and number of animals to be used.

6. Information about the microenvironment at the transplanting site.

7. Dose of cells to be transplanted.

8. Selection of a positive control cell and definition of positive tumor-forming event.

9. Monitoring periods.

10. Protocol for immunohistochemistry (IHC) to detect transplanted cells in host tissue.

11. Method to detect ectopic tumor formation.

3. Specification of Test Cells

Cells used in tumorigenic tests should be generated in a manner as close as possible to that intended for clinical use. In this context, it is preferable that cells used for all preclinical tests should be generated in a GMP-grade cell processing facility for clinical use. This approach would minimize bias originating from differences in cell production quality. Several types of data, including gene expression profiles obtained from gene chips or qRT-PCR to assess stem cell-like markers and differentiation markers, phenotypic analysis by flow cytometry, sterility tests, mycoplasma tests, exome sequencing, chromosomal stability tests with comparative genomic hybridization (CGH) array and karyotyping by multi-color banding (mBAND) or fluorescent *in situ* hybridization (FISH) would be valuable. For iPSC-derived cell products, EB formation assays would provide insights into differentiation potential. The results could be used to select "good" clones that demonstrate no differentiation bias or no differentiation resistance. These quality control tests and cell characterization tests are not a part of tumorigenicity testing *per se*. However, the information on starting material should be linked to the results of tumorigenicity testing to render the test results more informative.

In tumorigenicity testing of PSC-derived cell products, one can anticipate several tumor-forming events that include teratoma formation from residual "differentiation-resistant" PSC with normal karyotype, cancer-like progressive tumor formation from cells with abnormal karyotype or acquired genetic variation during culture and tumors with differentiation bias generated from imperfectly reprogrammed cells. To understand the nature of tumor-forming events, the link with results of these quality control tests is indispensable.

4. Selection of an Animal Model

In general, if one were to use "non-immunodeficient" healthy animals or "non-immunodeficient" disease model animals for tumorigenicity testing, one would have to administer a large amount of immunosuppressant for long-term monitoring. However, this approach will not always guarantee satisfactory engraftment of xeno-transplants. Primates can be used for tumorigenicity testing as models representative of humans, but this model is more useful for POC tests, not for tumorigenicity tests. Therefore, immunodeficient healthy rodents are widely used for tumorigenicity testing if human cells (final product) are to be used in the test. Large immunodeficient animals like the SCID pig [14] are also available. However, again, the SCID pig model would be useful to address transplantation efficiency of human cells, such as xeno-bone marrow transplantation of human hematopoietic stem cells as a part of a POC study in large animals. They are not cost-effective large scale statistical studies. To conduct tumorigenicity tests with a sufficient number of immunodeficient animals, a rodent model is a reasonable option for the preparation of test cells. Immunodeficient mice such as nude mice (BALB/cA, JCl-nu/nu), SCID mice (C.B-17/Icr-scid/scid), NOD-SCID mice (NOD/ShiJic-scid) and NOG mice (NOD/ShiJic-scid, IL-2Rγ KO) have been widely used for human cell transplantation studies. Prior to the design of tumorigenicity tests, one needs to evaluate the tumor-generating potential of these immunodeficient mouse strains by transplanting various dose of tumorigenic cell lines subcutaneously.

Another well-known transplantation site in rodents is beneath the testicular capsule space. This transplantation model is mainly used to test for satisfactory engraftment of test cells for POC tests, not for tumorigenicity tests. In our hands, it requires elaborate surgical skills and needs at least 10^4 iPSCs to generate tumors in NOG mice. In addition, tumor formation in the intraperitoneal space is hard to detect from the appearance of mice, thereby preventing statistical studies for tumor-forming events in a timely manner. In our case, the tumorigenic potential of immunodeficient mice was assessed by transplanting various doses of HeLa cells subcutaneously, following recommended procedure stated in WHO TRS 878 [11,12]. The mice were monitored over 12 months, and the TPD50 (minimum dose that can generate a tumor in 50% of transplanted mice) was calculated by the Trimmed Spearman-Karber method for each strain [9]. HeLa cells were used as a representative line of somatic tumorigenic cells with a genetic abnormality. For transplantation, a collagen-based gel lacking nutrients is sometime used to embed cells and to retain them at the designated transplantation site. Importantly, the gel *per se* does not support growth of the transplanted cells at the site. We have used Matrigel® (BD Biosciences, San Jose, CA, USA) to embed cells and to increase their tumor-forming potential [15]. We obtained the following values for the TPD50 for HeLa cells with Matrigel® via a subcutaneous route: Nude, $10^{3.5}$ ($n = 120$); SCID, $10^{2.5}$ ($n = 24$); NOD-SCID, $10^{2.17}$ ($n = 24$); NOG, $10^{1.1}$ ($n = 75$). It is notable that during the course of experiments covering 9 months of observation, we also observed spontaneous thymomas with a frequency of some 14% in NOD-SCID mice in agreement with previous reports [16], which makes interpretation of tumorigenicity tests with NOD-SCID mice complicated.

Based on the preceding data, we chose NOG mice for subcutaneous tumorigenicity testing of iPSC-derived RPE, assuming that NOG mice could generate tumors from the lowest number of residual PSC or tumorigenic non-terminally differentiated PSC-derived cells. We then subcutaneously transplanted various doses of iPSC (201B7, Riken CDB) with Matrigel® into NOG mice to determine TPD50 for iPSC. The TPD50 value for iPSC (201B7) via the subcutaneous route was $10^{2.12}$ ($n = 20$) over 84 weeks of observation [9] (Figure 1). Tumorigenicity tests via a subcutaneous route with NOG mice is a sensitive quality control test to detect a small number of remaining PSC in PSC-derived investigational product regardless of cell type. Of course, the TPD50 for iPSC transplanted via a clinical route can be checked independently. In our case, we used nude rats for tumorigenicity testing via a clinical route, as the subretinal space of mice is very small and transplanting cells via a clinical route requires outstanding technique by a skilled operator. Thus, we needed larger animals to avoid "false" negative results due to failure of transplantation, to transplant a clinically relevant dose of GMP-grade iPSC-derived RPE (without Matrigel) and to confirm that the transplantation of brown colored RPE was in the right position in the albino eye ball of nude rats [9]. We did not use any "AMD" disease model animals [17,18] because they will not recapitulate all the features of human AMD. In human AMD, the macular region is focally affected and the rest of the retinal area is intact. Treatment of human wet-type AMD with an iPSC-derived RPE sheet is conducted by transplanting the RPE sheet into the affected lesion after removal of choroidal neovascularization. Thus, we assumed that a transplanted RPE sheet would receive a trans-effect from the intact retina. For that reason, we transplanted the RPE sheets into nude rats with intact retinal function rather the recapitulate the microenvironment of the clinical setting. Thus, the choice of animal should be made depending on the degree of immunodeficiency, anatomical demands and planned clinical manipulation. The TPD50 value for iPSC or HeLa cells via the clinical route was $10^{4.74}$ ($n = 26$) or $10^{1.32}$ ($n = 37$) respectively (Figure 2). The large discrepancy between the TPD50 values for iPSC and that of HeLa prompted us to examine the effect of the microenvironment on iPSC-derived products to better design tumorigenicity tests via the clinical route (see below).

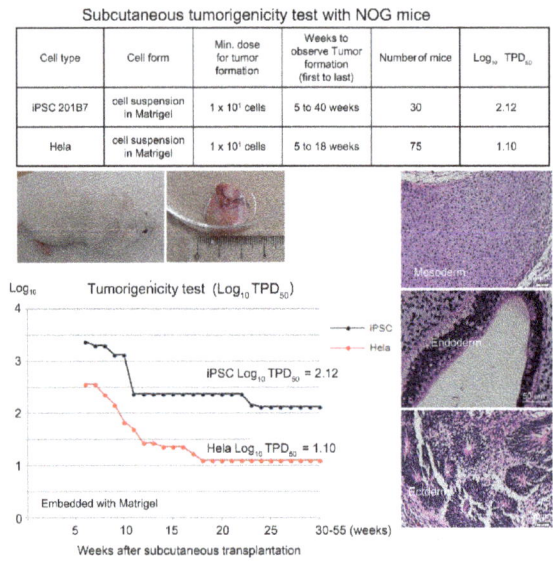

Figure 1. Subcutaneous tumorigenicity test with NOG mice. A table in above showed type of cells used as a positive control for tumorigenicity test (iPSC cell line 201B7 and tumor cell line HeLa), minimum dose for tumor formation and Log_{10} TPD50 for them when transplanted subcutaneously with Matrigel®. A line graph showed value for Log_{10} TPD50 for iPSC or HeLa at respective monitoring point (0–55 weeks). Photos (clock-wise); NOG mouse with tumor, teraoma from NOG mouse, Slice section of teratoma after HE staining; cartilage (mesoderm), intestinal tissue-like (endoderm) or neural rosette-like (ectoderm) tissue.

Tumorigenicity test via clinical route with Nude rats

Cell type	Cell form	Min. dose for tumor formation	Weeks to observe Tumor formation (first to last)	Number of rats	$Log_{10} TPD_{50}$
iPSC 201B7	cell suspension	1×10^4 cells	7 to 33 weeks	20	4.73
Hela	cell suspension	1×10^1 cells	5 to 33 weeks	13	1.32

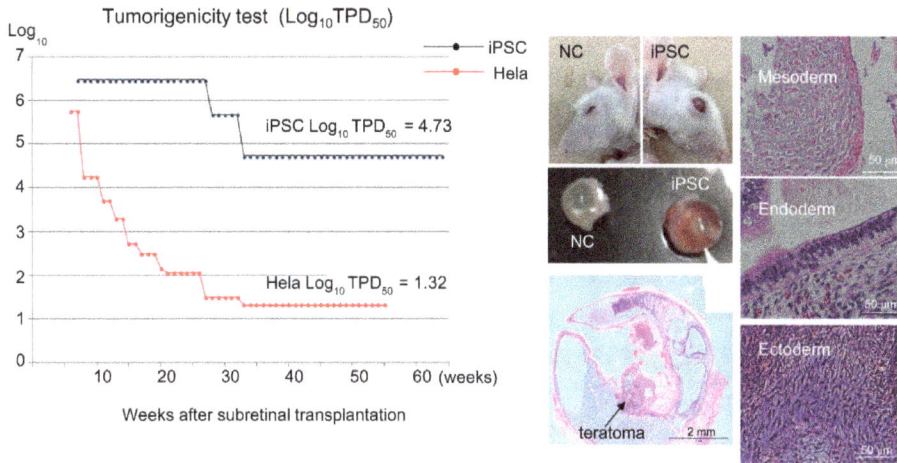

Figure 2. Tumorigenicity test via clinical route with Nude rats. A table in above showed type of cells used as a positive control for tumorigenicity test (iPSC cell line 201B7 and tumor cell line HeLa), minimum dose for tumor formation and Log_{10} TPD_{50} for them when transplanted via clinical route. A line graph showed value for Log_{10} TPD_{50} for iPSC or HeLa at respective monitoring point (0–55 or 64 weeks). Photos (left from top to bottom); NC: non-transplanted control, iPSC: iPSC transplanted mouse. iPSC-transplanted (iPSC) or non-treated control (NC) eye ball. HE staining of slice section of iPSC-transplanted eye ball. Photos (right top to bottom) histology of teratoma formed; cartilage (mesoderm), intestinal tissue-like (endoderm) or neuron-like (ectoderm) tissue.

Another option to address the tumorigenic potential of autologous iPSC-derived products is to transplant rodent cells into a rodent with same genetic background to evade immune rejection associated with xeno-transplantation. Of course, it will be necessary to accumulate sufficient data to demonstrate that rodent cells used in this test are equivalent to human investigational cell products before starting the test.

5. Administration Route and Microenvironment at the Transplantation Site

The administration route should mimic the clinical route as closely as possible to address the tumorigenic potential of investigational cells in the context of the microenvironment at the transplantation site. Therefore, evaluation of the microenvironment of the transplantation site including trans-effects from the microenvironment on investigational cells should be assessed prior to the commencement of large scale tumorigenicity testing. In the event of teratoma formation by residual undifferentiated PSCs, trans-effects of host tissue on PSC should be examined. Towards this end, we have established an *in vitro* co-culture system by placing PSC in culture inserts and culturing host or human primary tissue on the bottom of the dish. When iPSCs in culture inserts were co-cultured with cardiomyocytes or neural cells in the bottom of the dish, the growth of iPSC was not affected, but when they were co-cultured with RPE, the number of iPSCs was reduced drastically [19]. We found that RPE secreted Pigment Epithelium-derived Factor (PEDF). Addition of anti-PEDF antibody into the co-culture system blocked the reduction of iPSC cell number. Further addition of recombinant human PEDF (hrPEDF) induced apoptotic cell death and dramatically reduced ESC and iPSC cell number. hrPEDF did not show any reduction in the number of HeLa cells. Indeed, the TPD50 for iPSC was $10^{4.75}$ when transplanting into the subretinal space (clinical route), while that for HeLa was $10^{1.32}$. That means that approximately 20 HeLa cells could generate a tumor in the subretinal space in half of the rats transplanted, but more than 5×10^4 iPSCs were required to generate teratomas in the subretinal space in half of the rats transplanted. As we transplanted $0.8–1.5 \times 10^4$ iPSC-derived RPE cells in sheets via the clinical route in tumorigenicity tests, it is unlikely that we could observe teratomas from tumorigenicity tests via the clinical route. Further tests, such as transplanting serial dilutions of iPSC in the final product in the subretinal space would not be informative and cannot be justified if tried. However, tumorigenicity tests via the clinical route could be useful to address the tumorigenic potential of non-terminally differentiated tumorigenic cells in iPSC-derived RPE products. This test would be sensitive enough to detect tumors in half the rats transplanted with 20 HeLa cells. We conducted this test for this reason and observed no tumor-forming event ($n = 36$) during a 10–20 months monitoring period. The lack of tumor-forming events was eventually confirmed by IHC of transplanted cells in host tissue section.

We point out that the risk of teratoma formation by a small number of residual iPSC in iPSC-derived RPE in a clinical setting should be thoroughly addressed especially for autologous cell transplantation. Towards this end, subcutaneous tumorigenicity tests are being conducted concurrently with NOG mice wherein we transplant 1×10^6 cells embedded in Matrigel. This test is sensitive enough to detect as few as 10 iPSCs [8]. We have conducted this test with 71 animals that were monitored for 9 to 21 months and obtained negative result after examination of tissue sections by IHC.

In addition, we reported a highly sensitive residual hiPSC detection method based upon qRT-PCR using primers for the *LIN28A* transcript [20] in hiPSC-derived RPE. This method enabled us to detect residual hiPSCs down to 0.002% of differentiated RPE cells. These assays were effective quality control tests and test cells with negative results with this qRT-PCR test could be used for tumorigenicity testing and therapy. We conclude that even if a few (less than 10) autologous iPSCs are present in an iPSC-derived cell product, the chance of developing a teratoma is negligible when transplanted into the subretinal space.

6. Monitoring Period

We subcutaneously transplanted various doses of HeLa cells with or without Matrigel® into Nude, SCID, NDO-SCID and NOG mice and into the subretinal space of nude rats. We also subcutaneously transplanted various doses of iPSC with or without Matrigel® into NOG mice or into the subretinal space of NOG mice. As HeLa cells and iPSC can generate tumors in NOG mice with a relatively small number of cells, a long observation period can be required so that a tumorigenic event originating from a small number of transplanted cells is not overlooked. Ten HeLa cells needed 18 weeks and 10 iPSCs needed 40 weeks to generate tumors in NOG mice in the longest cases. Ten HeLa cells needed 33 weeks and 1×10^4 iPSCs required 33 weeks to generate tumors in the subretinal space of nude rats in the most protracted cases. Overall, it is recommended that the immunodeficient rodents be monitored up to 12 months so that a tumor formation event is not missed and to conduct satisfactory statistical analyses.

7. Detection of Transplanted Cells

Tumor formation by transplanted human cells can be detected regardless of cell type (teratoma or tumor) by staining tissue sections of the transplant site in host animal with human-specific antibody and Ki67. Nuclear staining with DAPI or Hoechst will not demonstrate that the cells in the tissue section were viable at the time of sacrifice, but sharp margins of the nuclear membrane will suggest that cells were alive and free from autophagy or necrotic events. Human-specific antibodies such as STEM121 (StemCells, AB-121-U-050), Lamin A + C (Abcam, AB108595), and HNA clone 3E1.3 Millipore MAB4383) can be used to identify human cells in host tissue. *In situ* hybridization with a species-specific (human, mouse, rat, *etc.*) probe may generate clear signals, but it may require elaborate sample preparation steps when a paraffin section is used. Tumor-forming cells with proliferation potentials were clearly distinguished by positive staining with Ki67 (MIB-1, Dako M7240) [9]. Further staining of human cells with antibodies specific for human differentiation markers will clearly identify the transplanted human cells.

8. Dose, Number and Sex of Immune Deficient Animals

The dose used in tumorigenicity tests should be determined in the context of the intended clinical use. In general, toxicology tests or POC tests require an escalation of doses to define the safety margin or the effective therapeutic margin. However, this may not be the case with tumorigenicity tests as they aim to address the tumorigenic potential of the maximum dose of the cell product that will be used in therapy. Considering the body size of the animal and anatomical space of the receptive transplant site in the animal, a relevant dose should be administered via the clinically route. In our case, we transplanted 0.8–1.5×10^4 iPSC-derived RPE cells into the subretinal space of nude rats and 1×10^6 iPSC-derived RPE cells with Matrigel® subcutaneously, based on the fact that we intended to transplant 4–8×10^4 iPSC-derived RPE in the clinic. We transplanted a maximum or supra-maximum test dose to minimize the risk of underestimating tumor-forming events in a clinical setting.

The number of rodents in each group should be more than 6 for statistical analysis to obtain significant results using the Clopper-Pearson method. If the cell therapy focuses on a single gender, the sex of mice should be matched in the tumorigenicity test. If not, female mice should be chosen to conduct the tests as stated in WHO TRS 878. Male mice attack cage mates, which leads to a reduction of animal number during long-term monitoring.

9. Conclusions

It is important to design animal tumorigenicity tests so that they do not underestimate the frequency of tumorigenic events in a clinical setting, based on risk assessment of the respective test. In this review, we have highlighted points to be considered by emphasizing the possible risks and the countermeasures we have taken against them. It is important to gather genetic information from the PSC-derived cell product by CGH array, mBAND and FISH analysis in a timely manner. We need to evaluate the effect of the microenvironment on test cells at the transplant site and the tumor-forming potential of test animals via both the clinical route and via the subcutaneous route. The latter would serve as a sensitive quality control test. This analysis must be mindful of the required dose, type and duration of monitoring and application of an effective IHC method to detect and evaluate the transplanted cells. Conducting pilot studies will help to obtain some of the information and design informative pivotal tests. Clinical researchers need to fully understand the scope and limit of each preclinical test to predict adverse events in the clinic.

Acknowledgments

We thank Chikako Morinaga of Laboratory for Retinal Regeneration, RIKEN Center for Developmental Biology for critical advising of the experiments, Yoji Sato of National Institute of Health Sciences, Tokyo for scientific discussion, Masayuki Shikamura of FBRI and Hiroyuki Kamao of Department of Ophthalmology, Kawasaki Medical School for rodent studies and Mamoru Ito of CIEA for supplying NOG mice.

Author Contributions

Conceived and designed the experiments: Hoshimi Kanemura, Masahiro J. Go and Shin Kawamata. Performed the experiments: Hoshimi Kanemura. Contributed reagents and materials/analysis tools: Noriko Sakai and Masayo Takahashi. Wrote the paper: Shin Kawamata, Hoshimi Kanemura and Masahiro J. Go.

Conflict of Interests

The authors declare no conflict of interest associated with this manuscript.

References

1. Strauss, S. Geron trial resumes, but standards for stem cell trials remain elusive. *Nat. Biotechnol.* **2010**, *28*, 989–990.

2. Schwartz, S.D.; Hubschman, J.P.; Heilwell, G.; Franco-Cardenas, V.; Pan, C.K. Embryonic stem cell trials for macular degeneration: A preliminary report. *Lancet* **2012**, *379*, 713–720.

3. Cyranoski, D. Stem cells cruise to clinic. *Nature* **2013**, *494*, doi:10.1038/494413a.

4. Reardon, S.; Cyranoski, D. Japan stem-cell trial stirs envy. *Nature* **2014**, *513*, 287–288.

5. Researchers Perform World's 1st iPS Cell Implant Surgery on Human. Available online: http://ajw.asahi.com/article/sci_tech/medical/AJ201409130015 (accessed on 13 September 2014).

6. Frey-Vasconcells, J.; Whittlesey, K.J.; Baum, E.; Feigal, E.G. Translation of stem cell research: Points to consider in designing preclinical animal studies. *Stem Cells Transl. Med.* **2012**, *1*, 353–358.

7. Lund, R.J.; Närvä, E.; Lahesmaa, R. Genetic and epigenetic stability of human pluripotent stem cells. *Nat. Rev. Genet.* **2012**, *13*, 732–744.

8. OECD. Guidelines for the Testing of Chemicals. Available online: http://www.oecd.org/chemicalsafety/testing/oecdguidelinesforthetestingofchemicals.htm (accessed on 17 December 2014).

9. Kanemura, H.; Go, M.J.; Shikamura, M.; Nishishita, N.; Sakai, N.; Kamao, H.; Mandai, M.; Morinaga, C.; Takahashi, M.; Kawamata, S. Tumorigenicity studies of induced pluripotent stem cell (iPSC)-derived retinal pigment epithelium (RPE) for the treatment of age-related macular degeneration. *PLoS One* **2014**, *9*, e85336.

10. Sykova, E.; Forostyak, S. Stem cells in regenerative medicine. *Laser Ther.* **2013**, *22*, 87–92.

11. World Health Organization. Recommendations for the Evaluation of Animal Cell Cultures as Substrates for the Manufacture of Biological Medicinal Products and for the Characterization of Cell Banks. Proposed Replacement of TRS 878, Annex 1. Available online: http://www.who.int/biologicals/Cell_Substrates_clean_version_18_April.pdf (accessed on 17 December 2014).

12. World Health Organization. Requirements for the Use of Animal Cells as *in Vitro* Substrates for the Production of Biologicals; WHO Technical Report Series No. 878, Annex 1. Available online: http://whqlibdoc.who. int/trs/WHO_TRS_878.pdf (accessed on 17 December 2014).

13. Bailey, A.M. Balancing tissue and tumor formation in regenerative medicine. *Sci. Transl. Med.* **2012**, *4*, doi:10.1126/scitranslmed.3003685.

14. Suzuki, S.; Iwamoto, M.; Saito, Y.; Fuchimoto, D.; Sembon, S.; Suzuki, M.; Mikawa, S.; Hashimoto, M.; Aoki, Y.; Najima, Y.; *et al*. *Il2rg* gene-targeted severe combined immunodeficiency pigs. *Cell Stem Cell* **2012**, *10*, 753–758.

15. Machida, K.; Suemizu, H.; Kawai, K.; Ishikawa, T.; Sawada, R.; Ohnishi, Y.; Tsuchiya, T. Higher susceptibility of NOG mice to xenotransplanted tumors. *J. Toxicol. Sci.* **2009**, *34*, 123–127.

16. Prochazka, M.; Gaskins, H.R.; Shultz, L.D.; Leiter, E.H. The nonobese diabetic scid mouse: Model for spontaneous thymomagenesis associated with immunodeficiency. *Proc. Natl. Acad. Sci. USA* **1992**, *89*, 3290–3294.

17. Ciulla, T.A.; Criswell, M.H.; Danis, R.P.; Hill, T.E. Intravitreal Triamcinolone Acetonide Inhibits Choroidal Neovascularization in a Laser-Treated Rat Model. *Arch. Ophthalmol.* **2001**, *119*, 399–404.

18. Ciulla, T.A.; Criswell, M.H.; Danis, R.P.; Fronheiser, M.; Yuan, P.; Cox, T.A.; Csaky, K.G.; Robinson, M.R. Choroidal neovascular membrane inhibition in a laser treated rat model with intraocular sustained release triamcinolone acetonide microimplants. *Br. J. Ophthalmol.* **2003**, *87*, 1032–1037.

19. Kanemura, H.; Go, M.J.; Nishishita, N.; Sakai, N.; Kamao, H.; Sato, Y.; Takahashi, M.; Kawamata, S. Pigment Epithelium-Derived Factor Secreted from Retinal Pigment Epithelium Facilitates Apoptotic Cell Death of iPSC. *Sci. Rep.* **2013**, *3*, doi:10.1038/srep02334.

20. Kuroda, T.; Yasuda, S.; Kusakawa, S.; Hirata, N.; Kanda, Y.; Suzuki, K.; Takahashi, M.; Nishikawa, S.; Kawamata, S.; Sato, Y. Highly sensitive *in vitro* methods for detection of residual undifferentiated cells in retinal pigment epithelial cells derived from human iPS cells. *PLoS One* **2012**, *7*, e37342.

Concise Review: Methods and Cell Types Used to Generate Down Syndrome Induced Pluripotent Stem Cells

Youssef Hibaoui and Anis Feki

Abstract: Down syndrome (DS, trisomy 21), is the most common viable chromosomal disorder, with an incidence of 1 in 800 live births. Its phenotypic characteristics include intellectual impairment and several other developmental abnormalities, for the majority of which the pathogenetic mechanisms remain unknown. Several models have been used to investigate the mechanisms by which the extra copy of chromosome 21 leads to the DS phenotype. In the last five years, several laboratories have been successful in reprogramming patient cells carrying the trisomy 21 anomaly into induced pluripotent stem cells, *i.e.*, T21-iPSCs. In this review, we summarize the different T21-iPSCs that have been generated with a particular interest in the technical procedures and the somatic cell types used for the reprogramming.

Reprinted from *J. Clin. Med.* Cite as: Youssef Hibaoui and Anis Feki. Concise Review: Methods and Cell Types Used to Generate Down Syndrome Induced Pluripotent Stem Cells. *J. Clin. Med.* **2015**, *4*, 696–714.

1. Introduction

Down syndrome (DS), caused by a trisomy of chromosome 21 (HSA21), is the most common genetic developmental disorder, with an incidence of 1 in 800 live births. DS individuals show cognitive impairment, learning and memory deficits, arrest of neurogenesis and synaptogenesis, and early onset of Alzheimer's disease [1,2]. They are also at greater risk of developing acute lymphoblastic leukemia (ALL) and acute myeloid leukemia (AML). The incidence of ALL, the most common leukemia in childhood, is approximately 20-fold higher in children with DS than in the general population. The incidence of AML is between 46- to 83-fold higher, with a particular susceptibility to acute megakaryoblastic leukemia [3]. The detailed pathogenetic mechanisms by which the extra copy of HSA21 leads to the DS phenotype remain unknown. However, there is evidence that several regions exist on HSA21 with various "dosage sensitive" genes contributing to a given phenotype, which could also be modified by other genes on HSA21 and in the rest of the genome [4,5].

Several models have been used to recapitulate the DS phenotype, such as mouse models [6]. However, they do not accurately recapitulate the specificities of the human phenotype. A new finding indicating that induced pluripotent stem cells (iPSCs) can be reprogrammed through the introduction of a few factors [7,8] has opened a new avenue for the investigation of neurological diseases (reviewed in [9]). The first application of this technology appeared only one year after the release of these articles, with the derivation of iPSC lines from patients affected by several diseases including trisomy 21 [10]. Since that research paper, a dozen other studies reporting the generation of trisomy 21 iPSCs (T21-iPSCs) have appeared in the last five years. In this concise review, we will summarize the T21-iPSCs that have been reported up to now with a particular focus on the origin of the somatic cells and the procedures used for the reprogramming.

2. Procedures Used for the Reprogramming of T21-iPSCs

Direct reprogramming into iPSCs involves the ectopic introduction of a set of core pluripotency-related transcription factors in a somatic cell. In the vast majority of iPSC studies, *OCT4* (also known as *POU5F1*), *SOX2*, *KLF4* and *MYC* (also known as *c-MYC*) are used for the reprogramming into pluripotency as in the original study by Yamanaka's team [7]. In addition to this so-called OSKM cocktail, Thomson and colleagues also proposed another reprogramming cocktail that comprises *OCT4* and *SOX2* but *NANOG* and *LIN28* instead of *KLF4* and *c-MYC*: the so-called OSNL cocktail [8]. When this process is successful, compacted colonies appeared in the culture dish that showed marked similarities to embryonic stem cells (ESCs) with respect to morphology, growth properties, expression of pluripotency factors, self-renewal and developmental potential [7,8,11]. The current published T21-iPSC lines have been all generated with the OSKM cocktail, except for one study where T21-iPSCs were derived with the OSNL cocktail [12]. Thus, these T21-iPSC lines were derived predominantly through integrative delivery systems and, to a lesser extent, through non-integrative delivery systems (Table 1).

Table 1. The different T21-iPSCs reprogrammed.

Type and Age of Donor Cells	Reprogramming Method	Characteristic of the iPSCs	DS Phenotype Investigated	References
Fibroblasts from patients (1 year, 1 month) with unrelated controls	Retrovirus with OSKM	The first T21-iPSCs generated		[10]
Fibroblasts from a DS patient (1 year) with unrelated controls	Retrovirus with OSKM		Neurons and AD associated phenotype	[10,13,14]
Skin fibroblasts from DS patients (childs) with no control	Lentivirus with OSKM	T21-iPSCs with different karyotypes for DS		[15]
Amniotic fluid cells (second trimester) with age match control	Lentivirus with OSKM		Reduced number of neurons	[16]
Fibroblasts from DS individuals	Retrovirus with OSKM	Isogenic iPSCs	Myeloid Leukemia	[10,17]
Neonatal fibroblasts Fetal stromal cells Fetal mononuclear cells	Doxycycline-induced Lentivirus with OSKM, Retrovirus with OSKM		Myeloid Leukemia	[18]
Fibroblasts from DS individuals	Lentivirus with OSNL	Trisomy 21 deletion through TKNEO	Proliferation and neurogenesis	[12]

Table 1. *Cont.*

Type and Age of Donor Cells	Reprogramming Method	Characteristic of the iPSCs	DS Phenotype Investigated	References
Fibroblasts from unrelated patients and controls Fibroblasts from a mosaic DS patient.	Episomal vectors with OSK or OSNLM	Non integrating procedures Isogenic iPSCs	Neurogenesis, gliogenic shift	[19]
Fibroblasts from unrelated patients and controls Fibroblasts from a mosaic DS patient	Retrovirus with OSKM Sendai virus with OSKM	Isogenic iPSCs	Neuron deficit	[20]
Fibroblasts from a DS patient (1 year)	Retrovirus with OSKM Sendai virus with OSKM	Trisomy 21 deletion through Xist	Proliferation and neurogenesis	[10,21]
Fetal skin fibroblasts from monozygotic twins discordant for trisomy 21	Lentivirus with OSKM	Monozygotic twins discordant for trisomy 21	Neurogenesis, gliogenic shift, rescue of the phenotype	[22–24]
Fibroblasts	Retrovirus with OSKM	Non-isogenic and isogenic iPSCs	Neurogenesis, gliogenic shift	[25]

DS: Down syndrome; iPSCs: induced pluripotent stem cells; reprogramming cocktails: O for OCT4, S for *SOX2*, K for *KLF4*, M for *c-MYC*, N for *NANOG*, L for *LIN28*.

2.1. Integrative Procedures Used for the Derivation of T21-iPSCs

The first T21-iPSC lines were generated with the OSKM cocktail using the Maloney murine leukemia virus (MMLV)-derived retroviruses pMXs [10]. MMLV-derived retroviruses have been used in more than half of the studies reporting the generation of T21-iPSCs (Table 1). In this respect, MMLV-derived retroviruses allow the delivery of genes into the genomes of dividing cells, and the efficiency of iPSC generation from human fibroblasts using MMLV-derived retroviruses is approximately 0.01%.

Lentiviral vectors have also been successfully used to reprogram T21-iPSCs (Table 1). They are generally derived from HIV. They exhibit higher infection efficiency than MMLV-derived retroviruses and allow the delivery of genes into the genome of dividing and non-dividing cells. The efficiency of iPSC generation from human fibroblasts using lentiviral vectors is comparable to those of MMLV-derived retroviruses (~0.01%). However, compared to MMLV-derived retroviruses, lentiviruses are less repressed in human pluripotent stem cells (hPSCs) [26]. In this respect, a major improvement has been seen in the method with the development of single polycistronic vectors containing all the reprogramming factors, which reduce multiple transgene insertion into the genome [27]. Moreover, in one study, T21-iPSCs were derived through doxycycline-induced lentiviral vectors with an OSKM cocktail [18]. The main advantage of this method is that it allows greater control over transgene expression; compared with constitutive lentivirus, in which the vector is integrated and then may or may not be silenced, the doxycycline-induced lentivirus is integrated and silenced when doxycycline is removed. A more recent improvement of the method has been the introduction of lentiviral vectors that incorporate loxP sites allowing their excision via Cre recombinase when pluripotency is achieved [28]. However, viral elements flanking the loxP sites still remain after excision.

The use of integrating vectors offers a more efficient means of reprogramming but also raises major drawbacks with the risk of (i) genetic and epigenetic aberrations; (ii) overexpression of potentially tumorigenic genes such as *c-MYC*; and (iii) incomplete silencing of reprogramming factors following differentiation. Also, the use of integrative approaches has been associated with genomic instability of the generated iPSCs. Genomic instability in iPSCs could come from various sources, which means karyotype analysis is one of the first verifications that has to be done when establishing an iPSC-based disease model. Mutations can originate from the parental somatic cells from which the iPSCs are derived or can be generated during the reprogramming process [29]. However, this is still debated, as growing evidence supports a similar frequency of genetic aberrations in iPSCs, independently of the reprogramming method (integrative or non-integrative) or the cell type used for the reprogramming [29–33]. Alternatively, it could be acquired after culture adaptation and passaging over time [34,35]. For example, mechanical passaging appears to produce more stable cells with a normal karyotype than enzymatic harvesting methods [36–38]. This genomic instability is not restricted to long-term culture, but can appear very rapidly, within five passages after switching human ESCs to enzymatic dissociation [39].

Another major concern of integrative delivery systems is related to a possible transgene reactivation that could lead to the overexpression of potentially tumorigenic genes such as *c-MYC* or *KLF4*. For instance, the presence of *c-MYC* is a major limitation, as chimeras derived from iPSCs frequently develop tumours due to the reactivation of *c-MYC* [40,41]. Therefore, transgene silencing has to be investigated after initial expansion of a few passages of the newly generated iPSCs. Moreover, early reports have proposed that residual transgene expression (of *c-MYC* or *KLF4* in particular), after using integrating viral approaches may affect pluripotency and differentiation states [8,11]. It is important to note, however, that reprogramming approaches that exclude *c-MYC* are more labor-intensive and less efficient. In fact, *c-MYC* is an important inducer of reprogramming [42–45], activating pluripotent genes and maintaining the pluripotent state of PSCs [46–48]. It is considered the driver of the first transcriptional wave during cellular reprogramming into iPSCs [49]. This could explain, at least in part, why the vast majority of the reported iPSC lines are achieved using *c-MYC*. Of note, other potential contributors of tumorigenicity of iPSCs have been reported; in particular, we highlighted the crucial role of *NANOG* during reprogramming into iPSCs with respect to germ cell tumor formation [50].

Regarding the impact of these methods on the differentiation potential of iPSC lines, Hu *et al.* reported variable potency of iPSCs to differentiate into neural cells independently of the set of reprogramming transgenes used to derive iPSCs as well as the presence or absence of the reprogramming transgenes in the generated iPSCs [51]. In line with this, in a study comparing the differentiation potential of iPSC lines derived from a single parental fibroblast line via several reprogramming strategies (+/− *c-MYC*, excised or non-excised transgene), neither the presence of *c-MYC* nor the presence of the transgene removed the *in vitro* potential of these iPSCs to differentiate into neuroprogenitor cells, neurons, astrocytes and oligodendrocytes [52]. Furthermore, it appears that omission in iPSCs of reprogramming factors, and of *c-MYC* in particular, compromises the efficiency of their subsequent differentiation into neuroprogenitor cells and neurons [53].

2.2. Non-Integrative Procedures Used for the Derivation of T21-iPSCs

Two non-integrative approaches have been used for the generation of T21-iPSCs: episomal vectors [19] and Sendai virus vectors [20]. Briggs *et al.* reported the first generation of T21-iPSCs free of vectors and transgenes [19]. This reprogramming was achieved by transfection with oriP/Epstein-Barr nuclear antigen-1 (oriP/EBNA1)-based episomal vectors [54]. These plasmids can be transfected without the need for viral delivery and can be removed from cells by culturing in the absence of selection. In other terms, the exogenous DNA is not integrated into the iPSC genome. However, the reprogramming efficiency of this approach for human fibroblasts is extremely low, ~0.0006% [54].

An alternative non-integrative method has been used for the generation of T21-iPSCs by the mean of Sendai virus [20]. Sendai virus, a member of the Paramyxovirus family is an enveloped virus with a nonsegmented negative-strand RNA genome. Modified Sendai virus (through the deletion in one of the two envelope glycoproteins) has emerged as an efficient and robust RNA-based gene delivery system. Since Sendai virus RNA replication occurs in cytoplasm of the infected cells without a DNA phase, there is no risk of vector genome integration into host genome [55]. Thus, the efficiency reached by this method is much higher than that achieved with episomal vectors for the reprogramming of human fibroblasts to iPSCs: ~1% [55].

3. Age and Type of the Donor Cells Used for the Reprogramming

Reprogramming into iPSCs requires the delivery of pluripotency factors into a somatic cell. This is achieved with different efficiencies and kinetics depending on the donor cell type. Therefore, the choice of the type of the donor cells is an important aspect to consider before the generation of disease-specific iPSCs. As for 80% of the studies reporting the derivation of human iPSCs, fibroblasts remain the cell type the most commonly used for the derivation of T21-iPSCs (Table 1). There are many reasons for this. Even though dermal fibroblasts are obtained from skin biopsies or neonatal foreskin biopsies, which require invasive procedures, they present several advantages. First, the culture of fibroblasts is relatively easy and cheap. In culture, fibroblasts also exhibit a high proliferation rate, viability and stability (at least in low passages, as the risk of accumulated genomic alteration increases with passaging). Moreover, the discovery of iPSC technology has been done initially in mouse fibroblasts [56] and subsequently adapted in human fibroblasts [7,8]. Then, most of the data available on the relative kinetics and efficiencies of the different methods used for the reprogramming have been characterized using fibroblasts as donor's cells (reviewed in [57]). In line with this, most of the iPSCs banked have been generated with fibroblasts as a starting material. All these considerations make fibroblasts as the main cell type used for the reprogramming in general as well as in DS research. However, other cell type has been used for the generation of T21-iPSCs such as cells from amniotic fluids which are more easily obtained and reprogrammed into iPSCs [16]. Indeed, second semester amniocenteses are routinely collected in the context of prenatal diagnosis screening. Also, compared with fibroblasts, cells from amniotic fluids transduced with OSKM exhibited higher efficiency (100 times more) and are reprogrammed into pluripotency more than twofold faster [58]. This makes cells from amniotic fluids as easy to reprogram as keratinocytes [59]. Similarly, fetal stromal cells and mononuclear cells have been used for the generation of T21-iPSCs [18].

During the reprogramming process, the epigenetic state of the donor's cells has to be reset to obtain a pluripotent state; this includes modification of the DNA methylation profile, and chromatine marks [60,61]. However, genome wide DNA methylation studies showed that iPSCs retain the DNA methylation signature of the donor's cells [60,62]. This so-called "epigenetic memory" consists of residual specific marks of the parental somatic cells that escape the reprogramming process, leading to a preferential differentiation potential of the generated iPSCs into the tissue of origin rather than other lineages [60,61]. For instance, iPSCs derived from cord blood display a higher capacity for hematopoietic differentiation than iPSCs derived from keratinocyte, and reciprocally [60]. However, it is important to note that studies investigating donor epigenetic memory of iPSCs have confounded the donor's cell type and the donor genetic background due to the practical difficulty of collecting various primary tissues from the same donor. Also, it has been reported that donor epigenetic memory appears to be gradually lost after prolonged iPSC culture [60,62,63], which supports the idea that the preferential differentiation potential due to epigenetic memory can be overcome. Moreover, there are some indications that non-coding RNAs such as miRNAs play a role in maintaining residual memory of donor cells in iPSC-derived cells [64,65]. For instance, miR-155 have been identified as a key player in somatic donor memory of iPSCs in the context of iPSC differentiation toward hematopoietic progenitors [64].

Another important factor that should be considered when deriving disease specific iPSCs is the age of the donor's cells. T21-iPSCs have been generated from DS tissue from fetal, neonatal and adult stages (Table 1). In this respect, embryonic tissue appears to be more prone to reprogramming into pluripotency than adult tissue. Barriers such as the age and the differentiation status of the donor's cells could explain this property [66–68]. For instance, it has been shown that the increased levels of the age-related genes *p16* (*INK4A*), *p19* (*ARF*) and *p15* (*INK4B*), which encodes two tumor suppressors, limit the efficiency and the fidelity of the reprogramming [67]. Also, the differentiation stage of the starting cell used for the reprogramming has a critical impact on the efficiency of reprogramming into iPSCs. Blood progenitors reprogram into iPSCs up to 300 times more efficiently than terminally differentiated blood cells [68]. Similarly, neural progenitor cells which express *SOX2* endogenously have only been successfully reprogrammed into iPSCs with *OCT4* [69]. Considering that donor cell type and age may affect the differentiation potential of the iPSCs, it is crucial to establish D21-iPSCs and T21-iPSCs from the same parental somatic cells at the same developmental age.

4. Isogenic D21-iPSCs and T21-iPSCs

Among the potential variables that must be considered when establishing an hPSC-based disease model, the definition of a non-disease control is of crucial importance [70,71]. The genetic background of both control and the affected cells has to be identical or similar in order to be sure that the differences observed in the studies are due only to the disease and not to the choice of either the control or the affected samples. Traditionally, iPSCs from unrelated healthy individuals together with ones from age-matched, unrelated affected patients are often used to decrease the variability of individual genetic background and the variability among the iPSC lines regarding their *in vitro* differentiation potential. To overcome these problems, several approaches have been developed to obtain isogenic D21-iPSCs and T21-iPSCs. This is particularly important as isogenic D21-iPSCs and T21-iPSCs represent an ideal situation for the investigation of the effect of the supernumerary HSA21 on the DS phenotype, since the rest of the genome is theoretically identical. It could also limit the need to generate several iPSC lines.

Chromosomal aberrations have been often observed after culture adaptation over time in hPSCs [34]. In particular, stable genomic aberrations that confer growth, self-renewal, and differentiation advantages for hPSCs are often selected over time [29,34,72]. In the study by MacLean *et al.*, one clone of T21-iPSCs lost one copy of HSA21 with culture passages leading to a mixed culture of isogenic D21-iPSCs and T21-iPSCs. Then, they succeeded in isolating isogenic D21-iPSCs and T21-iPSCs from this mixed culture by cultivating them as single cells and discriminating D21-iPSCs from T21-iPSCs by FISH analysis (Figure 1A) [17]. This event seemed to occur also for one clone of T21-iPSCs generated by Chen *et al.* [25].

In another study, Li *et al.* succeeded in deriving isogenic D21-iPSCs from T21-iPSCs. For this, they used an adeno-associated virus to introduce a *TKNEO* transgene into one copy of HSA21 of T21-iPSCs. When the T21-iPSCs were grown in a medium that selected against *TKNEO*, the only cells that survived were the ones that spontaneously lost the extra HSA21 (Figure 1B) [12].

In an elegant study, Lawrence *et al.* have shown that the extra copy of HSA21 in T21-iPSCs can be silenced through the insertion of the RNA gene called *XIST*, a gene responsible for the silencing of one of the two X-chromosomes in female cells. Interestingly, they demonstrated that the insertion of *XIST* gene at a specified location in the HSA21 using zinc finger nuclease technology effectively repressed genes across the supernumerary HSA21 in T21-iPSCs, leading to the generation of isogenic D21-iPSCs and T21-iPSCs (Figure 1B) [21].

It is well known that varying degrees of mosaicism for trisomy 21 may exist in the generation population; it represents 1%–3% of DS cases [73]. This leads to a combination of euploid cells and cells carrying trisomy 21 anomaly within individual tissues (reviewed in [74]). Taking advantage of this rare situation, two recent studies reported the derivation of isogenic D21-iPSCs and T21-iPSCs from fibroblasts from an individual mosaic for trisomy 21 (Figure 2A) [19,20].

378

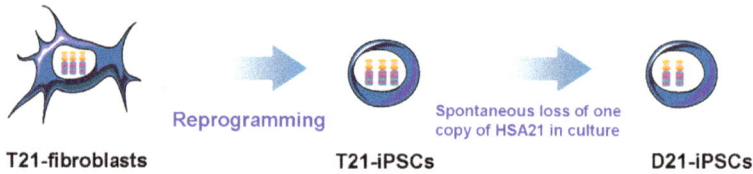

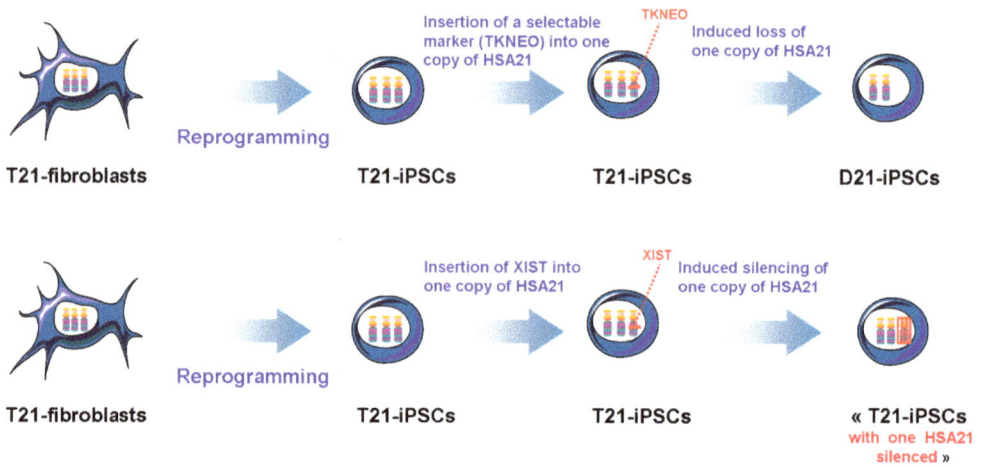

Figure 1. Isogenic iPSCs obtained through spontaneous or induced loss of trisomy 21. Isogenic D21-iPSCs and T21-iPSCs have been obtained either via spontaneous or induced loss of one copy of HSA21. (**A**) T21-iPSCs can lose one copy of HSA21 after culture adaptation and passaging over time [17,25]; (**B**) The loss of one copy of HSA21 in T21-iPSCs has been induced through the insertion of a foreign gene called *TKNEO* into one copy of HSA21 (within the *APP* gene) of T21-iPSCs. When these T21-iPSCs were grown in a medium that selected against *TKNEO*, the most common reason for the cells to survive was the loss of one copy of HSA21 [12]. The silencing of one copy of HSA21 in T21-iPSCs has been induced through the insertion of *XIST* into one copy of HSA21 of T21-iPSCs. This leads ultimately to the generation of isogenic D21-iPSCs [21].

Most monozygotic twins are "genetically identical" and are in general expected to be concordant for health, chromosomal abnormalities, and Mendelian disorders. However, in very rare cases, monozygotic twins can be discordant for the disease (reviewed in [75]). One example of this is monozygotic twins discordant for trisomy 21 [76]. We exploited this rare and unique situation by deriving iPSCs from fetal fibroblasts of monozygotic twins discordant for trisomy 21 [22–24] and thus confounding effects from genomic variability were theoretically eliminated (Figure 2B).

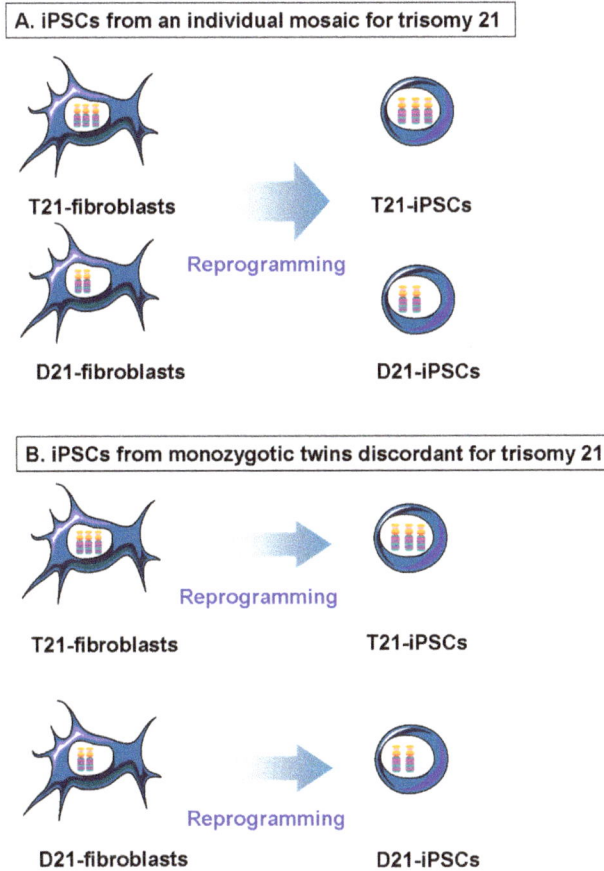

Figure 2. Isogenic iPSCs from individual mosaic for trisomy 21 or from monozygotic twins discordant for trisomy 21. (**A**) Isogenic D21-iPSCs and T21-iPSCs have been derived from mosaic patients for trisomy 21 [19,20]; (**B**) Isogenic D21-iPSCs and T21-iPSCs have been generated from monozygotic twins discordant for trisomy 21 [22–24].

5. Down Syndrome Phenotype Investigated

Among the phenotypes observed in DS individuals, only two have been explored using T21-iPSCs, namely brain-related defects and myeloid leukemia.

5.1. Brain-Related Defects

Five groups, including our own, have reported the recapitulation of the relevant DS phenotype using neurons derived from T21-iPSCs. Consistent with a DS post-mortem human brain, T21-iPSCs showed reduced neurogenesis when induced to differentiate into neuroprogenitor cells (NPCs) and further mature into neurons [19,21,23]. This effect was associated with a proliferation deficit and increased apoptosis of NPCs derived from T21-iPSCs [23]. Thus, together with the reduced neurogenesis, T21-iPSCs showed a greater propensity to generate both astroglial [19,23] and oligodendroglial cells [23] upon neural induction and differentiation. This gliogenic shift appeared early in development as it starts at the NPC level [23]. Moreover, neurons derived from T21-iPSCs exhibited not only a reduction of their population but also structural alterations compared to those derived from D21-iPSCs. They exhibited in particular reduced dendritic development [23] and reduced expression of synaptic proteins such as synapsin or SNAP25 [20,23]. In line with this, we found a lower proportion of excitatory glutamatergic synapses whereas the proportion of inhibitory GABA-ergic synapses was not substantially altered in neurons derived from T21-iPSCs [23]. Regarding the electrophysiological properties, neurons derived from T21-iPSCs displayed a significant synaptic deficit that affects excitatory glutamatergic synapses and inhibitory GABA-ergic synapses equally [20].

Furthermore, the increased proportion of astroglial cells at the expense of neurons upon neural induction and differentiation of T21-iPSCs [19,23] is of special interest as it has been shown that astrocytes derived from T21-iPSCs exhibited higher levels of reactive oxygen species (ROS) and lower levels of synaptogenic molecules than astrocytes derived from D21-iPSCs. This ultimately contributes to oxidative stress-mediated cell death and abnormal maturation of neurons derived from T21-iPSCs [25].

Finally, Shi *et al.* used T21-iPSCs as a PSC model of Alzheimer's disease pathology, given that DS individuals present early onset of Alzheimer's disease. They showed that cortical neurons derived from T21-iPSCs exhibited greater secretion of amyloid peptides, tau protein phosphorylation and cell death, supporting the notion that T21-iPSCs are an excellent model for AD study [13].

5.2. Myeloid Leukemia

Two recent studies have explored the potential of T21-iPSCs to model hematopoietic defects associated with trisomy 21 [17,18]. Using a differentiation protocol that mainly drives hPSCs towards primitive yolk sac-type hematopoietic progenitors, Chou *et al.* showed that hematopoietic progenitors derived from T21-iPSCs exhibit an increased propensity for erythropoiesis [18], similar to what it is observed in DS fetal liver hematopoiesis [77,78]. However, in contrast with DS fetal liver hematopoiesis, no difference was found between D21-iPSCs and T21-iPSCs in their capacity to generate megakaryocytes [18]. In the second study, MacLean and colleagues used a differentiation protocol that drives hPSCs towards definitive fetal-liver type progenitors. They found that hematopoietic progenitors derived from T21-iPSCs (and from T21-ESCs) exhibit higher multi-lineage colony-forming potential [17]. In particular, T21-iPSC-derived hematopoietic progenitors showed a greater colony-forming unit for erythroid, myeloid and megakaryocyte lineages [17], consistent with DS fetal liver hematopoiesis [77,78]. This indicates that trisomy 21 favours the expansion of hematopoietic progenitor cells. Altogether, these two studies point to different defects in primitive yolk sac-type hematopoietic progenitors and definitive fetal-liver type progenitors derived from T21-iPSCs and further suggest that the effects of trisomy 21 are likely specific to the developmental stages of the hematopoietic progenitors. Further studies using this iPSC-based model should provide important clues regarding the impact of trisomy 21 on hematopoietic development.

6. Conclusions and Perspectives

Since the first paper demonstrating that fibroblasts from DS patients can be reprogrammed into iPSCs by retroviral delivery of OSKM cocktail [10], several alternative methods and cell types have been used to generate T21-iPSCs (Table 1). At the moment, there is no consensus for the cell type that should be used for the reprogramming. The choice of the starting material depends not only on the availability of the cell type, but also on the ability and efficiency of these cells for reprogramming. With respect to the reprogramming method that should be used, this depends mostly on the priorities regarding the applications of the generated iPSCs. The priorities are not the same if the generated iPSCs aimed at investigating (i) the reprogramming mechanisms; (ii) disease modelling and drug screening and (iii) regenerative medicine. For the former aim, as the reprogramming approach needs to be efficient, the integrative inducible lentiviruses will meet most of the requirements. The safety of the generated iPSCs is a major requirement for clinical applications but less crucial for disease modelling and drug screening studies. In this respect, Sendai viruses and mRNA methods offer the advantage of generating iPSCs free of vectors and transgenes with a high efficiency [79].

Another major concern when generating iPSCs is the definition of a non-diseased control. In most of the studies reporting disease modelling using iPSCs, iPSC lines from unrelated healthy donors have been used as controls since genetically matched non-diseased controls are often difficult to obtain. In this respect, isogenic D21-iPSCs and T21-iPSCs offer the unique opportunity to study the effect of the supernumerary HSA21 on DS phenotype without the biological "noise" that could result from the variability of individual genetic background. These isogenic D21-iPSCs and T21-iPSCs has been achieved via several ways: (i) by spontaneous or induced loss of one copy of HSA21 in T21-iPSCs [12,17,21,25]; (ii) isogenic D21-iPSCs and T21-iPSCs from an individual mosaic for trisomy 21 [19,20]; (iii) isogenic D21-iPSCs and T21-iPSCs from monozygotic twins discordant for trisomy 21 [22–24]. Of note is the recent progress in genomic editing technologies such as transcription Activator-Like Effector Nucleases (TALEN), Zinc Finger Nucleases (ZFN) and Clustered Regularly Interspaced Short Palindromic Repeats (CRISPRs) (for review [80]) should provide opportunities to investigate genotype-phenotype correlations using "gene-edited" iPSC lines. For instance, it should allow the study of the contribution of candidate genes on DS phenotype by the investigation of the effect of genetic loss-of-function in T21-iPSCs and gain-of-function in D21-iPSCs of HSA21 genes in the target cell type of interest for DS.

A major drawback of iPSC technology is the variability that can appear at each step of the reprogramming and the differentiation processes. Reprogramming into iPSCs can give rise to unpredictable alterations of the genome such as copy number variants, karyotypic abnormalities, point mutations and deletions, epigenetic memory of the parental somatic cells [29–39,60–63]. Therefore, it is possible that such genetic and epigenetic alterations can affect the fidelity of the results regarding disease modeling and drug screening. Also, there is evidence that iPSC lines display variable potency to differentiate into the cell type of interest [51,60]. However, it is unclear what factors contribute to this variable efficiency of the iPSC differentiation, as it appears independent of the methods used for the reprogramming [51]. For this reasons, it is important to generate several iPSC lines from accurately chosen tissue of multiple normal and DS individuals, using them in priority non-integrative procedures. Such efforts will improve the identification of the pathogenetic mechanisms involved in DS by reducing the noise that could result from the variability of individual genetic background and from the experimental artifacts. At the same time, it will reduce the discovery of false pathogenetic mechanisms.

Another aspect that should be taken into account in DS modelling using iPSCs is the presence of a broad phenotypic variability among DS individuals. Even though DS individuals share some morphogenetic characteristics [1,4,5], trisomy 21 can have differential pathogenicity on individual genomes [81]. For example, brain-related defects are common traits in all DS individuals but other traits such as congenital heart defects only occur in ~40% of them. In line with this, cases of partial trisomy 21 and other HSA21 rearrangements associated with DS features have been reported [4,5]. Such cases could serve to link genomic regions of HSA21 with specific phenotypes given the possibility of generating the target cell type of interest for DS using T21-iPSCs.

Regarding the applications of T21-iPSCs, the abundance of studies reporting the generation of T21-iPSCs clearly shows that T21-iPSCs are reliable tool for DS modelling, given that the protocols for differentiation of iPSCs into neurons or hematopoietic cells are available. These protocols enable the production of large quantities of the target cell type for DS modelling. Some of these studies have been successful in recapitulating DS phenotypes using iPSCs (see Table 1). In this respect, transcriptional profiling of T21-iPSCs has proven extremely informative for the study of the pathogenetic mechanisms involved in DS phenotype [17–19,22–24]. For example, T21-iPSCs recapitulate the developmental disease transcriptional signature of DS [22–24]. Furthermore, T21-iPSCs allow the possibility of linking the genetic data to biological insights by deciphering the molecular changes in the target cell type of interest for DS (reviewed [82]). Then, the causal involvement of candidate HSA21 genes and pathways can be assayed by studies involving genetic loss-of-function in T21-iPSCs and gain-of-function in D21-iPSCs through genomic editing methods (for review [80]). Regarding DS modelling, only two phenotypes have been investigated so far: brain-related defects and myeloid leukemia (Table 1). However, other phenotypes associated with DS deserve investigations (heart defects, lymphoid leukemia and others). Moreover, modelling DS using iPSCs offers opportunities for drug screening. In concert with functional genomics, iPSCs form a powerful cellular model platform for drug screening assays with direct relevance to the DS phenotype. Integrating the genetic findings and the functional insights obtained from T21-iPSC-derived cells should provide a path to predict which drug might best counteract DS phenotype. Four studies have produced the proof of concept of such an application. Several proteins or pathways have been targeted and demonstrated beneficial effects on the DS phenotype, including oxidative stress-mediated cell death (with *N*-acetylcysteine, an antioxidant) [19], neurogenesis impairment (with epigallocatechine gallate, a DYRK1A inhibitor) [23], the gliogenic shift (with monocycline, an anti-inflammatory drug) [25] and AD-related phenotype (with inhibitors of gamma secretase) [13]. Finally, one promising aspect of iPSC technology is the potential use of these cells in cell replacement therapy to treat neurological diseases [9]. However, iPSCs have not been used until recently for clinical applications due to concerns over the immunogenicity and tumorigenicity of these cells [83,84]. Recently, iPSC technology has generated enthusiasm in the field of cell replacement therapy with the decision of Takahashi's team to treat a patient with a degenerative eye disease [85]. The possibility to induce the loss of one copy of HSA21 in T21-iPSCs and to produce subsequently isogenic D21-cells offers great hope for the treatment of some DS phenotypes (such as brain-related defects). However, numerous challenges remain for cell replacement therapy [9,86], and further studies are needed to address to which extent cells derived from iPSCs can be used for DS therapy. The coming years will tell whether these cells fulfil their potential.

In conclusion, we believe that T21-iPSC-derived cells are an invaluable resource for medical research. They will advance our understanding of the pathogenetic mechanism by which the extra copy of HSA21 leads to the DS phenotype. They have already offered the first opportunity to study the developmental events in the cell type of interest for DS: brain-related defects using iPSC-derived neurons and leukemia using iPSC-derived hematopoietic cells. IPSCs could also serve as a cellular platform for the evaluation of potential therapeutics.

Acknowledgments

This work was supported by grants from Dubois-Ferrière Dinu Lipatti, Gertrude Von Meissner and Novartis Foundations. The authors would like to especially thank Iwona Grad for useful comments and proofreading.

Author Contributions

Youssef Hibaoui and Anis Feki contributed to manuscript writing. Youssef Hibaoui prepared the figures and tables. Youssef Hibaoui and Anis Feki edited and revised the final manuscript.

Conflicts of Interest

The authors declare no conflict of interest.

References

1. Antonarakis, S.E.; Lyle, R.; Dermitzakis, E.T.; Reymond, A.; Deutsch, S. Chromosome 21 and down syndrome: From genomics to pathophysiology. *Nat. Rev. Genet.* **2004**, *5*, 725–738.
2. Lott, I.T.; Dierssen, M. Cognitive deficits and associated neurological complications in individuals with Down's syndrome. *Lancet Neurol.* **2010**, *9*, 623–633.
3. Lange, B. The management of neoplastic disorders of haematopoeisis in children with Down's syndrome. *Br. J. Haematol.* **2000**, *110*, 512–524.
4. Lyle, R.; Bena, F.; Gagos, S.; Gehrig, C.; Lopez, G.; Schinzel, A.; Lespinasse, J.; Bottani, A.; Dahoun, S.; Taine, L.; *et al.* Genotype-phenotype correlations in Down syndrome identified by array CGH in 30 cases of partial trisomy and partial monosomy chromosome 21. *Eur. J. Hum. Genet.* **2008**, *17*, 454–466.

5.   Korbel, J.O.; Tirosh-Wagner, T.; Urban, A.E.; Chen, X.-N.; Kasowski, M.; Dai, L.; Grubert, F.; Erdman, C.; Gao, M.C.; Lange, K.; *et al.* The genetic architecture of down syndrome phenotypes revealed by high-resolution analysis of human segmental trisomies. *Proc. Natl. Acad. Sci. USA* **2009**, *106*, 12031–12036.

6.   Das, I.; Reeves, R.H. The use of mouse models to understand and improve cognitive deficits in Down syndrome. *Dis. Model. Mech.* **2011**, *4*, 596–606.

7.   Takahashi, K.; Tanabe, K.; Ohnuki, M.; Narita, M.; Ichisaka, T.; Tomoda, K.; Yamanaka, S. Induction of pluripotent stem cells from adult human fibroblasts by defined factors. *Cell* **2007**, *131*, 861–872.

8.   Yu, J.; Vodyanik, M.A.; Smuga-Otto, K.; Antosiewicz-Bourget, J.; Frane, J.L.; Tian, S.; Nie, J.; Jonsdottir, G.A.; Ruotti, V.; Stewart, R.; *et al.* Induced pluripotent stem cell lines derived from human somatic cells. *Science* **2007**, *318*, 1917–1920.

9.   Hibaoui, Y.; Feki, A. Human pluripotent stem cells: Applications and challenges in neurological diseases. *Front. Physiol.* **2012**, *3*, doi:10.3389/fphys.2012.00267.

10.   Park, I.-H.; Arora, N.; Huo, H.; Maherali, N.; Ahfeldt, T.; Shimamura, A.; Lensch, M.W.; Cowan, C.; Hochedlinger, K.; Daley, G.Q.; *et al.* Disease-specific induced pluripotent stem cells. *Cell* **2008**, *134*, 877–886.

11.   Park, I.-H.; Zhao, R.; West, J.A.; Yabuuchi, A.; Huo, H.; Ince, T.A.; Lerou, P.H.; Lensch, M.W.; Daley, G.Q. Reprogramming of human somatic cells to pluripotency with defined factors. *Nature* **2008**, *451*, 141–146.

12.   Li, Li B.; Chang, K.-H.; Wang, P.-R.; Hirata, R.K.; Papayannopoulou, T.; Russell, D.W. Trisomy correction in Down syndrome induced pluripotent stem cells. *Cell Stem Cell* **2012**, *11*, 615–619.

13.   Shi, Y.; Kirwan, P.; Smith, J.; MacLean, G.; Orkin, S.H.; Livesey, F.J. A human stem cell model of early Alzheimer's disease pathology in Down syndrome. *Sci. Transl. Med.* **2012**, *4*, doi:10.1126/scitranslmed.3003771.

14.   Vallier, L.; Touboul, T.; Brown, S.; Cho, C.; Bilican, B.; Alexander, M.; Cedervall, J.; Chandran, S.; Ährlund-Richter, L.; Weber, A.; *et al.* Signaling pathways controlling pluripotency and early cell fate decisions of human induced pluripotent stem cells. *Stem Cells* **2009**, *27*, 2655–2666.

15.   Mou, X.; Wu, Y.; Cao, H.; Meng, Q.; Wang, Q.; Sun, C.; Hu, S.; Ma, Y.; Zhang, H. Generation of disease-specific induced pluripotent stem cells from patients with different karyotypes of Down syndrome. *Stem Cell Res. Ther.* **2012**, *3*, doi:10.1186/scrt105.

16.   Lu, H.-E.; Yang, Y.-C.; Chen, S.-M.; Su, H.-L.; Huang, P.-C.; Tsai, M.-S.; Wang, T.-H.; Tseng, C.-P.; Hwang, S.-M. Modeling neurogenesis impairment in Down syndrome with induced pluripotent stem cells from trisomy 21 amniotic fluid cells. *Exp. Cell Res.* **2013**, *319*, 498–505.

17.   MacLean, G.A.; Menne, T.F.; Guo, G.; Sanchez, D.J.; Park, I.-H.; Daley, G.Q.; Orkin, S.H. Altered hematopoiesis in trisomy 21 as revealed through *in vitro* differentiation of isogenic human pluripotent cells. *Proc. Natl. Acad. Sci. USA* **2012**, *109*, 17567–17572.

18. Chou, S.T.; Byrska-Bishop, M.; Tober, J.M.; Yao, Y.; VanDorn, D.; Opalinska, J.B.; Mills, J.A.; Choi, J.K.; Speck, N.A.; Gadue, P.; *et al.* Trisomy 21-associated defects in human primitive hematopoiesis revealed through induced pluripotent stem cells. *Proc. Natl. Acad. Sci. USA* **2012**, *109*, 17573–17578.

19. Briggs, J.A.; Sun, J.; Shepherd, J.; Ovchinnikov, D.A.; Chung, T.-L.; Nayler, S.P.; Kao, L.-P.; Morrow, C.A.; Thakar, N.Y.; Soo, S.-Y.; *et al.* Integration-free induced pluripotent stem cells model genetic and neural developmental features of Down syndrome etiology. *Stem Cells* **2013**, *31*, 467–478.

20. Weick, J.P.; Held, D.L.; Bonadurer, G.F.; Doers, M.E.; Liu, Y.; Maguire, C.; Clark, A.; Knackert, J.A.; Molinarolo, K.; Musser, M.; *et al.* Deficits in human trisomy 21 iPSCs and neurons. *Proc. Natl. Acad. Sci. USA* **2013**, *110*, 9962–9967.

21. Jiang, J.; Jing, Y.; Cost, G.J.; Chiang, J.-C.; Kolpa, H.J.; Cotton, A.M.; Carone, D.M.; Carone, B.R.; Shivak, D.A.; Guschin, D.Y.; *et al.* Translating dosage compensation to trisomy 21. *Nature* **2013**, *500*, 296–300.

22. Letourneau, A.; Santoni, F.A.; Bonilla, X.; Sailani, M.R.; Gonzalez, D.; Kind, J.; Chevalier, C.; Thurman, R.; Sandstrom, R.S.; Hibaoui, Y.; *et al.* Domains of genome-wide gene expression dysregulation in Down's syndrome. *Nature* **2014**, *508*, 345–350.

23. Hibaoui, Y.; Grad, I.; Letourneau, A.; Sailani, M.R.; Dahoun, S.; Santoni, F.A.; Gimelli, S.; Guipponi, M.; Pelte, M.-F.; Béna, F.; *et al.* Modelling and rescuing neurodevelopmental defect of Down syndrome using induced pluripotent stem cells from monozygotic twins discordant for trisomy 21. *EMBO Mol. Med.* **2014**, *6*, 259–277.

24. Hibaoui, Y.; Grad, I.; Letourneau, A.; Santoni, F.A.; Antonarakis, S.E.; Feki, A. Data in brief: Transcriptome analysis of induced pluripotent stem cells from monozygotic twins discordant for trisomy 21. *Genomics Data* **2014**, *2*, 226–229.

25. Chen, C.; Jiang, P.; Xue, H.; Peterson, S.E.; Tran, H.T.; McCann, A.E.; Parast, M.M.; Li, S.; Pleasure, D.E.; Laurent, L.C.; *et al.* Role of astroglia in Down's syndrome revealed by patient-derived human-induced pluripotent stem cells. *Nat. Commun.* **2014**, *5*, doi:10.1038/ncomms5430.

26. Yao, S.; Sukonnik, T.; Kean, T.; Bharadwaj, R.R.; Pasceri, P.; Ellis, J. Retrovirus silencing, variegation, extinction, and memory are controlled by a dynamic interplay of multiple epigenetic modifications. *Mol. Ther.* **2004**, *10*, 27–36.

27. Carey, B.W.; Markoulaki, S.; Hanna, J.; Saha, K.; Gao, Q.; Mitalipova, M.; Jaenisch, R. Reprogramming of murine and human somatic cells using a single polycistronic vector. *Proc. Natl. Acad. Sci. USA* **2009**, *106*, 157–162.

28. Sommer, C.A.; Sommer, A.G.; Longmire, T.A.; Christodoulou, C.; Thomas, D.D.; Gostissa, M.; Alt, F.W.; Murphy, G.J.; Kotton, D.N.; Mostoslavsky, G.; *et al.* Excision of reprogramming transgenes improves the differentiation potential of iPS cells generated with a single excisable vector. *Stem Cells* **2010**, *28*, 64–74.

29. Mayshar, Y.; Ben-David, U.; Lavon, N.; Biancotti, J.-C.; Yakir, B.; Clark, A.T.; Plath, K.; Lowry, W.E.; Benvenisty, N. Identification and classification of chromosomal aberrations in human induced pluripotent stem cells. *Cell Stem Cell* **2010**, *7*, 521–531.

30. Gore, A.; Li, Z.; Fung, H.-L.; Young, J.E.; Agarwal, S.; Antosiewicz-Bourget, J.; Canto, I.; Giorgetti, A.; Israel, M.A.; Kiskinis, E.; *et al.* Somatic coding mutations in human induced pluripotent stem cells. *Nature* **2011**, *471*, 63–67.

31. Taapken, S.M.; Nisler, B.S.; Newton, M.A.; Sampsell-Barron, T.L.; Leonhard, K.A.; McIntire, E.M.; Montgomery, K.D. Karyotypic abnormalities in human induced pluripotent stem cells and embryonic stem cells. *Nat. Biotechnol.* **2011**, *29*, 313–314.

32. Ben-David, U.; Benvenisty, N. High prevalence of evolutionarily conserved and species-specific genomic aberrations in mouse pluripotent stem cells. *Stem Cells* **2012**, *30*, 612–622.

33. Martins-Taylor, K.; Nisler, B.S.; Taapken, S.M.; Compton, T.; Crandall, L.; Montgomery, K.D.; Lalande, M.; Xu, R.-H. Recurrent copy number variations in human induced pluripotent stem cells. *Nat. Biotechnol.* **2011**, *29*, 488–491.

34. Baker, D.E.C.; Harrison, N.J.; Maltby, E.; Smith, K.; Moore, H.D.; Shaw, P.J.; Heath, P.R.; Holden, H.; Andrews, P.W. Adaptation to culture of human embryonic stem cells and oncogenesis *in vivo*. *Nat. Biotechnol.* **2007**, *25*, 207–215.

35. Hovatta, O.; Jaconi, M.; Töhönen, V.; Béna, F.; Gimelli, S.; Bosman, A.; Holm, F.; Wyder, S.; Zdobnov, E.M.; Irion, O.; *et al.* A teratocarcinoma-like human embryonic stem cell (hESC) line and four hESC lines reveal potentially oncogenic genomic changes. *PLoS ONE* **2010**, *5*, e10263.

36. Buzzard, J.J.; Gough, N.M.; Crook, J.M.; Colman, A. Karyotype of human ES cells during extended culture. *Nat. Biotechnol.* **2004**, *22*, 381–382.

37. Mitalipova, M.M.; Rao, R.R.; Hoyer, D.M.; Johnson, J.A.; Meisner, L.F.; Jones, K.L.; Dalton, S.; Stice, S.L. Preserving the genetic integrity of human embryonic stem cells. *Nat. Biotechnol.* **2005**, *23*, 19–20.

38. Olariu, V.; Harrison, N.J.; Coca, D.; Gokhale, P.J.; Baker, D.; Billings, S.; Kadirkamanathan, V.; Andrews, P.W. Modeling the evolution of culture-adapted human embryonic stem cells. *Stem Cell Res.* **2010**, *4*, 50–56.

39. Bai, Q.; Ramirez, J.-M.; Becker, F.; Pantesco, V.; Lavabre-Bertrand, T.; Hovatta, O.; Lemaître, J.-M.; Pellestor, F.; de Vos, J. Temporal analysis of genome alterations induced by single-cell passaging in human embryonic stem cells. *Stem Cells Dev.* **2015**, *24*, 653–662.

40. Markoulaki, S.; Hanna, J.; Beard, C.; Carey, B.W.; Cheng, A.W.; Lengner, C.J.; Dausman, J.A.; Fu, D.; Gao, Q.; Wu, S.; *et al.* Transgenic mice with defined combinations of drug-inducible reprogramming factors. *Nat. Biotechnol.* **2009**, *27*, 169–171.

41. Okita, K.; Ichisaka, T.; Yamanaka, S. Generation of germline-competent induced pluripotent stem cells. *Nature* **2007**, *448*, 313–317.

42. Sridharan, R.; Tchieu, J.; Mason, M.J.; Yachechko, R.; Kuoy, E.; Horvath, S.; Zhou, Q.; Plath, K. Role of the murine reprogramming factors in the induction of pluripotency. *Cell* **2009**, *136*, 364–377.

43. Nakagawa, M.; Koyanagi, M.; Tanabe, K.; Takahashi, K.; Ichisaka, T.; Aoi, T.; Okita, K.; Mochiduki, Y.; Takizawa, N.; Yamanaka, S.; *et al.* Generation of induced pluripotent stem cells without Myc from mouse and human fibroblasts. *Nat. Biotechnol.* **2008**, *26*, 101–106.

44. Judson, R.L.; Babiarz, J.E.; Venere, M.; Blelloch, R. Embryonic stem cell-specific microRNAs promote induced pluripotency. *Nat. Biotechnol.* **2009**, *27*, 459–461.

45. Araki, R.; Hoki, Y.; Uda, M.; Nakamura, M.; Jincho, Y.; Tamura, C.; Sunayama, M.; Ando, S.; Sugiura, M.; Yoshida, M.A.; *et al.* Crucial role of c-Myc in the generation of induced pluripotent stem cells. *Stem Cells* **2011**, *29*, 1362–1370.

46. Cartwright, P.; McLean, C.; Sheppard, A.; Rivett, D.; Jones, K.; Dalton, S. LIF/STAT3 controls ES cell self-renewal and pluripotency by a Myc-dependent mechanism. *Development* **2005**, *132*, 885–896.

47. Smith, K.N.; Singh, A.M.; Dalton, S. Myc represses primitive endoderm differentiation in pluripotent stem cells. *Cell Stem Cell* **2010**, *7*, 343–354.

48. Meyer, N.; Penn, L.Z. Reflecting on 25 years with Myc. *Nat. Rev. Cancer* **2008**, *8*, 976–990.

49. Polo, J.M.; Anderssen, E.; Walsh, R.M.; Schwarz, B.A.; Nefzger, C.M.; Lim, S.M.; Borkent, M.; Apostolou, E.; Alaei, S.; Cloutier, J.; *et al.* A molecular roadmap of reprogramming somatic cells into iPS cells. *Cell* **2012**, *151*, 1617–1632.

50. Grad, I.; Hibaoui, Y.; Jaconi, M.; Chicha, L.; Bergström-Tengzelius, R.; Sailani, M.R.; Pelte, M.F.; Dahoun, S.; Mitsiadis, T.A.; Töhönen, V.; *et al.* Nanog priming before full reprogramming may generate germ cell tumours. *Eur. Cells Mater.* **2011**, *22*, 258–274.

51. Hu, B.-Y.; Weick, J.P.; Yu, J.; Ma, L.-X.; Zhang, X.-Q.; Thomson, J.A.; Zhang, S.-C. Neural differentiation of human induced pluripotent stem cells follows developmental principles but with variable potency. *Proc. Natl. Acad. Sci. USA* **2010**, *107*, 4335–4340.

52. Major, T.; Menon, J.; Auyeung, G.; Soldner, F.; Hockemeyer, D.; Jaenisch, R.; Tabar, V. Transgene excision has no impact on *in vivo* integration of human iPS derived neural precursors. *PLoS ONE* **2011**, *6*, e24687.

53. Löhle, M.; Hermann, A.; Glaß, H.; Kempe, A.; Schwarz, S.C.; Kim, J.B.; Poulet, C.; Ravens, U.; Schwarz, J.; Schöler, H.R.; *et al.* Differentiation efficiency of induced pluripotent stem cells depends on the number of reprogramming factors. *Stem Cells* **2012**, *30*, 570–579.

54. Yu, J.; Hu, K.; Smuga-Otto, K.; Tian, S.; Stewart, R.; Slukvin, I.I.; Thomson, J.A. Human induced pluripotent stem cells free of vector and transgene sequences. *Science* **2009**, *324*, 797–801.

55. Fusaki, N.; Ban, H.; Nishiyama, A.; Saeki, K.; Hasegawa, M. Efficient induction of transgene-free human pluripotent stem cells using a vector based on Sendai virus, an RNA virus that does not integrate into the host genome. *Proc. Jpn. Acad. Ser. B Phys. Biol. Sci.* **2009**, *85*, 348–362.

56. Takahashi, K.; Yamanaka, S. Induction of pluripotent stem cells from mouse embryonic and adult fibroblast cultures by defined factors. *Cell* **2006**, *126*, 663–676.

57. González, F.; Boué, S.; Belmonte, J.C.I. Methods for making induced pluripotent stem cells: Reprogramming à la carte. *Nat. Rev. Genet.* **2011**, *12*, 231–242.

58. Li, C.; Zhou, J.; Shi, G.; Ma, Y.; Yang, Y.; Gu, J.; Yu, H.; Jin, S.; Wei, Z.; Chen, F.; *et al.* Pluripotency can be rapidly and efficiently induced in human amniotic fluid-derived cells. *Hum. Mol. Genet.* **2009**, *18*, 4340–4349.

59. Aasen, T.; Raya, A.; Barrero, M.J.; Garreta, E.; Consiglio, A.; Gonzalez, F.; Vassena, R.; Bilic, J.; Pekarik, V.; Tiscornia, G.; *et al*. Efficient and rapid generation of induced pluripotent stem cells from human keratinocytes. *Nat. Biotechnol.* **2008**, *26*, 1276–1284.

60. Kim, K.; Zhao, R.; Doi, A.; Ng, K.; Unternaehrer, J.; Cahan, P.; Hongguang, H.; Loh, Y.-H.; Aryee, M.J.; Lensch, M.W.; *et al*. Donor cell type can influence the epigenome and differentiation potential of human induced pluripotent stem cells. *Nat. Biotechnol.* **2011**, *29*, 1117–1119.

61. Bar-Nur, O.; Russ, H. A.; Efrat, S.; Benvenisty, N. Epigenetic memory and preferential lineage-specific differentiation in induced pluripotent stem cells derived from human pancreatic islet beta cells. *Cell Stem Cell* **2011**, *9*, 17–23.

62. Polo, J.M.; Liu, S.; Figueroa, M.E.; Kulalert, W.; Eminli, S.; Tan, K.Y.; Apostolou, E.; Stadtfeld, M.; Li, Y.; Shioda, T.; *et al*. Cell type of origin influences the molecular and functional properties of mouse induced pluripotent stem cells. *Nat. Biotechnol.* **2010**, *28*, 848–855.

63. Kim, K.; Doi, A.; Wen, B.; Ng, K.; Zhao, R.; Cahan, P.; Kim, J.; Aryee, M.J.; Ji, H.; Ehrlich, L.I.R.; *et al*. Epigenetic memory in induced pluripotent stem cells. *Nature* **2010**, *467*, 285–290.

64. Vitaloni, M.; Pulecio, J.; Bilic, J.; Kuebler, B.; Laricchia-Robbio, L.; Izpisua Belmonte, J.C. MicroRNAs contribute to induced pluripotent stem cell somatic donor memory. *J. Biol. Chem.* **2014**, *289*, 2084–2098.

65. Georgantas, R.W.; Hildreth, R.; Morisot, S.; Alder, J.; Liu, C.-G.; Heimfeld, S.; Calin, G.A.; Croce, C.M.; Civin, C.I. CD34+ hematopoietic stem-progenitor cell microRNA expression and function: A circuit diagram of differentiation control. *Proc. Natl. Acad. Sci. USA* **2007**, *104*, 2750–2755.

66. Marion, R.M.; Strati, K.; Li, H.; Murga, M.; Blanco, R.; Ortega, S.; Fernandez-Capetillo, O.; Serrano, M.; Blasco, M.A. A p53-mediated DNA damage response limits reprogramming to ensure iPS cell genomic integrity. *Nature* **2009**, *460*, 1149–1153.

67. Li, H.; Collado, M.; Villasante, A.; Strati, K.; Ortega, S.; Canamero, M.; Blasco, M.A.; Serrano, M. The INK4/ARF locus is a barrier for iPS cell reprogramming. *Nature* **2009**, *460*, 1136–1139.

68. Eminli, S.; Foudi, A.; Stadtfeld, M.; Maherali, N.; Ahfeldt, T.; Mostoslavsky, G.; Hock, H.; Hochedlinger, K. Differentiation stage determines potential of hematopoietic cells for reprogramming into induced pluripotent stem cells. *Nat. Genet.* **2009**, *41*, 968–976.

69. Kim, J.B.; Sebastiano, V.; Wu, G.; Araúzo-Bravo, M.J.; Sasse, P.; Gentile, L.; Ko, K.; Ruau, D.; Ehrich, M.; van den Boom, D.; *et al*. Oct4-induced pluripotency in adult neural stem cells. *Cell* **2009**, *136*, 411–419.

70. Inoue, H.; Yamanaka, S. The use of induced pluripotent stem cells in drug development. *Clin. Pharmacol. Ther.* **2011**, *89*, 655–661.

71. Zhu, H.; Lensch, M.W.; Cahan, P.; Daley, G.Q. Investigating monogenic and complex diseases with pluripotent stem cells. *Nat. Rev. Genet.* **2011**, *12*, 266–275.

72. Amps, K.; Andrews, P.W.; Anyfantis, G.; Armstrong, L.; Avery, S.; Baharvand, H.; Baker, J.; Baker, D.; Munoz, M.B.; Beil, S.; *et al.* Screening ethnically diverse human embryonic stem cells identifies a chromosome 20 minimal amplicon conferring growth advantage. *Nat. Biotechnol.* **2011**, *29*, 1132–1144.

73. Devlin, L.; Morrison, P.J. Mosaic Down's syndrome prevalence in a complete population study. *Arch. Dis. Child.* **2004**, *89*, 1177–1178.

74. Kovaleva, N. Germ-line transmission of trisomy 21: Data from 80 families suggest an implication of grandmaternal age and a high frequency of female-specific trisomy rescue. *Mol. Cytogenet.* **2010**, *3*, doi:10.1186/1755-8166-3-7.

75. Zwijnenburg, P.J.G.; Meijers-Heijboer, H.; Boomsma, D.I. Identical but not the same: The value of discordant monozygotic twins in genetic research. *Am. J. Med. Genet. B Neuropsychiatr. Genet.* **2010**, *153B*, 1134–1149.

76. Dahoun, S.; Gagos, S.; Gagnebin, M.; Gehrig, C.; Burgi, C.; Simon, F.; Vieux, C.; Extermann, P.; Lyle, R.; Morris, M.A.; *et al.* Monozygotic twins discordant for trisomy 21 and maternal 21q inheritance: A complex series of events. *Am. J. Med. Genet. A* **2008**, *146A*, 2086–2093.

77. Tunstall-Pedoe, O.; Roy, A.; Karadimitris, A.; de la Fuente, J.; Fisk, N.M.; Bennett, P.; Norton, A.; Vyas, P.; Roberts, I. Abnormalities in the myeloid progenitor compartment in Down syndrome fetal liver precede acquisition of GATA1 mutations. *Blood* **2008**, *112*, 4507–4511.

78. Chou, S.T.; Opalinska, J.B.; Yao, Y.; Fernandes, M.A.; Kalota, A.; Brooks, J.S.J.; Choi, J.K.; Gewirtz, A.M.; Danet-Desnoyers, G.-A.; Nemiroff, R.L.; *et al.* Trisomy 21 enhances human fetal erythro-megakaryocytic development. *Blood* **2008**, *112*, 4503–4506

79. Schlaeger, T.M.; Daheron, L.; Brickler, T.R.; Entwisle, S.; Chan, K.; Cianci, A.; DeVine, A.; Ettenger, A.; Fitzgerald, K.; Godfrey, M.; *et al.* A comparison of non-integrating reprogramming methods. *Nat. Biotechnol.* **2015**, *33*, 58–63.

80. Kim, H.S.; Bernitz, J.M.; Lee, D.-F.; Lemischka, I.R. Genomic editing tools to model human diseases with isogenic pluripotent stem cells. *Stem Cells Dev.* **2014**, *23*, 2673–2686.

81. Prandini, P.; Deutsch, S.; Lyle, R.; Gagnebin, M.; Vivier, C.D.; Delorenzi, M.; Gehrig, C.; Descombes, P.; Sherman, S.; Bricarelli, F.D.; *et al.* Natural gene-expression variation in Down syndrome modulates the outcome of gene-dosage imbalance. *Am. J. Hum. Genet.* **2007**, *81*, 252–263.

82. Briggs, J.A.; Mason, E.A.; Ovchinnikov, D.A.; Wells, C.A.; Wolvetang, E.J. Concise review: New paradigms for Down syndrome research using induced pluripotent stem cells: Tackling complex human genetic disease. *Stem Cells Transl. Med.* **2013**, *2*, 175–184.

83. Zhao, T.; Zhang, Z.-N.; Rong, Z.; Xu, Y. Immunogenicity of induced pluripotent stem cells. *Nature* **2011**, *474*, 212–215.

84. Ben-David, U.; Benvenisty, N. The tumorigenicity of human embryonic and induced pluripotent stem cells. *Nat. Rev. Cancer* **2011**, *11*, 268–277.

85. Reardon, S.; Cyranoski, D. Japan stem-cell trial stirs envy. *Nature* **2014**, *513*, 287–288.

86. Fox, I.J.; Daley, G.Q.; Goldman, S.A.; Huard, J.; Kamp, T.J.; Trucco, M. Use of differentiated pluripotent stem cells in replacement therapy for treating disease. *Science* **2014**, *345*.

Chapter 10:
Immune Response

The Possible Future Roles for iPSC-Derived Therapy for Autoimmune Diseases

Meilyn Hew, Kevin O'Connor, Michael J. Edel and Michaela Lucas

Abstract: The ability to generate inducible pluripotent stem cells (iPSCs) and the potential for their use in treatment of human disease is of immense interest. Autoimmune diseases, with their limited treatment choices are a potential target for the clinical application of stem cell and iPSC technology. IPSCs provide three potential ways of treating autoimmune disease; (i) providing pure replacement of lost cells (immuno-reconstitution); (ii) through immune-modulation of the disease process *in vivo*; and (iii) for the purposes of disease modeling *in vitro*. In this review, we will use examples of systemic, system-specific and organ-specific autoimmunity to explore the potential applications of iPSCs for treatment of autoimmune diseases and review the evidence of iPSC technology in auto-immunity to date.

Reprinted from *J. Clin. Med.* Cite as: Meilyn Hew, Kevin O'Connor, Michael J. Edel and Michaela Lucas. The Possible Future Roles for iPSC-Derived Therapy for Autoimmune Diseases. *J. Clin. Med.* **2015**, *4*, 1193–1206.

1. Introduction

Pluripotent stem cells have the ability to differentiate into all three of the embryonic germ layers, endoderm, mesoderm, or ectoderm. While these pluripotent cells may be of embryonic origin, somatic cells can be induced into this pluripotency state by transient ectopic expression of defined groups of transcription factors, hence the term "inducible" pluripotent stem cells (iPSCs). The advantages of inducing pluripotency includes the potential generation of unlimited numbers of required cells, deriving cells from hard-to-source tissues, reproduction of disease models, bypassing the ethical concerns regarding the use of embryonic stem cells and importantly provide an autologous cell therapy strategy that removes the need for immune suppression drugs.

2. Background

Following the seminal paper by Takahashi and Yamanaka [1], which reported using appropriate transcription factors, Oct4, Sox2, Klf4, and c-Myc, mouse fibroblasts could be reprogrammed into a pluripotent state, it has been demonstrated in human somatic cells. Furthermore, other combinations of transcription factors are able to induce pluripotency in human somatic cells as well [1–5].

Autoimmune diseases affect individual organs or a combination of organs, including the kidneys, brain, bone marrow, joints, or skin, however, the pathogenesis of most autoimmune diseases remains, at best, only partially delineated. IPSC technology has the potential to provide key cellular subsets which, given to patients, may alter their disease course by providing pure replacement of lost cells, may limit damage through immune-modulation of the disease process *in vivo*, and may provide substrates for the purposes of disease modeling *in vitro*. In this review, systemic lupus erythematosus (SLE) is taken as a prototypical example of a systemic auto-immune disease, along with rheumatoid arthritis (RA); diabetes mellitus (DM) as an example of organ specific autoimmunity; and multiple sclerosis (MS) as an example of system-specific neurological autoimmunity, to demonstrate the promising future research potential towards translational medicine of iPSC-derived treatment in a range of different contexts within Clinical Immunology.

3. Disease Immunomodulation and Potential Cellular Components—SLE and RA as Examples

The loss of tolerance to self is the fundamental basis of autoimmunity, with resultant aberrant immune responses of autoantibody formation and/or cellular immunity against self-tissue.

Systemic lupus erythematosus (SLE) is a prototypical systemic autoimmune disease. Usually affecting women of childbearing age, it is characterised by the production of multiple auto-antibodies directed against double-stranded DNA and other nuclear antigens, which are widely distributed throughout the body. The autoantibodies are produced by activated auto-reactive B cells following presentation of these self-antigens to self-reactive T cells. Along with autoantibody production are reduced populations of regulatory T cells (Tregs), reduced responses to regulation by these cells on effector T cells, immunological dysregulation and increased inflammation [6], immune complex formation and deposition, and end-organ damage, particularly if the disease affects the kidneys or central nervous system.

Rheumatoid arthritis is a symmetrical, inflammatory disease of synovial joints which also manifests extra-articular pathology in about 40% of patients. Affecting other parts of the musculoskeletal system, as well as the skin, eye, lung, heart, kidney, and vascular and nervous system tissues, it is likely that the inflammatory processes driving the synovial inflammation are also responsible for these extra-articular manifestations. RA patients develop autoantibodies to post-translationally modified synovial or stress-related proteins, which results in the conversion of arginine residues into citrulline (a process known as citrullination). In genetically susceptible individuals, preferential binding of these citrullinated self-peptides to MHC molecules may enable presentation to peripheral T cells, allowing expansion of potentially self-reactive T-cell populations. At the same time, if there is no presentation centrally in the thymus, there is no deletion or negative selection of autoreactive T cell populations, which is a possible mechanism for loss of self-tolerance in RA.

The mainstay of treatment, for both SLE and RA, is with immunosuppressive medications, however, true immunomodulation in the absence of toxicity is difficult to achieve.

There are a number of important cell populations that impact on systemic autoimmune disease course in which iPSC technology could potentially assist to model their effects and ideally contribute to regaining self-tolerance, such as regulatory T cells (Tregs) and dendritic cells. Targeting of particular cell lineages, rather than their end products, is also likely to be beneficial in the treatment of other autoimmunity diseases.

3.1. Regulatory T Cells (Tregs)

Regulatory T cells (Tregs), have an important role in the state of equilibrium that is immune tolerance, and are, therefore, also known as tolerogenic T cells. Tregs are CD4, CD25, and Foxp3 positive, and act to restrict the extent and duration of T cell mediated immune responses, and maintain peripheral tolerance by suppressing auto-reactive T cells that have escaped negative selection in the thymus. The mechanisms by which Tregs work continue to be discovered [7]. Most Tregs arise centrally in the thymus where cell lineage commitment is determined by T-cell receptor (TCR) specificity to self antigen. The transcription factor Foxp3 stabilises gene expression that specifies Treg differentiation while other transcription factors, including c-Rel, links TCR engagement and Foxp3 expression, within an appropriate cytokine and co-stimulatory molecule milieu, for Treg differentiation.

In the periphery, Tregs can be induced following repeated antigen exposure [8] under the influence of TGF-beta, converting Foxp3 negative T cells into Foxp3 positive induced Tregs (iTregs). Hence, this replaces T effector populations with regulatory populations, converting harmful responses to beneficial regulatory responses.

The list of potential defects in Tregs leading to autoimmune diseases are many (Table 1). Considering this extensive list, however, enables multiple potential targets for iPSC application and analysis of disease processes.

Table 1. Potential defects in regulatory T cells in autoimmune diseases [9,10].

Imbalances in peripheral effector and regulatory T cells due to defects in thymic selection
Genetic defects inducing failed Treg function or inadequate Treg activity
Overwhelming of Treg responses due to epitope spreading in autoimmune diseases,
Deficient IL-2 (required for Treg development)
Low CD25 expression (hence reduction of IL-2 signalling)
Defective conversion of naive T cells to adaptive Tregs (due to IL-10 or TGF-beta deficiency)
APC maturation defects leading to altered T cell activation and altered development of tolerogenic phenotype
Hyper-costimulation by APCs leading to pathogenic T cells rather than tolerogenic phenotype
Aberrant cytokine milieu leading to Treg suppression

The transfer of autologous Tregs to suppress immune responses has already been demonstrated experimentally in SLE and other autoimmune diseases such as diabetes mellitus [11,12]. Regulatory T cells are present at locations of inflammation (e.g., synovial fluid, mucosa) [13] though, if regulatory T cells are obtained from these sites, there may be inadvertent contamination of auto-reactive effector T cells, which could lead to unintended inflammatory consequences from therapeutic reinfusion of collected cells. Once isolated, it is technically challenging to induce these regulatory T cells to proliferate exogenously, which places limits on the application of harvested Tregs from patients for use in therapeutic treatments.

The ability to instead induce functional Tregs rather than needing to collect them, has been demonstrated from iPSCs *in vivo* [14]. These cells produced the immunoregulatory cytokines TGF beta and IL-10, thus producing a population of presumably functional Tregs. In a promising find, both allogeneic and autologous transfers of these iPSC derived Tregs demonstrated clinical efficacy, by reducing disease incidence and clinical severity scores in collagen-induced arthritis (CIA), an inducible mouse model of RA.

3.2. Dendritic Cells

Dendritic cells are highly proficient APCs that are potent in stimulating naive T cells during the primary immune response [15]. Numerous abnormalities in dendritic cells have been noted in patients with autoimmune diseases, including variations in cells proportions, differences in cytokine receptor expression particularly inhibitory receptors, and increased expression of costimulatory molecules [16,17].

Conventional dendritic cells (cDCs, previously known as myeloid DCs) are extremely efficient APCs, expressing several Toll-like receptors (TLRs) on their surface and producing TNF-alpha, IL-1, IL-6, IL-12, and IL-10 upon stimulation. Under different stimuli, cDCs can demonstrate different tolerogenic phenotypes, inducing antigen-specific unresponsiveness in central and peripheral lymphoid organs, and, therefore, have a crucial role in the induction of immune tolerance [18]. These tolerogenic dendritic cells are characteristically able to induce proliferation of Tregs (which then modulate immune responses to self-antigens), and to induce anergy in auto-reactive effector T cells [18,19]. Depending on the stimuli applied to the cDCs, different tolerogenic phenotypes are demonstrated, with functional differences in the Treg responses that are elicited [10]. Thus, depending on the desired Treg outcome, there is potential to preferentially select these outcomes by altering the particular phenotype of the applied tolerogenic dendritic cell in disease immunotherapy.

For example, Tregs can be induced *in vivo* by NFKB or CD40-deficient DCs. Conventional DCs require the transcription factor RelB to enable priming of the immune system through CD40 and MHC-molecule expression [20,21]. Blocking of RelB and other NFKB family members in cDCs results in induction of Tregs through modified cDC activity, therefore RelB activity is thought to determine the outcomes of antigen-presentation to cDCs. Methods to block RelB activity, and that of other NFKB family members have been developed to produce modified DCs that are consistently tolerogenic through the induction of Tregs [20,22,23]. In murine models of antigen-induced arthritis, modified DCs have been shown to suppress joint inflammation and erosion [24]. As tolerance induction by these DCs has been shown to be dose-dependent and route-independent [22], after induction of inflammatory arthritis by joint injection of methylated bovine serum albumin (mBSA), the mice were able to be subcutaneously injected with modified DCs exposed to mBSA, resulting in a suppression of inflammatory responses in the joints.

Given proof of concept studies using regulatory DCs in immunotherapy have demonstrated a reduction in effector T cell in other autoimmune diseases [25,26] the use of regulatory DCs as autologous immunotherapy is an exciting focus for possible future therapies [10,16,17], particularly in the immunomodulation of the inflammation noted in SLE and RA.

Plasmacytoid dendritic cells (pDCs) constitutively produce anti-viral Type 1 interferons as part of the immune response to viral infections. However, in patients with autoimmune diseases, such as SLE, pDCs are thought to instead make interferons following TLR ligation by endogenously derived nucleic acids [27]. The immune response is, thus, driven not by exogenous infection, but by activity against self-antigens.

Plasmacytoid dendritic cells that produce Type I interferons are found in the tissues of affected organs in SLE and other autoimmune conditions. Type I interferons have activity through several down-stream pathways to increase dendritic cell maturation and activation and, hence, antigen presentation to immune lymphocytes, and non-haematopoietic cell cytokine and MHC expression [6]. This immune activation results in up-regulated inflammation, and a positive-feedback loop with further dendritic cell production of interferon, and resultant anti-self T cell activation and B cell auto-antibody production.

In patients with active SLE, polymorphonuclear lymphocytes (PMNLs) have been shown to up-regulate interferon genes giving an interferon "signature", which correlates with disease severity, and high dose steroids which abrogate this signature induce clinical remission. Depletion of pDCs early in the course of SLE can reduce the clinical and serological evidence for autoimmunity [28]. This evidence indicates that the ability to model the interactions of pDCs would be beneficial to understanding more of the underlying pathogenesis in SLE.

The routine use of dendritic cells for research into the generation of immunomodulation, or for disease modeling *in vitro*, in SLE, RA and other autoimmune diseases is limited by the lack of plentiful and stable dendritic cells of the appropriate phenotype. Peripheral collection of precursors for autologous transfer through plasma exchange is not without morbidity, and the cost and logistics for wide-spread collection may not be feasible. Therefore, while able to be generated from haematopoietic stem cells, regulatory dendritic cells have recently been generated from murine iPSCs [19]. These iPSC-derived regulatory dendritic cells have been shown to have similar morphology to bone marrow derived regulatory DCs, and appeared to have similar activity to bone marrow derived regulatory DCs in not stimulating allogeneic CD4+ T cells, only weakly stimulating allogeneic CD8+ T cells and having similar efficient antigen uptake. What remains is to demonstrate stable phenotype and function, which can then enable comparison of results in clinical trials and other applications to be explored.

Once cells are generated from iPSCs, these need to have a valid functional assessment for tolerogenic properties. Similarly, as there is a theoretical risk for replication of the disease process with autologous transfer of cells, and a demonstrated risk for malignancy with iPSCs, appropriate monitoring and assessments will be required.

3.3. Disease Modelling in SLE or RA

Theoretically, the potential for disease modelling could be greatly expanded by generating and studying the different tissue lineages from patient-derived iPSCs [3]. While neurological tissue collection remains elusive, methods for expansion of renal specific cells into iPSCs through non-invasive urinary cell collection has been described [29]. Therefore *in vitro* examination of pathological processes using iPSCs derived from affected patients, and, possibly, regeneration of tissue from unaffected patients may both be possible. However, the end-organ damage of SLE is a manifestation of systemic immune dysregulation therefore the targets of therapy or investigation may be more well-focussed on the interactions between cellular populations and an examination of the matrix of effects on tolerance and auto-reactivity. Both SLE and RA are multifactorial in their pathogenesis with a complex interaction between environment and genetics, resulting in the loss of self-tolerance [30,31].

4. Generation of Reparative Tissue in Autoimmunity—Diabetes Mellitus

Diabetes mellitus is a significant clinical problem with high morbidity and mortality associated with microvascular and macrovascular complications of hyperglycaemia. Arising either from beta cell dysfunction and insulin resistance, or from autoimmune cell-mediated pancreatic islet cell destruction and resultant lack of insulin, treatments are usually aimed at glycaemic control, or reducing insulin resistance. Accurately and consistently replacing insulin at an amount appropriate for associated oral intake can be difficult for patients, with the risk for unstable sugars and hypoglycaemia.

Replacement of pancreatic tissue through tissue donation is in current use, however limited through lack of donors and restrictive through the requirement for life-long immunosuppression. It has been previously pointed out therefore, that treatment for diabetes would ideally renew beta cell function and, hence, insulin for glycaemic control, prevent repeat autoimmune destruction of the new pancreatic tissue, and repair the micro- and macrovascular complications that may have already occurred [32].

The current state of play with iPSCs and diabetes, also detailing concerns of immunogenicity, tumorigenicity, appropriate differentiation, full maturation, stability of function, and successful engraftment have recently been reviewed [33] with much work still required for understanding the basic biology of reprogrammed cells.

However, in terms of current research aspirations, there is great interest in attempting to recapitulate normal pancreatic development and generate pancreatic cell types from pluripotent cells [34]. This would encompass differentiating iPSCs into definitive endoderm, morphogenesis into a three-dimensional structure with contact with appropriate mesenchymal supportive cells to provide required growth and development signals, and then commitment of the pancreatic endoderm to endocrine precursor cells and thence to beta cells that produce the required insulin in a glucose-responsive fashion.

Thereafter, considerations need to be made on prevention of rejection of transplants, potentially preferring patient-specific iPSC generation and autologous transfer [35]. iPSC lines have so far been generated from patients with type 1 and type 2 diabetes, as well as maturity-onset diabetes of the young [36–38].

In terms of functional beta cell production, polyhormonal insulin-expressing cells have been derived from human embryonic stem cells and transplanted for some years now, though whether from insufficient cell volume transfer, or transfer of functionally immature beta cells, while helping fasted blood glucose states, they do not yet consistently ameliorate diabetes in non-fasted mice subjects, or tend to lose insulin-secretion capacity [39–41]. In an alternative line of investigation, when given enough time to develop *in vivo* (90–140 days post transplant), engraftment of pancreatic progenitor cells derived from human embryonic stem cells have been able to secrete insulin, and maintain normoglycaemia in a murine model of induced diabetes up until the grafts are removed [42].

Subsequently, glucose-responsive, insulin-producing cells have been generated from human iPSCs and also shown to have the ability in murine models to reverse hypoglycaemia [43], however, can lose insulin secretion over time [44]. While it is important to remember that there are differences between embryonic stem cells and iPSCs [45], potentially, progenitor pancreatic cells may be developed as well from iPSCs for trials in engraftment, but with the advantages inherent over requiring embryonic cell sources.

5. iPSCs in Autoimmune Neurological Disease—Multiple Sclerosis

Inducible pluripotent stem cells have been studied extensively in neurodegenerative and neurogenetic disorders, more so currently than for inflammatory neurological conditions, such as multiple sclerosis (MS), however, the final common pathway of neuronal injury and death is better understood in MS than for neurodegenerative conditions. IPSC technology allows potential avenues for therapeutics by regeneration of specific neuronal populations [46] or for exerting an immunomodulatory effect [47], but also allowing more accurate modelling of neurological disease than can be obtained through animal studies [46].

MS is the archetypal and most common disabling autoimmune condition of the central nervous system (CNS), which provides an ideal framework for research and understanding immune dysregulation. MS is a chronic condition, characterised by focal or multifocal inflammatory demyelinating episodes resulting in neurological disability depending on the area of the CNS involved. There are periods of quiescence and recovery in the most common phenotype, known as remitting relapsing MS [48].

The pathogenesis of MS and its triggers are multi-factorial with a complex interaction between genetic predisposition and environmental factors resulting in immune dysregulation. The first risk allele to be identified was the human leukocyte antigen (HLA) class II haplotype HLA-DRB*1501 in the 1970s [49]. The Genome-wide Association Study (GWAS) has since identified over 50 susceptibility loci [50], many of which encode for pro-inflammatory IL-2 and IL-7 [51], with others encoding for cytokines, such as CXCR5, IL-12A, IL-12β, and IL-12Rβ1 [48].

The genetic association alone does not explain fully the development of MS with vitamin D3 and Epstein-Barr virus (EBV) both being important environmental factors to consider in MS. Increased latitude is associated with lower serum levels of vitamin D3, due to lower levels of sun exposure, which corresponds with the higher incidence and prevalence of MS in these high latitude countries [48,52] though the effect of vitamin D3 deficiency on adaptive immunity is not yet fully understood. What has also been observed, is that individuals who are seronegative for EBV have almost no risk of developing MS [53], and it has been hypothesised that, through molecular mimicry, EBV may mimic myelin basic protein pathogenic antigens by presentation on HLA-DRB1*1501, therefore, providing links to both environmental and genetic risk factors [48,54]. Myelin reactive CD4+ T cells secreting interferon gamma are one of many T cell mediators in the pathogenesis of MS [55], with the role of other cell types and cell subsets being also involved, with a reduction in effector function of Tregs in MS patients [56], and a key role of pro-inflammatory T helper 17 (Th17) cells emerging [48,57]. Given the production of oligoclonal bands in CSF, there is a role of B cells in MS pathology, and the understanding of the part played by innate immunity by way of NK (natural killer) cells and dendritic cells in the pathogenesis is evolving [48].

Given the significant effects of MS on affected patients, efforts to provide regenerative or immunomodulatory therapy are highly sought.

Oligodendrocyte precursor cells (OPCs) derived from iPSCs, first described by Onorati *et al.* in 2010 [58], possibly provide an exogenous way in which to remyelinate axons as soon as possible after an episode of acute demyelination, to best protect axons from ongoing inflammation and eventual gliosis. Axonal loss is responsible for the most debilitating functional deficits in the more progressed stages of MS, with this loss followed by retrograde neuronal degeneration [59]. Axonal degeneration not only occurs in chronic lesions, with good evidence now showing axonal injury in acute lesions [60].

Cell replacement with OPCs derived from iPSCs have been shown to be successful in animal studies, with remyelination and amelioration of disability in experimental autoimmune encephalitis (EAE), an animal model of MS [61,62].

Neural precursor cells (NPCs) derived from iPSCs have also been shown in EAE to not only have a regenerative effect, but also an immunomodulatory effect. One study, in which mouse iPSC-derived NPCs were intrathecally transplanted in mice with EAE, exerted a neuroprotective effect, not by differentiating into myelin producing cells, but by producing the specific neurotrophin, leukaemia inhibitory factor (LIF), which supports the *in vivo* survival and differentiation of native oligodendrocytes [63]. LIF has been shown to inhibit the differentiation of Th17 cells through MAP kinase suppression of the cytokine signalling 3 (SOCS3) inhibitory signalling cascade, antagonising the interleukin 6 (IL-6)-mediated phosphorylation of signal transducer and activator of transcription 3 (STAT3) [64], which is essential for the differentiation of Th17 cells, thus limiting CNS inflammation and hence subsequent tissue damage.

Finally, the disease in a dish approach may give unique insights into the study of pathogenesis in neuronal disease and in particular to inflammatory diseases of the CNS, given its inaccessibility. IPSCs have been successfully derived from a MS patient's dermal fibroblasts, and differentiated into astrocytes, oligodendrocytes and neurons with a normal karyotype. The patient-derived neurons showed electrophysiological differences compared with the control cell line, paving the way for a novel approach to the study of MS pathogenesis [65].

6. Conclusions

Autoimmune diseases are the result of a combination of environmental influences acting on a susceptible genetic background. This causes significant aberrations of self-antigen recognition, lymphocyte activation and differentiation, production of pro-inflammatory cytokines and autoantibodies, and the final end product of tissue and organ damage. Induced pluripotent stem cells technology has the potential to create new safe treatment options, as well as better models to study disease and therapies *in vitro*. Here, we review the so far limited literature in this field. In addition to organ replacement strategies where iPSC technology has been applied, we propose that complex auto-immune diseases require unique immunomodulatory therapy strategies using cellular components and that these components could be made by iPSC technology. Importantly, iPSC technology enables us to produce, differentiate and genetically modify large numbers of immune cells that can be used therapeutically. Prior to the development of such technologies modification of small cell populations with limited *ex vivo* expansion potential was near impossible. Nevertheless, these novel approaches will need to have extensive functional and safety assessments prior to their use in a clinical setting.

Finally, iPSC technology allows for modelling of normal and diseased (based on genetic and epigenetic modifications) cellular growth and development, influences of mutations onto function and clinical phenotype. In the time of personalized medicine iPSC technologies are likely to feature as a key therapeutic tool in auto-immune diseases.

Acknowledgments

Michael J. Edel (RYC-2010-06512) is supported by the Program Ramon y Cajal, project grant BFU2011-26596 and UWA-CCTRM near miss grant.

Conflicts of Interest

The authors declare no conflict of interest and support free open access publishing.

References

1. Takahashi, K.; Yamanaka, S. Induction of pluripotent stem cells from mouse embryonic and adult fibroblast cultures by defined factors. *Cell* **2006**, *126*, 663–676.
2. Lowry, W.E.; Richter, L.; Yachechko, R.; Pyle, A.D.; Tchieu, J.; Sridharan, R.; Clark, A.T.; Plath, K. Generation of human induced pluripotent stem cells from dermal fibroblasts. *Proc. Natl. Acad. Sci. USA* **2008**, *105*, 2883–2888.
3. Lu, X.; Zhao, T. Clinical therapy using iPSCs: Hopes and challenges. *Genomics Proteomics Bioinform.* **2013**, *11*, 294–298.
4. Park, I.H.; Zhao, R.; West, J.A.; Yabuuchi, A.; Huo, H.; Ince, T.A.; Lerou, P.H.; Lensch, M.W.; Daley, G.Q. Reprogramming of human somatic cells to pluripotency with defined factors. *Nature* **2008**, *451*, 141–146.

5. Wernig, M.; Meissner, A.; Foreman, R.; Brambrink, T.; Ku, M.; Hochedlinger, K.; Bernstein, B.E.; Jaenisch, R. *In vitro* reprogramming of fibroblasts into a pluripotent ES-cell-like state. *Nature* **2007**, *448*, 318–324.

6. Wahren-Herlenius, M.; Dorner, T. Immunopathogenic mechanisms of systemic autoimmune disease. *Lancet* **2013**, *382*, 819–831.

7. Tang, Q.; Bluestone, J.A. The Foxp3+ regulatory t cell: A jack of all trades, master of regulation. *Nat. Immunol.* **2008**, *9*, 239–244.

8. Rosenblum, M.D.; Gratz, I.K.; Paw, J.S.; Lee, K.; Marshak-Rothstein, A.; Abbas, A.K. Response to self antigen imprints regulatory memory in tissues. *Nature* **2011**, *480*, 538–542.

9. Brusko, T.M.; Putnam, A.L.; Bluestone, J.A. Human regulatory T cells: Role in autoimmune disease and therapeutic opportunities. *Immunol. Rev.* **2008**, *223*, 371–390.

10. Gordon, J.R.; Ma, Y.; Churchman, L.; Gordon, S.A.; Dawicki, W. Regulatory dendritic cells for immunotherapy in immunologic diseases. *Front. Immunol.* **2014**, *5*, 7.

11. Bluestone, J.A.; Tang, Q. Therapeutic vaccination using CD4+CD25+ antigen-specific regulatory T cells. *Proc. Natl. Acad. Sci. USA* **2004**, *101 Suppl 2*, 14622–14626.

12. Scalapino, K.J.; Daikh, D.I. Suppression of glomerulonephritis in NZB/NZW lupus prone mice by adoptive transfer of *ex vivo* expanded regulatory T cells. *PLoS ONE* **2009**, *4*, e6031.

13. van Amelsfort, J.M.; Jacobs, K.M.; Bijlsma, J.W.; Lafeber, F.P.; Taams, L.S. CD4(+)cD25(+) regulatory T cells in rheumatoid arthritis: Differences in the presence, phenotype, and function between peripheral blood and synovial fluid. *Arthritis Rheum.* **2004**, *50*, 2775–2785.

14. Haque, R.; Lei, F.; Xiong, X.; Bian, Y.; Zhao, B.; Wu, Y.; Song, J. Programming of regulatory T cells from pluripotent stem cells and prevention of autoimmunity. *J. Immunol.* **2012**, *189*, 1228–1236.

15. Banchereau, J.; Briere, F.; Caux, C.; Davoust, J.; Lebecque, S.; Liu, Y.J.; Pulendran, B.; Palucka, K. Immunobiology of dendritic cells. *Annu. Rev. Immunol.* **2000**, *18*, 767–811.

16. Mackern-Oberti, J.P.; Llanos, C.; Vega, F.; Salazar-Onfray, F.; Riedel, C.A.; Bueno, S.M.; Kalergis, A.M. Role of dendritic cells in the initiation, progress and modulation of systemic autoimmune diseases. *Autoimmun. Rev.* **2015**, *14*, 127–139.

17. Mackern-Oberti, J.P.; Vega, F.; Llanos, C.; Bueno, S.M.; Kalergis, A.M. Targeting dendritic cell function during systemic autoimmunity to restore tolerance. *Int. J. Mol. Sci.* **2014**, *15*, 16381–16417.

18. Schmidt, S.V.; Nino-Castro, A.C.; Schultze, J.L. Regulatory dendritic cells: There is more than just immune activation. *Front. Immunol.* **2012**, *3*, 274.

19. Zhang, Q.; Fujino, M.; Iwasaki, S.; Hirano, H.; Cai, S.; Kitajima, Y.; Xu, J.; Li, X.K. Generation and characterization of regulatory dendritic cells derived from murine induced pluripotent stem cells. *Sci. Rep.* **2014**, *4*, 3979.

20. O'Sullivan, B.J.; MacDonald, K.P.; Pettit, A.R.; Thomas, R. RelB nuclear translocation regulates B cell MHC molecule, CD40 expression, and antigen-presenting cell function. *Proc. Natl. Acad. Sci. USA* **2000**, *97*, 11421–11426.

21. Pai, S.; O'Sullivan, B.J.; Cooper, L.; Thomas, R.; Khanna, R. RelB nuclear translocation mediated by C-terminal activator regions of Epstein-Barr virus-encoded latent membrane

protein 1 and its effect on antigen-presenting function in B cells. *J. Virol.* **2002**, *76*, 1914–1921.

22. Martin, E.; O'Sullivan, B.; Low, P.; Thomas, R. Antigen-specific suppression of a primed immune response by dendritic cells mediated by regulatory T cells secreting interleukin-10. *Immunity* **2003**, *18*, 155–167.

23. Li, M.; Zhang, X.; Zheng, X.; Lian, D.; Zhang, Z.X.; Ge, W.; Yang, J.; Vladau, C.; Suzuki, M.; Chen, D.; *et al.* Immune modulation and tolerance induction by RelB-silenced dendritic cells through rna interference. *J. Immunol.* **2007**, *178*, 5480–5487.

24. Martin, E.; Capini, C.; Duggan, E.; Lutzky, V.P.; Stumbles, P.; Pettit, A.R.; O'Sullivan, B.; Thomas, R. Antigen-specific suppression of established arthritis in mice by dendritic cells deficient in NF-kappaB. *Arthritis Rheum.* **2007**, *56*, 2255–2266.

25. Harry, R.A.; Anderson, A.E.; Isaacs, J.D.; Hilkens, C.M. Generation and characterisation of therapeutic tolerogenic dendritic cells for rheumatoid arthritis. *Ann. Rheum. Dis.* **2010**, *69*, 2042–2050.

26. Raiotach-Regue, D.; Grau-Lopez, L.; Naranjo-Gomez, M.; Ramo-Tello, C.; Pujol-Borrell, R.; Martinez-Caceres, E.; Borras, F.E. Stable antigen-specific T-cell hyporesponsiveness induced by tolerogenic dendritic cells from multiple sclerosis patients. *Eur. J. Immunol.* **2012**, *42*, 771–782.

27. Bave, U.; Nordmark, G.; Lovgren, T.; Ronnelid, J.; Cajander, S.; Eloranta, M.L.; Alm, G.V.; Ronnblom, L. Activation of the type I interferon system in primary Sjogren's syndrome: A possible etiopathogenic mechanism. *Arthritis Rheum.* **2005**, *52*, 1185–1195.

28. Rowland, S.L.; Riggs, J.M.; Gilfillan, S.; Bugatti, M.; Vermi, W.; Kolbeck, R.; Unanue, E.R.; Sanjuan, M.A.; Colonna, M. Early, transient depletion of plasmacytoid dendritic cells ameliorates autoimmunity in a lupus model. *J. Exp. Med.* **2014**, *211*, 1977–1991.

29. Chen, Y.; Luo, R.; Xu, Y.; Cai, X.; Li, W.; Tan, K.; Huang, J.; Dai, Y. Generation of systemic lupus erythematosus-specific induced pluripotent stem cells from urine. *Rheumatol. Int.* **2013**, *33*, 2127–2134.

30. Armstrong, D.L.; Zidovetzki, R.; Alarcon-Riquelme, M.E.; Tsao, B.P.; Criswell, L.A.; Kimberly, R.P.; Harley, J.B.; Sivils, K.L.; Vyse, T.J.; Gaffney, P.M.; *et al.* GWAS identifies novel SLE susceptibility genes and explains the association of the HLA region. *Genes Immun.* **2014**, *15*, 347–354.

31. Orozco, G.; Barton, A. Update on the genetic risk factors for rheumatoid arthritis. *Expert Rev. Clin. Immunol.* **2010**, *6*, 61–75.

32. Liew, A.; O'Brien, T. The potential of cell-based therapy for diabetes and diabetes-related vascular complications. *Curr. Diabetes Rep.* **2014**, *14*, 469.

33. Giannoukakis, N.; Trucco, M. A 2015 reality check on cellular therapies based on stem cells and their insulin-producing surrogates. *Pediatric Diabetes* **2015**.

34. Schiesser, J.V.; Wells, J.M. Generation of beta cells from human pluripotent stem cells: Are we there yet? *Ann. N. Y. Acad. Sci.* **2014**, *1311*, 124–137.

35. Araki, R.; Uda, M.; Hoki, Y.; Sunayama, M.; Nakamura, M.; Ando, S.; Sugiura, M.; Ideno, H.; Shimada, A.; Nifuji, A.; *et al.* Negligible immunogenicity of terminally differentiated cells derived from induced pluripotent or embryonic stem cells. *Nature* **2013**, *494*, 100–104.

36. Teo, A.K.; Windmueller, R.; Johansson, B.B.; Dirice, E.; Njolstad, P.R.; Tjora, E.; Raeder, H.; Kulkarni, R.N. Derivation of human induced pluripotent stem cells from patients with maturity onset diabetes of the young. *J. Biol. Chem.* **2013**, *288*, 5353–5356.

37. Kudva, Y.C.; Ohmine, S.; Greder, L.V.; Dutton, J.R.; Armstrong, A.; De Lamo, J.G.; Khan, Y.K.; Thatava, T.; Hasegawa, M.; Fusaki, N.; *et al.* Transgene-free disease-specific induced pluripotent stem cells from patients with type 1 and type 2 diabetes. *Stem Cells Transl. Med.* **2012**, *1*, 451–461.

38. Maehr, R.; Chen, S.; Snitow, M.; Ludwig, T.; Yagasaki, L.; Goland, R.; Leibel, R.L.; Melton, D.A. Generation of pluripotent stem cells from patients with type 1 diabetes. *Proc. Natl. Acad. Sci. USA* **2009**, *106*, 15768–15773.

39. Basford, C.L.; Prentice, K.J.; Hardy, A.B.; Sarangi, F.; Micallef, S.J.; Li, X.; Guo, Q.; Elefanty, A.G.; Stanley, E.G.; Keller, G., *et al.* The functional and molecular characterisation of human embryonic stem cell-derived insulin-positive cells compared with adult pancreatic beta cells. *Diabetologia* **2012**, *55*, 358–371.

40. Eshpeter, A.; Jiang, J.; Au, M.; Rajotte, R.V.; Lu, K.; Lebkowski, J.S.; Majumdar, A.S.; Korbutt, G.S. *In vivo* characterization of transplanted human embryonic stem cell-derived pancreatic endocrine islet cells. *Cell Prolif.* **2008**, *41*, 843–858.

41. Phillips, B.W.; Hentze, H.; Rust, W.L.; Chen, Q.P.; Chipperfield, H.; Tan, E.K.; Abraham, S.; Sadasivam, A.; Soong, P.L.; Wang, S.T.; *et al.* Directed differentiation of human embryonic stem cells into the pancreatic endocrine lineage. *Stem Cells Dev.* **2007**, *16*, 561–578.

42. Kroon, E.; Martinson, L.A.; Kadoya, K.; Bang, A.G.; Kelly, O.G.; Eliazer, S.; Young, H.; Richardson, M.; Smart, N.G.; Cunningham, J.; *et al.* Pancreatic endoderm derived from human embryonic stem cells generates glucose-responsive insulin-secreting cells *in vivo*. *Nat. Biotechnol.* **2008**, *26*, 443–452.

43. Van Hoof, D.; Liku, M.E. Directed differentiation of human pluripotent stem cells along the pancreatic endocrine lineage. *Methods Mol. Biol.* **2013**, *997*, 127–140.

44. Pellegrini, S.; Ungaro, F.; Mercalli, A.; Melzi, R.; Sebastiani, G.; Dotta, F.; Broccoli, V.; Piemonti, L.; Sordi, V. Human induced pluripotent stem cells differentiate into insulin-producing cells able to engraft *in vivo*. *Acta Diabetol.* **2015**, doi:10.1007/s00592-015-0726-z.

45. Yamanaka, S. Induced pluripotent stem cells: Past, present, and future. *Cell Stem Cell* **2012**, *10*, 678–684.

46. Mattis, V.B.; Svendsen, C.N. Induced pluripotent stem cells: A new revolution for clinical neurology? *Lancet Neurol.* **2011**, *10*, 383–394.

47. De Feo, D.; Merlini, A.; Laterza, C.; Martino, G. Neural stem cell transplantation in central nervous system disorders: From cell replacement to neuroprotection. *Curr. Opin. Neurol.* **2012**, *25*, 322–333.

48. Hoglund, R.A.; Maghazachi, A.A. Multiple sclerosis and the role of immune cells. *World J. Exp. Med.* **2014**, *4*, 27–37.

49. Svejgaard, A. The immunogenetics of multiple sclerosis. *Immunogenetics* **2008**, *60*, 275–286.

50. Sawcer, S.; Hellenthal, G. The major histocompatibility complex and multiple sclerosis: A smoking gun? *Brain: J. Neurol.* **2011**, *134*, 638–640.

51. International Multiple Sclerosis Genetics Consortium; Hafler, D.A.; Compston, A.; Sawcer, S.; Lander, E.S.; Daly, M.J.; De Jager, P.L.; de Bakker, P.I.; Gabriel, S.B.; Mirel, D.B.; *et al.* Risk alleles for multiple sclerosis identified by a genomewide study. *N. Engl. J. Med.* **2007**, *357*, 851–862.

52. Simpson, S., Jr.; Blizzard, L.; Otahal, P.; Van der Mei, I.; Taylor, B. Latitude is significantly associated with the prevalence of multiple sclerosis: A meta-analysis. *J. Neurol. Neurosurg. Psychiatry* **2011**, *82*, 1132–1141.

53. Ascherio, A.; Munger, K.L. Environmental risk factors for multiple sclerosis. Part I: The role of infection. *Ann. Neurol.* **2007**, *61*, 288–299.

54. Lang, H.L.; Jacobsen, H.; Ikemizu, S.; Andersson, C.; Harlos, K.; Madsen, L.; Hjorth, P.; Sondergaard, L.; Svejgaard, A.; Wucherpfennig, K.; *et al.* A functional and structural basis for TCR cross-reactivity in multiple sclerosis. *Nat. Immunol.* **2002**, *3*, 940–943.

55. Compston, A.; Coles, A. Multiple sclerosis. *Lancet* **2008**, *372*, 1502–1517.

56. Viglietta, V.; Baecher-Allan, C.; Weiner, H.L.; Hafler, D.A. Loss of functional suppression by CD4+CD25+ regulatory T cells in patients with multiple sclerosis. *J. Exp. Med.* **2004**, *199*, 971–979.

57. McFarland, H.F.; Martin, R. Multiple sclerosis: A complicated picture of autoimmunity. *Nat. Immunol.* **2007**, *8*, 913–919.

58. Onorati, M.; Camnasio, S.; Binetti, M.; Jung, C.B.; Moretti, A.; Cattaneo, E. Neuropotent self-renewing neural stem (NS) cells derived from mouse induced pluripotent stem (IPS) cells. *Mol. Cell. Neurosci.* **2010**, *43*, 287–295.

59. Tallantyre, E.C.; Bo, L.; Al-Rawashdeh, O.; Owens, T.; Polman, C.H.; Lowe, J.S.; Evangelou, N. Clinico-pathological evidence that axonal loss underlies disability in progressive multiple sclerosis. *Mult. Scler.* **2010**, *16*, 406–411.

60. Filippi, M.; Bozzali, M.; Rovaris, M.; Gonen, O.; Kesavadas, C.; Ghezzi, A.; Martinelli, V.; Grossman, R.I.; Scotti, G.; Comi, G.; *et al.* Evidence for widespread axonal damage at the earliest clinical stage of multiple sclerosis. *Brain: J. Neurol.* **2003**, *126*, 433–437.

61. Czepiel, M.; Balasubramaniyan, V.; Schaafsma, W.; Stancic, M.; Mikkers, H.; Huisman, C.; Boddeke, E.; Copray, S. Differentiation of induced pluripotent stem cells into functional oligodendrocytes. *Glia* **2011**, *59*, 882–892.

62. Sher, F.; Balasubramaniyan, V.; Boddeke, E.; Copray, S. Oligodendrocyte differentiation and implantation: New insights for remyelinating cell therapy. *Curr. Opin. Neurol.* **2008**, *21*, 607–614.

63. Laterza, C.; Merlini, A.; De Feo, D.; Ruffini, F.; Menon, R.; Onorati, M.; Fredrickx, E.; Muzio, L.; Lombardo, A.; Comi, G., *et al.* IPSC-derived neural precursors exert a neuroprotective role in immune-mediated demyelination via the secretion of LIF. *Nat. Commun.* **2013**, *4*, 2597.

64. Cao, W.; Yang, Y.; Wang, Z.; Liu, A.; Fang, L.; Wu, F.; Hong, J.; Shi, Y.; Leung, S.; Dong, C.; *et al.* Leukemia inhibitory factor inhibits T helper 17 cell differentiation and confers treatment effects of neural progenitor cell therapy in autoimmune disease. *Immunity* **2011**, *35*, 273–284.

65. Song, B.; Sun, G.; Herszfeld, D.; Sylvain, A.; Campanale, N.V.; Hirst, C.E.; Caine, S.; Parkington, H.C.; Tonta, M.A.; Coleman, H.A.; *et al.* Neural differentiation of patient specific IPS cells as a novel approach to study the pathophysiology of multiple sclerosis. *Stem Cell Res.* **2012**, *8*, 259–273.

MDPI AG
Klybeckstrasse 64
4057 Basel, Switzerland
Tel. +41 61 683 77 34
Fax +41 61 302 89 18
http://www.mdpi.com/

JCM Editorial Office
E-mail: jcm@mdpi.com
http://www.mdpi.com/journal/jcm